Ocular Syndromes and Systemic Diseases

DECLARATION

Care has been taken to confirm the accuracy of the information presented and to describe generally accepted practices. However, the author and publisher are not responsible for errors or omissions or for any consequences from application of the information in a particular situation which remains the professional responsibility of the practitioner.

The author and publisher have exerted every effort to ensure that drug selection and dosage set forth in this text are in accordance with current recommendations and practice at the time of publication. However, in view of ongoing research, changes in government regulations and the constant flow of information relating to drug therapy and drug reactions, the reader is urged to check the package insert for each drug for any change in indications and dosage, and for added warnings and precautions. This is particularly important when the recommended agent is a new or infrequently employed drug.

Some drugs and medical devices presented in this publication have Food and Drug Administration (FDA) clearance for limited use in restricted research settings. It is the responsibility of the health care provider to ascertain the FDA status of each drug or device planned for use in their clinical practice.

This text would not have been possible without the superb efforts of Renee Tindall.

Ocular Syndromes and Systemic Diseases

FIFTH EDITION

Frederick Hampton Roy MD FACS

Little Rock, Arkansas, USA

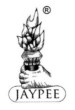

JAYPEE BROTHERS MEDICAL PUBLISHERS (P) LTD

New Delhi • London • Philadelphia • Panama

Jaypee Brothers Medical Publishers (P) Ltd

Headquarters
Jaypee Brothers Medical Publishers (P) Ltd
4838/24, Ansari Road, Daryaganj
New Delhi 110 002, India
Phone: +91-11-43574357
Fax: +91-11-43574314
Email: jaypee@jaypeebrothers.com

Overseas Offices

J.P. Medical Ltd
83, Victoria Street, London
SW1H 0HW (UK)
Phone: +44-2031708910
Fax: +02-03-0086180
Email: info@jpmedpub.com

Jaypee-Highlights Medical Publishers Inc.
City of Knowledge, Bld. 237, Clayton
Panama City, Panama
Phone: +507-301-0496
Fax: +507-301-0499
Email: cservice@jphmedical.com

Jaypee Medical Inc.
The Bourse
111 South Independence Mall East
Suite 835, Philadelphia, PA 19106, USA
Phone: + 267-519-9789
Email: jpmed.us@gmail.com

Jaypee Brothers
Medical Publishers (P) Ltd
17/1-B Babar Road, Block-B
Shaymali, Mohammadpur
Dhaka-1207, Bangladesh
Mobile: +08801912003485
Email: jaypeedhaka@gmail.com

Jaypee Brothers
Medical Publishers (P) Ltd
Shorakhute, Kathmandu
Nepal
Phone: +00977-9841528578
Email: jaypee.nepal@gmail.com

Website: www.jaypeebrothers.com
Website: www.jaypeedigital.com

Inquiries for bulk sales may be solicited at: jaypee@jaypeebrothers.com

This book has been published in good faith that the contents provided by the author contained herein are original, and is intended for educational purposes only. While every effort is made to ensure accuracy of information, the publisher and the author specifically disclaim any damage, liability, or loss incurred, directly or indirectly, from the use or application of any of the contents of this work. If not specifically stated, all figures and tables are courtesy of the author. Where appropriate, the readers should consult with a specialist or contact the manufacturer of the drug or device.

Ocular Syndromes and Systemic Diseases

Previous Editions: 1992, 1997, 2002, 2007

Fifth Edition: **2014**

ISBN 978-93-5025-520-9

Printed at Ajanta Offset & Packagings Ltd, New Delhi, India.

Dedicated to

Kay

My Children:
Helena, Robert, Kimberly, Frederick Jr, Charles and Nichols

Dr Bruce Herndon, who daily throughout our joint eye
residency stumped me with another "weird" syndrome

Renee Tindall for her hard work and diligence.

Preface

Ocular Syndromes and Systemic Diseases was my second book. My fellow eye resident Dr Bruce Herndon would stump me daily with another "weird" syndrome. I have always been troubled with a poor memory. Being compulsive, I felt it is important to compile a book of *Ocular Syndromes and Systemic Diseases*, so that I would not have to try to remember all of them.

This is a companion text to Ocular Differential Diagnosis (ODDX). ODDX has many lists of causes of diseases like ptosis, strabismus and others.

I am fortunate that Renee Tindall, who has worked with me for many years, has provided valuable aid on this and all the other editions.

Frederick Hampton Roy

Contents

(For a complete alphabetic list of all included syndromes see the index)

1. A-ESOTROPIA SYNDROME

General

Esotropia greater looking up by 15 prism diopters than looking down; an overaction of superior oblique muscles or underaction of inferior rectus muscles; fusion may be obtained by chin elevation; mongoloid (upward) slant of lid fissures; may be accommodative, nonaccommodative or paralytic esotropia components.

Laboratory

Diagnosis is made by clinical findings.

Treatment

Recess the medial rectus bilaterally with a half tendon upshift. If unilateral surgery recess medial rectus with upshift and resect the lateral rectus (LR) with a half tendon downshift. With significant oblique overaction—recess the medial rectus bilaterally or recess the medial rectus and resect the LR unilaterally for esotropia in primary position weaken the superior oblique bilaterally if 25 diopters from up to down.

Bibliography

1. Beyer-Machule C, von Noorden GK. Atlas of Ophthalmic Surgery. New York: Thieme; 1984.
2. Hwang J, Wright KW. Strabismus syndromes. In: Wright KW (Ed). Pediatric Ophthalmology and Strabismus. St. Louis: Mosby; 1995. p. 223.
3. Roy FH. Practical Management of Eye Problems: Glaucoma, Strabismus, Visual Fields. Philadelphia: Lea & Febiger; 1975. pp. 32-134.

2. A-EXOTROPIA SYNDROME

General

Exotropia greater looking down by 15 prism diopters than looking up; mongoloid (upward) slant of lid fissures; alternating sursumduction and associated vertical divergence; overaction of superior oblique muscles or underaction of inferior oblique or inferior rectus muscles; fusion obtained by chin depression.

Laboratory

Diagnosis is made by clinical findings.

Treatment

Recess the lateral rectus with downshift. If unilateral surgery recess the lateral rectus with downshift and resect the medial rectus with upshift. With oblique dysfunction—recess the rectus bilateral and weaken the superior oblique bilaterally.

Bibliography

1. Hardesty HH. Superior oblique tenotomy. Arch Ophthalmol. 1972;88:181-4.
2. Hwang J, Wright KW. Strabismus syndromes. In: Wright KW (Ed). Pediatric Ophthalmology and Strabismus. St. Louis: Mosby; 1995. p. 223.
3. Roy FH. Practical Management of Eye Problems: Glaucoma, Strabismus, Visual Fields. Philadelphia: Lea & Febiger; 1975. pp. 144-5.

3. A-PATTERN STRABISMUS

General

Visual axis greater in upgaze than downgaze by at least 15 prism diopters.

Clinical

None

Ocular

A-esotropia; A-exotropia; amblyopia.

Laboratory

Diagnosis is made by clinical findings.

Treatment

A-pattern esotropia without oblique dysfunction—recess medial rectus bilateral with upshift or recess the medial rectus with upshift and resect lateral rectus with downshift in one eye. A-pattern esotropia with superior oblique overaction—recess the medial rectus bilaterally or recess medial rectus and resect lateral rectus unilaterally and weaken superior oblique by tenectomy. A-pattern exotropia without oblique dysfunction—recess the lateral rectus bilaterally with downshift or unilaterally recess the lateral rectus with a downshift and resect the medial rectus with a upshift. A-pattern exotropia with superior oblique overaction—recess the lateral rectus bilaterally or unilaterally recess the lateral rectus and resect the medial rectus and weaken the superior oblique bilaterally by tenectomy.

Additional Resource

1. Plotnik JL (2011). A-Pattern Esotropia and Exotropia. [online] Available from http://www.emedicine.com/oph/TOPIC560.HTM [Accessed April, 2012].

4. AARSKOG-SCOTT SYNDROME (FACIOGENITAL DYSPLASIA)

General

Sex-linked; characterized by ocular hypertelorism, anteverted nostrils, broad upper lip and saddle-bag scrotum.

Ocular

Ptosis; hypertelorism.

Clinical

Hyperextensibility of fingers; genu recurvatum; flat feet; hypermobility in cervical spine with neurologic deficit; cleft lip and palate; anteverted nostrils; broad upper lip; abnormal penoscrotal relations; "saddle-bag scrotum".

Laboratory

For full and detailed physical examination, a radiologic evaluation is essential. Standard posteroanterior and lateral views are used for the initial evaluation.

Treatment

Primary goal is to prevent the development of a severe deformity rather than treating the current deformity.

Bibliography

1. Bowle E, Tyrkus M, Lipman S, et al. Aarskog syndrome: full male and female expression associated with an X-autosome translocation. Am J Med Genet. 1984;17:595-602.
2. McKusick VA. Mendelian Inheritance in Man: A Catalog of Human Genes and Genetic Disorders, 12th edition. Baltimore: The Johns Hopkins University Press; 1998.
3. Scott CI. Unusual facies, joint hypermobility, genital anomaly and short stature: a new dysmorphic syndrome. Birth Defects Orig Artic Ser. 1971;7:240-6.

5. AARSKOG SYNDROME (FACIAL-DIGITAL-GENITAL SYNDROME)

General

X-linked recessive; males fully affected; females exhibit partial features; normal birth weight and length.

Ocular

Telecanthus; hypertelorism; unilateral or bilateral blepharoptosis; strabismus; hyperopic astigmatism; large cornea.

Clinical

Short stature; triangular facies; deformity of hands and feet; anomalies of external genitalia; inguinal hernia; protruding umbilicus; abnormal cervical vertebrae; cryptorchidism.

Laboratory

For full and detailed physical examination, a radiologic evaluation is essential. Standard posteroanterior and lateral views are used for the initial evaluation.

Treatment

Primary goal is to prevent the development of a severe deformity rather than treating the current deformity.

Bibliography

1. Kirkham TH, Milot J, Berman P. Ophthalmic manifestations of Aarskog (facial-digital-genital) syndrome. Am J Ophthalmol. 1975;79:441-5.

6. ABDOMINAL TYPHUS (ENTERIC FEVER; TYPHOID FEVER)

General

Causative agent is *Salmonella typhi*.

Ocular

Conjunctivitis; chemosis; corneal ulcer; tenonitis; paralysis of extraocular muscles; endophthalmitis; panophthalmitis; optic neuritis; retinal detachment; central scotoma; central retinal artery emboli; iritis with or without hypopyon; choroiditis; retinal hemorrhages; bilateral optic neuritis; abnormal ocular motility (likely secondary to thrombotic infarcts affecting the ocular motor nerve nuclei, fascicles, brainstem or cerebral hemispheres).

Clinical

Fever; headache; bradycardia; splenomegaly; maculopapular rash; leukopenia; encephalitis. Salmonella may produce an illness characterized by fever and bacteremia without any other manifestations of enterocolitis or enteric fever, which is particularly common in patients with acquired immunodeficiency syndrome (AIDS).

Laboratory

Gram-negative bacillis isolation from blood culture (50–70% of cases). Stool culture positive less frequent.

Treatment

Early detection, antibiotic therapy, adequate fluids, electrolytes, and nutrition reduce the rate of complications and reduce the case-fatality rate.

Additional Resource

1. Brusch JL (2011). Typhoid Fever. [online] Available from http://www.emedicine.com/med/TOPIC2331.HTM [Accessed April, 2012].

7. ABDUCENS PARALYSIS (SIXTH NERVE)

General

Unilateral or bilateral, multiple etiologies because of long course of sixth nerve.

Clinical

Childhood neoplasm, raised intracranial pressure, hypertension, diabetes.

Ocular

Inability to turn the eye laterally.

Laboratory

Diagnosis is made by clinical findings.

Treatment

Tape or base-out prism on one eyeglass may be useful, botulinum toxin type A into the antagonist medial recturs muscle, if no improvement after 6–12 months—recess/resect of medial and lateral rectus.

Additional Resource

1. Ehrenhaus MP (2012). Abducens Nerve Palsy. [online] Available from http://www.emedicine.com/oph/TOPIC158.HTM [Accessed April, 2012].

8. ABERFELD SYNDROME (CONGENITAL BLEPHAROPHIMOSIS ASSOCIATED WITH GENERALIZED MYOPATHY SYNDROME; OCULAR AND FACIAL ABNORMALITIES SYNDROME; SCHWARTZ-JAMPEL SYNDROME)

General

Etiology not known; autosomal recessive inheritance, although there are reports of dominant inheritance; progressive disorder.

Ocular

Blepharophimosis; exotropia; myopia; congenital cataracts; microcornea.

Clinical

Myopathy; bone deformities; arachnodactyly; dwarfism; hypoplastic facial bones; hypertrichosis; kyphoscoliosis.

Laboratory

Physicians might consider referring suspected cases to genetic clinics that have affiliations with groups actively research so that genetic studies can be performed. Muscle biopsy findings are consistent with a myopathy.

Treatment

The goal is to reduce the abnormal muscle activity that causes stiffness. Botulinum toxin therapy may be considered for the treatment of blepharospasm. However, if ptosis is present, this is contraindicated. Some medications that have been found useful in myotonic disorders such as the anticonvulsants and the antiarrhythmics.

Additional Resource

1. Ault J (2012). Schwartz-Jampel Syndrome. [online] Available from http://www.emedicine. com/neuro/TOPIC337.HTM [Accessed April, 2012].

9. ABSENCE OF FOVEAL REFLEX

The absence of foveal reflex is caused by drugs, including amodiaquine, chloroquine, diiodohydroxyquin, hydroxychloroquine, iodochlorhydroxyquin or quinine.

Bibliography

1. Fraunfelder FT. Drug-Induced Ocular Side Effects and Drug Interactions. Philadelphia: Lea & Febiger; 1982.

10. ACANTHAMOEBA

General

Caused by *Acanthamoeba polyphaga* and *Acanthamoeba cartel* (see Herpes Simplex Masquerade Syndrome); all types of contact lenses have been associated with acanthamoeba keratitis, particularly daily-wear soft contact lenses.

Ocular

Hypopyon; uveitis; conjunctivitis and chemosis; keratitis; pannus; corneal ring abscess; papillitis; vitreitis; retinal perivasculitis; secondary glaucoma; postkeratoplasty acanthamoeba keratitis may present as an infectious crystalline keratopathy in the periphery of the graft.

Clinical

Meningoencephalitis; meningitis; hemorrhagic encephalitis.

Laboratory

Polygonal double-walled cysts, under brightfield or phase-contrast microscopy or stained with hematoxylin and eosin, Gram, Giemsa or celluflor white.

Treatment

Medical therapy for Acanthamoeba infection is not well established. Topical antimicrobial agents that achieve high concentrations at the site of the infection can be considered. Treatment of keratitis consists of early diagnosis and aggressive surgical and medical therapies.

Additional Resources

1. Crum-Cianflone NF (2011). Acanthamoeba. [online] Available from http://www.emedicine. com/med/TOPIC10.HTM [Accessed April, 2012].
2. Wang JC (2010). Ophthalmologic Manifestations of Herpes Simplex Keratitis. [online] Available from http://www.emedicine.com/oph/TOPIC100. HTM [Accessed April, 2012].

11. ACANTHOSIS NIGRICANS

General

Rare skin disease of unknown etiology; occurs at any age; equal frequency in males and females; thickening and hyperpigmentation of the skin of the entire body, especially in flexural areas; autosomal dominant inheritance.

Ocular

Conjunctivitis; pigmentation of palpebral conjunctiva; tumors on lids and lid margins; madarosis; trichiasis.

Clinical

Hyperkeratotic lesions on face, neck, oral mucosa, axillae, groin, antecubital fossae and umbilicus.

Laboratory

Basic workup for underlying malignancy and screen for insulin resistance.

Treatment

The goal of therapy is to correct the underlying disease process. Treatment of the lesions of acanthosis nigricans (AN) is for cosmetic reasons only.

Additional Resource

1. Miller JH (2010). Acanthosis Nigricans. [online] Available from http://www.emedicine.com/derm/TOPIC1.HTM [Accessed April, 2012].

12. ACCOMMODATIVE ESOTROPIA

General

Hereditary, onset between the ages of 6 months and 5 years.

Clinical

None

Ocular

Uncorrected hyperopia with insufficient fusional divergence. The hyperopia averages 5 diopters. The esotropia is equal distance and near.

Laboratory

Diagnosis is made by clinical findings.

Treatment

Amblyopia therapy: Spectacle correction—full cycloplegic refraction if esotropia is at same distance and near, greater near than distant esotropia—bifocals up to +3.50 diopters set high at mid-pupil, gradually reduce the power to maintain fusion, contact lens if patient is capable, echothiopate iodine use to reduce the use of spectacles and if residual esotropia after full correction consider strabismus surgery.

Additional Resource

1. Noyes C (2012). Accommodative Esotropia. [online] Available from http://www.emedicine.com/oph/TOPIC554.HTM [Accessed April, 2012].

13. ACCOMMODATIVE INSUFFICIENCY (ACCOMMODATIVE EFFORT SYNDROME)

General

Male or female, 10–35 years of age.

Ocular

Asthenopia with near vision appearing within a few minutes after reading, sewing or observing a near object; increased amplitude of accommodative adduction; abnormal relaxation of accommodation induced by relative divergence at close distances; latent convergence insufficiency; may result secondary to ciliary dysfunction associated with Adie's pupil.

Clinical

It may be secondary to a systemic disorder such as Parkinson disease or oral lithium.

Laboratory

Accommodation testing are the basic tests that used to help diagnose this condition.

Treatment

Convergence exercises including orthoptics, vision therapy and/or base-in prisms are the mainstays of treatment of convergence insufficiency.

Additional Resource

1. Bartiss MJ (2011). Convergence Insufficiency. [online] Available from http://www.emedicine.com/oph/TOPIC553.HTM [Accessed April, 2012].

14. ACCOMMODATIVE SPASM (SPASM OF THE NEAR REFLEX)

General

Episodic excessive contraction of the ciliary muscle.

Clinical

Posterior fossa tumor, central nervous system (CNS) infection, head trauma, cerebrovascular injuries.

Ocular

Diplopia, esotropia, accommodation, convergence, miosis.

Laboratory

Computed tomography (CT) and magnetic resonance imaging (MRI).

Treatment

Cycloplegics to break the accommodative component, refractive correction for distance with reading addition.

Bibliography

1. Roy FH, Fraunfelder FW, Fraunfelder FT. Roy and Fraunfelder's Current Ocular Therapy, 6th edition. Philadelphia: WB Saunders; 2008.

15. ACERULOPLASMINEMIA

General

Autosomal recessive, adult-onset.

Ocular

Maculopathy which resembles aging macular degeneration.

Clinical

Associated with increased levels of copper in the retina.

Laboratory

Increased urinary copper level, greater than 100 mcg/24 hours (normal, 10–80 mcg/24 h).

Treatment

A low copper diet is recommended. Foods that are high in copper content include shellfish, liver, mushrooms, broccoli, chocolate and nuts.

Bibliography

1. Miyajima H. Aceruloplasminemia, an iron metabolic disorder. Neuropathology. 2003;23:345-50.

16. ACHARD SYNDROME

General

All features of Marfan syndrome, with the addition of dysostosis mandibulofacialis; arachnodactyly; receding lower jaw; joint laxity limited to the hands and feet; differs from Marfan syndrome in that the skull is broad and brachycephalic with small mandible.

Ocular

Myopia; lens dislocation; spherophakia.

Clinical

Mandibulofacial dysostosis; skeletal anomalies; arachnodactyly; high-arched palate; heart disease.

Laboratory

Genetic testing, molecular studies.

Treatment

Dislocated lens can be treated with careful phacoemulsification, topical steroids to control ocular inflammation.

Bibliography

1. Achard D. Arachnodactylie. Bull Mem Soc Med Hop Paris. 1902;19:834.
2. Jackson LG. Genetic principles for the ophthalmologist. Trans Pa Acad Ophthalmol Otolaryngol. 1974;27:20-8.
3. Magalini SI, Scrascia E. Dictionary of Medical Syndromes, 2nd edition. Philadelphia: JB Lippincott; 1981.
4. McKusick VA. Mendelian Inheritance in Man: A Catalog of Human Genes and Genetic Disorders, 12th edition. Baltimore: The Johns Hopkins University Press; 1998.
5. McKusick-Nathans Institute for Genetic Medicine, Johns Hopkins University and National Center for Biotechnology Information, National Library of Medicine. (2007). Online Mendelian Inheritance in Man (OMIM). [online] Available from http://www.ncbi.nlm.nih.gov/omim [Accessed April, 2012].

17. ACHONDROPLASIA

General

Dwarfism; etiology unknown; occurs in both sexes; inheritance is autosomal dominant with almost complete penetrance; characterized by rhizomelic dwarfism (reduction most marked in the proximal limbs); mid-face hypoplasia; exaggerated lumbar lordosis; limitation of hip and elbow expansion; location of achondroplastic gene reported to be in the short arm of chromosome 1.

Ocular

Strabismus; optic atrophy; hypermetropia.

Clinical

Osseous impingement upon cranial nerves; rhizomelic short stature; facial features include frontal bossing, depressed nasal bridge, relative mandibular prognathism; connective tissue dysplasia; hypotonic in infancy; paraplegia may develop in the second or third decade.

Laboratory

Plasma can be analyzed for the fibroblast growth factor receptor 3 (FGFR3) mutation in the mother when a short-limb skeletal dysplasia is diagnosed prenatally on ultrasound. This can be confirmatory for achondroplasia.

Treatment

Growth hormone is currently being used to augment the height of patients with achondroplasia. Orthopedic physician will need to be consulted concerning problems related to the spine.

Additional Resource

1. Parikh S (2012). Achondroplasia. [online] Available from http://www.emedicine.com [Accessed April, 2012].

18. ACHOO SYNDROME (AUTOSOMAL DOMINANT COMPELLING HELIO-OPHTHALMIC OUTBURST SYNDROME; PEROUTKA SNEEZE; PHOTIC SNEEZE REFLEX; SNEEZING FROM LIGHT EXPOSURE)

General

Autosomal dominant; sneezing in response to bright light, especially sunlight; association between photic sneeze and nephropathic cystinosis has been reported.

Ocular

Photic sneeze reflex by sudden exposure of dark-adapted subject to bright light.

Clinical

Successive sneezing, as many as 43 in a row.

Laboratory

Diagnosis is made by clinical findings.

Treatment

None

Bibliography

1. Collie WR, Pagon RA, Hall JG, et al. ACHOO syndrome. Birth Defects Orig Artic Ser. 1978;14:361-3.
2. Katz B, Melles RB, Swenson MR, et al. Photic sneeze reflex in nephropathic cystinosis. Br J Ophthalmol. 1990;74:706-8.
3. McKusick VA. Mendelian Inheritance in Man: A Catalog of Human Genes and Genetic Disorders, 12th edition. Baltimore: The Johns Hopkins University Press; 1998.
4. McKusick-Nathans Institute for Genetic Medicine, Johns Hopkins University and National Center for Biotechnology Information, National Library of Medicine. (2007). Online Mendelian Inheritance in Man (OMIM). [online] Available from http://www.ncbi.nlm.nih.gov/omim [Accessed April, 2012].

19. ACID BURNS OF THE EYE

General

Acid injuries of the eyes are characterized by protein coagulation and precipitation with the anion. Direct tissue damage produced by the hydrogen ion.

Clinical

None

Ocular

Chemosis, corneal epithelial defects, limbal blanching, corneal clouding, photophobia, corneal neovascularization, symblepharon formation.

Laboratory

Diagnosis is made from clinical history and findings.

Treatment

Immediate irrigation. Topical antibiotics for bacterial infection if needed. Contact lenses aid in re-epithelialization of the cornea.

Bibliography

1. Roy FH, Fraunfelder FW, Fraunfelder FT. Roy and Fraunfelder's Current Ocular Therapy, 6th edition. Philadelphia: WB Saunders; 2008.

20. ACINETOBACTER (ACINETOBACTER IWOFFI; MIMA POLYMORPHA)

General

Gram-negative pleomorphic bacillus *Mima*; generally occurs in patient with lowered resistance.

Ocular

Conjunctivitis and chemosis; corneal ulcer; blepharitis; iris prolapse; endophthalmitis.

Clinical

Meningitis; pneumonitis; endocarditis; urethritis; vaginitis; arthritis; dermatitis; intracranial abscess; subdural empyema.

Laboratory

Culture of the appropriate body fluid that is properly transported, plated and incubated grows *A. baumannii*.

Treatment

An infectious disease specialist should be consulted to differentiate colonization from infection and for antibiotic recommendations. Fluoroquinolone is the treatment of choice.

Additional Resource

1. Cunha BA (2011). Acinetobacter. [online] Available from http://www.emedicine.com/med/TOPIC3456. HTM [Accessed April, 2012].

21. ACKERMAN SYNDROME

General

Autosomal recessive; characterized by pyramidal molar roots.

Ocular

Juvenile glaucoma.

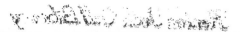

Clinical

Unusual upper lip and dental roots; pyramidal molar roots.

Laboratory

Diagnosis is made by clinical findings.

Treatment

Congenital glaucoma: Primary congenital glaucoma almost always is managed surgically, both goniotomy and trabeculectomy may be useful. When multiple goniotomies and/or trabeculectomies fail, the surgeon usually resorts to a filtering procedure.

Bibliography

1. Antine BE, Brown FM, Arisco MJ. Fibroma of the cornea. Arch Ophthalmol. 1974;91:278-80.
2. Kenyon KR. Mesenchymal dysgenesis in Peter's anomaly, sclerocornea and congenital endothelial dystrophy. Exp Eye Res. 1975;21:125-42.

22. ACL SYNDROME (ACROMEGALOID; CORNEAL LEUKOMA SYNDROME; CUTIS VERTICIS GYRATA)

General

Autosomal dominant; rare; three features include: (1) cutis verticis, (2) associated with acromegaly and (3) corneal leukoma; onset by age 1 year.

Ocular

Bilateral corneal leukoma; keratitis.

Clinical

Unusually tall; large hands, feet and chin; skin of hands very soft; skin of scalp lies in folds; frontal bosses; ear calcification; pituitary tumors; abnormal dermal ridge patterns; enlargement of supraorbital arch of frontal bone.

Laboratory

Anticardiolipin (aCL) antibodies react primarily to membrane phospholipids, such as cardiolipin and phosphatidylserine. Of the three known isotypes of aCL [i.e. immunoglobulin G (IgG), IgM, IgA], IgG correlates most strongly with thrombotic events.

Treatment

Ocular—patients with bilateral and visually disabling corneal opacity, penetrating keratoplasty (PK) is recommended.

Bibliography

1. Antine BE, Brown FM, Arisco MJ. Fibroma of the cornea. Report of a case associated with congenital generalized fibromatosis. Arch Ophthalmol. 1974; 91:278-80.

23. ACNE ROSACEA (ACNE ERYTHEMATOSA; OCULAR ROSACEA)

General

Etiology unknown; usually occurs in women 30-50 years of age; pathogenetic mechanism remains unclear.

Ocular

Conjunctivitis; corneal neovascularization (wedge-shaped); keratitis; meibomianitis; blepharitis; recurrent chalazion; conjunctival hyperemia; superficial punctate keratopathy; corneal vascularization, thinning, perforation and scarring; episcleritis; scleritis; iritis; nodular conjunctivitis.

Clinical

Symmetrical erythema; papules; pustules; telangiectasia; sebaceous gland hypertrophy of the forehead, malar eminences and nose.

Laboratory

Diagnosis is made by clinical findings.

Treatment

Systemic antibiotics are useful in most cases.

Additional Resource

1. Banasikowska AK (2011). Rosacea. [online] Available from http://www.emedicine.com/derm/TOPIC377.HTM [Accessed April, 2012].

24. ACOSTA SYNDROME (MOUNTAIN CLIMBER SYNDROME; MOUNTAIN SICKNESS; MONGE SYNDROME; SOROCHE SYNDROME)

General

Cause is cerebral hypoxia at high altitudes; Monge syndrome is the chronic form of mountain sickness.

Ocular

Acute blurred vision; difficulties in color discrimination; impaired light adaptation; retinal hemorrhage; chronic lid edema; bluish scleral injection; decreased visual acuity.

Clinical

Restlessness and irritability; headaches; impaired judgment at approximately 15,000 feet; confusion, cyanosis, muscular incoordination and possible loss of consciousness at approximately 18,000–20,000 feet; exertional dyspnea; epistaxis; gum bleeding; hemoptysis; anorexia; nausea; vomiting; tinnitus; cough; loss of libido; paresthesian extremities; coma; clubbing of fingers; hepatosplenomegaly.

Laboratory

Computed tomography (CT) is useful in patients with focal neurologic findings or in atypical cases of suspected high altitude disease.

Treatment

The symptoms improve dramatically with descent, and by the time a patient reaches the emergency department, further treatment is rarely indicated. Oxygen 4 L/min or to keep SaO_2 above 90% should be used in patients who continue to be acutely ill. Dexamethasone should be continued in symptomatic patients.

Additional Resource

1. Kale R (2012). Altitude-Related Disorders. [online] Available from http://www.emedicine.com/med/TOPIC3225.HTM [Accessed April, 2012].

25. ACQUIRED EXOTROPIA

General

Exodeviation characterized by visual axes that form a divergent angle. Intermittent exotropia, sensory exotropia and exotropia with neurologic causes are all types of acquired exotropia. More common in Middle East, Africa and Asia.

Clinical

Neurological issues.

Ocular

Exophoria, intermittent exotropia, diplopia, bitemporal suppression, asthenopia, and closing of one eye in bright light, amblyopia.

Laboratory

Diagnosis is made by clinical findings.

Treatment

Nonsurgical treatment involves correction of refractive error occlusion therapy for amblyopia, orthoptics and botulinum toxin injections. Treatment of neurologic defect is also important. Surgery is only considered when the patient has poor control of the deviation, diplopia and severe asthenopia.

Additional Resource

1. Thacker N (2012). Acquired Exotropia. [online] Available from http://www.emedicine.medscape.com/article/1199004-overview [Accessed April, 2012].

---

26. ACQUIRED IMMUNODEFICIENCY SYNDROME (ACQUIRED CELLULAR IMMUNODEFICIENCY; ACQUIRED IMMUNODEFICIENCY; AIDS)

General

Acquired breakdown of the immune system followed by disease that takes advantage of the body's collapsed defenses; acquired by shared drug needles or sexual intercourse; occurs most frequently in homosexually active men (75%), intravenous drug abusers (13%) and Haitian immigrants (6%).

Ocular

Retinal cotton-wool spots; cytomegalovirus (CMV) retinitis; retinal periphlebitis; conjunctival Kaposi sarcoma; necrotizing retinitis; retinal hemorrhages; conjunctivitis sicca; orbital Burkitt lymphoma; peripheral retinochoroiditis; vitreitis; fungal corneal ulcer; hypopyon; acute glaucoma; III nerve palsy; anterior uveitis; atypical retinitis; orbital pseudotumor; herpes zoster ophthalmicus; herpes simplex keratitis; bacterial keratitis; molluscum contagiosum; CMV retinitis; toxoplasma retinitis; acute retinal necrosis; human immunodeficiency virus (HIV) retinitis; syphilitic retinitis; pneumocystis carinii choroiditis; fungal and bacterial endophthalmitis; fungal choroiditis; conjunctival microvasculopathy; keratitis sicca; subconjunctival hemorrhage.

Clinical

Because of lowered immunity, one-third of individuals develop Kaposi sarcoma; pneumonia caused by *Pneumocystis carinii*; death.

Laboratory

Enzyme-linked immunosorbent assay (ELISA) test is used for screening while other tests are used to evaluate false-positive and false-negative test results.

Treatment

Medical consultations are required for systemic treatment. The treatment of CMV retinitis can include drugs such as ganciclovir, valganciclovir, fomivirsen, foscarnet and cidofovir. All of these drugs have specific adverse effects and complicate the decision to use for treatment.

Additional Resources

1. Dubin J (2011). Rapid Testing for HIV. [online] Available from http://www.emedicine.com/emerg/TOPIC253.HTM [Accessed April, 2012].
2. Copeland R (2011). Ocular Manifestations of HIV Infection. [online] Available from http://www.emedicine.com/oph/TOPIC417.HTM [Accessed April, 2012].

27. ACQUIRED LUES (ACQUIRED SYPHILIS; LUES VENEREA; MALUM VENEREUM; SYPHILIS)

General

Causative agent, *Treponema pallidum,* usually transmitted sexually.

Ocular

Conjunctival chancroid; conjunctivitis; keratitis; blepharitis; ptosis; iris atrophy; hippus; dacryocystitis; optic nerve atrophy; optic neuritis; periostitis; episcleritis; scleritis; nystagmus; uveitis; vitreous hemorrhages; paralysis of sixth nerve; papilledema; retinal hemorrhages; retinitis proliferans; oculogyric crisis; neuroretinitis; papilledema (associated with aseptic meningitis); diffuse or multifocal chorioretinitis; vertical supranuclear gaze palsy; Benedikt syndrome.

Clinical

Primary lesion associated with regional lymphadenopathy; secondary bacteremic stage associated with generalized mucocutaneous lesions; tertiary stage characterized by destructive mucocutaneous, musculoskeletal, or parenchymal lesions, aortitis, or central nervous system disease; syphilis and HIV infection often coexist in the same patient who experiences a higher incidence and greater severity of neurologic and ocular manifestations; a significant percentage of patients infected with HIV-I and *T. pallidum* become seronegative to syphilis testing.

Laboratory

Serologic nontreponemal tests include Venereal Disease Research Laboratory (VDRL) and rapid plasma reagin (RPR).

Treatment

The goals are to reduce morbidity and to prevent complications. Penicillin is the antibiotic of choice for treating syphilis. Ocular syphilis should be treated the same as patients with neurosyphilis.

Additional Resources

1. Majmudar PA (2011). Interstitial Keratitis Overview of Interstitial Keratitis. [online] Available from http://www.emedicine.com/oph/TOPIC453.HTM [Accessed April, 2012].
2. Euerle B (2012). Syphilis. [online] Available from http://www.emedicine.com/med/TOPIC2224.HTM [Accessed April, 2012].

28. ACQUIRED NONACCOMMODATIVE ESOTROPIA

General

Convergent deviation with onset after age of 6 months, unaffected by accommodation.

Clinical

None

Ocular

Esotropia same in all fields of gaze, amblyopia.

Laboratory

Diagnosis is made by clinical findings.

Treatment

Amblyopia therapy, eyeglasses if significant refractive error, orthoptics, unilateral surgery—recess medial rectus and resect lateral rectus or bilateral—recess both medial rectus.

Additional Resource

1. Pascotto A (2010). Acquired Esotropia. [online] Available from http://www.emedicine.com/oph/TOPIC327.HTM [Accessed April, 2012].

29. ACRODERMATITIS CHRONICA ATROPHICANS

General

Rare familial skin disorder; autosomal recessive; both sexes equally affected; occurs in infants; not present at birth but develops during the first few weeks; zinc deficiency; there are reports of improvement following treatment with zinc suggesting an abnormality in the zinc-binding factor.

Ocular

Scarring of the conjunctiva; recurrent iridocyclitis; keratomalacia; cataracts; photophobia; blepharitis; punctal stenosis; corneal opacification.

Clinical

Vesiculobullous eruption around body orifices, skin of knees, elbows and paronychial areas; complete alopecia; erythematous psoriasiform plaques.

Laboratory

Diagnose is based on evaluation of the history, including epidemiologic data, signs, and symptoms of early and late infection; on a detailed physical examination; and on the specific serologic tests results and histopathologic picture of skin biopsy specimens.

Treatment

The goals of pharmacotherapy are to eradicate the infection, to reduce morbidity and to prevent complications with the use of antibiotics.

Additional Resource

1. Chodynicka B (2011). Acrodermatitis Chronica Atrophicans. [online] Available from http://www.emedicine.com/derm/TOPIC4.HTM [Accessed April, 2012].

30. ACROPACHY (HYPERTROPHIC PULMONARY OSTEOARTHROPATHY)

General

Three separate components: (1) clubbing of fingers, (2) periosteal proliferation of distal ends of long bones and (3) arthritis; symptoms disappear with control of disease.

Ocular

Exophthalmos

Clinical

Finger edema; fibrous overgrowth to fingertips; nail deformity; elevated hormone levels; periosteal bone changes which affect distal radius, ulna, tibia, fibula, metacarpals and phalanges.

Laboratory

Because clubbing typically is secondary to an underlying pathological process, perform pertinent laboratory studies for primary medical disorders that are suggested clinically.

Treatment

Clubbing is a clinical sign of many pathological processes; therefore, consultation with specialists may be necessary to diagnose the underlying disease.

Additional Resource

1. Schwartz RA (2012). Clubbing of the Nails. [online] Available from http://www.emedicine. com/derm/TOPIC780.HTM [Accessed April, 2012].

31. ACRORENO-OCULAR SYNDROME

General

Autosomal dominant; Duane syndrome with radial defects.

Ocular

Complete coloboma; coloboma of optic nerve; ptosis and Duane anomaly.

Clinical

Renal anomalies; hypoplasia of distal part of thumb with lack of motion at phalangeal joint; renal ectopia without fusion; bladder diverticula; malrotation of both kidneys; absence of kidney; clubhand or absence of thumb.

Laboratory

Diagnosis is made by clinical findings.

Treatment

Ptosis: If visual acuity is affected most cases require surgical correction, and there are several procedures that may be used including levator resection, repair or advancement and Fasanella-Servat.

Bibliography

1. Halal F, Homsy M, Perreault G. Acro-renal-ocular syndrome: autosomal dominant thumb hypoplasia, renal ectopia, and eye defect. Am J Med Genet. 1984;17:753-62.
2. McKusick VA. Mendelian Inheritance in Man: A Catalog of Human Genes and Genetic Disorders, 12th edition. Baltimore: The Johns Hopkins University Press; 1998.
3. McKusick-Nathans Institute for Genetic Medicine, Johns Hopkins University and National Center for Biotechnology Information, National Library of Medicine. (2007). Online Mendelian Inheritance in Man (OMIM). [online] Available from http://www.ncbi.nlm.nih.gov/omim [Accessed April, 2012].

32. ACTINIC AND SEBORRHEIC KERATOSIS

General

Actinic is a precancerous lesion that occurs most commonly on sunlight-exposed areas of the skin. Seborrheic keratosis is a benign epithelial tumor that appears predominantly on the trunk and head.

Clinical

Lupus

Ocular

Eyebrow and eyelids lesions.

Laboratory

Diagnosis is made by clinical findings.

Treatment

Cryosurgery is the treatment of choice.

Bibliography

1. Roy FH, Fraunfelder FW, Fraunfelder FT. Roy and Fraunfelder's Current Ocular Therapy, 6th edition. Philadelphia: WB Saunders; 2008.

33. ACTINOMYCOSIS

General

Caused by Gram-positive *Actinomyces israelii.*

Ocular

Hypopyon; conjunctivitis; keratitis; corneal ulcer; proptosis; uveitis; dacryocystitis; yellow nodules on conjunctiva and eyelids; occlusion of nasolacrimal canaliculi; canaliculitis; orbital abscess; endophthalmitis (rare).

Clinical

Chronic inflammatory induration and sinus formation.

Laboratory

Canalicular discharge may be sent for Gram stain/Giemsa stain, cultures and sensitivities (i.e. blood agar, Sabouraud, anaerobic), and special stains (i.e. calcofluor white).

Treatment

Penicillins and cephalosporins are useful. Subconjunctival penicillin coadministered with systemic iodides and topical sulfacetamide or penicillin can be used.

Additional Resource

1. Roque MR (2010). Actinomycosis in Ophthalmology. [online] Available from http://www.emedicine.com/oph/TOPIC491.HTM [Accessed April, 2012].

34. ACUTE FOLLICULAR CONJUNCTIVITIS (ADENOVIRAL CONJUNCTIVITIS; PHARYNGOCONJUNCTIVAL FEVER; SYNDROME OF BEAL)

General

Infectious disease produced by adenovirus; serotypes 3, 4, 7, 8, 19, 37 and several others may cause acute conjunctivitis with or without upper respiratory tract involvement; epidemic keratoconjunctivitis has been reported worldwide associated with 11 virus serotypes, with serotypes 8, 11 and 19 being the most commonly responsible.

Ocular

Conjunctivitis; chemosis; keratitis; blepharitis; blepharospasm.

Clinical

Fever; pharyngitis; lymph node enlargement; malaise; myalgia; headache; diarrhea.

Laboratory

Lab tests generally are not useful. Cell cultures from infected areas and adenoviral antibody titer allows for precise identification of serotype.

Treatment

Symptomatic control may include cold compresses and artificial tears; nonsteroidal and occasionally steroidal drops to relieve itching.

Additional Resource

1. Scott IU (2012). Pharyngoconjunctival Fever. [online] Available from http://www.emedicine. com/oph/TOPIC501.HTM [Accessed April, 2012].

---

35. ACUTE FROSTED RETINAL PERIPHLEBITIS

General

Etiology unknown, virus suspected; involvement of veins and arteries; veins more severely affected.

Ocular

Vascular sheathing; retinal hemorrhages; exudative detachment; retinal neovascularization; thick, inflammatory infiltrates around retinal veins; macular detachment; retinal tears associated with posterior vitreous detachment; peripheral uveitis; retinal periphlebitis; associated cytomegalovirus retinitis in HIV-seropositive patients; observed as an idiopathic finding in a child.

Clinical

Associated with tuberculosis; syphilis; sarcoidosis; multiple sclerosis; HIV infection.

Laboratory

Diagnosis is made by clinical findings.

Treatment

Retinal detachment: Scleral buckle, pneumatic retinopexy and vitrectomy may be used to close all the breaks.

Bibliography

1. Kleiner RC, Kaplan HJ, Shakin JL, et al. Acute frosted retinal periphlebitis. Am J Ophthalmol. 1988;106:27-34.
2. Mansour AM, Li HK. Frosted retinal periphlebitis in the acquired immunodeficiency syndrome. Ophthalmologica. 1993;207:182-6.
3. Nakai A, Saika S. A case of frosted-branch retinal angiitis in a child. Ann Ophthalmol. 1992;24:415-7.
4. Secchi AG, Tognon MS, Turrini B, et al. Acute frosted retinal periphlebitis associated with cytomegalovirus retinitis. Retina. 1992;12:245-7.
5. Watanabe Y, Takeda N, Adachi-Usami E. A case of frosted branch angiitis. Br J Ophthalmol. 1987;71:553-8.

36. ACUTE HEMORRHAGIC CONJUNCTIVITIS (APOLLO 11 DISEASE; AHC; EPIDEMIC HEMORRHAGIC KERATOCONJUNCTIVITIS)

General

First reported in 1969, first epidemic in the United States in 1981; enterovirus; explosive onset; usually bilateral; coxsackievirus A24 and enterovirus 70 have been implicated in the most recent outbreaks.

Ocular

Chemosis; follicular conjunctivitis; petechial bulbar hemorrhages; seromucous discharge; keratitis; lacrimation; lid edema; photophobia; preauricular lymphadenopathy.

Clinical

Systemic symptoms are rare, although several cases of lumbosacral radiculomyelitis have occurred late in the course of the disease; polio-like paralysis (associated with enterovirus 70).

Laboratory

Antisera have been used with good results. These are being supplanted by polymerase chain reaction (PCR) methods, which reduce the time needed for viral typing.

Treatment

Very contagious with transmitted eye to hand to eye contact. Self-limited course generally no treatment is necessary.

Additional Resource

1. Plechaty G (2011). Acute Hemorrhagic Conjunctivitis. [online] Available from http://www.emedicine.com/oph/TOPIC492.HTM [Accessed April, 2012].

37. ACUTE MULTIFOCAL PLACOID PIGMENT EPITHELIOPATHY

General

Acquired inflammatory disorder of the retina; seen in healthy adults; characterized by placoid subretinal lesions; self-limited disease that resolve in weeks to months; frequently bilateral; cause is unknown but may be a hypersensitivity-induced vasculitis.

Clinical

Microvascular nephropathy; thyroiditis; hearing loss; cerebral angiitis; headache; flu-like symptoms.

Ocular

Yellow-white placoid subretinal lesions; retinal pigment epithelial disturbance; decreased visual acuity; episcleritis; optic neuritis; photophobia; photopsia.

Laboratory

Diagnosis is made from typical clinical appearance.

Treatment

No treatment is normally necessary because the lesions appear to run a relatively short self-limited course and generally have little residual effect. In complicated cases laser photo-coagulation may be useful.

Additional Resource

1. Kooragayala LM (2011). Acute Multifocal Placoid Pigment Epitheliopathy. [online] Available from http://www.emedicine.medscape.com/article/1225531-overview [Accessed April, 2012].

38. ACUTE ORBITAL COMPARTMENT SYNDROME

General

Increased pressure within the confined orbital space generally secondary to facial trauma or surgery; blindness can occur without prompt treatment.

Clinical

Facial trauma; head trauma.

Ocular

Decreased visual acuity; ischemic optic neuropathy; retrobulbar hematoma; diplopia; proptosis; eye pain; reduction of ocular motility; papilledema; cherry-red macula; ecchymosis of lids; chemosis; increased intraocular pressure; afferent pupillary defect; ophthalmoplegia.

Laboratory

Computed tomography (CT) or MRI may be useful to identify the etiology of compression.

Treatment

Immediate osmotic agents and carbonic anhydrase inhibitors should be used; lateral orbital canthotomy should be used as soon as diagnosis is made and life-threatening injuries are stabilized to prevent permanent visual loss.

Additional Resource

1. Peak DA (2011). Acute Orbital Compartment Syndrome. [online] Available from http://www.emedicine.medscape.com/article/799528-overview [Accessed April, 2012].

39. ACUTE POSTERIOR MULTIFOCAL PLACOID PIGMENT EPITHELIOPATHY (WHITE DOT SYNDROME)

General

Inflammatory chorioretinopathy etiology unknown but can be associated with systemic conditions such as viral disease, thyroiditis, Lyme disease, tuberculosis and nephritis.

Clinical

Thyroiditis; erythema nodosum; Wegener granulomatosis; polyarteritis nodosa; nephritis; sarcoidosis; CNS vasculitis.

Ocular

Blurred vision; central and paracentral scotomas.

Laboratory

Clinical observation by funduscopic examination and fluorescein angiography.

Treatment

There is no current consensus on treatment and most resolve without treatment. Systemic and intravitreal steroids may be beneficial to shorten the duration and for those cases involving the fovea.

Additional Resource

1. Mansour SE (2010). Multifocal Choroidopathy Syndromes. [online] Available from http://www.emedicine.medscape.com/article/1190935-overview [Accessed April, 2012].

40. ACUTE RETINAL NECROSIS SYNDROME (ARN SYNDROME; BARN SYNDROME; BILATERAL ACUTE RETINAL NECROSIS SYNDROME)

General

Evidence of association with herpes-type deoxyribonucleic acid (DNA) virus; occurs both unilaterally and bilaterally; includes varicella zoster virus and herpes simplex virus type 1.

Ocular

Uveitis; vasculitis; vitreitis; retinal detachment; vitreous opacification; retinal periarteritis; exudates of peripheral retina; retinal necrosis; optic nerve enlargement; papillitis; arcuate neuroretinitis; arteritis and phlebitis (affecting the retinal vasculature); necrotizing retinitis; moderate to severe vitreitis; anterior segment inflammation; optic neuritis; late retinal detachment.

Clinical

None

Laboratory

Diagnosis is made by clinical findings.

Treatment

Antiviral therapy, anti-inflammatory therapy, antithrombotic therapy and retinal detachment prophylaxis. Vitrectomy may be necessary.

Bibliography

1. Tibbetts MD, Shah CP, Young LH, et al. Treatment of acute retinal necrosis. Ophthalmology. 2010; 117:818-24.
2. Wong R, Pavesio CE, Laidlaw DA, et al. Acute retinal necrosis: the effects of intravitreal foscarnet and virus type on outcome. Ophthalmology. 2010;117:556-60.

Additional Resource

1. Dahl AA (2011). Acute Retinal Necrosis. [online] Available from http://www.emedicine.com/oph/TOPIC377.HTM [Accessed April, 2012].

41. ADDISON PERNICIOUS ANEMIA SYNDROME (BIERMER SYNDROME; MACROCYTIC ANEMIA; PERNICIOUS ANEMIA SYNDROME; VITAMIN B$_{12}$ DEFICIENCY ANEMIA)

General

Autosomal dominant; female preponderance; onset between the ages of 30 and 50 years; lack of intrinsic factor normally produced in the fundus of stomach and important for absorption of vitamin B$_{12}$ in the intestinal tract; infrequent ocular involvement.

Ocular

Central scotoma, centrocecal scotomata and field contractions in a few cases; retinal hemorrhages (round with white center) at the posterior pole; both retina and disk may have a whitish, hazy appearance; optic neuritis (ischemic); optic atrophy; palsies of extraocular muscles; ocular hypotony; cataract; bilateral, slowly progressive optic neuropathy and unclear etiology.

Clinical

Megaloblastic anemia (chronic and progressive); hypochlorhydria; glossitis; stomatitis; constipation or diarrhea; paresthesias and numbness; incoordination; ataxia; sphincter malfunction.

Laboratory

The peripheral blood usually shows a macrocytic anemia with a mild leukopenia and thrombocytopenia.

Treatment

The cause of the failure to absorb cobalamin (Cbl) should be determined. Vitamin B_{12} is available as either cyanocobalamin or hydroxocobalamin and each are useful in the treatment of vitamin B_{12} deficiency.

Additional Resource

1. Schick P (2011). Pernicious Anemia. [online] Available from http://www.emedicine.com/med/TOPIC1799.HTM [Accessed April, 2012].

42. ADDISON SYNDROME (ADDISON DISEASE; ADRENAL CORTICAL INSUFFICIENCY; IDIOPATHIC HYPOPARATHYROIDISM; MONILIASIS-IDIOPATHIC HYPOPARATHYROIDISM)

General

Familial occurrence; association with moniliasis; onset during end of first and beginning of second decade of life; atrophy of adrenal cortex; prognosis for life is poor, with death in adrenal crisis.

Ocular

Ptosis; blepharitis; blepharospasm; keratoconjunctivitis with extreme photophobia; corneal ulcers; episcleritis; keratitic moniliasis; cataracts; papilledema.

Clinical

Moniliasis; tetany; progressive weakness; anorexia; progressive skin pigmentation; dry skin; brittle fingernails and toenails; sparse pubic and axillary hair or total alopecia; impotence.

Laboratory

Diagnosis made rests on the functional capacity of the adrenal cortex to synthesize cortisol. This is accomplished primarily by use of the rapid adrenocorticotropic hormone (ACTH) stimulation test (Cortrosyn, Cosyntropin or Synacthen).

Treatment

Endocrinologist should be consulted the acute care and chronic care.

Additional Resources

1. Griffing GT (2010). Addison Disease. [online] Available from http://www.emedicine.com/med/TOPIC42.HTM [Accessed April, 2012].
2. Liotta EA (2010). Addison Disease. [online] Available from http://www.emedicine.medscape.com/article/1096911-overview [Accessed April, 2012].

43. ADIE SYNDROME (HOLMES-ADIE SYNDROME; IRIDOPLEGIA INTERNA; MARKUS SYNDROME; MYOTONIC PUPIL; PSEUDOTONIC PUPILLOTONIA; ROSS SYNDROME; SAENGER SYNDROME; TONIC PUPIL; WEILL-REYE'S SYNDROME)

General

Cause unknown; more frequent in females; manifested in the second and third decades; abnormal sensitivity to 2.5% solution of methacholine; segmental compensatory hyperhidrosis; tonic pupil constricts, whereas normal pupils are unaffected; tonic pupil, hyporeflexia and segmental hypohidrosis are manifestations of Ross syndrome.

Ocular

Slightly enlarged pupils; delayed or diminished direct and consensual reaction to light; usually unilateral; consensual reflex is abolished on the affected side but normal on the other; amblyopia.

Clinical

Loss of tendon reflexes, particularly ankle and knee jerk (partial or total).

Laboratory

Diagnosis is made by clinical findings.

Treatment

None

Bibliography

1. Agbeja AM, Dutton GN. Adie's syndrome as a cause of amblyopia. J Pediatr Ophthalmol Strabismus. 1987;24:176-7.

44. ADRENOLEUKODYSTROPHY (MELANODERMIC LEUKODYSTROPHY; SUDANOPHILIC LEUKODYSTROPHY)

General

Degenerative metabolic disease in which cholesterol with long-chain fatty acids accumulates in affected cells; symptoms usually begin between the ages of 3 and 12 years but may have their onset in adulthood; X-linked recessive with predominantly central nervous system and adrenal dysfunction.

Ocular

Optic atrophy; retinal ganglion cell degeneration; exotropia; esotropia; cataracts; optic pallor; optic nerve hypoplasia; visual field defects; macular pigmentary changes; progressive visual loss.

Clinical

Central nervous system manifestations consisting of behavioral changes, disturbance of gait, dysarthria and dysphagia; seizures; spastic quadriparesis; decorticate posturing; one-third of patients show adrenal insufficiency.

Laboratory

A cosyntropin stimulation test will confirm the diagnosis of adrenocortical insufficiency.

Treatment

Once electrolytes, blood sugar, cortisol, 17-hydroxyprogesterone and ACTH concentrations are obtained treatment with glucocorticoids can be used. This therapy is based on suspicion of adrenal insufficiency, since it may be life preserving.

Additional Resource

1. Wilson TA (2012). Adrenal Hypoplasia. [online] Available from http://www.emedicine.com/ped/TOPIC45.HTM [Accessed April, 2012].

45. ADULT CATARACTS

General

Cataract is a disorder in which the crystalline lens becomes opacified.

Clinical

None

Ocular

Glare, monocular diplopia, changes in refractive error, decreased visual acuity.

Laboratory

Diagnosis is made by clinical findings.

Treatment

Change in glasses can sometimes improve a patient's visual function temporarily; however, the most common treatment is cataract surgery.

Bibliography

1. Roy FH, Fraunfelder FW, Fraunfelder FT. Roy and Fraunfelder's Current Ocular Therapy, 6th edition. Philadelphia: WB Saunders; 2008.

46. AFRICAN EYE WORM DISEASE (LOIASIS)

General

Caused by the filarial nematode *Loa loa*; transmitted to humans by diurnally biting flies (deerflies) of the *Chrysops* species that live in the rainforests of West and Central Africa.

Ocular

Parasites of anterior chamber, conjunctiva, eyelid, vitreous and choroid; conjunctivitis; keratitis; optic nerve atrophy; white, cottony mass of vitreous; central retinal artery occlusion; macular hemorrhages; paralysis of extraocular muscles; nystagmus; uveitis.

Clinical

Transient erythematous swelling; pruritus; eosinophilia; fever; urticaria; rarely neurologic involvement.

Laboratory

Diagnosis is made by clinical findings.

Treatment

Remove surgically when possible.

Additional Resource

1. Hökelek M (2011). Nematode Infections. [online] Available from http://www.emedicine.medscape.com/article/224011-overview [Accessed April, 2012].

47. AFTER CATARACTS

General

After cataract is a term originally used to describe lens epithelial cell proliferation following cataract surgery.

Clinical

None

Ocular

Posterior capsule opacification, delayed endophthalmitis.

Laboratory

Diagnosis is made by clinical findings.

Treatment

Laser posterior capsulotomy.

Bibliography

1. Roy FH, Fraunfelder FW, Fraunfelder FT. Roy and Fraunfelder's Current Ocular Therapy, 6th edition. Philadelphia: WB Saunders; 2008.

48. AGE-RELATED MACULAR DEGENERATION

General

Pathologic changes of this chronic degenerative condition occur primarily in the retinal pigment epithelium, Bruch's membrane and the choriocapillaris of the macular region.

Clinical

Hypertension, high cholesterol level.

Ocular

Vision loss, choroidal neovascularization.

Laboratory

Diagnosis is made by clinical findings.

Treatment

No treatment available for non-neovascular age-related macular degeneration (AMD). Preventative therapy includes no smoking, control of hypertension, cholesterol and blood sugar, exercise and vitamins. Neovascular AMD treatment consists of laser, Avastin and Lucentis.

Bibliography

1. Lima LH, Schubert C, Ferrara DC, et al. Three major loci involved in age-related macular degeneration are also associated with polypoidal choroidal vasculopathy. Ophthalmology. 2010;117:1567-70.

Additional Resources

1. Prall FR (2012). Exudative ARMD. [online] Available from http://www.emedicine.com/oph/TOPIC653.HTM [Accessed April, 2012].
2. Maturi RK (2011). Nonexudative ARMD. [online] Available from http://www.emedicine.com/oph/TOPIC383.HTM [Accessed April, 2012].

49. AGRANULOCYTOSIS SYNDROME (AGRANULOCYTIC ANGINA SYNDROME; MALIGNANT NEUTROPENIA SYNDROME; PERNICIOUS LEUKOPENIA SYNDROME; SCHULTZ SYNDROME)

General

Caused by hypersensitivity reaction to chemicals, drugs and ionizing radiation; may be idiopathic; more frequent in adults; female preponderance (3:1); acute onset.

Ocular

Scleral and conjunctival icterus; conjunctival hemorrhages; retinal hemorrhages.

Clinical

Swollen, painful joints; malaise; sore throat with mucous membrane ulceration; sepsis.

Laboratory

Evaluation of the peripheral blood smear provides information about RBC and platelet morphology.

Treatment

Indentify etiology and discontinue the offending agent. If the identity of the causative agent is not known, stop administration of all drugs until the etiology is established.

Additional Resource

1. Godwin JE (2011). Neutropenia. [online] Available from http://www.emedicine.com/med/TOPIC82. HTM [Accessed April, 2012].

50. AICARDI SYNDROME

General

All symptoms present at birth; cause unknown; all findings progress with age; shows X-linked dominant inheritance.

Ocular

Microphthalmia; lid twitching; absent pupillary reflexes; round retinal lacunae up to disk size look like holes with retinal vessels crossing over them; funnel-shaped disk; chorioretinitis.

Clinical

Infantile spasms (tonic seizures in flexion); epileptic seizures; cyanosis; mental anomaly; vertebral anomalies; telangiectasia; hypotonia; head deformities with biparietal bossing, occipital flattening and plagiocephaly; defects of corpus callosum; cortical heterotopia; characteristic electroencephalogram; dilated intracranial ventricle with leukomalacia.

Laboratory

Generally diagnosis is made by clinical findings. Neuroimaging can delineate the degree of CNS dysgenesis and help evaluate other potential etiologies of intractable epilepsy and developmental delay.

Treatment

Consultation with a child neurologist is recommended. Use of traditional epilepsy therapies for seizure manifestations is recommended.

Additional Resource

1. Davis RG (2012). Aicardi Syndrome. [online] Available from http://www.emedicine.com/ped/ TOPIC58.HTM [Accessed April, 2012].

51. ALACRIMA

General

Autosomal recessive; wide spectrum of lacrimal secretory disorders that are mostly congenital in origin; symptoms of these disorders can range from a complete absence of tears to hyposecretion of tears; symptoms of rarer disorders include a selective absence of tearing in response to emotional stimulation but a normal secretory response to mechanical stimulation; may be associated with syndromes such as Riley-Day, anhidrotic ectodermal dysplasia, Sjögren and Allgrove.

Clinical

Decreased salivation and sweating; osteoporosis; short stature; adrenocortical insufficiency.

Ocular

Foreign body sensation; photophobia, decreased visual acuity; absence of tears; chronic blepharoconjunctivitis; hyperemia; thick mucoid discharge; keratinization; pannus; corneal ulcers or perforation; tonic pupils; optic atrophy.

Laboratory

Computed tomography (CT) scan of orbits to determine aplastic lacrimal glands; schirmer testing; conjunctival and lacrimal gland biopsy.

Treatment

Artificial tears, gels and ointments are used as the primary treatment. Permanent or temporary punctal occlusion can be effective. Tarsorrhaphy may be necessary if the cornea becomes compromised.

Additional Resource

1. DeAngelis DD (2010). Alacrima. [online] Available from http:// www. emedicine.medscape.com/ article/1210539-overview [Accessed April, 2012].

52. ALAGILLE SYNDROME (AGS; ALAGILLE-WATSON SYNDROME, AWS; CHOLESTASIS WITH PERIPHERAL PULMONARY STENOSIS; ARTERIOHEPATIC DYSPLASIA, AHD; HEPATIC DUCTULAR HYPOPLASIA, SYNDROMATIC)

General

Alagille syndrome may be associated with 20p 11.2 deletion and four distinct coding mutations in *JAG1* gene.

Ocular

Posterior embryotoxon and retinal pigmentary changes; anterior chamber anomalies, associated with eccentric or ectopic pupils.

Clinical

Neonatal jaundice; prominent forehead and chin; pulmonic valvular stenosis as well as peripheral arterial stenosis; abnormal vertebrae ("butterfly" vertebrae) and decrease in interpediculate distance in the lumbar spine; absent deep tendon reflexes and poor school performance; in the facies, broad forehead, pointed mandible and bulbous tip of the nose; and in the fingers, varying degrees of foreshortening.

Laboratory

Liver biopsy specimens typically exhibit features suggestive of chronic cholestasis and paucity of interlobular bile ducts. The majority of biopsies (wedge or needle) reveal features of bile duct paucity.

Treatment

Subspecialty consultation may facilitate diagnosis and provide long-term care. Consultation with an ophthalmologist may provide the diagnosis. A pediatric hepatologist can assist with management of chronic cholestatic liver disease. Cardiology consultation can assist with the diagnosis and therapy for intracardiac disease, as well as other vascular abnormalities. Nephrology consultation is useless when structural renal disease is present or if suspicions of evolving renal insufficiency arise.

Additional Resource

1. Scheimann A (2012). Alagille Syndrome. [online] Available from http://www.emedicine.com/ped/TOPIC60.HTM [Accessed April, 2012].

53. ALBERS-SCHONBERG DISEASE (MARBLE BONE DISEASE; OSTEOPETROSIS; OSTEOPOIKILOSIS; OSTEOSCLEROSIS CONGENITA DIFFUSA; OSTEOSCLEROSIS FRAGILIS GENERALISATA)

General

Simple recessive inheritance, also dominant transmission; benign form is asymptomatic in about 50% of cases and known under the synonym Henck-Assmann syndrome; prognosis is poor for malignant form, with death usually in infancy.

Ocular

Oculomotor paralysis; cranial nerve VII (facial) palsy; optic atrophy; ptosis; exophthalmos; papilledema; nystagmus; anisocoria; congenital cataracts; hypertelorism; visual loss in infancy; nasolacrimal duct obstruction; keratoconus.

Clinical

Cartilage and bone thickening; multiple fractures; hyperchromic anemia; osteomyelitis; severe forms: jaundice, hepatosplenomegaly, skeleton sclerosis, lymphadenopathy and hydrocephalus in infants; mild forms: nerve compression, fractures and milder form of anemia; pancytopenia from marrow obliteration; low serum calcium; elevated phosphorus.

Laboratory

Radiologic features are usually diagnostic. Patients usually have generalized osteosclerosis. Bones may be uniformly sclerotic, but alternating sclerotic and lucent bands may be noted in iliac wings and near ends of long bones. The bones might be clublike or appear like a bone within bone.

Treatment

Infantile therapy: Vitamin D appears to help by stimulating dormant osteoclasts and thus stimulate bone resorption. Large doses of calcitriol, along with restricted calcium intake, sometimes improve osteopetrosis dramatically.

Adult treatment: No specific medical treatment exists for the adult type.

Additional Resource

1. Blank R (2012). Osteopetrosis. [online] Available from http://www.emedicine.com/med/TOPIC1692.HTM [Accessed April, 2012].

54. ALBINISM (BROWN OCULOCUTANEOUS ALBINISM; NETTLESHIP-FALLS SYNDROME)

General

Congenital hypopigmentation.

1. Complete.

Ocular

Iris thin, pale blue; prominent choroidal vessels with poorly defined fovea; nystagmus; head nodding; frequently myopic astigmatism and strabismus; marked photophobia; eyelashes and eyebrows are white; optic atrophy; cataract; abnormal decussation of retinogeniculate axons at the chiasm.

Clinical

White hair, eyebrows and skin; autosomal recessive.

2. Modified complete.

Ocular

Slight pigmentation at pupillary border; may be nystagmus, photophobia and myopia; choroidal vessels prominent.

Clinical

Negroes; slight pigmentation; golden hair; tendency to hyperkeratoses; freckling in exposed areas of skin; autosomal recessive.

3. Ocular.

Ocular

Marked deficiency of pigment in iris and choroid; nystagmus and myopic astigmatism; iris of female carrier frequently is translucent; macular hypoplasia; photophobia; pigmentation of retinal pigment epithelium.

Clinical

Normal pigmentation elsewhere; autosomal recessive.

4. Amish.

Ocular

At birth, complete albinism with blue translucent irides and albinotic fundal reflex; nystagmus; photophobia; increasing pigmentation with age; abnormal decussation of retinogeniculate axons at the chiasm.

Clinical

White hair and skin at birth; increasing pigmentation with yellow hair and normal skin that tans; autosomal recessive.

Laboratory

The most definitive test in determining the albinism type is genetic sequence analysis. This test is useful only for families with individuals who have albinism. The test cannot be used as a screening tool.

Treatment

Currently, there is no therapy for albinism. Sunglasses to reduce photophobia, low-vision aids and treatment for strabismus might be useful.

Additional Resource

1. Bashour M (2010). Albinism. [online] Available from http://www.emedicine.com/oph/TOPIC315. HTM [Accessed April, 2012].

55. ALBRIGHT SYNDROME (FIBROUS DYSPLASIA; FULLER ALBRIGHT SYNDROME; JAFFE-LICHTENSTEIN SYNDROME; MCCUNE-ALBRIGHT SYNDROME; OSTEITIS FIBROSA DISSEMINATA; OSTEODYSTROPHIA FIBROSA; POLYOSTOTIC FIBROUS DYSPLASIA)

General

Etiology unknown; disease rare; manifested in children and young adults; found predominantly in females.

Ocular

Unilateral proptosis; papilledema; optic atrophy; lacrimal fossa mass; acute or chronic monocular visual loss.

Clinical

Medullary structures replaced by fibrous dysplasia; pelvic bones and lower extremities most frequently involved (spontaneous fractures); brown pigmented areas of skin, from small, freckle-like dots to large, flat patches on thighs, sacrum, upper spine, neck and scalp; endocrine dysfunction (precocious puberty in females) with early menarche, adolescent external genitalia and breast enlargement; loss of hearing; convulsions; mental retardation.

Laboratory

A highly sensitive polymerase chain reaction test can find activating mutations of the *GNAS1* gene in peripheral blood cells of patients with McCune-Albright syndrome (MAS) or isolated fibrous dysplasia. Full endocrine studies should be performed, arterial blood gas determination can be performed to evaluate for acidosis and a complete metabolic profile can be performed to screen for hyperbilirubinemia.

Treatment

Endocrinology consultation is indicated to manage endocrine defects. Orthopedist consultation is helpful for pathologic fractures.

Additional Resource

1. Scheinfeld NS (2011). Albright Syndrome. [online] Available from http://www.emedicine.com/derm/TOPIC13.HTM [Accessed April, 2012].

56. ALCOHOLISM

General

Classified into three groups: (1) symptoms of mental disease, (2) physiologic poison or (3) result of social drinking; addiction compounds other health disorders.

Ocular

Congestion of conjunctiva; amblyopia; diplopia; night blindness; nystagmus; cataracts; paralysis of accommodation; paralysis of extraocular muscles; esophoria for distance fixation; acute visual loss; cotton-wool spots; cherry-red spot (associated with pancreatitis).

Clinical

Tremors; seizures; delirium; alcoholic hepatitis; cirrhosis; gastritis; pancreatitis; cancer of mouth and esophagus; peripheral neuropathy; organic brain disease; hypertension; cardiomyopathy; hypoglycemia; anemia; hyperuricemia; susceptibility to infections; skeletal myopathies.

Treatment

Address the issue, strongly encourage AA and encourage family members to contact Al-Anon and Alateen.

Additional Resource

1. Thompson W (2012). Alcoholism. [online] Available from http://www.emedicine.com/med/TOPIC98.HTM [Accessed April, 2012].

---

57. ALEXANDER DISEASE

General

Rare degenerative neurologic disorder characterized by diffuse demyelination in the presence of Rosenthal fibers; cases may resemble multiple sclerosis; neuroradiological findings include increased cerebellar white matter hyperintensity and diffuse periventricular signal hyperintensities.

Ocular

Impaired smooth pursuit; gaze-evoked horizontal nystagmus; slowed saccades; ocular myoclonus.

Clinical

In infants, hydrocephalus, spasticity and seizures; in juveniles and adults, bulbar palsy and hyperreflexia, intermittent neurologic dysfunction.

Laboratory

Diagnosis is made by clinical findings.

Treatment

None

Bibliography

1. Reichard EA, Ball WS, Bove KE. Alexander disease: a case report and review of the literature. Pediatr Pathol Lab Med. 1996;16:327-43.
2. Russo LS, Aron A, Anderson PJ. Alexander's disease: a report and reappraisal. Neurology. 1976;26:607-14.

---

58. ALKALINE INJURY OF THE EYE

General

A splash of alkaline solution causes the pH to rise and results in immediate damage to the external ocular tissues. These injuries are frequently seen from household chemicals or farming injuries from liquid ammonia used as fertilizer.

Ocular

Pain; lacrimation; blepharospasm; rise in intraocular pressure; rapid penetration of the cornea and sclera; chemical injury to iris, lens or ciliary body; symblepharon; phthisis bulbi; ankyloblepharon.

Laboratory

Diagnosis is made by clinical findings and history.

Treatment

Immediate copious irrigation, sticky paste of lime should be removed with a cotton-tipped applicator, mydriasis and topical antibiotics, pain medications, treatment of glaucoma with carbonic anhydrase inhibitors, patching and soft contact lenses may facilitate re-epithelialization, insertion of a methylmethacrylate ring may prevent fibrinous adhesions, lysis of adhesions with or without mucous membrane grafts, corneal stem cell transplantation, corneal transplantation, keratoprosthesis and conjunctival autographs.

Bibliography

1. Roy FH, Fraunfelder FW, Fraunfelder FT. Roy and Fraunfelder's Current Ocular Therapy, 6th edition. Philadelphia: WB Saunders; 2008.

59. ALKAPTONURIA (GARROD SYNDROME; OCHRONOSIS)

General

Rare autosomal recessive metabolic disease; enzyme homogentisic acid oxidase missing; both sexes affected; onset in the first few days of life; manifestations more severe in males.

Ocular

Pigmentation of cornea, sclera and conjunctiva; ochronosis of sclera; oil globulation within Bowman's membrane.

Clinical

Black-colored urine on standing; osteoarthritis; valvular heart disease; atherosclerosis (homogentisic acid oxidase deficiency); pigmentation of cartilage and other connective tissues.

Laboratory

Homogentisic acid can be identified in urine using gas chromatography—mass spectroscopy.

Treatment

Reduction of phenylalanine and tyrosine reduced homogentisic acid excretion in the urine of a child. Vitamin C, up to 1 g/d, is recommended for older children and adults.

Additional Resource

1. Roth KS (2011). Alkaptonuria. [online] Available from http://www.emedicine.com/ped/TOPIC64.HTM [Accessed April, 2012].

60. ALLERGIC CONJUNCTIVITIS (ALLERGIC RHINOCONJUNCTIVITIS; ATOPIC KERATOCONJUNCTIVITIS; GIANT PAPILLARY CONJUNCTIVITIS; HAY FEVER CONJUNCTIVITIS)

General

Exposure of sensitive individuals to specific allergens, recurrent, seasonal (spring and summer due to pollens) or house dust and animal dander.

Clinical

None

Ocular

Itching, conjunctival erythema and chemosis, papillary hypertrophy.

Laboratory

Diagnosis is made by clinical findings.

Treatment

Artificial tears, cool compresses, vasoconstrictors, antihistamines, mast cell stabilizers, nonsteroidal anti-inflammatories, steroids and systemic antihistamine.

Additional Resource

1. Ventocilla M (2012). Allergic Conjunctivitis [online] Available from http://www.emedicine.com/oph/TOPIC85.HTM [Accessed April, 2012].

61. ALLERGIC TO EVERYTHING SYNDROME

General

"Environmentally ill" or allergic to unusual or common substances in the environment; females affected most frequently.

Ocular

Transient visual loss.

Clinical

Stupor; lethargy; memory loss; depression; gastrointestinal dysfunction; rashes; migraine headache; hearing loss.

Laboratory

Diagnosis is made by clinical findings.

Treatment

Adequate hygiene and avoidance of the contactant may be helpful. Many cases of localized mild contact dermatitis respond well to cool compresses and adequate wound care. Antibiotic therapy may be necessary for secondary infection. Low-strength topical steroids, such as hydrocortisone, may be effective in decreasing inflammation and symptoms associated with very mild contact dermatitis. Systemic steroids are the mainstay of therapy in acute episodes of severe extensive allergic contact dermatitis.

Additional Resource

1. Elston DM (2011). Pediatric Contact Dermatitis. [online] Available from http://www.emedicine.com/ped/TOPIC2569.HTM [Accessed April, 2012].

62. ALLGROVE SYNDROME

General

Autosomal recessive.

Ocular

Distichiasis, conjuncitivitis, keratitis, congenital alacrima.

Clinical

Adrenocorticotropic hormone (ACTH) insensitivity, achalasia.

Laboratory

Lacrimal gland biopsy is examined with an electron microscope. Evidence of neuronal degeneration associated with depletion of secretory granules in the acinar cells are present. The reduced or absent lacrimation that accompanies this change frequently leads to the dehydration-induced keratopathy observed with rose Bengal staining. CT demonstrates atrophic adrenal glands. As with all states of ACTH unresponsiveness, one may expect to see atrophy of the zona fasciculata.

Treatment

Replacement of glucocorticoids in patients with known adrenal insufficiency is critical to avoid an adrenal crisis. The symptoms of alacrima can be handled with topical lubricants or punctal occlusion. Achalasia is best managed with surgical correction either pneumatic dilatation or anterior cardiomyotomy.

Additional Resource

1. Boston BA (2012). Allgrove (AAA) Syndrome. [online] Available from http://www.emedicine. com/ped/TOPIC71.HTM [Accessed April, 2012].

---

63. ALOPECIA AREATA

General

Unknown etiology; increased incidence of autoimmune disease, Addison disease, diabetes mellitus and vitiligo; initially occurs episodically; most commonly in patients between the ages of 5 and 40 years; most cases repopulate with normal hair in 6–12 months without any specific treatment.

Ocular

Loss of eyelashes and eyebrows; cataract.

Clinical

Circumscribed patches of hair loss on scalp and all body hair areas; fingernail changes.

Laboratory

Diagnosis usually can be made on clinical findings; a scalp biopsy seldom is necessary.

Treatment

The condition is benign, and spontaneous remissions and recurrences are common. Generally treatments used are to stimulate hair growth.

Additional Resource

1. Bolduc C (2010). Alopecia Areata. [online] Available from http://www.emedicine.com/derm/TOPIC14. HTM [Accessed April, 2012].

---

64. ALPORT SYNDROME (FAMILIAL NEPHRITIS; HEREDITARY FAMILIAL CONGENITAL HEMORRHAGIC NEPHRITIS; HEREDITARY NEPHRITIS)

General

Autosomal dominant inheritance; early death in males; normal life span in females.

Ocular

Anterior lenticonus (bilateral progressive); subcapsular cataracts; thinning of lens capsule; fundus albipunctatus; retinopathy similar to juvenile macular degeneration; hyaline bodies of optic nerve head; vesicles in Descemet's membrane affecting basement membrane collagen; anterior and polar cataracts.

Clinical

Hemorrhagic nephritis; progressive nerve deafness; deafness (high tone, sensorineural); most often transmitted as an X-linked dominant trait, although dominant and recessive transmission has been reported.

Laboratory

Urinalysis reveals microscopic or gross hematuria. Renal ultrasonography is indicated for children with persistent microscopic hematuria.

Treatment

There is no treatment to prevent progression. Renal transplantation is the treatment of choice.

Additional Resource

1. Prasad D (2011). Pediatric Alport Syndrome. [online] Available from http://www.emedicine.com/ped/TOPIC74.HTM [Accessed April, 2012].

65. ALSTROM DISEASE (CATARACT AND RETINITIS PIGMENTOSA)

General

Retinal lesion associated with deafness; severe visual loss in the first decade.

Ocular

Cataract; retinitis pigmentosa; optic atrophy; salt and pepper pigment epithelial abnormalities. Electroretinogram pathognomonic findings include initially normal rod component, which can become undetectable as early as 5 years of age; undetectable cone activity at 18 months.

Clinical

Nerve deafness; diabetes mellitus in childhood; obesity; renal disease; baldness; hyperuricemia; hypogenitalism; acanthosis nigricans; skeletal anomalies; diabetes mellitus; deafness.

Laboratory

Diagnosis is made by clinical observation.

Treatment

Vitamin A 15,000 IU/day is thought to slow the decline of retinal function, dark sunglasses for outdoor use, surgery for cataract, genetic counseling.

Bibliography

1. Geeraets WJ. Ocular Syndromes, 3rd edition. Philadelphia: Lea & Febiger; 1976.
2. Harley RD (Ed). Pediatric Ophthalmology, 4th edition. Philadelphia: WB Saunders; 1998.
3. Konigsmark BW, Knox DL, Hussels IE, et al. Dominant congenital deafness and progressive optic nerve atrophy. Occurrence in four generations of a family. Arch Ophthalmol. 1974;91:99-103.
4. Millay RH, Weleber RG, Heckenlively JR. Ophthalmologic and systemic manifestations of Alstrom's disease. Am J Ophthalmol. 1986;102:482-90.
5. Tremblay F, LaRoche RG, Shea SE, et al. Longitudinal study of the early electroretinographic changes in Alstrom's syndrome. Am J Ophthalmol. 1993;115:657-65.

66. ALZHEIMER DISEASE (DEMENTIA)

General

Diffuse brain atrophy coming on well before the senile period of life; progressive; etiology currently unknown but hereditary disorder suspected; terminally, nearly decorticate, with loss of all ability to think, perceive, speak or move.

Ocular

Fixed dilated pupil; optic atrophy; decreased contrast sensitivity, color vision and stereo vision; abnormalities of the optic nerve head and nerve fiber layer; controversy exists regarding the ability to diagnose patients with Alzheimer disease by their marked hypersensitivity in pupil dilation response to tropicamide.

Clinical

Emotional disturbances; depression; anxiety; antisocial behavior; aphasia; apraxic disturbances; abnormalities of space perception; shuffling gait; generalized shuffling gait with short steps; disturbances in thought process.

Laboratory

Brain MRI or CT scans show diffuse cortical and/ or cerebral atrophy.

Treatment

Medical treatments include psychotropic medications and behavioral interventions, cholinesterase inhibitors and the avoidance of centrally acting anticholinergic medications, N-methyl-D-aspartate antagonists, and other and new therapeutic interventions.

Additional Resource

1. Anderson HS (2012). Alzheimer Disease. [online] Available from http://www.emedicine.com/ neuro/TOPIC13.HTM [Accessed April, 2012].

---

67. AMANTADINE-ASSOCIATED CORNEAL EDEMA

General

Onset from 2 months to several years following the start of the drug amantadine. Most corneal edema resolves after the discontinuation of therapy; however, some cases do not and result in the need for surgical correction. Amantadine is an antiviral agent used for the treatment of Parkinson or multiple sclerosis.

Clinical

Multiple sclerosis, Parkinson disease.

Ocular

Corneal edema, loss of endothelial cells, loss of visual acuity.

Laboratory

Diagnosis is made by clinical findings.

Treatment

Most cases resolve by stopping the use of amantadine. If corneal decompensation is persistent after discontinuation a penetrating keratopathy may be necessary.

Bibliography

1. Jeng BH, Galor A, Lee MS, et.al. Amantadine-associated corneal edema potentially irreversible even after cessation of the medication. Ophthalmology. 2008;115:1540-4.

68. AMAUROSIS FUGAX SYNDROME

General

Caused by malignant hypertension; often occurs in association with heavy smoking; may indicate vascular insufficiency of the vertebrobasilar arterial system; may precede a cerebrovascular accident and not infrequently seen in vascular insufficiency problems of the carotid arterial system; the cause, if found, is commonly an abnormality in the ipsilateral carotid artery or a cardiac source of embolism.

Ocular

Partial blindness in short attacks to permanent complete blindness; scintillating scotoma; teichopsia; retinal arteriolar spasm; signs of arteriolar sclerosis.

Clinical

Malignant hypertension; atherosclerosis; expanding lesions of the frontal or temporal lobe; vascular insufficiency.

Laboratory

There is no specific test but is essential to evaluate the erythrocyte sedimentation rate (ESR) and C-reactive protein (CRP) levels to rule out other causes. Doppler test may be useful.

Treatment

No specific treatment, except when the Doppler test is positive, carotid surgery may be indicated.

Additional Resource

1. Leibovitch I (2011). Ocular Ischemic Syndrome. [online] Available from http://www.emedicine. com/oph/TOPIC487.HTM [Accessed April, 2012].

69. AMBLYOPIA (FUNCTIONAL AMBLYOPIA; LAZY EYE)

General

Reduction of best-corrected visual acuity that cannot be explained by structural abnormalities. Usually associated with strabismus or anisometropic. Onset in childhood.

Clinical

None

Ocular

Decreased central visual acuity, decreased contrast sensitivity, strabismus, anisometropic.

Laboratory

Diagnosis is made by clinical findings.

Treatment

If there is a obstacle to vision such as cataract, corneal opacity, ptosis or refractive error, this must be treated first. Occlusion of the sound eye is the mainstay of treatment and the success depends on the compliance. Atropine ophthalmic drops can be used in the sound eye in mild or moderate cases of amblyopia. Early diagnosis and treatment provide the best chance of regaining useful vision.

Additional Resource

1. Yen KG (2011). Amblyopia. [online] Available from http://www.emedicine.com/oph/TOPIC316.HTM [Accessed April, 2012].

70. AMBLYOPIC SCHOOLGIRL SYNDROME

General

Etiology unknown.

Ocular

Amblyopia; changes in visual fields; abnormal dark adaptation curve; visual field defects usually are tubular or spiral but also include central, paracentral and ring scotomas; hemianopsias and superior and inferior field defects reported.

Clinical

Psychogenic disorder: affective and hysterical.

Laboratory

Organic cause for decreased vision and the ocular examination is normal, then further investi-gations into retinal or optic nerve causes should be initiated. Studies to perform include imaging of the visual system through CT scan, MRI and fluorescein angiography to assess the retina.

Treatment

Organic cause should be determined and treated. Occlusion therapy, forcing the use of the amblyopic eye, has been the mainstay of treatment.

Additional Resource

1. Yen KG (2011). Amblyopia. [online] Available from http://www.emedicine.com/oph/TOPIC316.HTM [Accessed April, 2012].

71. AMEBIASIS (AMEBIC DYSENTERY)

General

Caused by *Entamoeba histolytica; E. histolytica* cysts in stools are diagnostic.

Ocular

Conjunctivitis; iridocyclitis; hypopyon; central choroiditis; retinal hemorrhages; retinal perivasculitis; macular edema; corneal ulceration; granulomatous and nongranulomatous uveitis; vitreous hemorrhage.

Clinical

Chronic dysentery; abscesses of liver and brain; toxic megacolon.

Laboratory

Enzyme immunoassay (EIA) is the best test for making the specific diagnosis of *E. histolytica*.

Treatment

Metronidazole is considered the drug of choice for symptomatic, invasive disease. Asymptomatic intestinal infection may be treated with iodo-quinol, paromomycin or diloxanide furoate.

Additional Resource

1. Dhawan VK (2010). Pediatric Amebiasis. [online] Available from http://www.emedicine.com/ped/TOPIC80.HTM [Accessed April, 2012].

72. AMENDOLA SYNDROME

General

Observed in Sao Paulo, Brazil; all ethnic groups are affected; endemic form of pemphigus foliaceus; possibly caused by environmental agents; autoimmune disease mediated by autoantibodies of the immunoglobulin G (IgG) class, IgG4 subclass.

Ocular

Blisters around eyebrows; entropion; ectropion; trichiasis; iritis.

Clinical

Brazilian pemphigus (fogo selvagem, "wild fire"), which resembles, because of its appearance, pemphigus foliaceus; fever; chills.

Laboratory

Diagnosis is made by clinical findings.

Treatment

Entropion: Topical antibiotics and lubricants, temporary sutures to evert the eyelid, lateral cantholysis with subconjunctival incision just inferior to the tarsus. Inferior retractors are isolated and reattached to anteroinferior portion of tarsus with multiple interrupted sutures.

Ectropion: Topical ocular lubricants. Congenital-full thickness skin graft with canthal tendon tightening. Involutional-tighten lid by resecting full thickness wedge-medial spindle procedure for punctal eversion. Paralytic may require a fascia lata sling procedure if it does not resolve in 3–6 months.

Iritis: Oral steroids if not responsive to topical steroids, immunosuppressants if bilateral disease that does not respond to oral steroids, periocular steroids for unilateral or posterior uveitis. Vitrectomy can be used for severe vitreous opacification. Cryotherapy and laser photocoagulation may be used for localized pars plana exudates.

Bibliography

1. Amendola F. Cataracta no pemfigo foliaceo (nota previa). Rev Paul Med. 1945;26:286.
2. Korting GW. The skin and the eye: a dermatologic correlation of diseases of the periorbital region. Philadelphia: WB Saunders; 1973. p. 82.
3. Magalini SI, Scrascia E. Dictionary of Medical Syndromes, 2nd edition. Philadelphia: JB Lippincott; 1981.
4. Sampaio SA, Rivitti EA, Aoki V, et al. Brazilian pemphigus foliaceus, endemic pemphigus foliaceus, or fogo selvagem (wild fire). Dermatol Clin. 1994;12:765-76.

73. AMERICAN MUCOCUTANEOUS LEISHMANIASIS (CUTANEOUS LEISHMANIASIS; ORIENTAL SORE)

General

Causative agent is protozoal parasite *Leishmania braziliensis*.

Ocular

Keratitis; eyelid edema; conjunctival ulcer; vascular sclerosis of choroid; granulomata of eyelid and conjunctiva; blepharoconjunctivitis.

Clinical

Ulcerating granulomas of the skin, nasal septum, nasopharynx, lips, soft palate, larynx and genitals.

Laboratory

The parasite can be detected through direct evidence from peripheral blood, bone marrow or splenic aspirates. The smears are stained in Leishman, Giemsa or Wright stains and examined under oil immersion microscope.

Treatment

Sodium stibogluconate, a pentavalent antimonial compound, is the drug of choice in the treatment of visceral leishmaniasis except for in Europe and Sbv-unresponsive regions of India.

Additional Resource

1. Vidyashankar C (2011). Pediatric Leishmaniasis. [online] Available from http://www.emedicine.com/ped/TOPIC1292.HTM [Accessed April, 2012].

74. AMINOPTERIN-INDUCED SYNDROME

General

Teratogenic effect of aminopterin and derivatives on fetus; present at birth; usually fetal or postnatal death.

Ocular

Hypertelorism

Clinical

Small body; microcephaly; hypoplasia of cranial bones; broad nasal bridge; micrognathia; cleft palate; low-set ears; mesomelic; hypodactyly; talipes equinovarus.

Laboratory

Diagnosis is made by clinical findings.

Treatment

None

Additional Resource

1. Draper JC (2011). Teratology and Drug Use During Pregnancy. [online] Available from http://www.emedicine.com/med/TOPIC3242.HTM [Accessed April, 2012].

75. AMNIOGENIC BAND SYNDROME (RING CONSTRICTION; STREETER DYSPLASIA)

General

Caused by fetus swallowing one or more of the free-floating strands that result from amniotic rupture; the tension of these strands intraorally and extraorally produces secondary tears and deformations; no hereditary factor known.

Ocular

Upward slant of palpebral fissures; bilateral upper and lower lid colobomas; telecanthus; bilateral corneal opacities; microphthalmos; strabismus; hypertelorism; epibulbar choristoma; unilateral chorioretinal defects or lacuna (rare).

Clinical

Craniofacial and limb abnormalities.

Laboratory

Diagnosis is made by clinical findings.

Treatment

Esotropia: Equalized vision with correct refractive error; surgery may be helpful in patient with diplopia.

Bibliography

1. Braude LS, Miller M, Cuttone J, et al. Ocular abnormalities in the amniogenic band syndrome. Br J Ophthalmol. 1981;65:299-303.

2. Hashemi K, Traboulsi EI, Chavis R, et al. Chorio-retinal lacuna in the amniotic band syndrome. J Pediatr Ophthalmol Strabismus. 1991;28:238-9.

3. Miller MT, Deutsch TA, Cronin C, et al. Amniotic bands as a cause of ocular anomalies. Am J Ophthalmol. 1987;104:270-9.

4. Murata T, Hashimoto S, Ishibashi T, et al. A case of amniotic band syndrome with bilateral epibulbar choristoma. Br J Ophthalmol. 1992;76:685-7.

5. Streeter GL. Focal deficiencies in fetal tissues and their relation to intrauterine amputation. Contrib Embryol Carney Inst. 1930;22:1-44.

76. AMYLOIDOSIS OF GINGIVA AND CONJUNCTIVA, WITH MENTAL RETARDATION (PRIMARY SYSTEMIC AMYLOIDOSIS)

General

Autosomal recessive; primary amyloidosis differs from secondary by the mesodermal tissues being affected and nodular form of deposits; no preexisting medical condition; preferential involvement of mesenchymal tissues; variable staining of deposits.

Ocular

Conjunctivitis with deposits; corneal leukoma; waxy eyelid papules with purpura; proptosis; diplopia; decreased vision; ptosis; keratitis sicca; upper lid mass; tonic pupil; accommodative paresis; diffuse yellow conjunctival mass.

Clinical

Hyperplastic gingivitis, tongue, skin and muscles; lungs with icing-like coating; mental retardation; peripheral neuropathy; congestive heart failure; polyarthropathy; spontaneous, incidental purpura; macroglossia; bleeding diathesis; idiopathic carpal tunnel syndrome.

Laboratory

Echocardiography is valuable in the evaluation of amyloid heart disease. Doppler studies are useful and may show abnormal relaxation early in the course of the disease. Advanced involvement is characterized by restrictive hemodynamics.

Treatment

The treatment is often unsatisfactory. No reliable method for the accurate assessment of the total amount of amyloid in the body exists. The similarity with multiple myeloma suggests that chemotherapy may be useful. Using different regimens of intermittent oral melphalan and prednisone may also be useful.

Additional Resource

1. Nyirady J (2011). Primary Systemic Amyloidosis. [online] Available from http://www.emedicine.com/derm/TOPIC19.HTM [Accessed April, 2012].

77. ANDERSEN-WARBURG SYNDROME (ATROPHIA OCULI CONGENITAL FETAL IRITIS SYNDROME; CONGENITAL PROGRESSIVE OCULO-ACOUSTICO-CEREBRAL DYSPLASIA; NORRIE DISEASE; OLIGOPHRENIA MICROPHTHALMOS SYNDROME; WHITNALL-NORMAN SYNDROME)

General

Sex-linked inheritance; gross deformation of both eyes; only males affected; onset at birth; putative gene for Norrie disease has been isolated and mapped to Xp11.3.

Ocular

Bilateral microphthalmos with extensive destruction of all ocular structures often resembling a pseudotumor; blindness at birth; iris atrophy; iritis; corneal opacification and lenticular destruction with a mass visible behind the lens as long as the lens is still clear; malformed retina and choroid with retinal pseudotumors; retinal detachment; retrolental vascular mass.

Clinical

Mental retardation ranging from imbecility to idiocy (may begin at any age) in about two-thirds of cases; deafness of differing severity with onset between the ages of 9 and 45 years.

Laboratory

Diagnosis is made by clinical findings.

Treatment

Topical treatment for iritis, retinal detachment surgery and vitrectomy may be neccesary.

Immediate laser treatment is recommended following birth.

Bibliography

1. Andersen SR, Warburg M. Norrie's disease: congenital bilateral pseudotumor of retina with recessive X-chromosomal inheritance; preliminary report. Arch Ophthalmol. 1961;66:614-8.
2. Black G, Redmond RM. The molecular biology of Norrie's disease. Eye (Lond). 1994;8(Pt 5):491-6.
3. Chow CC, Kiernan DF, Chau FY, et al. Laser photocoagulation at birth prevents blindness in Norrie's disease diagnosed using amniocentesis. Ophthalmology. 2010;117:2402-6.
4. Enyedi LB, de Juan E, Gaitan A. Ultrastructural study of Norrie's disease. Am J Ophthalmol. 1991;111:439-45.
5. Liberfarb RM, Eavey RD, De Long GR, et al. Norrie's disease: a study of two families. Ophthalmology. 1985;92:1445-51.
6. Norrie G. Causes of blindness in children. Twenty-five years' experience of Danish Institutes for the Blind. Acta Ophthalmol (Copenh). 1927;5:357-86.
7. Warburg M. Norrie's disease: differential diagnosis and treatment. Acta Ophthalmol (Copenh). 1975;53:217-36.
8. Wong F, Goldberg MF, Hao Y. Identification of a nonsense mutation at codon 128 of the Norrie's disease gene in a male infant. Arch Ophthalmol. 1993;111:1553-7.

78. ANDOGSKY SYNDROME (ATOPIC CATARACT SYNDROME; DERMATOGENOUS CATARACT)

General

Inherited abnormality involving the skin and lens with an altered reactivity to antigen.

Ocular

Atopic keratoconjunctivitis; keratoconus; uveitis; dense subcapsular cataract developing to a complete dense opacification.

Clinical

Atopic dermatitis as erythematous thickening of the skin with papular hyperpigmented and scaly changes, most frequently found in regions of the wrist, popliteal fossa, neck and sometimes forehead.

Laboratory

Diagnosis is made by clinical findings.

Treatment

Uveitis: Topical steroids and cycloplegic medication should be the initial treatment of choice. Oral steroids if not responsive to topical steroids, immunosuppressants if bilateral disease that does not respond to oral steroids, periocular steroids for unilateral or posterior uveitis. Vitrectomy can be used for severe vitreous opacification. Cryotherapy and laser photocoagulation may be used for localized pars plana exudates.

Cataract: It can be treated by a change in glasses which can sometimes improve a patient's visual function temporarily; however, the most common treatment is cataract surgery.

Bibliography

1. Andogsky N. Cataracts dermatogenes. Ein beitrag zur aetiologieder linsentrubung. Klin monatsbl Augennheilk. 1914;52:824.
2. Coles RS, Laval J. Retinal detachments occurring in cataract associated with neurodermatitis. AMA Arch Ophthalmol. 1952;48:30-9.
3. Geeraets WJ. Ocular Syndromes, 3rd edition. Philadelphia: Lea & Febiger; 1976.
4. Magalini SI, Scrascia E. Dictionary of Medical Syndromes, 2nd edition. Philadelphia: JB Lippincott; 1981.

79. ANEMIA

General

Ocular complications generally only seen in severe anemia.

Ocular

Palpebral conjunctival pallor; retinal hemorrhages; cotton-wool spots; retinal vein dilation; papilledema; ischemic optic neuropathy.

Clinical

Blood loss; excessive red blood cell destruction; inadequate red blood cell production; thrombocytopenia; leukemia.

Laboratory

Complete blood count (CBC), reticulocyte count and review of the peripheral smear.

Treatment

Medical care consists of establishing the diagnosis and reason for the iron deficiency. In most patients, the iron deficiency should be treated with oral iron therapy, and the underlying etiology should be corrected so the deficiency does not recur.

Additional Resource

1. Inoue S (2011). Pediatric Acute Anemia. [online] Available from http://www.emedicine.com/ped/ TOPIC98.HTM [Accessed April, 2012].

---

80. ANENCEPHALY

General

Congenital neural tube defect that affects the formation of the brain and skull bones. Lethal in all cases.

Ocular

Anophthalmos

Clinical

Absence of bony covering over the back of the head, cleft palate, heart defects.

Laboratory

Flattened head may be detected by prenatal ultrasound. Alpha-fetoprotein levels are elevated and can be detected in the amniotic fluid. Amniocentesis can be used to determine the chromosomal and genetic disorder.

Treatment

There is no treatment. Grief and genetic counseling should be offered to the parents.

Additional Resource

1. Best RG (2011). Anencephaly. [online] Available from http://www.emedicine.medscape.com/article/ 1181570-overview [Accessed April, 2012].

---

81. ANGELUCCI SYNDROME (CRITICAL ALLERGIC CONJUNCTIVITIS SYNDROME)

General

Etiology unknown; pruriginous cutaneous and mucous reactions that appear and cease rather suddenly.

Ocular

Chemosis; conjunctivitis (papillary type); severe itching and burning; photophobia.

Clinical

Tachycardia; vasomotor lability; excitability; allergies (asthma, urticaria, edema); dystrophic conditions and endocrine disorders are frequently associated findings.

Laboratory

Diagnosis is made by clinical findings.

Treatment

Symptomatic control may include cold compresses and artificial tears; nonsteroidal and occasionally steroidal drops to relieve itching.

Bibliography

1. Angelucci A. Di una Sindrome Sconoscita Negli Infermi di Cattarro Primaverile. Arch Ottal Palermo. 1897-1898;4:270.

2. Geeraets WJ. Ocular Syndromes, 3rd edition. Philadelphia: Lea & Febiger; 1976.

3. Magalini SI, Scrascia E. Dictionary of Medical Syndromes, 2nd edition. Philadelphia: JB Lippincott; 1981.

82. ANGIONEUROTIC EDEMA (GIANT EDEMA; GIANT URTICARIA; HIVES; NETTLE RASH; QUINCKE DISEASE)

General

Vascular reaction involving subcutaneous tissues or submucosa; both sexes affected; allergy to various agents, including medications; emotional factor may be involved; recurrent.

Ocular

Optic neuritis; papilledema; central serous retinopathy; corneal edema; exophthalmos; nystagmus; secondary glaucoma; uveitis; periorbital and lid edema.

Clinical

Transient erythema; angioneurotic edema of loose subcutaneous tissue; sporadic urticaria; nausea; vomiting; diarrhea; cephalalgia; severe respiratory distress; polyuria.

Laboratory

Plasma levels for the diagnosis include the following: C4 level less than 104 mg/L (diagnostic).

Treatment

The goal is to prevent episodes of swelling. Minor episodes of subepithelial swelling need no treatment, but the patient with edema of the face and neck should be closely observed for spread of edema and signs of airway involvement. When hoarseness or other signs of a compromised airway occur, an otolaryngologist should be consulted for possible tracheostomy.

Additional Resource

1. Shih-Wen Huang (2012). Pediatric Angioedema. [online] Available from http://www.emedicine.com/ped/TOPIC101.HTM [Accessed April, 2012].

83. ANGIOID STREAKS

General

Irregular, jagged lines that radiate from the optic nerve in all directions.

Clinical

Paget's disease, sickle cell anemia, hypertensive cardiovascular disorders.

Ocular

Choroidal neovascularization, retinal pigment epithelial detachment and macular degeneration.

Laboratory

Fluorescein angiography and indocyanine green angiography.

Treatment

Laser photocoagulation may be of benefit with juxtafoveal choroidal neovascularization associated with angioid streaks. Avastin injections have shown some promise for the control of choroidal neovascular membrane.

Additional Resource

1. Abusamak M (2011). Angioid Streaks. [online] Available from http://www.emedicine.com/oph/TOPIC378.HTM [Accessed April, 2012].

84. ANGLE RECESSION GLAUCOMA

General

Manifestation of blunt ocular trauma.

Clinical

None

Ocular

Angle recession involves rupture of the face of the ciliary body, resulting in a tear between the longitudinal and circular fibers of the ciliary muscle, which may cause glaucoma.

Laboratory

Diagnosis is made by clinical findings.

Treatment

Topical steroids with cycloplegic agents for inflammation. Antiglaucoma agents for IOP control. Surgical-filtration surgery with the use of antimetabolites appears to be the most effective technique.

Additional Resource

1. Sullivan BR (2010). Glaucoma, Angle Recession. [online] Available from http://www.emedicine.com/oph/TOPIC121.HTM [Accessed April, 2012].

85. ANGULAR CONJUNCTIVITIS (MORAX-AXENFELD BACILLUS)

General

Caused by *Moraxella lacunata*, which frequently inhabits the nose.

Ocular

Conjunctivitis; hypopyon; keratitis; uveitis; corneal marginal ulcer.

Laboratory

Diagnosis is made by clinical findings.

Treatment

Conjunctivitis: Antibiotic medication should be used to treat the infection.

Corneal ulcer: Corneal cultures may be taken and treatment initiated. Treatment includes a broad spectrum of antibiotics and cycloplegic drops.

Uveitis: Topical steroids and cycloplegic medication should be the initial treatment of choice. Oral steroids if not responsive to topical steroids, immunosuppressants if bilateral disease that does not respond to oral steroids, periocular steroids for unilateral or posterior uveitis. Vitrectomy can be used for severe vitreous opacification. Cryotherapy and laser photocoagulation may be used for localized pars plana exudates.

Bibliography

1. Jones DB. Early diagnosis and therapy of bacterial corneal ulcers. Int Ophthalmol Clin. 1973;13:1-29.
2. Marioneaux SJ, Cohen EJ, Arentsen JJ, et al. Moraxella keratitis. Cornea. 1991;10:21-4.
3. Van Bijsterveld OP. Bacterial proteases in Moraxella angular conjunctivitis. Am J Ophthalmol. 1971; 72:181-4.

86. ANIRIDIA (CONGENITAL ANIRIDIA, HEREDITARY ANIRIDIA)

General

Hereditary, recessive (two-thirds of cases), can be dominant, sporadic or traumatic; absence of the iris; rare; usually bilateral unless due to trauma.

Ocular

Absence of iris; subluxed lens; iridodialysis; cataract; glaucoma; corneal scarring, vascularization and edema; iris colobomata; round eccentric pupils; keratoconus.

Clinical

Cerebellar ataxia; mental retardation; Wilms tumor.

Laboratory

Chromosomal deletion, cytogenic analysis, submicroscopic deletions of Wilms' tumor gene with FISH technique, PCR genotyping halotypes across PAX6-WT1 region provides evidence of a chromosomal deletion.

Treatment

Systemic or topical antiglaucoma therapy.

Bibliography

1. Francois J, Coucke D, Coppieters R. Aniridia-Wilms' tumour syndrome. Ophthalmologica. 1977;174:35-9.
2. Johns KJ, O'Day DM. Posterior chamber intraocular lenses after extracapsular extraction in patients with aniridia. Ophthalmology. 1991;98:1698-702.
3. Kremer I, Rajpal RK, Rapuano CJ, et al. Results of penetrating keratoplasty in aniridia. Am J Ophthalmol. 1993;115:317-20.
4. Magalini SI, Scrascia E. Dictionary of Medical Syndromes, 2nd edition. Philadelphia: JB Lippincott; 1981.
5. Mintz-Hittner HA, Ferrell RE, Lyons LA, et al. Criteria to detect minimal expressivity within families with autosomal dominant aniridia. Am J Ophthalmol. 1992;114:700-7.
6. Nelson LB, Spaeth GL, Nowinski TS, et al. Aniridia. A review. Surv Ophthalmol. 1984;28:621-42.

87. ANIRIDIA AND ABSENT PATELLA

General

Autosomal dominant; rare.

Ocular

Absence of iris; cataracts; glaucoma.

Clinical

Absence of knee cap, hypoplastic or aplastic.

Laboratory

Chromosomal deletion is detected by cytogenetic testing with the use of high-resolution banding.

Treatment

The goal is directed toward control of intraocular pressure with the use of topical drops. Frequently, this goal is not met. Photophobia can be treated with tinted glasses. Strabismus, amblyopia, refractive errors and nystagmus may also require treatment with traditional methods.

Additional Resource

1. Singh D (2010). Aniridia. [online] Available from http://www.emedicine.com/oph/TOPIC43.HTM [Accessed April, 2012].

88. ANIRIDIA, CEREBELLAR ATAXIA AND MENTAL DEFICIENCY (GILLESPIE SYNDROME)

General

Autosomal recessive; onset at birth.

Ocular

Congenital cataracts; incomplete formation of iris; bilateral congenital mydriasis.

Clinical

Cerebellar ataxia; mental deficiency; delayed developmental milestones; persistent hypotonia of muscles; gross incoordination; attention tremor; scanning speech.

Laboratory

Chromosomal deletion is detected by cytogenetic testing with the use of high-resolution banding.

Treatment

The goal is directed toward control of intraocular pressure with the use of topical drops. Frequently, this goal is not met. Photophobia can be treated with tinted glasses. Strabismus, amblyopia, refractive errors and nystagmus may also require treatment with traditional methods.

Additional Resource

1. Singh D (2010). Aniridia. [online] Available from http://www.emedicine.com/oph/TOPIC43.HTM [Accessed April, 2012].

89. ANIRIDIA, PARTIAL WITH UNILATERAL RENAL AGENESIS AND PSYCHOMOTOR RETARDATION

General

Autosomal recessive.

Ocular

Congenital glaucoma; telecanthus; absence of iris; hypertelorism.

Clinical

One kidney absent or in failure; motor effects of cerebral or psychic activity retarded or slowed.

Laboratory

Chromosomal deletion is detected by cytogenetic testing with the use of high-resolution banding.

Treatment

The goal is directed toward control of intraocular pressure with the use of topical drops. Frequently, this goal is not met. Photophobia can be treated with tinted glasses. Strabismus, amblyopia, refractive errors and nystagmus may also require treatment with traditional methods.

Additional Resource

1. Singh D (2010). Aniridia. [online] Available from http://www.emedicine.com/oph/TOPIC43.HTM [Accessed April, 2012].

90. ANISOCORIA

General

Unequal pupil size which can be caused by a variety of pathophysiological processes.

Clinical

Horner syndrome; carotid dissection; III nerve palsy; aneurysmal expansion.

Ocular

Ptosis; miosis; anhidrosis; pupillary size difference; diplopia; photophobia; proptosis.

Laboratory

Topical anesthetic drops are used for diagnostic testing to detect Horner syndrome. Cholinergic agents are used for testing related to tonic pupil. Sympathomimetric agents are useful to test integrity of the third-order sympathetic neuron. MRI may be useful to detect Horner syndrome and cerebral aneurysm.

Treatment

Medical and surgical care depends upon the specific etiology.

Additional Resource

1. Eggenberger ER (2010). Anisocoria Treatment & Management. [online] Available from http://www.emedicine.medscape.com/article/1158571-treatment [Accessed April, 2012].

91. ANKYLOBLEPHARON FILIFORME ADNATUM AND CLEFT PALATE (AEC SYNDROME; HAY-WELLS SYNDROME)

General

Autosomal dominant; cleft palate and/or cleft lip; congenital filiform fusion of eyelids.

Ocular

Filiform fusion of eyelids; pterygium; keratoconus.

Clinical

Cleft lip and palate; paramedian mucous pits of lower lip; ectodermal dysplasia; infrequent association with trisomy 18; partial thickness fusion of central portion of lid margins.

Laboratory

Generally, laboratory studies are not useful in the diagnosis.

Treatment

Dermatologists are useful in the management of patients with chronic eczematous dermatitis or scalp erosions. General dentists or periodontal dentists can provide regular preventative dental care and restorative service as indicated. Plastic surgeons can provide evaluation and management of cleft lip and/or palate defects, other facial defects, and hand and foot defects. Speech and physical or occupational therapists can assist patients with cleft lip and/or palate with feeding and speech difficulties and can provide therapy to assist patients with hand and foot defects.

Additional Resource

1. Shah KN (2012). Ectodermal Dysplasia. [online] Available from http://www.emedicine.com/derm/TOPIC114.HTM [Accessed April, 2012].

92. ANKYLOSTOMIASIS (HOOKWORM DISEASE)

General

Causative agents include *Necator americanus, Ancylostoma duodenale, Ancylostoma braziliense* and *Ancylostoma caninum*; final diagnosis depends upon finding eggs in feces.

Ocular

Retinal hemorrhages around optic disk; diplopia; conjunctival xerosis; visual field defects; cataract.

Clinical

Maculopapules; localized erythema; microcytic hypochromic anemia.

Laboratory

Stool examination for ova and parasites usually reveals oval eggs with thin, colorless shells that can be seen 2 months after exposure.

Treatment

Imidazoles are the most effective drugs to treat hookworm. Albendazole or mebendazole is the drug of choice.

Additional Resource

1. Haburchak DR (2011). Hookworms. [online] Available from http://www.emedicine.com/med/TOPIC1028.HTM [Accessed April, 2012].

93. ANNETTE VON DROSTE-HULSHOFF SYNDROME

General

Premature birth; pseudostrabismus due to macular ectopia in retinopathy of prematurity.

Ocular

Myopia; retinal detachment; negative and positive angle kappa; esotropia; temporal macular ectopia; chorioretinal colobomata; falciform folds; persistent hyaloids artery; abnormal position of blind spot; epicanthus; telecanthus; blepharophimosis; hypertelorism; asymmetrical orbits; exophthalmos; enophthalmos.

Clinical

Face turn; angioma; neoplasia.

Laboratory

Diagnosis is made by clinical findings.

Treatment

Retinal detachment: Scleral buckle, pneumatic retinopexy and vitrectomy may be used to close all the breaks.

Esotropia: Equalized vision with correct refractive error; surgery may be helpful in patient with diplopia.

Bibliography

1. Alfieri MC, Magli A, Chiosi E, et al. The Annette von Droste-Hulshoff syndrome. Pseudostrabismus due to macular ectopia in retinopathy of prematurity. Ophthalmic Paediatr Genet. 1988;9:13-6.
2. Meyer-Schwickerath G. The Annette von Droste-Hulshoff syndrome. Klin Monbl Augenheilkd. 1984;184:574-7.

94. ANOPHTHALMOS

General

Primary optic vesicle fails to develop.

Clinical

None

Ocular

Small orbit with narrowed palpebral fissure and shrunken fornix.

Laboratory

Computed tomography (CT) and MRI of orbit and brain, B-scan ultrasound imaging.

Treatment

Orbital expansion with serial implants in the growing orbit, increase horizontal length of palpebral fissure, dermis fat graft, inflatable silicone expander.

Additional Resource

1. Mamalis N (2010). Anophthalmos. [online] Available from http://www.emedicine.com/oph/TOPIC572.HTM [Accessed April, 2012].

95. ANOREXIA NERVOSA (APEPSIA HYSTERICCI)

General

Compulsive neurosis; refusal to eat; occurs in adolescent to young adult females; symptomatic recovery or chronic course.

Ocular

Cataract; central retinal vein occlusion; myopathy of orbicularis oculi (weakness of eye closure).

Clinical

Severe cachexia; loss of hair; nausea; constipation; diarrhea; depression; vigorous activity; weight loss; menstrual disturbance.

Laboratory

No definitive diagnostic tests are available; however, given the multiorgan system effects of starvation, a thorough medical evaluation is warranted.

Treatment

Initial therapy should be stabilization for any life-threatening conditions. Metabolic abnormalities should be corrected as needed, with oral or parenteral treatment depending on the patient's mental status and decision to cooperate.

Additional Resource

1. Waldrop RD (2011). Emergent Management of Anorexia Nervosa. [online] Available from http://www.emedicine.com/emerg/TOPIC34.HTM [Accessed April, 2012].

96. ANOXIC OVERWEAR SYNDROME

General

Caused by a reduction in oxygen supply due to continuously worn hydrogel lenses; allergic or toxic reactions to preservatives used in the cleaning process.

Ocular

Refractive error changes; endothelial cell changes; physical trauma to the anterior surface of the cornea; corneal neovascularization; giant papillary conjunctivitis; contact lens deposits; acute red eye syndrome.

Laboratory

Diagnosis is made by clinical findings.

Treatment

Observation, topical steroid drops, reduce time individual uses contact lens, corneal laser photocoagulation.

Bibliography

1. Binder PS. The physiologic effects of extended wear soft contact lenses. Ophthalmology. 1980;87: 745-9.
2. Sarver MD, Baggett DA, Harris MG, et al. Corneal edema with hydrogel lenses and eye closure: effect of oxygen transmissibility. Am J Optom Physiol Opt. 1981;58:386-92.

97. ANTERIOR CHAMBER CLEAVAGE SYNDROME
(PETERS-PLUS SYNDROME; REESE-ELLSWORTH SYNDROME)

General

Abnormalities in the embryologic development of the anterior chamber due to failure of normal migration of mesodermal cells across the anterior segment of the eye or failure of later differentiation of the mesodermal elements; various conditions described as congenital: central anterior synechiae, persistent mesenchymal tissue in the chamber angle, posterior embryotoxon, congenital corneal hyaline membrane, posterior marginal dysplasia, prominent Schwalbe line, mesodermal dysgenesis, and internal corneal ulcer seem all to fall in this same category of the anterior chamber cleavage syndrome; condition is present at birth; about 80% are bilateral; autosomal dominant inheritance; may be associated with congenital sensory neuropathy and ichthyosis.

Ocular

Increased intraocular pressure; adhesions between the iris and cornea; persistence of mesenchymal tissue in the chamber angle; usually shallow anterior chamber; iris coloboma and hypoplasia; prominent Schwalbe ring; contiguous hyaloid membrane; corneal opacities of various density with or without edema, usually at the site of iris adhesion; anterior pole cataract; remains of hyaloid artery.

Clinical

Dental anomalies; mental retardation; cleft palate; syndactyly; craniofacial dysostosis; myotonic dystrophy.

Laboratory

Diagnosis is made by clinical findings.

Treatment

Glaucoma: Its medication should be the first plan of action. If medication is unsuccessful, a filtering surgical procedure with or without antimetabolites may be beneficial.

Cataract: Change in glasses can sometimes improve a patient's visual function temporarily; however, the most common treatment is cataract surgery.

Additional Resource

1. Giri G (2012). Peters Anomaly. [online] Available from http://www.emedicine.com/oph/TOPIC112. HTM [Accessed April, 2012].

98. ANTERIOR SEGMENT ISCHEMIA SYNDROME

General

Occasional complication of strabismus surgery; usually occurs in adult patients who have paretic strabismus after extensive transposition procedures; also may be secondary to giant cell arteritis or develop following trabeculectomy or strabismus surgery.

Ocular

Corneal edema; corneal ulceration; uveitis; iris atrophy; ectopic pupil; posterior synechiae; cataract; hypotony; phthisis bulbi.

Laboratory

Diagnosis is made by clinical findings.

Treatment

Uveitis: Topical steroids and cycloplegic medication should be the initial treatment of choice. Oral steroids if not responsive to topical steroids, immunosuppressants if bilateral disease that does not respond to oral steroids, periocular steroids for unilateral or posterior uveitis. Vitrectomy can be used for severe vitreous opacification. Cryotherapy and laser photocoagulation may be used for localized pars plana exudates.

Cataract: Change in glasses can sometimes improve a patient's visual function temporarily; however, the most common treatment is cataract surgery.

Bibliography

1. Birt CM, Slomovic A, Motolko M, et al. Anterior segment ischemia in giant cell arteritis. Can J Ophthalmol. 1994;29:93-4.
2. Hiatt RL. Production of anterior segment ischemia. J Pediatr Ophthalmol Strabismus. 1978;15:197-204.
3. Saunders RA, Sandall GS. Anterior segment ischemia syndrome following rectus muscle transposition. Am J Ophthalmol. 1982;93:34-8.
4. Saunders RA, Bluestein EC, Wilson ME, et al. Anterior segment ischemia after strabismus surgery. Surv Ophthalmol. 1994;38:456-66.
5. Watson NJ. Anterior segment ischemia. Ophthalmic Surg. 1992;23:429-31.

99. ANTERIOR SPINAL ARTERY SYNDROME (BECK SYNDROME; MEDULLARY SYNDROME; MYELOMALACIA SYNDROME; VENTRAL MEDULLARY SYNDROME)

General

Impaired blood supply to the anterior two-thirds of the spinal cord, which includes the corticospinal and lateral spinothalamic tracts and anterior horns of the gray matter; caused by thrombosis, aneurysms, or extramedullary tumors; onset is sudden, and symptoms are preceded by pain and paresthesias.

Ocular

Nystagmus

Clinical

Quadriplegia (usually sudden with cervical lesions) with loss of sense of position; arms may be unimpaired with thoracic location of the lesion; anesthesia for determination of sensations; disturbed intestinal and bladder function with incontinence; disturbed sense for temperature and pain.

Laboratory

Imaging can identify a mass or space-occupying lesion that is compressing or compromising the circulation of the spinal cord (extra-axial) or is within the cord tissue (intra-axial).

Treatment

The standard drug therapy is aspirin.

Additional Resource

1. Scott TF (2012). Spinal Cord Infarction. [online] Available from http://www.emedicine.com/neuro/TOPIC348.HTM [Accessed April, 2012].

100. ANTERIOR VITREOUS DETACHMENT

General

Vitreous cortex is separated from the posterior lens or zonular fibers; usually caused by vitreous shrinkage.

Ocular

Vitreous floaters, peripheal flashes of light

Laboratory

Diagnosis is made by clinical observation.

Treatment

No treatment is necessary unless the detachment causes a retinal detachment or macular hole. It is important to be followed by an ophthalmologist so that if complications occur they can be treated promptly.

Bibliography

1. Tolentino FI, Schepens CL, Freeman HM. Vitreoretinal Disorders: Diagnosis and Management. Philadelphia: WB Saunders; 1976.

101. ANTHRAX

General

Disease of wild and domestic animals; transmitted to humans by contact with animals or their products; causative agent is *Bacillus anthracis*.

Ocular

Pustules and edema of lids; phlebitis of ophthalmic veins; optic neuritis; optic atrophy; panophthalmitis; itchy erythematous papule of the eyelids.

Clinical

Necrotic cutaneous ulcer.

Laboratory

The preferred diagnostic procedure for cutaneous anthrax is staining the ulcer exudate with methylene blue or Giemsa stain. *B. anthracis* readily grows on blood agar, and staining will microbiologically differentiate the organism and nonanthracis bacilli species.

Treatment

The goals of pharmacotherapy are to eradicate the infection, reduce morbidity, and prevent complications. The preferred agent used to treat anthrax is penicillin.

Additional Resource

1. Cunha BA (2011). Anthrax. [online] Available from http://www.emedicine.com/med/TOPIC148.HTM [Accessed April, 2012].

102. ANTIMONGOLISM SYNDROME (CHROMOSOME 21 PARTIAL DELETION SYNDROME; G-DELETION SYNDROME; MONOSOMY 21 PARTIAL SYNDROME)

General

Partial monosomy of chromosome 21 with absence of the short arm and part of the long arm of this chromosome.

Ocular

Antimongoloid slant of lid fissures; blepharochalasis; sclerocornea.

Clinical

Hypertony; large ear lobes; prominent nasal bridge; mental retardation; pyloric stenosis; dystrophic nails; retarded growth; heart disease; hemivertebrae; micrognathia.

Laboratory

Diagnosis is made by clinical findings.

Treatment

Blepharochalasis: Surgical-excise the redundant skin, reposition the ectopic lacrimal gland and reconstruct lateral canthal tendon.

Bibliography

1. Lejeune J, Berger R, Rethore MO, et al. Monosomie partielle pour un petit acrocentrique. C R Acad Sci (Paris). 1964;259:4187-90.
2. Magalini SI, Scrascia E. Dictionary of Medical Syndromes, 2nd edition. Philadelphia: JB Lippincott; 1981.
3. Penrose LS. Antimongolism [Letter]. Lancet. 1966;1:497.

103. ANTIPHOSPHOLIPID ANTIBODY SYNDROME (HUGHES SYNDROME)

General

Recurrent arterial and venous thrombosis.

Ocular

Subconjunctival hemorrhage, hyphema, vitreous hemorrhage, central retinal vein and artery occlusions.

Laboratory

Evaluate for anticardiolipin, antiphosphatidylethanolamine, antiphosphatidylinositol, antiphosphatidylserine, antiphosphatidylglycerol, and antiphosphatidic acid. These antibodies are primarily of the IgG and IgM isotypes, although evidence is mounting for the clinical significance of IgA antibodies as well treatment. In asymptomatic patients with no risk factors no treatment is necessary. In asymptomatic patients who are positive for arterial or venous thrombosis or fetal loss antiplatelet prophylaxis, such as aspirin may be useful.

Treatment

Vitreous hemorrhage: If possible the source of the bleeding needs to be isolated and treated with laser. Vitrectomy may be necessary.

Central artery occlusion: Intraocular pressure lowering medications, carbogen therapy, hyperbaric oxygen. Vitrectomy may be necessary.

Additional Resource

1. Myones BL (2009). Pediatric Antiphospholipid Antibody Syndrome. [online] Available from http://www.emedicine.com/ped/TOPIC118.HTM [Accessed April, 2012].

104. ANTON SYNDROME (DENIAL-VISUAL HALLUCINATION SYNDROME)

General

Cause unknown, but isolation of diencephalon from occipital lobe would be necessary to result in the features of the syndrome; lesions of the calcarine-thalamic connections or bilateral destruction of the occipital regions have been claimed to cause denial of blindness; the disease is rare and little understood; has been reported in association with blindness from a peripheral lesion such as bifrontal contusions and optic nerve damage.

Ocular

Denial of blindness; patients may persistently deny having any loss of visual perception; the objects the patient describes and claims to see are regarded as visual hallucinations; visual field hemianopsia.

Clinical

Confabulation; allocheiria (reference of a sensation is made to the opposite side to which the stimulus is applied).

Laboratory

Diagnosis is made by clinical findings.

Treatment

None

Bibliography

1. Anton G. Ueber die Selbstwahrnehmung der Herderkrankung des Gehirns durch den Kranken bei Rindentaubheit. Arch Psychiatr Nervenkr. 1899;32:86-127.
2. Magalini SI, Scrascia E. Dictionary of Medical Syndromes, 2nd edition. Philadelphia: JB Lippincott; 1981.
3. McDaniel KD, McDaniel LD. Anton's syndrome in a patient with post-traumatic optic neuropathy and bifrontal contusions. Arch Neurol. 1991; 48:101-5.
4. Tyler HR. Cerebral disorders of vision. In: Smith JL (Ed). Neuro-Ophthalmology. St. Louis: CV Mosby; 1968.

105. APERT SYNDROME (ABSENT-DIGITS-CRANIAL-DEFECTS SYNDROME; ACROCEPHALOSYNDACTYLISM SYNDROME; ACROCRANIO-DYSPHALANGIA; ACRODYSPLASIA; SPHENOACROCRANIO-SYNDACTYLY)

General

Inherited; most often recessive, sometimes dominant; an extreme form of Apert syndrome has been described as Carpenter syndrome, with the latter being familial and transmitted as an autosomal recessive.

Ocular

Shallow orbit; exophthalmos; hypertelorism; ptosis; strabismus; nystagmus; ophthalmoplegia; hyperopia; exposure keratitis; cataracts; ectopia lentis; medullated nerve fibers; retinal detachment; papilledema with subsequent optic atrophy; keratoconus.

Clinical

Oxycephaly ("tower skull"); syndactyly (symmetrically); synostoses and synarthroses of shoulder and elbows frequent; agenesis of spinal bones and limbs; headaches; hypertelorism; hypoplastic maxilla; acrocephaly; abnormality of sutures.

Laboratory

Computed tomography (CT) is the most useful radiological examination in identifying skull shape and presence or absence of involved sutures. MRI reveals the anatomy of the soft-tissue structures and associated with brain abnormalities.

Treatment

Medical treatment involves fitting patient with hearing aids, providing airway management and psychological counseling. Surgical care involves early release of the coronal suture and fronto-orbital advancement and reshaping to reduce dysmorphic and unwanted skull growth changes.

Additional Resource

1. Chen H (2011). Apert Syndrome. [online] Available from http://www.emedicine.com/ped/TOPIC122. HTM [Accessed April, 2012].

106. APHAKIC AND PSEUDOPHAKIC GLAUCOMA

General

Increased intraocular pressure following cataract surgery. Pathophysiology may include distortion of chamber angle, retained viscoelastics, inflammation, hemorrhage, ghost cell, vitreous in the anterior chamber, pigment dispersion, aqueous misdirection syndrome and pupillary block.

Clinical

None

Ocular

Elevated intraocular pressure; uveitis; hyphema; retained cortical lens material; shallow anterior chamber; vitreous in anterior chamber.

Laboratory

Imaging studies include ultrasound biomicro-scopy; gonioscopy.

Treatment

Mydriasis is the initial treatment to break the block. Iridotomy, trabeculoplasty, cyclophoto-coagulation and pars plana vitrectomy may be necessary.

Additional Resource

1. Graham RH (2012). Aphakic and Pseudophakic Glaucoma. [online] Available from http://www. emedicine.medscape.com/article/1207170-overview [Accessed April, 2012].

107. ARGININOSUCCINIC ACIDURIA (TRICHORRHEXIS NODOSA)

General

Argininosuccinase (A Sase) deficiency; both sexes affected; prevalent in females; autosomal recessive inheritance.

Ocular

Friable tufted eyelashes and eyebrows; visual field defects; cataract.

Clinical

Clinical findings vary widely; mental retardation; seizures; ataxia; hepatomegaly; friable hair (trichorrhexis nodosa); may have citrullinemia; hyperammonemia; increased argininosuccinic acid (most pronounced in the cerebrospinal fluid).

Laboratory

Computed tomography or MRI of the brain may show cerebral edema. Plasma and urinary organic acid tests screen for the presence of an organic academia. Arterial blood gas analysis determines acid-base status; respiratory alkalosis strongly suggests a urea cycle defect.

Treatment

Correct biochemical abnormalities and ensure adequate nutritional intake. Treatment involves compounds that increase the removal of nitrogen waste.

Additional Resource

1. Crisan E (2010). Hyperammonemia. [online] Available from http://www.emedicine.com/neuro/TOPIC162.HTM [Accessed April, 2012].

---

108. ARGYLL ROBERTSON SYNDROME (SPINAL MIOSIS)

General

Caused by syphilis or, rarely, epidemic encephalitis; disseminated sclerosis; diabetes; brain tumor; syringomyelia; syringobulbia; chronic alcoholism; injury; encephalitis lethargica, Guillain-Barré syndrome, Lyme disease, multiple sclerosis, polyarteritis nodosa, and sarcoidosis have been associated with this condition.

Ocular

No direct or consensual pupil reaction to light but to normal accommodation (except in terminal stages, when pupil is fixed to all stimuli); pupil contraction with eserine but poor dilation with atropine; miosis (generally); irregular pupil; occurs unilaterally and bilaterally; anisocoria or discoria frequent.

Clinical

Syphilis of central nervous system; general paresis; tabes dorsalis.

Laboratory

Rapid plasma reagin (RPR) test is preferred to the Venereal Disease Research Laboratory (VDRL) test in an office setting; however, laboratory study has proven sufficiently sensitive or specific to serve as a single test for the definitive diagnosis of neurosyphilis

Treatment

Drug of choice is penicillin. Adequate treatment is based largely on achieving treponemicidal levels of PCN.

Additional Resource

1. Knudsen RP (2011). Neurosyphilis Overview of Syphilis of the CNS. [online] Available from http://www.emedicine.com/neuro/TOPIC684.HTM [Accessed April, 2012].

109. ARNDT-GOTTRON SYNDROME (SCLEROMYXEDEMA)

General

Etiology unknown; rare cutaneous disease of hyaluronic acid deposits in dermis; variant of lichen myxedematosus (papular mucinosis); progressive disease commonly involving the face, neck, upper trunk, forearms, and hands, producing thickening of the skin with overlying fine papules.

Ocular

Corneal opacities of amyloid deposits; thickening of eyelids; lagophthalmos; ectropion; thickened eyebrow or eyelid skin; corneal opacities.

Clinical

Exaggerated facial folds impair opening of the mouth; flexion contractures from poor joint mobility; erythema; scaling of skin; phimosis; urethral stenosis.

Laboratory

Complete blood count to rule out significant anemia; EKG, chest X-ray, venous pressure and circulation time can be helpful

Treatment

High doses of thalidomide may help some patients for a period of time but symptoms often reoccur.

Bibliography

1. Goldin HM, Axelrod AJ, Bronson DM, et al. Scleromyxedema with corneal deposits. Ophthalmology. 1987;94:1334-8.
2. Pusateri TJ, Margo CE, Groden LR. Corneal manifestations of scleromyxedema. Ophthalmology. 1987;94:510-3.

110. ARNOLD-CHIARI SYNDROME (BASILAR IMPRESSIONS; CEREBELLOMEDULLARY MALFORMATION SYNDROME; PLATYBASIA SYNDROME)

General

Malformation of the hindbrain; developmental deformity of the occipital bone and upper cervical spine; recognized in children or adults; clinical picture may be indistinguishable from that of Dandy-Walker syndrome in infants.

Ocular

Horizontal, vertical, and rotary forms of nystagmus; vertical nystagmus in both up gaze and down gaze is most common; papilledema; esotropia; Duane retraction syndrome (association); oscillopsia.

Clinical

Hydrocephalus; cerebellar ataxia; bilateral pyramidal tract signs.

Laboratory

Computed tomography scans are used most commonly for the diagnosis of hydrocephalus and for the evaluation of suspected shunt malfunction.

Treatment

Early recognition and treatment is important because of the potential life-threatening symptoms. Early surgical intervention, especially in infants may prevent irreversible changes and death.

Additional Resource

1. Incesu L (2011). Imaging in Chiari II Malformation. [online] Available from http://www.emedicine.com/radio/TOPIC150.HTM [Accessed April, 2012].

111. ARNOLD PICK SYNDROME (APHASIA-AGNOSIA-APRAXIA SYNDROME; PICK DISEASE OF THE BRAIN; PICK SYNDROME 2)

General

Widespread cortical atrophy; manifested between the ages of 40 and 70 years; pathogenesis remains unknown; cannot be consistently differentiated from Alzheimer disease on clinical grounds alone.

Ocular

Apperceptive blindness (inability of patient to fix upon objects within his or her gaze); visual agnosia (inability to recognize familiar objects by sight); visual field defects due to atrophy in occipital lobe.

Clinical

Presenile or progressive dementia; patient is unaware of his or her surroundings; poor insight; loss of words and utterance of stereotyped phrases; aphasia (motor type); apathy and indifference.

Laboratory

Initial workup includes a vitamin B_{12} level, thyroid function studies, fluorescent treponemal antibody testing for syphilis, and antinuclear antibodies.

Treatment

Referral to a case manager, geriatric nurse practitioner or other dementia specialists for social-family issues.

Additional Resource

1. Barrett AM (2012). Pick Disease. [online] Available from http://www.emedicine.com/neuro/TOPIC311. HTM [Accessed April, 2012].

112. ARTERIAL OCCLUSIVE RETINOPATHY AND ENCEPHALOPATHY SYNDROME

General

Rare; etiology unknown but may be virally induced, immune-mediated disease; most frequent in women; mechanism could be related to microangiopathy secondary to immunologically mediated vasculitis, although an abnormal coagulation system or microembolisms have been proposed to explain this condition.

Ocular

Multiple branch retinal arterial occlusions; rotary nystagmus; retinal hemorrhage; visual field defects; bilateral gaze palsy.

Clinical

Encephalopathy; behavior and memory disturbances; hearing loss; paranoid psychosis; neurologic dysfunction; seizures; headache; spasticity and hyperreflexia.

Laboratory

Diagnosis is made by clinical findings.

Treatment

Branch artery occlusion: Intraocular pressure lowering medications, carbogen therapy, hyperbaric oxygen.

Retinal hemorrhage: Vitrectomy may be necessary.

Bibliography

1. Bonamo J, Gregori CA, Breen JL. Anencephaly: an overview. J Med Soc N J. 1980;77:439-41.
2. Cappeto JR, Currie JN, Monteiro ML, et al. A syndrome of arterial occlusive retinopathy and encephalopathy. Am J Ophthalmol. 1984;98:189-202.
3. Gordon DL, Hayreh SS, Adams HP. Microangiopathy of the brain, retina, and ear: improvement without immunosuppressive therapy. Stroke. 1991;22:933-7.
4. Nicolle MW, McLachlan RS. Microangiopathy with retinopathy, encephalopathy, and deafness (RED-M) and systemic features. Semin Arthritis Rheum. 1991;21:123-8.

113. ARTERIOSCLEROSIS

General

Thickening and induration of the arterial wall; prominent in the elderly.

Ocular

Increased arterial light reflex, copper/silver wire arteries; arteriovenous crossing changes; arterial caliber variation/irregularity; arterial straightening or tortuosity; intimal hyperplasia, medial atrophy, atherosclerotic fibrous plaques and calcifications of the internal elastic lamina observed in aged human orbital arteries.

Clinical

Increased collagen deposition in small- and medium-sized arteries with progressive replacement of the smooth muscle in the vessel walls; arterial wall changes at arteriovenous crossings.

Laboratory

Diagnosis is made by clinical findings.

Treatment

None

Bibliography

1. Buchi ER, Schiller P, Felice M, et al. Common histopathological changes in aged human orbital arteries. Int Ophthalmol. 1993;17:37-42.
2. Collins JF. Handbook of Clinical Ophthalmology. New York: Masson; 1982. p. 269.

114. ARTERIOVENOUS FISTULA (ARTERIOVENOUS ANEURYSM; ARTERIOVENOUS ANGIOMA; ARTERIOVENOUS MALFORMATION; CIRSOID ANEURYSM; RACEMOSE HEMANGIOMA; VARICOSE ANEURYSM)

General

Abnormal communications between arteries and veins that allow arterial blood to enter the vein directly without traversing a capillary network; may be congenital or secondary to penetrating trauma or blunt trauma.

Ocular

Uveitis; chemosis and neovascularization of conjunctiva; bullous keratopathy; eyelid edema; ptosis; exophthalmos; iris atrophy; papilledema; retinal hemorrhages; cataract; paresis of third or sixth nerves; glaucoma; upper lid tumor;

total choroidal detachment; leaking retinal macroaneurysms; central retinal vein occlusion; iris neovascularization.

Clinical

Cerebral hemorrhage; death; substernal pain; dyspnea; varicose veins.

Laboratory

Orbital ultrasonography, computed tomography and six-vessel cranial digital subtraction angiography.

Treatment

Obtain emergent neurosurgical consultation for definitive treatment.

Additional Resource

1. Zebian RC (2011). Emergent Management of Subarachnoid Hemorrhage. [online] Available from http://www.emedicine.com/emerg/TOPIC559. HTM [Accessed April, 2012].

---

115. ARTHROGRYPOSIS MULTIPLEX CONGENITA

General

Heterogeneous group of disorders of multiple proposed etiologies; often one manifestation of a complex of congenital anomalies; probable autosomal recessive transmission; found in Eskimos; affects more males than females; characterized by decreased fetal joint mobility secondary to neuropathic disease, myopathic disease, or some other cause.

Ocular

Congenital bilateral cataract; associated with ophthalmoplegia, retinopathy, goniodysgenesis, and infantile glaucoma, as well as Duane retraction syndrome.

Clinical

Multiple articular rigidities; hypoplasia of adjacent muscle groups; soft tissue shortening; duck-like waddle; muscle atrophy.

Laboratory

In general, laboratory tests are not extremely useful.

Treatment

Goals include lower-limb alignment and establishment of stability for ambulation and upper-limb function for self-care. Early vigorous physical therapy to stretch contractures is very important to promote active range of motion.

Additional Resource

1. Chen H (2011). Arthrogryposis. [online] Available from http://www.emedicine.com/ped/TOPIC142. HTM [Accessed April, 2012].

116. ARYLSULFATASE A DEFICIENCY (GREENFIELD DISEASE; FAMILIAL PROGRESSIVE CEREBRAL SCLEROSIS; INFANTILE METACHROMATIC LEUKODYSTROPHY; INFANTILE PROGRESSIVE CEREBRAL SCLEROSIS; LEUKODYSTROPHIA CEREBRI PROGRESSIVA METACHROMATICA DIFFUSA; METACHROMATIC LEUKODYSTROPHY; OPTICOCHLEODENTATE DEGENERATION; SCHOLZ SYNDROME; SCHOLZ-BIELSCHOWSKY-HENNEBERG SYNDROME; SULFATIDE LIPOIDOSIS SYNDROME; VAN BOGAERT-NYSSEN DISEASE; VAN BOGAERT-NYSSEN-PEIFFER DISEASE)

General

Accumulation of sulfatide caused by deficient activity of arylsulfatase A; autosomal recessive; familial form of metachromatic leukodystrophy; Greenfield disease (late infantile form); van Bogaert-Nyssen-Peiffer syndrome (adult form); affects central and peripheral nervous systems by demyelination and by accumulation of metachromatic material.

Ocular

Visual loss in association with optic atrophy; strabismus; macular cherry-red spot; corneal opacification; oculomotor disorders (nystagmus, strabismus); optic nerve and retinal demyelination.

Clinical

Motor and mental deterioration with spasticity; paralysis; seizures; dementia; death in early childhood, although attenuated and adult forms of the disease occur; schizophrenia; temporo-occipital demyelination; unreactive to visual and auditory stimuli; adult form: moodiness, withdrawal, megalomania, hallucinations, violent reactions and dementia.

Laboratory

Arylsulfatase A enzyme activity may be decreased in leukocytes or in cultured skin fibroblasts. Brain MRI may identify white matter lesions and atrophy.

Treatment

There is no effective treatment to reverse the deterioration and loss of function. Bone marrow or cord blood transplantation may be useful in individuals with asymptomatic late infantile and early juvenile forms of the disease.

Additional Resource

1. Ikeda AK (2010). Metachromatic Leukodystrophy. [online] Available from http://www.emedicine. com/ped/TOPIC2893.HTM [Accessed April, 2012].

117. ASCARIASIS

General

Roundworm infection caused by *Ascaris lumbricoides*.

Ocular

Conjunctivitis; xerosis; periphlebitis; pigmentation of macular lesion; papilledema; uveitis; subluxation of lens; scotoma; secondary glaucoma; vitreal hemorrhages; possible association with phlyctenular eye disease.

Clinical

Occasional colicky abdominal pain; slight abdominal distention; pneumonitis; intestinal obstruction.

Laboratory

Stool examination for ova and parasites almost always discloses large, brown trilayered eggs.

Treatment

Albendazole 400 mg one dose orally is the drug of choice.

Additional Resource

1. Haburchak DR (2011). Ascariasis. [online] Available from http://www.emedicine.com/med/TOPIC172. HTM [Accessed April, 2012].

---

118. ASCHER SYNDROME (BLEPHAROCHALASIS WITH STRUMA AND DOUBLE LIP)

General

Rare occurrence; blepharochalasis transmitted as a simple dominant; related to development of thyroid gland; symptoms usually start around puberty.

Ocular

"Bulging" of orbital fat; blepharochalasis; protrusion of lacrimal gland; entropion (rare).

Clinical

Goiter; reduplication of upper lip; hypothyroidism; alopecia areata totalis.

Laboratory

Lateral cephalometric evaluation is indicated to rule out dento-osseous causes of lip protrusion.

Treatment

Lip reduction surgery is the most common treatment.

Additional Resource

1. Dev VR (2011). Lip Reduction. [online] Available from http://www.emedicine.com/plastic/TOPIC66. HTM [Accessed April, 2012].

---

119. ASPERGILLOSIS

General

Systemic infection common in poultry farmers, feeders or breeders of pigeons, and persons who work with grains; should be considered in immunocompromised patients.

Ocular

Corneal ulcer; blepharitis; keratitis; scleritis; endophthalmitis; exophthalmos; retinal hemorrhages; retinal detachment; vitreitis; cataract; conjunctivitis; orbital cellulitis; paresis of extraocular muscles; secondary glaucoma; scleromalacia perforans; endogenous endophthalmitis; anterior chamber mass; invasion of choroid and anterior optic nerve.

Clinical

Pulmonary infections; invasive fungal disease.

Laboratory

Cuture from superfical scrapings from bed of infection.

Treatment

Voriconazole is the drug of choice. Although disease outcomes substantially improve with antifungal treatment, patient survival and infection resolution depend on improved immunosuppression.

Additional Resource

1. Batra V (2011). Pediatric Aspergillosis. [online] Available from http://www.emedicine.com/ped/ TOPIC148.HTM [Accessed April, 2012].

120. ASTHMA (HAY FEVER)

General

Asthma characterized by paroxysms of expiratory dyspnea and wheezing, overinflation of the lungs, cough, and rhonchi; causes include allergy to external inhaled allergens, respiratory infections, and psychophysiologic reaction to stress. Hay fever (allergic asthma) characterized by sneezing, rhinorrhea, swelling of nasal mucosa, and itchy eyes; caused by spread of pollens in air or exposure to antigens; seasonal; occurs most frequently in young persons.

Ocular

Lacrimation; allergic conjunctivitis; periocular xanthogranulomas.

Clinical

Rhinorrhea; sneezing; mucosal swelling with occlusion of airway; insomnia; nasal polyps; wheezing; cough; headache; rhinitis.

Laboratory

Testing for reaction to specific allergens can be helpful to confirm the diagnosis of allergic rhinitis and to determine specific allergic triggers.

Treatment

The management involves allergen avoidance, pharmacological management, and immuno-therapy. Symptoms can be treated with oral antihistamines, decongestants or both.

Additional Resource

1. Morris MJ (2012). Asthma. [online] Available from http://www.emedicine.com/emerg/TOPIC43. HTM [Accessed April, 2012].

121. ASTIGMATISM, LASIK AND PRK

General

Astigmatism, a refractive condition where the surface of the cornea is not spherical, can decrease visual acuity by forming a distorted image because light images focus on two separate points in the eye. Correction of astigmatism by means of surgery is indicated when the degree of the astigmatism impacts visual acuity. Typically, visually significant astigmatism is roughly defined as being more than 1.00 D, although many patients may experience symptoms from lower amounts. May be due to wound dehiscence and postoperative complications; injury or hereditary and other disease processes such as diabetes mellitus.

Clinical

None

Ocular

Blurred vision, streak phenomena around light sources, diplopia.

Laboratory

Corneal topography and tomography.

Treatment

The excimer laser corrects simple myopia by applying a greater amount of laser energy to the central cornea than to the peripheral cornea.

LASIK—a refractive laser procedure combining the use of ALK and photorefractive keratectomy in reshaping the central cornea to treat refractive errors. An automated microkeratome, similar to that used in ALK, is used to fashion a flap with a hinge. Subsequent ablation is performed on the corneal stromal bed with stitchless replacement of the corneal flap.

PRK is the application of ultraviolet high-energy photons (193-nm wavelength) of the ultraviolet range generated by an argon fluoride excimer laser to the anterior corneal stroma to change its curvature and, thus, to correct a refractive error. The physical process of remodeling by PRK is called photoablation. This surgical procedure reshapes the central cornea to a flatter shape for people who are nearsighted and a more curved surface for people who are farsighted. Several techniques are being used to correct for astigmatism.

Recent advances in techniques used to gather refractive data allow for correction of not only myopia, hyperopia and astigmatism but also higher order aberrations. This wavescan digital technology was originally developed for astrophysics to reduce atmospheric distortions when viewing distant objects in space through high-powered telescopes.

Additional Resources

1. Hardten DR (2012). LASIK Astigmatism. [online] Available from http://www.emedicine.medscape.com/article/1220489-overview [Accessed April, 2012].
2. Roque MR (2012). PRK Astigmatism. [online] Available from http://www.emedicine.medscape.com/article/1220845-overview [Accessed April, 2012].

---

122. ATAXIA, SPASTIC, WITH CONGENITAL MIOSIS

General

Autosomal dominant.

Ocular

Congenital miosis; nystagmus; small, nonreacting pupils.

Clinical

Symmetrical ataxia of gait and limb movement; dysarthria; late in walking; slurred speech; increased deep tendon reflexes; extensor plantar reflexes.

Laboratory

Diagnosis is made by clinical findings.

Treatment

None/Ocular.

Additional Resource

1. Prasad A (2010). Ataxia with Identified Genetic and Biochemical Defects. [online] Available from http://www.emedicine.com/neuro/TOPIC556.HTM [Accessed April, 2012].

123. ATHEROSCLEROSIS

General

Etiologic importance of lipid infiltration; cholesterol; patchy nodular form of arteriosclerosis.

Clinical

Angina pectoris, myocardial infarct, coronary heart disease.

Ocular

Central retinal artery obstruction; branch retinal artery obstruction; most common cause is embolization from carotid plaques.

Laboratory

Elevated LDL cholesterol is a risk factor for atherosclerotic vascular disease. High triglycerides are associated with low high-density lipoprotein (HDL) cholesterol and are a probable risk factor for vascular disease. Ultrasonography aids in evaluating brachial artery reactivity and carotid artery intima-media thickness.

Treatment

The prevention and treatment of atherosclerosis requires control of the known modifiable risk factors for this disease. This includes the medical treatment of hypertension, hyperlipidemia, diabetes mellitus, and cigarette habituation.

Additional Resource

1. Boudi FB (2011). Noncoronary Atherosclerosis Overview of Atherosclerosis. [online] Available from http://www.emedicine.com/med/TOPIC182.HTM [Accessed April, 2012].

124. ATOPIC DERMATITIS (ATOPIC ECZEMA; BESNIER PRURIGO)

General

Highly specific disease resulting from a hereditary determined lowered cutaneous threshold to pruritus and characterized by intense itching; elevated total and specific immunoglobulin E.

Ocular

Keratoconjunctivitis; keratoconus; cataract; atopic dermatitis of lid; secondary glaucoma; uveitis; possible association with retinal detachment; pannus; blepharoconjunctivitis; corneal scarring; suppurative keratitis.

Clinical

In infants it involves the face with dry or oozing erythematous patches; in children and adolescents itching localized in the neck, antecubital spaces, popliteal folds, and ears; seborrheic changes.

Laboratory

Diagnosis is made by clinical findings.

Treatment

Topical corticosteroids are the mainstay of treatment. Adequate rehydration will minimize the direct effects of irritants and allergens on the skin and maximize the effect of topically applied therapies, thus decreasing the need for topical steroids.

Additional Resource

1. Schwartz RA (2011). Pediatric Atopic Dermatitis. [online] Available from http://www.emedicine.com/ped/TOPIC2567.HTM [Accessed April, 2012].

125. AUTOIMMUNE CORNEAL ENDOTHELIOPATHY

General

Etiology unknown; associated with implantation of an intraocular lens (IOL), pars planitis, iritis, secondary herpetic keratitis and corticosteroid use; rare.

Ocular

Stromal edema; migrating line of keratic precipitates; iritis; clouding of the cornea; lymphocytes and macrophages in anterior chamber; linear pigmented endothelial line; evidence supports that herpes simplex virus can be isolated in the aqueous humor of patients with this condition.

Clinical

Autoimmune disease, nonspecific.

Laboratory

Diagnosis is made by clinical findings.

Treatment

Check for elevated intraocular pressure. Medical treatment includes the use of hyperosmotic drops, nonsteroidal and steroid eye drops. Corneal transplant may be necessary.

Bibliography

1. Ohashi Y, Yamamoto S, Nishida K, et al. Demonstration of herpes simplex virus DNA in idiopathic corneal endotheliopathy. Am J Ophthalmol. 1991;112:419-23.

126. AUTOIMMUNOLOGICALLY MEDIATED SYNDROME (LYMPHOCYTIC HYPOPHYSITIS ASSOCIATED WITH DACRYOADENITIS SYNDROME)

General

Lymphocytes infiltrate the hypophysis.

Ocular

Dacryoadenitis

Clinical

Lymphocytic infiltration of the hypophysis by CD3 cells, T cells and CD20+ B cells is an autoimmune process that may rarely cause lacrimal gland swelling.

Laboratory

Computed tomography scan of the orbits with contrast can be helpful. The affected lacrimal gland shows diffuse enlargement, oblong shape, and marked enhancement with contrast.

Treatment

Warm compresses, oral nonsteroidal anti-inflammatories are useful. Treat the underlying systemic condition. If the enlargement does not subside after 2 weeks, consider lacrimal gland biopsy.

Additional Resource

1. Singh GJ (2011). Dacryoadenitis. [online] Available from http://www.emedicine.com/oph/TOPIC594.HTM [Accessed April, 2012].

127. AVITAMINOSIS B₂ (ARIBOFLAVINOSIS; PELLAGRA)

General

Niacin deficiency.

Ocular

Conjunctivitis; corneal vascularization; keratitis; pupillary dilation; optic atrophy; optic neuritis; cataract; blepharitis; central scotoma; marked photophobia.

Clinical

Occasional cranial nerve palsies; dermatitis; glossitis; gastrointestinal and nervous system dysfunction; mental deterioration; diarrhea; stomatitis.

Laboratory

Therapeutic response to niacin in a patient with the typical symptoms and signs of pellagra establishes the diagnosis.

Treatment

Niacin taken orally is usually effective in reversing the clinical manifestations.

Additional Resource

1. Rabinowitz SS (2010). Pediatric Pellagra. [online] Available from http://www.emedicine.com/ped/TOPIC1755.HTM [Accessed April, 2012].

128. AVITAMINOSIS C (SCURVY; VITAMIN C DEFICIENCY)

General

Vitamin C deficiency.

Ocular

Hemorrhages of lids, anterior chamber, vitreous cavity, retina, subconjunctival space, and orbit (most prominent, with resulting exophthalmos); keratitis, corneal ulcer; cataract.

Clinical

Increased capillary fragility with a tendency to hemorrhage in tissues throughout the body; poor wound healing; loose teeth; purpuric rash.

Laboratory

Laboratory tests are usually not helpful to ascertain a diagnosis of scurvy. Diagnosis is generally made by clinical findings and history.

Treatment

Dietary or pharmacologic doses of vitamin C are the standard treatment. Orange juice is a good choice to add to the diet.

Additional Resource

1. Goebel L (2011). Scurvy. [online] Available from http://www.emedicine.com/ped/TOPIC2073.HTM [Accessed April, 2012].

129. AVULSED RETINAL VESSEL SYNDROME

General

Visual prognosis good; reports of avulsed retinal vessels not associated with retinal breaks.

Ocular

Recurrent vitreous hemorrhages caused by an avulsed retinal vessel, during retinal tear formation; vitreous hemorrhages may recur until interruption of vessel occurs.

Laboratory

Diagnosis is made by clinical findings.

Treatment

Retinal detachment: Scleral buckle, pneumatic retinopexy and vitrectomy may be used to close all the breaks.

Bibliography

1. de Bustros S, Welch RB. The avulsed retinal vessel syndrome and its variants. Ophthalmology. 1984;91:86-8.
2. Uto M, Kaminagayoshi T, Uemura A. Two cases of isolated avulsed retinal vessels. Nihon Ganka Gakkai Zasshi. 1992;96:541-5.

130. AXENFELD-RIEGER SYNDROME (AXENFELD SYNDROME; POSTERIOR EMBRYOTOXON)

General

Dominant inheritance; occasionally sporadic; variable in expression.

Ocular

Posterior embryotoxon: ring-like opacity of cornea; long trabecula; prominent Schwalbe line; iris adhesions to Schwalbe line and cornea with large abnormal iris processes or broad sheets of tissues of varying size and location; anterior layer of iris may appear hypoplastic; ectopia of the pupil not uncommon; polycoria occurs; ring-like opacity of the deep corneal layers extending several millimeters from the limbus in continuity with the sclera; keratoconus.

Laboratory

Patients may need workup for associated systemic abnormalities.

Treatment

Patients may need workup for associated systemic abnormalities, so referring to a pediatrician or an internist is important.

Additional Resource

1. Irak-Dersu I (2010). Glaucoma, Secondary Congenital. [online] Available from http://www.emedicine.com/oph/TOPIC141.HTM [Accessed April, 2012].

131. AXENFELD-SCHÜRENBERG SYNDROME (CYCLIC OCULOMOTOR PARALYSIS)

General

Congenital manifestation; frequently unilateral.

Ocular

Cyclic oculomotor paralysis (paralysis alternating with spasm); during periods of paralysis, lid exhibits ptosis and affected eye is abducted; during spasm, lid is raised, deviation of affected eye is either inward or outward, and pupil is fixed and contracted.

Laboratory

Diagnosis is made by clinical findings.

Treatment

Prism therapy, surgical—muscle surgery on the affected muscle, occlusion of the involved eye to relieve diplopia.

Bibliography

1. Axenfeld T, Schurenberg L. Beitrage zur Kenntnis der Angeborenen Beweglichkeitsdefekte des Auges. Klin Monastbl Augenheilkd. 1901;39:64.
2. Hamed LM. Oculomotor palsy with cyclic spasm. In: Margo CE, Mames R, Hamed LM (Eds). Diagnostic Problems in Clinical Ophthalmology. Philadelphia: WB Saunders; 1994. p. 712.
3. Levy MR. Cyclic oculomotor paralysis with optic atrophy. Am J Ophthalmol. 1968;65:766-9.

132. B-K MOLE SYNDROME (DYSPLASTIC NEVUS SYNDROME, DNS; FAMILIAL ATYPICAL MULTIPLE MOLE MELANOMA SYNDROME)

General

Autosomal dominant.

Ocular

Ocular melanoma; metastasis to the anterior segment of the eye; occurs much less often than metastases to the choroid; iris nevi; choroidal nevi; conjunctival nevi.

Clinical

Many large, irregular, variable nevi predominantly occurring on the upper part of the trunk and extremities; atypical melanocytic hyperplasia; lymphocyte infiltration of the dermis and neovascularization; cutaneous melanoma (possible association).

Laboratory

Examination of the entire cutaneous surface. Biopsy if a recent change in a pigmented lesion is noted to rule out the development of malignant melanoma.

Treatment

Patients with unusual nevi, or many nevi, usually benefit from consultation with a dermatologist. Narrow-margin excisional biopsy or saucerization may be appropriate and can produce adequate tissue for histologic examination.

Additional Resource

1. Wenner KA (2012). Atypical Mole (Dysplastic Nevus). [online] Available from http://www.emedicine.com/derm/TOPIC42.HTM [Accessed April, 2012].

133. 3B TRANSLOCATION SYNDROME

General

Chromosomal anomaly transmitted by the female but not the male carrier.

Ocular

Iris coloboma; corneal opacity; proptosis; strabismus.

Clinical

Low birth weight; micrognathia; small ears; cleft lip and palate; cardiac defects; ventricular septal defect; atrial septal defect; absent ductus arteriosus; pulmonary arterial diverticulum; right aortic arch; absent pulmonic valve.

Laboratory

Diagnosis is made by clinical findings.

Treatment

Proptosis: Ocular lubricants are beneficial for control of the corneal exposure. Strabismus: Equalized vision with correct refractive error; surgery may be helpful in patient with diplopia.

Corneal opacity: Medical treatment includes the use of hyperosmotic drops, nonsteroidal and steroid eye drops. Corneal transplant may be necessary.

Bibliography

1. Magalini SI, Scrascia E. Dictionary of Medical Syndromes, 2nd edition. Philadelphia: JB Lippincott; 1981.
2. Walzer S, Favara B, Ming PM, et al. A new translocation syndrome (3/B). N Engl J Med. 1966;275:290-8.

134. BABINSKI-NAGEOTTE SYNDROME (MEDULLARY TEGMENTAL PARALYSIS)

General

Lesion in pontobulbar transitional region (corpus restiforme, Deiters nucleus, sympathetic fibers); Horner triad is always part of this syndrome; the findings are similar to Cestan-Chenais syndrome and Wallenberg syndrome; rare condition caused by ischemic lesion of the medulla oblongata involving the unilateral and medial areas of the medulla.

Ocular

Enophthalmos; ptosis; nystagmus; miosis.

Clinical

Contralateral hemiparesis and disturbance of sensibility; ipsilateral cerebellar hemiataxia; perhaps ipsilateral analgesia of the face, vocal cord and soft palate; adiadochokinesis; lateral pulsion; dysmetria.

Laboratory

Diagnosis is made by clinical observation.

Treatment

Cerebral infarction requires antiplatelet or warfarin therapy; brain abscess requires antibiotics and drainage; cerebral aneurysm requires surgical clipping and embolization; spinal cord injury requires conservative treatment and physical therapy.

Additional Resource

1. Bruno-Petrina A (2012). Motor Recovery In Stroke. [online] Available from http://www.emedicine.com/pmr/TOPIC189.HTM [Accessed April, 2012].

135. BACILLUS CEREUS

General

Highly virulent pathogen; most common contaminant of drug injection paraphernalia; usually enters the body as a result of penetrating trauma with a contaminated metallic foreign object; cause of food poisoning is toxin induced.

Ocular

Hypopyon; ring abscess of cornea; panophthalmitis; phthisis bulbi; orbital cellulitis; proptosis; vitreous abscess; necrosis of retina; endophthalmitis; keratitis.

Clinical

Fever; leukocytosis; septicemia; meningitis; endocarditis; osteomyelitis; wound infection.

Treatment

Most cases are self-limited and treatment is not necessary. Oral rehydration is achieved by administering clear liquids and sodium-containing and glucose-containing solutions. Intravenous solutions are indicated in patients who are severely dehydrated or who have intractable vomiting. Ocular treatment includes antibiotics (intravitreal, topical and systemic) and vitrectomy surgery.

Additional Resource

1. Gamarra RM (2012). Food Poisoning. [online] Available from http://www.emedicine.com/med/TOPIC807.HTM [Accessed April, 2012].

136. BACILLUS SPECIES INFECTIONS

General

Aerobic, Gram-positive spore-forming rods which are the cause of many ocular infections. Most common cause of post-traumatic endophthalmitis in rural settings. Most commonly enters the eye as a result of penetrating trauma with a contaminated foreign body but can be related to intravenous drug use. Extremely poor visual outcome is associated with this infection.

Clinical

Fever; leukocytosis.

Ocular

Corneal ring infiltrate; diffuse subepithelial infiltrates; hypopyon; vitreitis.

Laboratory

Gram stain reveals a Gram-positive rod.

Treatment

Antibiotic (generally vancomycin) should be given intravitreal, topical and systemic. Due to the aggressive nature of *Bacillus cereus* a vitreous tap with antibiotic injection alone is not recommended. Pars plana vitrectomy with intravitreal injection of vancomycin is the treatment of choice.

Additional Resource

1. Egan DJ (2011). Endophthalmitis. [online] Available from http://www.emedicine.com/emerg/TOPIC880.HTM [Accessed April, 2012].

137. BACILLUS SUBTILIS (HAY BACILLUS)

General

Gram-positive rod found in air, soil, dust, water, milk and hay; frequently seen in people who work near hay.

Ocular

Conjunctivitis; ring abscess of cornea; corneal ulcer; endophthalmitis; panophthalmitis; dacryocystitis; orbit abscess.

Clinical

Fever; leukocytosis.

Laboratory

Diagnosis is made by clinical examination.

Treatment

Conjunctivitis: Symptomatic control may include cold compresses and artificial tears; nonsteroidal and occasionally steroidal drops to relieve itching; bacterial—antibiotic medication should be used to treat the infection.

Corneal ulcer: Corneal cultures may be taken and treatment initiated. Treatment includes a broad spectrum of antibiotics and cycloplegic drops.

Additional Resource

1. Farber HJ (2010). Pediatric Hypersensitivity Pneumonitis. [online] Available from http://www.emedicine.com/ped/TOPIC2577.HTM [Accessed April, 2012].

138. BACTERIAL CONJUNCTIVITIS (INFECTIVE CONJUNCTIVITIS AND MUCOPURULENT CONJUNCTIVITIS)

General

Most common in children and occasionally seen in elderly, usually acute and hand to eye. Most important—*Streptococcus pneumoniae*, *Staphylococcus aureus* and *Haemophilus influenzae*.

Clinical

None

Ocular

Conjunctival erythema, mattering of the conjunctiva, chemosis.

Laboratory

Swab for blood agar plate, chocolate agar plate and Gram stain. Antimicrobial susceptibility testing.

Treatment

Systemic gonococcus, single intramuscular (IM) dose of ceftriaxone, *Haemophilus*, oral amoxicillin for children and adults. Topical Gram-positive use bacitracin ointment, and Gram-negative use gentamicin or tobramycin drops.

Additional Resource

1. Yeung KK (2011). Bacterial Conjunctivitis. [online] Available from http://www.emedicine.com/oph/TOPIC88.HTM [Accessed April, 2012].

139. BACTERIAL ENDOCARDITIS

General

Inflammation of the lining on the heart caused by an infective agent.

Ocular

Conjunctival petechial hemorrhages; retinal hemorrhages; Roth spots; cotton-wool spots; branch or central retinal arterial occlusion; metastatic endophthalmitis; iridocyclitis; optic disk edema; cranial nerve palsies; diplopia; nystagmus; choroidal abscess; choroidal neovascular membrane; anterior segment necrosis.

Clinical

Emboli of the central nervous system; fever; splenomegaly; heart murmur; embolic episodes.

Laboratory

The most definitive laboratory tests are blood cultures that grow an organism known to cause endocarditis.

Treatment

Therapy is tailored according to the etiologic agent. Consultants should include an infectious disease specialist, a cardiologist and a cardiac surgeon.

Additional Resource

1. Gewitz MH (2011). Pediatric Bacterial Endocarditis. [online] Available from http://www.emedicine.com/ped/TOPIC2511.HTM [Accessed April, 2012].

140. BACTERIAL ENDOPHTHALMITIS

General

Rare, intraocular bacteria infection which can follows intraocular surgery or penetrating injury.

Clinical

None

Ocular

Photophobia, pain, hypopyon, decreased vision.

Laboratory

Vitreous and anterior chamber specimens to determine organism.

Treatment

Systemic steroids, topical, intravitreal and subconjunctival antibiotics and vitrectomy.

Additional Resource

1. Graham RH (2012). Bacterial Endophthalmitis. [online] Available from http://www.emedicine.com/oph/TOPIC393.HTM [Accessed April, 2012].

141. BALINT SYNDROME (PSYCHIC PARALYSIS OF VISUAL FIXATION SYNDROME)

General

Bilateral lesion of parieto-occipital region; rare occurrence; affected patients are unaware of objects otherwise familiar to them. Inability to perceive the visual field as a whole, ocular apraxia and the inability to move the hand to a specific object by usning vision (optic ataxia).

Ocular

Psychic paralysis of visual fixation; lack of full voluntary control of eye movements; unstable visual fixation.

Clinical

Tonic and motor phenomena of upper limbs; loss of body coordination (bilateral); optic ataxia; it has been reported to occur in association with human immunodeficiency virus (HIV) encephalitis and with presenile-onset cerebral adrenoleukodystrophy.

Laboratory

Diagnosis is made by clinical observation.

Treatment

Rehabilitation is the best method of treatment and includes learning and using the person's capabilities as best can be.

Additional Resource

1. Helseth EK (2011). Posterior Cerebral Artery Stroke Overview of PCA Stroke. [online] Available from http://www.emedicine.medscape.com/article/2128100-overview [Accessed April, 2012].

142. BALLER-GEROLD SYNDROME (CRANIOSYNOSTOSIS RADIAL APLASIA)

General

Autosomal recessive inheritance.

Ocular

Ocular hypertelorism; epicanthal folds.

Clinical

High nasal bridge; low philtrum; dysplastic ears; radius hypoplastic or absent; ulna short and bowed; carpal bones missing or fused; thumb hypoplastic or missing; craniosynostosis; anal, urogenital, cardiac, central nervous system, and vertebral defects; agenesis of frontal and parietal bones; midline facial angioma; scrotally positioned anus; microcephaly; erythroblastosis of the liver; pancreatic islet cell hypertrophy.

Laboratory

Diagnosis is made by clinical findings.

Treatment

Surgery before age of 6 months to repair bilateral craniosynostosis.

Bibliography

1. Baller F. Radiuasaplasie und Inzucht. Z Mensch Vererb Konstitutionsl. 1950;29:782-90.
2. Dallapiccola B, Zelante L, Mingarelli R, et al. Baller-Gerold syndrome: case report and clinical and radiological review. Am J Med Genet. 1992; 42:365-8.
3. Lin AE, McPherson E, Nwokoro NA, et al. Further delineation of the Baller-Gerold syndrome. Am J Med Genet. 1993;45:519-24.
4. Magalini SI, Scrascia E. Dictionary of Medical Syndromes, 2nd edition. Philadelphia: JB Lippincott; 1981.
5. Van Maldergem L, Verloes A, Lejeune L, et al. The Baller-Gerold syndrome. J Med Genet. 1992; 29:266-8.

143. BAMATTER SYNDROME (OSTEOPLASTIC GERODERMA; WALT DISNEY DWARFISM)

General

Hereditary X-linked; rare; onset in early childhood; precocious aging; osteoporosis; autosomal recessive inheritance.

Ocular

Glaucoma; microphthalmia; microcornea; corneal opacities.

Clinical

Senile changes in skin; stunted growth; articular hypertrophy; multiple fractures and bone malformations; osteodysplasia; osteoporosis; dwarfism.

Laboratory

Test for metabolic alkalosis, levels of potassium, calcium and chloride in the urine.

Treatment

Keeping the blood potassium level above 3.5 mEg/L. High doses of NSATD's may also be used.

Bibliography

1. Bamatter F, Franceschetti A, Klein D, et al. Gerodermie os-theodysplastique hereditaire. Ann Pediatr. 1950;174:126-7.
2. Hunter AG. Is geroderma osteodysplastica underdiagnosed? J Med Genet. 1988;25:854-7.
3. Magalini SI, Scrascia E. Dictionary of Medical Syndromes, 2nd edition. Philadelphia: JB Lippincott; 1981.
4. McKusick VA. Mendelian Inheritance in Man: A Catalog of Human Genes and Genetic Disorders, 12th edition. Baltimore: The Johns Hopkins University Press; 1998.

144. BANG DISEASE (BRUCELLOSIS; GIBRALTAR FEVER; MALTA FEVER; MEDITERRANEAN FEVER; PIG BREEDER DISEASE; UNDULANT FEVER)

General

Transmitted to man from animals or animal products containing bacteria of the genus *Brucella*; human infection results from ingestion of infected animal tissue and milk products or through skin wounds directly bathed in freshly killed animal tissues.

Ocular

Conjunctivitis; punctate keratitis; optic neuritis; swollen optic nerves; chorioretinitis; extraocular muscle palsies; phlyctenules; dacryoadenitis; papilledema; episcleritis; macular edema; phthisis bulbi; uveitis; vitreous opacities; changes in intraocular pressure (early decrease or late increase).

Clinical

Fever; icterus; weakness; sweats; general malaise; mammary abscess.

Laboratory

Increasing serum agglutination test.

Treatment

The goal of medical therapy is to prevent complications and relapses. Multidrug antimicrobial regimens are the mainstay of therapy. Ocular treatment includes topical steroids and cycloplegics for uveitis.

Additional Resource

1. Al-Nassir W (2011). Brucellosis. [online] Available from http://www.emedicine.com/med/TOPIC248.HTM [Accessed April, 2012].

145. BANTI DISEASE (CHRONIC CONGESTIVE SPLENOMEGALY; FIBROCONGESTIVE SPLENOMEGALY; HEPATOLIENAL FIBROSIS; SPLENIC ANEMIA)

General

Etiology portal hypertension due to thrombosis, compression, or aneurysm; insidious or sudden onset; most frequently occurs before age 35 years; slowly evolving.

Ocular

Subconjunctival hemorrhage.

Clinical

Pallor; mild jaundice or brown pigmentation of skin; enlarged liver; weakness; melena; flatulence; diarrhea; epistaxis; vomiting of blood.

Laboratory

Spleen scan is useful for detecting lesions in the splenic substance, evaluating loss of spleen functions, assessing for the absence of a spleen or determining the presence of an accessory spleen.

Treatment

Successful medical treatment of the primary disorder can lead to regression without the need for surgery. Splenectomy is also indicated for the treatment of chronic, severe hypersplenism.

Additional Resource

1. Khan AN (2011). Portal Hypertension Imaging. [online] Available from http://www.emedicine.com/radio/TOPIC570.HTM [Accessed April, 2012].

146. BARAITSER-WINTER SYNDROME

General

X-linked mental retardation, macrosomia, macrocephaly, and obesity syndrome.

Ocular

Ptosis; hypertelorism; down-slanting palpebral fissures.

Clinical

May be confused with Noonan syndrome; phenotypic features appear to be variable.

Laboratory

Diagnosis is made by clinical findings.

Treatment

Ptosis: If visual acuity is affected most cases require surgical correction, and there are several proce-dures that may be used including levator resection, repair or advancement and Fasanella-Servat.

Bibliography

1. Megarbane A, Le Merrer M, el Kallab K. Ptosis, down-slanting palpebral fissures, hypertelorism, seizures and mental retardation: a possible new MCA/MR syndrome. Clin Dysmorphol. 1997;6: 239-44.
2. Verloes A. Iris coloboma, ptosis, hypertelorism, and mental retardation: Baraitser-Winter syn-drome or Noonan syndrome? J Med Genet. 1993; 30:425-6.

147. BARDET-BIEDL SYNDROME

General

Polydactyly; obesity; cognitive delay; retinal degeneration; nystagmus.

Ocular

Approximately 30–65% of patients have clinical nystagmus that may mimic spasmus nutans but either lacks head nodding or is not suppressed by head nodding; retinal degeneration with attenuated retinal vessels and pale optic disks.

Clinical

Nystagmus may be a presenting sign, but patients will have polydactyly, obesity, and motor/cognitive delay.

Laboratory

None

Treatment

Retinitis pigmentosa: Vitamin A 15,000 IU/day is thought to slow the decline of retinal function, dark sunglasses for outdoor use, surgery for cataract, genetic counseling.

Additional Resource

1. Schwarz SM (2012). Obesity in Children. [online] Available from http://www.emedicine.com/ped/TOPIC1699.HTM [Accessed April, 2012].

148. BARE LYMPHOCYTE SYNDROME

General

Rare, severe combined immunodeficiency characterized by the lack of expression of human leukocyte antigen (HLA) A, B and C antigens with severe T and B deficiency.

Ocular

Horizontal nystagmus; candida retinitis.

Clinical

Recurrent pulmonary infections; bronchiectasis; gastroenteritis; hepatomegaly; developmental delay; respiratory failure; death.

Laboratory

Lymphopenia is the classic hallmark; however, normal or even elevated lymphocyte counts can be seen in a significant proportion of patients.

Treatment

Bone marrow or other stem cell reconstitution is first-line emergent therapy.

Additional Resource

1. Schwartz RA (2011). Pediatric Severe Combined Immunodeficiency. [online] Available from http://www.emedicine.com/ped/TOPIC2083.HTM [Accessed April, 2012].

149. BARLOW SYNDROME (MITRAL VALVE PROLAPSE)

General

Common; usually benign; asymptomatic; predominant in females; vague with psychoneurotic basis.

Ocular

Retinal branch arterial occlusion; retinal emboli; keratoconus; ophthalmic migraine; amaurosis fugax; bilateral retinal artery occlusion.

Clinical

Myxomatous degeneration of the mitral valve; palpitation; chest pain; dyspnea; hyperventilation.

Laboratory

Echocardiography

Treatment

Most patients are asymptomatic and no treatment is necessary. Patients with symptoms should avoid stimulants such as caffeine and may need a beta-blocker. Cardiology consultation is recommended.

Additional Resource

1. Thakkar BV (2011). Mitral Valve Prolapse. [online] Available from http://www.emedicine.com/med/TOPIC1484.HTM [Accessed April, 2012].

150. BARRE-LIEOU SYNDROME (POSTERIOR CERVICAL SYMPATHETIC SYNDROME)

General

Irritation of the vertebral nerve causing circulatory disturbance in the area of the cranial nuclei; fifth and eighth nerves mainly involved; trauma and arthritic changes involving the third and fourth cervical vertebrae or cervical disk pathology may be etiologic factor; course chronic; occurrence in older patients.

Ocular

Reduced vision (transitory); corneal hypesthesia in association with persistent corneal ulcers confined to the lid fissure.

Clinical

Headache; vertigo; mild dizziness; vasomotor disturbances of face and facial pain; laryngeal and pharyngeal paresthesia; chronic cervical arthritis; ear noises are frequent; anxiety; depression; impaired memory; difficulty in thinking.

Laboratory

Diagnosis is made by clinical findings.

Treatment

Corneal ulcer: Corneal cultures may be taken and treatment initiated. Treatment includes a broad spectrum of antibiotics and cycloplegic drops.

Bibliography

1. Barre JA. Chronic vertebral arthritis and medullar disturbances: chronic vertebral arthritis and tumor of spinal cord. Paris Med. 1925;2:226.

2. Geeraets WJ. Ocular Syndromes, 3rd edition. Philadelphia: Lea & Febiger; 1976.
3. Magalini SI, Scrascia E. Dictionary of Medical Syndromes, 2nd edition. Philadelphia: JB Lippincott; 1981.

151. BARRIER DEPRIVATION SYNDROME (BINKHORST MEMBRANE DEPRIVATION SYNDROME; WORST DECOMPARTMENTALIZATION OF EYE SYNDROME)

General

Intracapsular cataract extraction; trauma to posterior capsule with extracapsular cataract extraction; more frequent in blue-eyed patients; often bilateral; cause thought to be increased pigment loss, which releases prostaglandins, creating allergic reaction.

Ocular

Cystoid macular edema; corneal endothelial dystrophy; retinal detachment; leakage in peripheral retina and macula; iris pigment loss; uveitis; vitreous in anterior chamber; retinal holes; band keratopathy; glaucoma; iritis.

Clinical

None

Treatment

Treatment varies depending on the etiology. Steroids or nonsteroidal anti-inflammatory drops are the most common form of treatment. Avastin injections have shown some promise for the control of macular edema that does not respond to traditional treatment.

Bibliography

1. Alpar JJ. Contribution to Binkhorst's membrane deprivation and Worst's decompartmentalization of the eye syndromes. Ann Ophthalmol. 1980;12:1399-5.
2. Waitzman MB. Topical indomethacin in treatment and prevention of intraocular inflammation with special reference to lens extraction and cystoid macular edema. Ann Ophthalmol. 1979;11: 489-91.

152. BARTSOCAS-PAPAS SYNDROME

General

A rare autosomal recessive variant of popliteal pterygium syndrome (PPS).

Ocular

Ptergium

Clinical

Popliteal webbing; cleft lip; cleft palate; lower lip pits; syndactyly; genital and nail abnormalities; equinus feet.

Laboratory

Diagnosis is made by clinical findings.

Treatment

Patients with pterygia can be observed unless the lesions exhibit growth toward the center of the cornea or the patient exhibits symptoms of significant redness, discomfort or alterations in visual function. Surgery for excision of pterygia is beneficial if visual function is disturbed.

Bibliography

1. Papadia F, Zimbalatti F, La Rosa CG. The Bartsocas-Papas syndrome: autosomal recessive form of popliteal pterygium syndrome in a male infant. Am J Med Genet. 1984;17:841-7.

153. BASAL CELL CARCINOMA

General

Most common malignant neoplasm of lids; it can occasionally occur as a primary basal cell cancer of the conjunctiva and in the lacrimal canaliculus.

Ocular

Neoplasm most common on lower lid and medial canthus; lacrimation.

Clinical

Tumors of skin and other regions, including sinuses.

Laboratory

Typical histological findings. Imaging studies only for invading or deep tumor in the medial canthus.

Treatment

Surgery involves local excision. Advanced and recurrent tumors are best managed by a multidisciplinary approach involving head and neck surgical oncologists. Photodynamic therapy and cryo surgery are also effective.

Additional Resource

1. Bader RS (2012). Basal Cell Carcinoma. [online] Available from http://www.emedicine.com/ent/TOPIC722.HTM [Accessed April, 2012].

154. BASAL CELL NEVUS SYNDROME (GORLIN SYNDROME; GORLIN-GOLTZ SYNDROME; MULTIPLE BASAL CELL NEVI SYNDROME; NEVOID BASAL CELL CARCINOMA SYNDROME; NEVOID BASALIOMA SYNDROME)

General

Autosomal dominant; onset of skin lesions in childhood, usually at puberty.

Ocular

Basal cell carcinomas of eyelids; strabismus; hypertelorism; congenital cataracts; choroidal colobomas; glaucoma; medullated nerve fibers; prominence of supraorbital ridges; corneal leukoma; basalioma of the skin; coloboma of the choroid and optic nerve.

Clinical

Basal cell tumors with facial involvement; shallow pits of the skin of the hands and feet; jaw cysts; rib anomalies; kyphoscoliosis and fusion of vertebrae; medulloblastoma; frontal and temporoparietal bossing; broad nasal root.

Laboratory

CT scanning, ultrasonography or MRI to evaluate neoplasms. Endoscopy to evaluate for the degree of polyposis and survey for malignant transformation.

Treatment

Patients may require medical attention for craniofacial, vertebral, dental and ophthalmologic abnormalities, in addition to diagnosis and treatment of potential neoplasia.

Additional Resource

1. Hsu EK (2011). Intestinal Polyposis Syndromes. [online] Available from http://www.emedicine. com/ped/TOPIC828.HTM [Accessed April, 2012].

155. BASEDOW SYNDROME (EXOPHTHALMIC GOITER; GRAVES' DISEASE; HYPERTHYROIDISM; PARRY DISEASE; THYROTOXICOSIS)

General

Diffuse toxic goiter; inherited as a simple autosomal recessive; penetrance greater in females; however, dominant mode of inheritance and variable penetrance are possible; uncommon in either sex before age 15 years.

Ocular

Exophthalmos; swelling of eyelids and discoloration of upper eyelids; lid lag (von Graefe); globe lag (Koeber); lid trembling on gentle closure (Rosenbach sign); reduced blinking (Stellwag); retraction of upper lid; difficulty in everting upper lid (Gifford sign); convergence weakness (Möbius); impaired fixation on extreme lateral gaze (Suker); possible external ophthalmoplegia (Ballet); Dalrymple sign (staring appearance); tearing; photophobia; epiphora; prolapse of lacrimal gland; neuroretinal edema; tortuous vessels; papilledema and papillitis; anisocoria; keratitis; increased intraocular pressure; increased intraocular pressure on upgaze; decreased visual acuity; enlargement of the extraocular muscles; increased volume of the extraorbital fat; superior rectus muscle enlargement; decreased venous outflow.

Clinical

Tachycardia; anxiety; insomnia; loss of weight; hyperhidrosis; restlessness; myocarditis (toxic); atrial fibrillation.

Laboratory

Visual field testing, forced duction testing for restrictive myopathy, CT, MRI, T4 and thyroid-stimulating hormone, thyroid-stimulating immunoglobulins.

Treatment

There is no immediate treatment the disease is self-limited but prolonged course over 1 or more years. Five percent of patients may require surgical intervention which could be orbital decompression, strabismus surgery, lid-lengthening surgery or blepharoplasty.

Bibliography

1. Regensburg NI, Wiersinga WM, Berendschot TT, et al. Do subtypes of Graves' orbitopathy exist? Ophthalmology. 2011;118:191-6.

Additional Resource

1. Ing E (2012). Thyroid-Associated Orbitopathy. [online] Available from http://www.emedicine. com/oph/TOPIC237.HTM [Accessed April, 2012].

156. BASIC AND INTERMITTENT EXOTROPIA

General

Divergent misalignment of visual axis.

Clinical

None

Ocular

Exotropias more frequent with visual field defects and craniofacial syndromes, amblyopia.

Laboratory

Diagnosis is made by clinical findings.

Treatment

Minus lenses, prisms, orthoptic exercises and occlusion. Surgical-recession of lateral recession or recess lateral rectus and resection of medial rectus.

Additional Resources

1. Thacker N (2012). Acquired Exotropia. [online] Available from http://www.emedicine.com/oph/TOPIC329.HTM [Accessed April, 2012].
2. Bashour M (2011). Congenital Exotropia. [online] Available from http://www.emedicine.com/oph/TOPIC330.HTM [Accessed April, 2012].

157. BASSEN-KORNZWEIG SYNDROME (ABETALIPOPROTEINEMIA; ACANTHOCYTOSIS; FAMILIAL HYPOLIPOPROTEINEMIA)

General

Inability to absorb and transport lipids; predominant in males; autosomal recessive inheritance; acanthocytosis, a peculiar burr cell malformation of the red blood cells; the basic defect is thought to be an inability to synthesize the apolipoprotein B peptide of low-density and very-low-density lipoproteins.

Ocular

Ptosis (may be present); nystagmus; progressive external ophthalmoplegia; retinitis pigmentosa (usually atypical); retinopathy develops with age after 10–14 years; optic atrophy occasionally; epicanthal folds; cataract; optic nerve pallor; hypopigmentation of retina; macular degeneration; dyschromatopsia.

Clinical

Steatorrhea; hypocholesterolemia; neurologic disorder with ataxia (similar to Friedreich ataxia); areflexia; Babinski sign; muscle weakness (facial, lingual; proximal and distal); slurred speech; lordosis; kyphosis.

Laboratory

Most patients will exhibit acanthocytosis on peripheral blood smear.

Treatment

Medical care is symptomatic and supportive.

Additional Resource

1. Gross KV (2010). Neuroacanthocytosis Syndromes. [online] Available from http://www.emedicine.com/neuro/TOPIC502.HTM [Accessed April, 2012].

158. BATTEN-MAYOU SYNDROME (BATTEN DISEASE; CEREBRORETINALDEGENERATION; CEREBROMACULAR DYSTROPHY; JUVENILE AMAUROTIC FAMILY IDIOCY; JUVENILE GANGLIOSIDE LIPIDOSIS; MAYOU-BATTEN DISEASE; MYOCLONIC VARIANT OF CEREBRAL LIPIDOSIS; NEURONAL CEROID LIPOFUSCINOSIS; PIGMENTARY RETINAL LIPOID NEURONAL HEREDODEGENERATION; SPIELMEYER-SJÖGREN SYNDROME; SPIELMEYERVOGT SYNDROME; STOCK-SPIELMEYER-VOGT SYNDROME; VOGT-SPIELMEYER SYNDROME)

General

Autosomal recessive; some cases of autosomal dominant; possible disturbance in lipid metabolism; most common in Jewish families; onset between the ages of 5 and 8 years; mean age at death is 17 years; poor prognosis (see Tay-Sachs Disease; Dollinger-Bielschowsky Syndrome). The lipopigment storage diseases are divided into four types based on clinical and electron microscopic features: (1) infantile (Hagberg-Santavuori syndrome), (2) late infantile (Jansky-Bielschowsky disease), (3) juvenile (Spielmeyer-Vogt disease) and (4) adult (Kufs disease).

Ocular

Vision initially reduced, progressing to total blindness; fat deposition in the retina with gradual development of pigment disturbances resembling retinitis pigmentosa; progressive primary optic atrophy; granular pigmentary change of macula; there is clinical evidence supporting the idea that the primary lesion of the retina is in the inner layers.

Clinical

Mental disturbances; convulsions (later); apathy; irritability; ataxia; upper and lower motor neuron palsies; rigidity; complete paralysis and dementia in terminal stage; hypertonus; death from intercurrent infection.

Laboratory

Palmitoyl protein thioesterase (PPT) levels can be measured in leukocytes, cultured fibroblasts, dried blood spots and saliva. Tripeptidyl peptidase 1 (TTP1) levels can be measured in leukocytes, cultured fibroblasts, dried blood spots and saliva. Fibroblast TTP1 activity is approximately 17,000 micromoles of amino acids produced per hour per milligram of protein. The TTP1 activity in LICNL is less than 4% of normal.

Treatment

No specific treatment is available for these diseases.

Additional Resource

1. Chang CH (2009). Neuronal Ceroid Lipofuscinoses. [online] Available from http://www.emedicine. com/neuro/TOPIC498.HTM [Accessed April, 2012].

159. BAYLISASCARIS (UNILATERAL SUBACUTE NEURORETINITIS AND OCULAR LARVA MIGRANS)

General

A diffuse unilateral subacute neuroretinitis caused by *Baylisascaris procyonis* which is the common raccoon roundworm or *Ancylostoma caninum*.

Clinical

Eosinophilic meningoencephalitis.

Ocular

Retinal or subretinal tracks, optic disk edema, pallor, vitreitis, snowbanking in pars plana and iritis.

Laboratory

Antibiotics to *B. procyonis* by indirect immunofluorescence and *Toxocara canis* by enzyme-linked immunosorbent assay (ELISA).

Treatment

Prompt laser photocoagulation of the motile worm in the retina is the preferred and most effective treatment.

Bibliography

1. Roy FH, Fraunfelder FW, Fraunfelder FT. Roy and Fraunfelder's Current Ocular Therapy, 6th edition. Philadelphia: WB Saunders; 2008.

160. BAZZANA SYNDROME (ANGIOSPASTIC OPHTHALMOAURICULAR SYNDROME)

General

Rare

Ocular

Visual fields have concentric contraction; retinal vascular tortuosity and irregular contours.

Clinical

Progressive deafness (bilateral), caused by otosclerosis.

Laboratory

Visual fields testing.

Treatment

See specific type visual field.

Bibliography

1. Bazzana E, Lombardo LE, Montanelli M. Otosclerosis and visual field. Arch Ital Otol Rinol Laringol. 1950;61:620-8.
2. Magalini SI, Scrascia E. Dictionary of Medical Syndromes, 2nd edition. Philadelphia: JB Lippincott; 1981.
3. Miller NR: Walsh & Hoyt's Clinical Neuro-Ophthalmology 6th ed. Lippincott, Williams and Wilkins, Baltimore: 2004.

161. BBB SYNDROME (HYPERTELORISM-HYPOSPADIAS SYNDROME; OPITZ SYNDROME)

General

X-linked inheritance possible; differentiated from G syndrome by facial features and onset in late childhood (see G Syndrome). This disorder is compatible with normal intelligence and life span. The abnormal gene may be located in the duplicated region 5p13-p12.

Ocular

Epicanthal folds; strabismus; blepharophimosis; telecanthus; widely spaced eyebrows.

Clinical

High nasal bridge; hypospadias; cryptorchidism; cleft palate and lip; urinary malformations; mental retardation; osteochondritis dissecans; congenital heart defects; upper urinary tract anomalies.

Laboratory

Skeletal radiography, MRI and echocardiography.

Treatment

Care is supportive. No treatment exists for the underlying disorder.

Bibliography

1. Leichtman LG, Werner A, Bass WT, et al. Apparent Opitz BBBG syndrome with a partial duplication of 5p. Am J Med Genet. 1991;40:173-6.
2. McKusick VA. Mendelian Inheritance in Man: A Catalog of Human Genes and Genetic Disorders, 12th edition. Baltimore: The Johns Hopkins University Press; 1998.
3. McKusick-Nathans Institute for Genetic Medicine, Johns Hopkins University and National Center for Biotechnology Information, National Library of Medicine. (2007). Online Mendelian Inheritance in Man (OMIM). [online] Available from http://www.ncbi.nlm.nih.gov/omim/ [Accessed April, 2012].
4. Stoll C, Geraudel A, Berland H, et al. Male-to-male transmission of the hypertelorism-hypospadias (BBB) syndrome. Am J Med Genet. 1985;20:221-5.

162. BEAL SYNDROME

General

Transient unilateral disease; becoming bilateral later, then resolving within 2 weeks.

Ocular

Acute follicular conjunctivitis (lymphoid follicles; cobblestoning of conjunctiva with rapid onset).

Clinical

No purulent discharge; associated with regional adenitis.

Laboratory

Diagnosis is made by clinical findings.

Treatment

Symptomatic control may include cold compresses and artificial tears; nonsteroidal and occasionally steroidal drops to relieve itching.

Bibliography

1. Ostler HB, Schachter J, Dawson CR. Acute follicular conjunctivitis of epizootic origin. Arch Ophthalmol. 1969;82:587-91.
2. Thygeson P. Follicular conjunctivitis: infectious diseases of the conjunctiva and cornea. In: Symposium of the New Orleans Academy of Ophthalmology. St. Louis: CV Mosby; 1965. p. 103.

163. BEARD DISEASE (NERVOUS EXHAUSTION; NEURASTHENIA)

General

Predominantly in women who are overworked or emotionally strained; occurs usually in the fourth or fifth decade; onset gradual; episodic recurrence.

Ocular

Hippus (visible, rhythmic but irregular pupillary oscillation, deliberate in time, and 2 mm or more excursion; it has no localizing significance).

Clinical

Muscle spasms; bodyaches; autonomic nervous system involvement; tiredness; insomnia; impotence; dyspepsia; phobic neurosis.

Laboratory

Diagnosis is made by clinical findings.

Treatment

Reassurance

Bibliography

1. Duke-Elder S, Scott GI. System of Ophthalmology. St. Louis: CV Mosby; 1971. pp. 637-8.
2. Magalini SI, Scrascia E. Dictionary of Medical Syndromes. 2nd edition. Philadelphia: JB Lippincott; 1981.

164. BEE STING OF THE EYE (BEE STING OF THE CORNEA)

General

Occurs when the toothed lancet of the stinging apparatus penetrates the cornea.

Ocular

Conjunctival hemorrhage, chemosis, and hyperemia; corneal abscess; keratitis; lid edema; iris depigmentation; iridoplegia; iritis; lacrimation; apoplectic visual loss; acute disk swelling secondary to acute demyelination.

Clinical

Laryngeal edema; anaphylaxis; death; localized tissue edema; fever.

Laboratory

Diagnosis usually is confirmed by patient's history.

Treatment

Remove foreign body from the eye.

Additional Resource

1. de Moor C (2010). Hymenoptera Stings. [online] Available from http://www.emedicine.com/emerg/TOPIC55.HTM [Accessed April, 2012].

165. BEHÇET SYNDROME (DERMATO-STOMATO-OPHTHALMIC SYNDROME; GILBERT SYNDROME; OCULOBUCCOGENITAL SYNDROME)

General

Virus infection; occurs in adults; chronic disease; complete remission is rare; etiology is unknown.

Ocular

Muscle palsies (occasional); nystagmus (occasional); conjunctivitis; hypopyon; iritis; recurrent uveitis; keratoconjunctivitis sicca; keratitis; vitreous hemorrhages; thrombophlebitis retinal veins (occasional); retinal hemorrhages; optic neuritis (occasional); macular edema; optic nerve atrophy; retinitis; secondary glaucoma; retinal vasculitis; disk edema; panophthalmitis; optic neuropathy; skin lesions, posterior uveitis and systemic complications have been associated with loss of vision with this disorder; corneal immune ring opacity.

Clinical

Aphthous lesions of mucous membranes of the mouth and genitalia; cerebellar signs; convulsions; paraplegia; skin erythema (multiforme, bullosum); arthritis; urethritis; glossitis; recurrent fever.

Laboratory

HLA-B51 positive may help to support diagnosis.

Treatment

The goals of therapy are to suppress inflammation, to reduce the frequency and severity of recurrences, and to minimize involvement of the retina. To be effective, treatment must be started early. Extent of involvement and severity of disease determine the choice of medication. Treatment options include corticosteroids, cytotoxic agents, cyclosporine and colchicine.

Additional Resource

1. Bashour M (2010). Ophthalmologic Manifestations of Behcet Disease. [online] Available from http://www.emedicine.com/oph/TOPIC425.HTM [Accessed April, 2012].

166. BEHR SYNDROME (OPTIC ATROPHY ATAXIA SYNDROME)

General

Infantile form of heredofamilial optic atrophy and hereditary ataxia; autosomal recessive; rare; temporary progression that after some years leads to a static condition; both sexes equally affected, although transmission of pure hereditary optic atrophy shows marked predominance in males; in most cases, the abnormalities do not progress after childhood.

Ocular

Nystagmus; central scotoma; severe progressive temporal atrophy of the optic nerve; bilateral retrobulbar neuritis; horizontal nystagmus.

Clinical

Pyramidal tract signs (increased tendon reflexes and positive Babinski sign); ataxia and disturbance of coordination; mental deficiency; vesical sphincter muscle weakness; muscular hypertonia; clubfoot; progressive spastic paraplegia; dysarthria; head nodding.

Laboratory

Visual field and fundus photography.

Treatment

Intravenous steroids may be used with optic neuritis or ischemic neuropathy. Stem cell treatment may be the future treatment of choice.

Bibliography

1. Behr C. Die Komplizierte, Hereditarfamiliare Optikusatrophie des Kindesalters; ein Fisher Nicht Beschriebener Symptomenkomplex. Klin Monatsbl Augenheilkd. 1909;47:136.
2. Landrigan PJ, Berenberg W, Bresnan M. Behr's syndrome: familial optic atrophy, spastic diplegia and ataxia. Dev Med Child Neurol. 1973;15:41-7.
3. Magalini SI, Scrascia E. Dictionary of Medical Syndromes, 2nd edition. Philadelphia: JB Lippincott; 1981.
4. Sheffer RN, Zlotogora J, Elpeleg ON, et al. Behr's syndrome and 3-methylglutaconic aciduria. Am J Ophthalmol. 1992;114:494-7.
5. Miller NR: Walsh & Hoyt's Clinical Neuro-Ophthalmology 6th ed. Lippincott, Williams and Wilkins, Baltimore: 2004.

167. BELL PALSY (IDIOPATHIC FACIAL PARALYSIS)

General

Unilateral facial nerve paralysis of sudden onset and gradual recovery involving the nerve as it runs through the fallopian canal; etiology unknown; more common in adults.

Ocular

Corneal ulcer; paralysis of seventh nerve; ectropion; lagophthalmos; ptosis; epiphora; decreased visual acuity; diplopia; ocular irritation; exposure keratitis.

Clinical

Aching in the ear or mastoid; tingling or numbness of cheek or mouth; alteration of taste; hyperacusis; epiphora; facial weakness; most commonly and frequently affected cranial nerve with herpes zoster is the facial nerve.

Laboratory

Diagnosed by clinical findings.

Treatment

Most patients recover without treatment. If spontanenous recovery does not occur the most widely accepted treatment is corticosteroids.

Additional Resource

1. Taylor DC (2011). Bell Palsy. [online] Available from http://www.emedicine.com/neuro/TOPIC413. HTM [Accessed April, 2012].

168. BENEDIKT SYNDROME (TEGMENTAL SYNDROME)

General

Lesion of the inferior nucleus tuber with obstruction of the third nerve; arteriosclerotic occlusion of branches of the basilar artery, trauma and hemorrhages in the midbrain, and neoplasm most common causes.

Ocular

Homolateral paralysis of cranial nerve III (oculomotor); involves associated movements of convergence, elevation, and depression of the eyes; loss of reflex to light and accommodation, diplopia.

Clinical

Unilateral hyperkinesis; contralateral hemiparesis, coarse tremor of upper extremity (greatly increased during movement), hemihypoesthesia, and absent deep sensibility; ipsilateral ataxia. There is at least one reported case of an HIV-positive patient with Benedikt syndrome who had elevated immunoglobulin G (IgG) toxoplasma IgG titers.

Laboratory

Computed tomography (CT), MRI, transcranial Doppler.

Treatment

Ocular—patients who do not recover from III cranial nerve palsy after 6–12 months may become candidates for eye muscle resection or recession to treat persistent and stable-angle diplopia.

Additional Resources

1. Kaye V (2011). Vertebrobasilar Stroke Overview of Vertebrobasilar Stroke. [online] Available from http://www.emedicine.com/pmr/TOPIC143.HTM [Accessed April, 2012].
2. Goodwin J (2012). Oculomotor Nerve Palsy. [online] Available from http://www.emedicine.com/oph/TOPIC183.HTM [Accessed April, 2012].

169. BENIGN MUCOSAL PEMPHIGOID (CHRONIC CICATRICIAL CONJUNCTIVITIS; CICATRICIAL PEMPHIGOID; ESSENTIAL SHRINKAGE OF THE CONJUNCTIVA; MEMBRANE PEMPHIGUS; OCULAR PEMPHIGOID)

General

Etiology unknown; involving older age group, especially over 70 years; chronic autoimmune disorder characterized by fibrosis beneath the conjunctival epithelium; associated with the major histocompatibility complex class I alleles, which confer susceptibility to the disease; likely due to a multigene effect and associated with environmental factors; incidence in women is twice as frequent as men, no geographic or racial predilection.

Ocular

Conjunctivitis; absence of goblet cells of conjunctiva; conjunctival ulcer; pannus and keratitis; corneal opacity; entropion; trichiasis; cicatrization of lacrimal ducts; corneal perforation; symblepharon; dry eyes; bilateral involvement (may be asymmetrical); ocular shrinkage; xerosis; conjunctival and corneal bullae.

Clinical

Subepidermal and subepithelial blistering of mucous membranes; blisters may occur in pharyngeal, laryngeal, nasal, anal, and genital mucosa.

Laboratory

Diagnosis is made by clinical observation.

Treatment

Subconjunctival injections of steroid or mitomycin may be helpful. Systemic immunmodulators is the major therapeutic plan.

Additional Resource

1. Foster CS (2011). Ophthalmologic Manifestations of Cicatricial Pemphigoid. [online] Available from http://www.emedicine.com/oph/TOPIC83.HTM [Accessed April, 2012].

170. BENJAMIN-ALLEN SYNDROME

General

Branchial arch syndrome; not hereditary.

Ocular

Bilateral dermoids of conjunctiva; marked follicular hyperplasia of conjunctiva.

Clinical

Lymphadenopathy; cutaneous nevoid lesions; incomplete alopecia; mental retardation; growth retardation.

Laboratory

Diagnosis is made by clinical findings.

Treatment

Symptomatic control may include cold compresses and artificial tears; nonsteroidal and occasionally steroidal drops to relieve itching.

Bibliography

1. Benjamin SN, Allen HF. Classification of limbal dermoid choristomas and branchial arch anomalies. Presentation of an unusual case. Arch Ophthalmol. 1972;87:305-14.
2. Mattos J, Contreras F, O'Donnell FE, et al. Ring dermoid syndrome. Arch Ophthalmol. 1980;98:1059-61.

171. BENSON DISEASE (ASTEROID BODIES OF THE VITREOUS; ASTEROID HYALITIS; SCINTILLATIO ALBESCENS; SNOWBALL OPACITIES OF THE VITREOUS)

General

Etiology unknown; occurs in people of advanced age who have been asymptomatic.

Ocular

Small, solid, stellate, spherical bodies in an otherwise normal vitreous; creamy, flat white, or shiny when viewed with an ophthalmoscope; may interfere with accurate measurement of axial length.

Clinical

Increased prevalence of diabetes mellitus, hypertension, atherosclerosis, and hyperopia.

Laboratory

Test for diabetes, hypertension and atherosclerosis.

Treatment

Diseases found—no effect on vitreous opacities.

Bibliography

1. Allison KL, Price J, Odin L. Asteroid hyalosis and axial length measurement using automated biometry. J Cataract Refract Surg. 1991;17:181-6.
2. Benson AH. Diseases of the vitreous: a case of monocular asteroid hyalitis. Trans Ophthalmol Soc UK. 1894;14:101-4.
3. Bergren RL, Brown GC, Duker JS. Prevalence and association of asteroid hyalosis with systemic diseases. Am J Ophthalmol. 1991;111:289-93.
4. Gartner J. Whipple's disease of the central nervous system, associated with ophthalmoplegia externa and severe asteroid hyalitis. A clinicopathologic study. Doc Ophthalmol. 1980;49:155-87.

172. BERARDINELLI-SEIP SYNDROME (CONGENITAL GENERALIZED LIPODYSTROPHY)

General

Autosomal recessive; disorder of the hypothalamus.

Ocular

Punctate corneal infiltrations (lipodystrophia cornea).

Clinical

Advanced bone age; dilation of the third ventricle and basal cistern; frequent elevation of growth hormone; severe lipid levels; enlarged liver; diabetes mellitus; hyperpigmentation of axillae and chest wall; phlebomegaly.

Laboratory

Radiographic features include advanced skeletal age, bone cysts, and dilated cerebral ventricles and basal cisterns on pneumoencephalography.

Treatment

Leptin, an adipocyte hormone, which may improve insulin resistance, hyperglycemia, dyslipidemia and hepatic steatosis. Surgical intervention may be helpful for patients with deformities.

Additional Resource

1. Janniger CK (2011). Dermatologic Manifestations of Generalized Lipodystrophy. [online] Available from http://www.emedicine.com/derm/TOPIC688.HTM [Accessed April, 2012].

173. BEST DISEASE (BEST MACULAR DEGENERATION; POLYMORPHIC MACULAR DEGENERATION OF BRALEY; VITELLIFORM DYSTROPHY; VITELLIRUPTIVE MACULAR DYSTROPHY)

General

Up to 7 years of age; a type of heredomacular dystrophy; autosomal dominant with variable expressivity.

Ocular

Egg yolk lesion at macula, later absorbed to leave atrophic scar; hemorrhagic or serous exudates beneath pigment epithelium; hyperopia; esotropia; strabismic amblyopia; unusual associations with full-thickness macular hole and extramacular multifocal vitelliform disease have been reported.

Laboratory

Fluorescein angiogram reveals blockage of choroidal fluorescence by the vitelliform lesion.

Treatment

No treatment exists. Secondary choroidal neovascularization can be managed with direct laser treatment.

Additional Resource

1. Altaweel M (2010). Best Disease. [online] Available from http://www.emedicine.com/oph/TOPIC700.HTM [Accessed April, 2012].

174. BETA-GLUCURONIDASE DEFICIENCY
(MUCOPOLYSACCHARIDOSIS VII; MPS VII)

General

Autosomal recessive disorder associated with enzyme deficiency of beta-glucuronidase; disorder combines clinical and biochemical features of the Morquio and Sanfilippo syndromes.

Ocular

Clouding of the cornea.

Clinical

Dwarfism; hepatosplenomegaly; skeletal deformity; mental retardation; hernias; unusual facies; delayed psychomotor development; frequent symptomatic pulmonary infections.

Laboratory

Urine-elevated glycosaminoglycans and oligosaccharides; blood-vacuoles in lymphocytes and fibroblasts. Metachromatic granular inclusions (Alder bodies) in leukocytes.

Treatment

No treatment is available for the underlying disorder, and care must be supportive.

Additional Resource

1. Banikazemi M (2011). Genetics of Mucopolysaccharidosis Type VII. [online] Available from http://www.emedicine.com/ped/TOPIC858.HTM [Accessed April, 2012].

175. BIEBER SYNDROME

General

X-linked recessive inheritance.

Ocular

Microphthalmos; corneal pannus; cataracts; uveal hypoplasia; retinal dysplasia; optic nerve hypoplasia; congenital blepharoptosis.

Clinical

Microencephaly; mental retardation; agenesis of corpus callosum; hypospadias; cryptorchidism.

Laboratory

Diagnosis is made by clinical findings.

Treatment

Ptosis: If visual acuity is affected most cases require surgical correction, and there are several procedures that may be used including levator resection, repair or advancement and Fasanella-Servat.

Cataract: Change in glasses can sometimes improve a patient's visual function temporarily; however, the most common treatment is cataract surgery.

Bibliography

1. Bieber FR, et al. Prenatal detection of a new form of X-linked microencephaly. Am J Hum Genet. 1983;35:81.
2. Duker JS, Weiss JS, Siber M, et al. Ocular findings in a new heritable syndrome of brain, eye, and urogenital abnormalities. Am J Ophthalmol. 1985;99:51-5.
3. Howard RO. Classification of chromosomal eye syndromes. Int Ophthalmol. 1981;4:77-91.

176. BIELSCHOWSKY-LUTZ-COGAN SYNDROME (INTERNUCLEAR OPHTHALMOPLEGIA)

General

Lesion in the medial longitudinal fasciculus; anterior internuclear ophthalmoplegia consists of paresis of convergence with paresis of homolateral medial rectus muscle during lateral gaze toward opposite side of the lesion; in posterior internuclear ophthalmoplegia, convergence is not affected, while the homolateral medial rectus muscle is paralytic on lateral gaze; the most common causes in young patients include a demyelinating process such as multiple sclerosis, whereas an ischemic process is more common in the elderly; other reported causes of brainstem infarction associated with internuclear ophthalmoplegia include sickle cell trait, periarteritis nodosa, Wernicke encephalopathy, "crack" cocaine smoking.

Ocular

Unilateral or bilateral palsy of the medial rectus muscle during conjugate lateral gaze but with or without normal function of this muscle during convergence, depending on the type of internuclear ophthalmoplegia; dissociated nystagmus in the maximal abducted contralateral eye.

Laboratory

Computed tomography (CT) and MRI.

Treatment

Intravenous and oral steroids may be beneficial.

Additional Resources

1. Luzzio C (2012). Multiple Sclerosis. [online] Available from http://www.emedicine.com/emerg/TOPIC321.HTM [Accessed April, 2012].
2. Lee AG (2012). Ophthalmologic Manifestations of Multiple Sclerosis. [online] Available from http://www.emedicine.com/oph/TOPIC179.HTM [Accessed April, 2012].

177. BIEMOND SYNDROME

General

Simple recessive; hypophyseal infantilism.

Ocular

Night blindness in the presence of retinal pigment degeneration; iris coloboma (occasionally); retinal pigmentary degeneration.

Clinical

Mental retardation; polydactyly; genital dystrophia (genital organs may have been arrested in their development; absence of secondary sex characteristics); obesity; hypogenitalism; postaxial polydactyly; hydrocephalus; hypospadias.

Laboratory

Diagnosis is made by clinical findings.

Treatment

Consult child endocronologist.

Bibliography

1. Biemond A. Infantilisme Hypophysaire Avec Colobome Irien, Polydactylie et Anomalies Physiques et Sequelettiques. Ned Tijdschr Geneeskd. 1934;78:1801.
2. Duke-Elder S (Ed). System of Ophthalmology. St. Louis: CV Mosby; 1964.
3. McKusick VA. Mendelian Inheritance in Man: A Catalog of Human Genes and Genetic Disorders, 12th edition. Baltimore: The Johns Hopkins University Press; 1998.
4. McKusick-Nathans Institute for Genetic Medicine, Johns Hopkins University and National Center for Biotechnology Information, National Library of Medicine. (2007). Online Mendelian Inheritance in Man (OMIM). [online] Available from http://www.ncbi.nlm.nih.gov/omim [Accessed April, 2012].

178. BIETTI DISEASE (BIETTI MARGINAL CRYSTALLINE DYSTROPHY)

General

Autosomal recessive; metabolic disturbance; histopathologic studies demonstrated advanced panchorioretinal atrophy with crystals and complex lipid inclusions seen in choroidal fibroblasts.

Ocular

Marginal corneal crystalline dystrophy with retinitis punctata albescens; panchorioretinal atrophy.

Clinical

Asymptomatic

Laboratory

Diagnosis is made by clinical findings.

Treatment

Mild cases can be observed and soft contact lenses are helpful, penetrating keratoplasty may be necessary, graft recurrences treated by superficial keratectomy, phototherapeutic keratectomy or repeat penetrating keratoplasty.

Bibliography

1. Bernauer W, Daicker B. Bietti's corneal-retinal dystrophy. A 16-year progression. Retina. 1992;12: 18-20.
2. Kaiser-Kupfer MI, Chan CC, Markello TC, et al. Clinical biochemical and pathologic correlations in Bietti's crystalline dystrophy. Am J Ophthalmol. 1994;118:569-82.
3. Mauldin WM, O'Connor PS. Crystalline retinopathy (Bietti's tapetoretinal degeneration without marginal corneal dystrophy). Am J Ophthalmol. 1981; 92:640-6.
4. Welch RB. Bietti's tapetoretinal degeneration with marginal corneal dystrophy crystalline retinopathy. Trans Am Ophthalmol Soc. 1977;75: 164-79.

179. BILATERAL TRANSIENT LOSS OF VISION (TRANSIENT DARKENING OF VISION AND AMAUROSIS FUGAX)

General

Caused by malignant hypertension; often occurs in association with heavy smoking; may indicate vascular insufficiency of the vertebrobasilar arterial system; may precede a cerebrovascular accident and not infrequently seen in vascular insufficiency problems of the carotid arterial system; the cause, if found, is commonly an abnormality in the ipsilateral carotid artery or a cardiac source of embolism.

Ocular

Partial blindness in short attacks to permanent complete blindness; scintillating scotoma; teichopsia; retinal arteriolar spasm; signs of arteriolar sclerosis.

Clinical

Malignant hypertension; atherosclerosis; expanding lesions of the frontal or temporal lobe; vascular insufficiency.

Laboratory

There is no specific test but is essential to evaluate the erythrocyte sedimentation rate (ESR) and C-reactive protein (CRP) levels to rule out other causes. Doppler test may be useful.

Treatment

No specific treatment, except when the Doppler test is positive, carotid surgery may beindicated.

Additional Resource

1. Leibovitch I (2011). Ocular Ischemic Syndrome. [online] Available from http://www.emedicine.com/oph/TOPIC487.HTM [Accessed April, 2012].

180. BING-NEEL SYNDROME

General

Association of macroglobulinemia and central nervous system symptoms; excessive production of gamma M globulin; over 50 years of age; anoxia secondary to blood sludging from increased viscosity is explanation for peripheral retinal vascular changes.

Ocular

Ptosis; paralysis of extraocular muscles; glaucoma; chorioretinitis; dilated and segmented retinal veins; vascular tortuosity; retinal hemorrhages; peripheral microaneurysms; mild papilledema.

Clinical

Chronic encephalopathy; peripheral neuropathy; strokes; subarachnoidal hemorrhages; weakness; fatigability; weight loss; splenomegaly; anemia.

Laboratory

Serum viscosity is diagnostic.

Treatment

Plasmapheresis is the treatment of choice for initial treatment and stabilization. A hematologist should be consulted to arrange plasma/cellular pheresis and plan for interval chemotherapy as indicated.

Additional Resource

1. Hemingway TJ (2010). Hyperviscosity Syndrome. [online] Available from http://www.emedicine. com/emerg/TOPIC756.HTM [Accessed April, 2012].

181. BIPOLARIS

General

Dematiaceous septate fungus found in dust, soil and decaying matter; associated with acquired immunodeficiency syndrome (AIDS).

Ocular

Gradual progressive visual loss; afferent pupillary defect; proptosis; corneal ulcers; optic disk pallor; orbital cellulitis; ophthalmoplegia; endophthalmitis.

Clinical

Pansinusitis; sinusitis; headaches; nosebleeds; mucoid rhinorrhea; allergic rhinitis; nasal stuffiness; allergic fungal sinusitis.

Laboratory

Computed tomography (CT) and MRI of sinsus.

Treatment

Medical control of the disease involves the use of antifungal medications, corticosteroids, and immunotherapy. Surgical removal of the fungal allergic mucin of the involved sinuses is usually necessary.

Bibliography

1. Pavan PR, Margo CE. Endogenous endophthalmitis caused by Bipolaris hawaiiensis in a patient with acquired immunodeficiency syndrome. Am J Ophthalmol. 1993;116:644-5.

182. BIRDSHOT RETINOPATHY (VITILIGINOUS CHORIORETINITIS)

General

Uncommon; may relate to an inherited immune dysregulation but exact cause is unknown; average presenting age is 50 years; spots in the retina resemble the pattern seen with birdshot scatter from the shotgun.

Clinical

None

Ocular

Gradual painless loss of vision; vitreous floaters; photopsia; vitreitis; multiple ovoid spots that are orange to cream in color and hypopigmented in the posterior pole and in the mid periphery of the retina.

Laboratory

HLA-A29 blood testing; fluorescein angiography; indocyanine green angiography; optical coherence tomography; electrophysiologic testing.

Treatment

Topical, systemic and regional steroids may be useful. Cyclosporine, ketoconazole and other immunomodulatory therapies may also be necessary.

Additional Resource

1. Samson CM (2011). Birdshot Retinopathy. [online] Available from http://www.emedicine.medscape.com/article/1223257-overview [Accessed April, 2012].

183. BLACKWATER FEVER

General

Usually occurs in association with malaria, *Plasmodium falciparum* infection; mortality 20–30%; recurrent hemolytic episodes with subsequent malarial infections.

Ocular

Scleral icterus; cotton-wool spots; retinal edema; optic disk edema; conjunctival calcium deposits; band keratopathy; cortical blindness; epibulbar hemorrhage of conjunctiva and episclera; retinal hemorrhages.

Clinical

Fever; hemolysis; icterus; hemoglobinuria; malaria; uremia; nausea; vomiting; vertigo; convulsions; coma; acute renal failure; hypertension, azotemia; hypervolemia; metabolic disturbances; hyponatremia; hypercalcemia.

Laboratory

Complete blood count, electrolyte panel, renal function tests, pregnancy test, urinalysis, free serum haptoglobin, urine and blood cultures, and thick and thin blood smears are useful.

Treatment

If the patient is experiencing life-threatening complications (i.e. coma, respiratory failure, coagulopathy, fulminant kidney failure), then investigate exchange transfusion as a treatment option.

Additional Resource

1. Fernandez MC (2011). Emergent Management of Malaria. [online] Available from http://www.emedicine.com/emerg/TOPIC305.HTM [Accessed April, 2012].

184. BLASTOMYCOSIS

General

Chronic fungal disease caused by *Blastomyces dermatitidis*.

Ocular

Hypopyon; mycotic keratitis; corneal ulcer; choroidal granuloma; nodules of iris; cicatrization of eyelid; ectropion; descemetocele; panophthalmitis; recurrent papillomatous lesion upper lid; granulomatous conjunctivitis.

Clinical

Granulomatous lesions of skin, lung, bone or any part of the body.

Laboratory

Periodic acid-Schiff and Gonosia methenamine silver stains.

Treatment

Therapeutic approaches involve the use of oral azoles, primarily itraconazole. Ocular treatment may include surgical draining of the lid in addition to antifungal therapy.

Additional Resource

1. Steele RW (2011). Pediatric Blastomycosis. [online] Available from http://www.emedicine.com/ped/TOPIC254.HTM [Accessed April, 2012].

185. BLATT SYNDROME (CRANIO-ORBITO-OCULAR DYSRAPHIA)

General

Autosomal dominant; characterized by distichiasis and anisometropia; both sexes affected; present from birth.

Ocular

Hypertelorism; microphthalmos; distichiasis with the meibomian glands usually absent; anisometropia.

Clinical

Meningocele or meningoencephalocele; cranial deformities; malformations of facial bones.

Laboratory

Diagnosis is made by clinical findings.

Treatment

Distichiasis: Symptomatic—therapeutic contact lenses as well as lubricating drops and ointments. Epilation with electrolysis cryosurgery, double freeze-thaw down to -20°F, lid splitting procedure.

Bibliography

1. Blatt N. Cranio-orbito-ocular dysrhaphia and meningocele. Rev Otoneuroophthalmol. 1961;33: 185-232.
2. Duke-Elder S (Ed). System of Ophthalmology. St. Louis: CV Mosby; 1976.
3. Magalini SI, Scrascia E. Dictionary of Medical Syndromes, 2nd edition. Philadelphia: JB Lippincott; 1981.

186. BLAU SYNDROME

General

Rare, autosomal dominant.

Ocular

Iris bombe, uveitis, secondary angle-closure glaucoma.

Clinical

Skin rash, camptodactyly, early-onset granulomatous arthritis, flexion deformity.

Laboratory

Diagnosis is made by clinical findings.

Treatment

Uveitis: Topical steroids and cycloplegic medication should be the initial treatment of choice. Oral steroids if not responsive to topical steroids, immunosuppressants if bilateral disease that does not respond to oral steroids, periocular steroids for unilateral or posterior uveitis. Vitrectomy can be used for severe vitreous opacification. Cryotherapy and laser photocoagulation may be used for localized pars plana exudates.

Angle-closure glaucoma: Iridotomy is the treatment of choice. Argon laser peripheral iridoplasty and goniosynechialysis may be necessary.

Bibliography

1. Kurokawa T, Kikuchi T, Ohta K, et al. Ocular manifestations in Blau syndrome associated with CARD15/Nod 2 mutation. Ophthalmology. 2003;110:2040-4.
2. Latkany P. Blau syndrome. Ophthalmology. 2004; 111:853-4.

---

187. BLEPHARITIS (ADULT BLEPHARITIS, MEIBOMIAN GLAND DYSFUNCTION, SEBORRHEIC BLEPHARITIS)

General

Common eyelid inflammation, seen frequently with seborrheic dermatitis.

Clinical

None

Ocular

Ocular symptoms—discharge, foreign body sensation, dryness, uncomfortable sensation, sticky sensation, pain, epiphora, itching, redness, heavy sensation, glare, excessive blinking, history of chalazion or hordeolum. Lid margin abnormalities—irregular lid margin, vascular engorgement, plugged meibomian gland, anterior or posterior replacement of the mucocutaneous junction. (Meibomian score is graded 1–3: 1 is less than one-third lid; 2 is from one-third to two-thirds lid; 3 is over two-thirds lid).

Laboratory

Diagnosis is made by clinical findings. Swab of lids usually is *Staphylococcus aureus*.

Treatment

Blepharitis: Oral tetracyclines, omega-3 fatty acids, flax seed oil or fish oil. Ocular therapy includes eyelid scrubs, warm compresses, bacitracin ointment to lid margins, topical cyclosporine A and preservative-free lubricants.

Bibliography

1. Ibrahim OM, Matsumoto Y, Dogru M, et al. The efficacy, sensitivity, and specificity of in vivo laser confocal microscopy in the diagnosis of meibomian gland dysfunction. Ophthalmology. 2010;117:665-72.

Additional Resource

1. Lowery RS (2011). Adult Blepharitis. [online] Available from http://www.emedicine.com/oph/ TOPIC81.HTM [Accessed April, 2012].

188. BLEPHARO-NASO-FACIAL MALFORMATION SYNDROME

General

Autosomal dominant.

Ocular

Telecanthus; lateral displacement of lacrimal puncta; lacrimal excretory obstruction.

Clinical

Mask-like face; bulky nose; weak facial muscles; torsional dystonia; mental retardation.

Laboratory

Diagnosis is made by clinical findings.

Treatment

Lacrimal excretory obstruction: It may spontaneously resolve during the first year of life with massage if not probing and irrigation of the nasolacrimal duct can be done.

Additional Resource

1. Tewfik TL (2010). Congenital Malformations of the Nose. [online] Available from http://www.emedicine.com/ent/TOPIC320.HTM [Accessed April, 2012].

189. BLEPHAROCHALASIS

General

Rare, with recurrent episodic painless periorbital edema.

Clinical

None

Ocular

Skin of the lids is thin and baggy.

Laboratory

Diagnosis is made by clinical findings.

Treatment

Cold compress may be of some use. Surgical-excise the redundant skin, reposition the ectopic lacrimal gland and reconstruct lateral canthal tendon.

Bibliography

1. Roy FH, Fraunfelder FW, Fraunfelder FT. Roy and Fraunfelder's Current Ocular Therapy, 6th edition. Philadelphia: WB Saunders; 2008.

190. BLEPHAROCONJUNCTIVITIS

General

Chronic blepharitis caused by staphylococcal, seborrheic, mebomian seborrhea or seborrheic with secondary meibomianitis.

Clinical

Sebprrheic dermatitis.

Ocular

Bleparitis, keratoconjunctivitis.

horizontal nystagmus from stroke, tumor, multiple sclerosis, trauma, infection and drug intoxication. Can occur from cataract, vitreous hemorrhage or optic atrophy.

Additional Resource

1. Bardorf CM (2012). Acquired Nystagmus. [online] Available from http://www.emedicine.com/oph/TOPIC339.HTM [Accessed April, 2012].

195. BLOOM SYNDROME (BLOOM-TORRE-MACHACEK SYNDROME; FACIAL DWARFISM; LEVI-TYPE DWARFISM; TELANGIECTASIS)

General

Autosomal recessive inheritance; male preponderance; usually low birth weight following full-term gestation; full-term, abnormally small children.

Ocular

Erythema of the lower eyelids.

Clinical

Facial rash; erythema of any part of the body; hypersensitivity to light; failure to grow; microcephaly; dolichocephaly; abnormalities of ears, extremities, digits and nose; facial rash from sensitivity to sunlight; predisposition to neoplasia (especially leukemia) and diabetes mellitus; multiple chromosomal breaks have been observed in DNA from these patients.

Laboratory

Chromosome study; blood and skin cells show a characteristic pattern of chromosome breakage and rearrangement.

Treatment

No specific treatment available. Avoiding sun exposure and using sunscreens can help prevent some of the cutaneous changes associated with photosensitivity.

Additional Resource

1. Bajoghli AA (2012). Bloom Syndrome (Congenital Telangiectatic Erythema). [online] Available from http://www.emedicine.com/derm/TOPIC54.HTM [Accessed April, 2012].

196. BLUE RUBBER BLEB NEVUS SYNDROME (BEAN SYNDROME)

General

Onset after birth; autosomal dominant.

Ocular

Subconjunctival hemangioma with overlying fibrosis; raised hemorrhagic lesion near macula suggestive of a small arteriovenous malformation.

Clinical

Vascular lesions; cutaneous lesions found anywhere on the body; profuse sweating may occur over the skin lesions with pain or tenderness on palpation; visceral lesions are common; tender bluish papules on the trunk and extremities; colonic hemangiomas.

Laboratory

Magnetic resonance imaging (MRI) is a useful tool for detecting extracutaneous lesions. Histopathologic examination of skin lesions reveals vascular tissue with tortuous, blood-filled ectatic vessels, lined by a single layer of endothelium, with surrounding thin connective tissue.

Treatment

No systemic therapy is a standard of care. Bleeding from GI lesions usually is managed conservatively with iron supplementation and blood transfusions when necessary. Cutaneous lesions do not need to be treated, unless they are cosmetically unacceptable or functionally troublesome.

Additional Resource

1. Cherpelis BS (2010). Blue Rubber Bleb Nevus Syndrome. [online] Available from http://www.emedicine.com/derm/TOPIC56.HTM [Accessed April, 2012].

197. BLUE SCLERA

General

Blue sclera is characterized by localized or generalized blue coloration of sclera because of thinness and loss of water content, which allow underlying dark choroid to be seen.

Clinical

Associated with high urine secretion, skeletal disorders and chromosome disorders.

Ocular

Congenital glaucoma, myopia, scleromalacia (perforans) and staphyloma.

Laboratory

Diagnosis is made by clinical findings.

Treatment

Identify and treat the cause.

Bibliography

1. Cameron JA, Cotter JB, Risco JM, et al. Epikeratoplasty for keratoglobus associated with blue sclera. Ophthalmology. 1991;98:446-52.
2. Fraunfelder FT, Randall JA. Minocycline-induced scleral pigmentation. Ophthalmology. 1997;104:936-8.

198. BOBBLE-HEAD DOLL SYNDROME

General

Caused by massive dilation of the third ventricle; occurs in childhood.

Ocular

Pallor of the optic disk or optic atrophy; visual loss.

Clinical

Flexion extension movements of the head and neck on the trunk at a rate of 2 or 3 per second; pendular movements also may involve the trunk and upper limbs; hydrocephalus; obesity; head bobbing ceases during sleep; mental retardation.

Laboratory

Check for hydrocephalus.

Treatment

Consult neurologist.

Bibliography

1. Benton JW, Nellhaus G, Huttenlocher PR, et al. The bobble-head doll syndrome. Neurology. 1966;16:725-9.
2. Kirkham TH. Optic atrophy in the bobble-head doll syndrome. J Pediatr Ophthalmol. 1977;14:299-301.
3. Magalini SI, Scrascia E. Dictionary of Medical Syndromes, 2nd edition. Philadelphia: JB Lippincott; 1981.

199. BOGORAD SYNDROME (CROCODILE TEAR SYNDROME; PAROXYSMAL LACRIMATION SYNDROME)

General

Subsequent to facial palsy if the lesion is proximal to the geniculate ganglion; during regeneration, fibers supposed to reinnervate the sublingual and submandibular glands are partly interchanged with fibers innervating the lacrimal gland and, hence, gustatory stimulation causes lacrimation.

Ocular

Unilateral lacrimation while eating or drinking due to misdirected nerve fiber regeneration.

Clinical

Excessive salivation (occasionally); diffuse facial muscle response or facial contracture with lacrimation.

Laboratory

Diagnosis is made by clinical findings.

Treatment

None

Bibliography

1. Bogorad FA. Symptoms of crocodile tears. Vrach Delo. 1928;11:1328.
2. McGovern FH. Paroxysmal lacrimation during eating following recovery from facial paralysis: syndrome of crocodile tears. Am J Ophthalmol. 1954;23:1388.

200. BONNET-DECHAUME-BLANC SYNDROME (CEREBRORETINAL ARTERIOVENOUS ANEURYSM SYNDROME; NEURORETINOANGIOMATOSIS SYNDROME; WYBURN-MASON SYNDROME)

General

Dominant inheritance; unilateral or bilateral arteriovenous aneurysm of the midbrain with ipsilateral retinal angioma and skin nevi; severity and extent of symptoms depend on location of cerebral aneurysm and structures it may involve; not regarded as hereditary; incidence is equal in men and women; usually becomes symptomatic at age 30 years.

Ocular

Exophthalmos; ptosis; strabismus; nystagmus; hemianopsia due to lesion in optic tract or pulvinar; sluggish pupils; anisocoria; retinal arteriovenous aneurysm; varicosity of retinal veins; arteriovenous angiomas; papilledema; optic atrophy of fellow eye; vitreous hemorrhage; rubeosis iridis; optic neuropathy secondary to compression by vascular malformation; proptosis; partial ophthalmoplegia.

Clinical

Arteriovenous angiomas of the thalamus and mesencephalon; facial vascular and pigmented nevi, usually in the trigeminal distribution; psychic disturbances; slow and scanning speech; hydrocephalus; headache; dizziness; hemiplegia; congenital defects of bone, muscle, kidneys and gastrointestinal tract.

Laboratory

Magnetic resonance imaging, magnetic resonance angiography (MRA), fluorescein angiography.

Treatment

Referral for neurologic evaluation is indicated since intracranial vascular malformations are associated more commonly with larger retinal vascular lesions. Stability of the retinal lesions limit the need for ocular treatment.

Additional Resource

1. Bidwell AE (2010). Wyburn-Mason Syndrome. [online] Available from http://www.emedicine.com/oph/TOPIC357.HTM [Accessed April, 2012].

201. BORNHOLM DISEASE (EPIDEMIC PLEURODYNIA)

General

Associated with group B coxsackievirus; epidemic occurrence in summer and early fall; person-to-person contact; incubation 3–5 days; affects both sexes; prevalent in children and young adults; recurrent episodes of sudden excruciating pain in abdominal or thoracic regions, increased by movement and respiration.

Ocular

Optic neuritis.

Clinical

Malaise; sore throat; anorexia; muscle pain; abdominal pain; cutaneous hyperesthesia and paresthesia over affected area; meningitis; myocarditis; hepatitis; orchitis.

Laboratory

Serological tests, viral isolation by cell culture and polymerase chain reaction (PCR).

Treatment

Treatment is symptomatic, using analgesics and heat application for pain relief. Severe pain may require opiate analgesics.

Additional Resource

1. Velazquez A (2010). Enteroviruses. [online] Available from http://www.emedicine.com/med/TOPIC681. HTM [Accessed April, 2012].

202. BOTULISM

General

Caused by a toxin-producing strain of *Clostridium botulinum*; occurs primarily after the ingestion of contaminated food; the organism can produce a neurotoxin, the effect of which can be life threatening.

Ocular

Absent optokinetic nystagmus, absent vertical gaze; marked limitation of horizontal gaze; ptosis; diplopia; decreased tear secretion; mydriasis; paralysis of accommodation; nystagmus; optic atrophy; optic neuritis; extraocular muscle paresis.

Clinical

Dizziness; severe respiratory impairment; gastrointestinal disturbances; dysphagia; dysarthria; postural hypotension.

Laboratory

Toxin assay for early diagnosis, whereas later cases are more likely to yield a positive specimen culture.

Treatment

Antitoxin appears to be the only effective medication. Supportive care such as ventilation and parenteral nutrition are necessary for the duration of the paralytic illness.

Additional Resource

1. Patel B (2012). Ophthalmologic Manifestations of Botulism. [online] Available from http://www. emedicine.com/oph/TOPIC493.HTM [Accessed April, 2012].

203. BOURNEVILLE SYNDROME (BOURNEVILLE-PRINGLE SYNDROME; EPILOIA; TUBEROUS SCLEROSIS)

General

Irregular dominant inheritance; more frequent in females; most patients die before age 24 years.

Ocular

Vitreous often cloudy; lens opacities; retinal mushroom-like tumor of grayish-white color; yellowish-white plaques with small hemorrhages and cystic changes in retina; papilledema; disk drusen; cerebral astrocytoma; 40–50% of patients have normal intelligence.

Clinical

Grand mal, petit mal or jacksonian seizures (manifest first 2 years of life); mental changes from feeblemindedness to imbecility and idiocy; skin changes arranged usually about nose and cheeks (adenoma sebaceum); congenital tumors of kidney (hypernephroma or tubular adenoma) and heart (rhabdomyoma); cerebral astrocytoma.

Laboratory

Brain MRI is recommended for the detection and follow-up imaging of cortical tubers.

Treatment

A neurologist should be consulted to assist with seizure management and anticonvulsant medication.

Additional Resource

1. Schwartz RA (2011). Genetics of Tuberous Sclerosis. [online] Available from http://www.emedicine.com/ped/TOPIC2796.HTM [Accessed April, 2012].

204. BOUTONNEUSE FEVER (MARSEILLES FEVER)

General

Caused by *Rickettsia conorii* and transmitted by ticks.

Ocular

Conjunctivitis; central serous retinopathy; retinal detachment; perivasculitis; uveitis; papillitis; keratitis.

Clinical

Fever; lymph node enlargement; papular rash.

Laboratory

Serology is usually a confirmatory method; however, these tests are useful only after an acute infection. Culture of the organism may be used for diagnosis early in the course of the disease.

Treatment

Tetracyclines with chloramphenicol and quinolones may be considered first-line antibiotics. Patients with the benign form are usually treated with antibiotics for 7 days. Patients with the malignant form are usually treated with antibiotics for 2 weeks.

Additional Resource

1. Zalewska A (2011). Boutonneuse Fever. [online] Available from http://www.emedicine.com/derm/TOPIC759.HTM [Accessed April, 2012].

205. BOWEN DISEASE (CARCINOMA IN SITU; DYSKERATOSIS; INTRAEPITHELIAL EPITHELIOMA)

General

Squamous cell carcinomas in situ of the skin or conjunctiva.

Ocular

Dysplastic epithelium, intraepithelial epithelioma or invasive squamous cell carcinoma of conjunctiva or cornea; infiltration of lacrimal system and sclera.

Laboratory

Ocular—full thickness conjunctival biopsy which should include basement membrane.

Treatment

The goals of therapy are to reduce morbidity and to prevent complications. Simple excision with conventional margins surgery is the most common and preferred treatment for smaller lesions and those not in problematic areas.

Additional Resource

1. Eid MP (2012). Bowen Disease. [online] Available from http://www.emedicine.com/derm/TOPIC59. HTM [Accessed April, 2012].

206. BRACHYMETAPODY-ANODONTIA-HYPOTRICHOSIS ALBINOIDISM SYNDROME (ANODONTIA-HYPOTRICHOSIS SYNDROME)

General

Autosomal recessive.

Ocular

Strabismus; nystagmus; distichiasis; cataracts; high myopia.

Clinical

Congenital anodontia; small maxilla; short stature; shortening of metacarpals and metatarsals; little hair growth; albinoidism.

Laboratory

Diagnosis is made by clinical findings.

Treatment

Cataract: Change in glasses can sometimes improve a patient's visual function temporarily; however, the most common treatment is cataract surgery.

Strabismus: Equalized vision with correct refractive error; surgery may be helpful in patient with diplopia.

Bibliography

1. McKusick VA. Mendelian Inheritance in Man: A Catalog of Human Genes and Genetic Disorders, 12th edition. Baltimore: The Johns Hopkins University Press; 1998.
2. McKusick-Nathans Institute for Genetic Medicine, Johns Hopkins University and National Center for Biotechnology Information, National Library of Medicine. (2007). Online Mendelian Inheritance in Man (OMIM). [online] Available from http://www.ncbi.nlm.nih.gov/omim [Accessed April, 2012].
3. Taumaala P, Haapanen E. Three siblings with similar anomalies in the eyes, bones and skin. Acta Ophthalmol. 1968;46:365-71.

207. BRAIN DYSFUNCTION SYNDROME (DYSCONTROL SYNDROME)

General

Suspected causes include tumors of the limbic system and/or localized atrophy of the brain.

Ocular

Visual field defects.

Clinical

Manic behavior; physical brutality without motive; sexual assaults; seizures; lack of memory; hallucinations; temporal lobe seizures; depression; speech difficulties.

Laboratory

Computed tomography (CT) and MRI.

Treatment

Consult neurologist.

Additional Resource

1. Benbadis SR (2012). Encephalopathic EEG Patterns. [online] Available from http://www.emedicine.com/neuro/TOPIC700.HTM [Accessed April, 2012].

208. BRANCHED-CHAIN KETOACIDURIA (MAPLE SYRUP URINE DISEASE)

General

Deficiency in the oxidative decarboxylation of the corresponding alpha-ketoacids; possibly autosomal recessive inheritance; both sexes affected; onset in the first week of life.

Ocular

Ptosis; epicanthal folds; hypertelorism; prominence of supraorbital ridges; cataract; strabismus; decreased or absent pupillary reaction to light; horizontal nystagmus; optic atrophy; ophthalmoplegia.

Clinical

Maple syrup odor of urine; neurologic symptoms; death may follow promptly or the patient may live for a decade during which severe mental retardation is apparent; vomiting; failure to thrive; absence of grasping reflex; generalized rigidity; hypoglycemic crisis; cortical blindness.

Laboratory

Plasma amino acids (elevation of branched-chain amino acids, detection of alloisoleucine)—the detection of alloisoleucine is diagnostic.

Treatment

The mainstay in the treatment is dietary restriction of branched-chain amino acids.

Additional Resource

1. Bodamer OA (2012). Maple Syrup Urine Disease. [online] Available from http://www.emedicine.com/ped/TOPIC1368.HTM [Accessed April, 2012].

209. BRANCHIAL CLEFTS WITH CHARACTERISTIC FACIES, GROWTH RETARDATION, IMPERFORATE NASOLACRIMAL DUCT AND PREMATURE AGING

General

Autosomal dominant.

Ocular

Strabismus; obstructed nasolacrimal ducts.

Clinical

Low birth weight; retarded growth; bilateral bronchial cleft sinuses; broad nasal bridge; protruding upper lip; carp mouth; premature aging; malformed ears; linear skin lesions behind the ears.

Laboratory

Diagnosis is made by clinical findings.

Treatment

Strabismus: Equalized vision with correct refractive error; surgery may be helpful in patient with diplopia.

Obstructed nasolacrimal ducts: May spontaneously resolve during the first year of life with massage if not probing and irrigation of the nasolacrimal duct can be done.

Additional Resource

1. Tewfik TL (2011). Manifestations of Craniofacial Syndromes. [online] Available from http://www.emedicine.medscape.com/article/844209-overview [Accessed April, 2012].

210. BRILL-SYMMERS DISEASE (GIANT FOLLICULAR LYMPHOMA; LYMPHOSARCOMA)

General

Occurs primarily in older patients.

Ocular

Unilateral or bilateral lid swelling; orbital masses with exophthalmos; lacrimal gland infiltration.

Clinical

Patients survive 6–7 years; special form of lymphoma.

Laboratory

Computed tomography (CT) scan of orbit, lacrimal gland biopsy.

Treatment

Local debulking of the orbital mass and adjunctive radiotherapy and chemotherapy.

Bibliography

1. Duane TD. Clinical Ophthalmology. Philadelphia: JB Lippincott; 1987.
2. Roy FH, Fraunfelder FW, Fraunfelder FT. Roy and Fraunfelder's Current Ocular Therapy, 6th edition. Philadelphia: WB Saunders; 2008.
3. Pau H. Differential Diagnosis of Eye Diseases. New York: Thieme; 1988.

211. BRITTLE CORNEA SYNDROME (BRITTLE CORNEA; BLUE SCLERA AND RED HAIR SYNDROME; BLUE SCLERA SYNDROME)

General

Autosomal recessive; rare.

Ocular

Spontaneous perforation of cornea (brittle cornea); blue sclera; acute hydrops; microcornea; sclerocornea; cornea plana; keratoconus; keratoglobus.

Clinical

Red hair; associated with Ehlers-Danlos syndrome, osteogenesis imperfecta and Marfan syndrome.

Laboratory

Diagnosis is made by clinical findings.

Treatment

Surgical correction of deformities, physiotherapy, and the use of orthotic support and devices to assist mobility were the primary means of treatment for osteogenesis imperfecta. With the more recent understanding of the molecular mechanisms of the disease, medical treatment to increase bone mass and strength are gaining popularity.

Additional Resource

1. Ramachandran M (2012). Osteogenesis Imperfecta. [online] Available from http://www.emedicine.com/orthoped/TOPIC530.HTM [Accessed April, 2012].

212. BROWN-MARIE SYNDROME (BROWN-MARIE ATAXIC SYNDROME; HEREDITARY ATAXIA SYNDROME; MARIE HEREDITARY ATAXIA; SANGER BROWN SYNDROME)

General

Cause unknown; simple recessive inheritance, although irregular dominant transmission has been observed.

Ocular

Nystagmus; strabismus; ophthalmoplegia; anisocoria; Argyll Robertson pupil; retinitis pigmentosa; optic nerve atrophy; retrobulbar optic neuritis.

Clinical

Hereditary ataxia; choreiform movements; athetosis; pyramidal tract paresis; speech difficulties; hyperreflexia.

Laboratory

Computed tomography (CT) and MRI.

Treatment

Treatment is directed to symptoms. Pharmacologic therapy has provided only minimal benefits.

Additional Resource

1. Azevedo CJ (2010). Olivopontocerebellar Atrophy. [online] Available from http://www.emedicine.com/neuro/TOPIC282.HTM [Accessed April, 2012].

213. BROWN-McLEAN SYNDROME

General

Following cataract surgery photophobia, posterior staphyloma, peripheral corneal edema with underlying endothelial pigment, iridonesis.

Ocular

Foreign body sensation.

Laboratory

Diagnosis is made by clinical findings.

Treatment

Control IOP, hypertonic salt solution or ointment, soft contact lens, anterior stromal puncture or conjunctival flap, PTK, hairdryer held at arms length and posterior lamellar keratoplasty.

Additional Resource

1. Wright KW (2010). Brown Syndrome. [online] Available from http://www.emedicine.com/oph/TOPIC552.HTM [Accessed April, 2012].

214. BROWN-SEQUARD SYNDROME

General

Caused by lesion (injury, tumor pressure) of spinal cord.

Ocular

Nystagmus (if lesion in upper cervical area); sluggish pupillary reaction to light (occasional finding); optic atrophy.

Clinical

Homolateral spastic paralysis with: (1) loss of ipsilateral deep joint, tendon and vibratory sensations below level of the lesion; (2) loss of contralateral pain and temperature sensations and (3) sphincteral disturbances. Cases of this syndrome caused by meningomyelitis secondary to syphilis, herpes zoster and multiple sclerosis have been reported.

Laboratory

Diagnosis is made on the basis of history and physical examination.

Treatment

Neurosurgical or orthopedic consultation is recommended.

Additional Resource

1. Beeson MS (2011). Brown-Sequard Syndrome in Emergency Medicine. [online] Available from http://www.emedicine.com/emerg/TOPIC70.HTM [Accessed April, 2012].

215. BROWN SYNDROME (SUPERIOR OBLIQUE TENDON SHEATH SYNDROME)

General

Etiology unknown; affects both sexes; present from birth; may be congenital or acquired (secondary to trauma, orbital surgery, or injections, or following delivery).

Ocular

Bilateral ptosis with associated backward head tilt; widening of palpebral fissure with attempted upward gaze; ocular movements show failure in direction of superior oblique action; may be associated with underaction of the inferior oblique; adduction or abduction restricted or completely abolished; choroidal coloboma.

Laboratory

Diagnosis is made by clinical findings.

Treatment

Once systemic disease is excluded, patients who have acquired Brown syndrome with signs of inflammation can be treated with anti-inflammatory medication. Oral ibuprofen is a good first-line choice. Local steroid injections in the area of the trochlea and oral corticosteroids can be used for inflammation. Once the inflammatory disease process is controlled, patients

with inflammatory Brown syndrome may show spontaneous resolution. Congenital Brown syndrome is unlikely to improve spontaneously; therefore, surgery is important to consider as an option.

Bibliography

1. Suh DW, Oystreck DT, Hunter DG. Long-term results of an intraoperative adjustable superior oblique tendon suture spacer using nonabsorbable sutrue for Brown syndrome. Ophthalmology. 2008;115:1800-4.

Additional Resource

1. Wright KW (2010). Brown Syndrome. [online] Available from http://www.emedicine.com/oph/TOPIC552.HTM [Accessed April, 2012].

---

216. BRUCH MEMBRANE DRUSEN

General

Autosomal dominant; round or oval lesions in grape like clusters in the posterior polar region; found on the vitreal side of Bruch membrane, secreted by the retinal pigment epithelial cells, apparently secondary to an inborn error of metabolism localized in the retinal pigment epithelium.

Ocular

Crystalline retinal degeneration; Doyne honey-comb choroiditis; fleck retina disease; macular edema; macular hemorrhage; pigmentary disturbances with secondary calcifications; central scotomata.

Clinical

None

Laboratory

Diagnosis is made by clinical findings.

Treatment

Thermal laser destruction might be considered for macular hemorrhage.

Additional Resource

1. Abusamak M (2011). Angioid Streaks. [online] Available from http://www.emedicine.com/oph/TOPIC378.HTM [Accessed April, 2012].

217. BRUNS SYNDROME (POSTURAL CHANGE SYNDROME)

General

Caused by tumors of the third, fourth or lateral ventricle, or by lesions of the midline in the brain. foramen obstruction and Bruns syndrome; Kramer reported a patient with a free-floating cysticercus cyst with this condition.

Ocular

Partial ophthalmoplegia (third nerve paralysis) and gaze paralysis; oculomotor paresis associated with postural change of head or body; amaurosis or transient blindness; flashes of light.

Clinical

Severe paroxysmal headache; nausea and vomiting; vertigo; irregular respiration; apnea; syncope; tachycardia; free-floating cysts within the fourth ventricle may produce intermittent

Laboratory

Computed tomography (CT) scan of the head.

Treatment

Consultation with a neurologist.

Bibliography

1. Geeraets WJ. Ocular Syndromes, 3rd edition. Philadelphia: Lea & Febiger; 1976.
2. Bruns O. Neuropathologische Demonstrationen. Neurol Centralbl. 1902;21:561-7.

218. BUERGER DISEASE (THROMBOANGIITIS OBLITERANS)

General

Unknown etiology; males who smoke and are under age 35 years; affects small- and medium-sized arteries and veins of the extremities; segmented episodic inflammatory panarteritis with associated thrombosis.

Ocular

Exudative retinopathy; occlusion of retinal vessels; retinal hemorrhages; perivasculitis and endovasculitis; blindness; cataract.

Clinical

Intermittent claudication; coolness; paresthesia; hyperemia; cyanosis and gangrene may be present in the lower extremities.

Laboratory

No specific laboratory tests confirm or exclude the diagnosis of Buerger disease.

Treatment

Except for absolute tobacco avoidance, no forms of therapy are definitive.

Additional Resource

1. Meireles OR (2012). Buerger Disease (Thromboangiitis Obliterans). [online] Available from http://www.emedicine.com/med/TOPIC253.HTM [Accessed April, 2012].

219. BULLOUS ICHTHYOSIFORM ERYTHRODERMA (COLLODION BABY; CONGENITAL ICHTHYOSIS; EPIDERMOLYTIC HYPERKERATOSIS; ICHTHYOSIS; ICHTHYOSIS VULGARIS; LAMELLAR ICHTHYOSIS; NONBULLOUS ICHTHYOSIFORM ERYTHRODERMA; X-LINKED ICHTHYOSIS; XERODERMA)

General

Autosomal inherited disorder; affects both sexes; normal at birth; onset within first 7 days; X-linked; pathogenesis may be secondary to physicochemical changes of corneal tissues including accumulation of cholesterol sulfate.

Ocular

Keratopathy; corneal scarring; keratitis; conjunctivitis; lagophthalmos; photophobia; ectropion; lid erythema; lacrimation; keratoconus; deep corneal punctate/filiform lesions.

Clinical

At birth, the skin surface is moist, red and tender; within several days, thick verrucous scales form.

Laboratory

Diagnosis is made by clinical findings.

Treatment

Genetic counseling and prenatal diagnosis also can be offered. Newborns with denuded skin are at increased risk for infection, secondary sepsis and electrolyte imbalance and should be transferred to the neonatal ICU to be monitored and treated as needed.

Additional Resource

1. Chen TS (2010). Epidermolytic Hyperkeratosis (Bullous Congenital Ichthyosiform Erythroderma). [online] Available from http://www.emedicine.com/derm/TOPIC590.HTM [Accessed April, 2012].

220. BURNETT SYNDROME (MILK DRINKER SYNDROME; MILK-ALKALI SYNDROME)

General

Characterized by alkalosis, hypercalcemia and transient renal insufficiency with azotemia; develops during milk-alkali therapy for peptic ulcer; seen in excessive intake of milk or soluble alkali, as in therapy for peptic ulcer.

Ocular

Band-shaped keratopathy; conjunctivitis with calcification.

Clinical

Nausea; vomiting; headache; irritability; dizziness; depression; confusion.

Laboratory

Diagnosing the etiology of hypercalcemia is difficult. Much of the laboratory workup should be guided by the history and physical examination and may include renal imaging, X-ray and serology.

Treatment

Initial treatment involves hydration to improve urinary calcium output. The addition of diuretics inhibits tubular reabsorption of calcium.

Additional Resource

1. Claudius IA (2009). Pediatric Hypercalcemia. [online] Available from http://www.emedicine.com/ped/TOPIC1062.HTM [Accessed April, 2012].

221. C SYNDROME (OPITZ TRIGONOCEPHALY SYNDROME; TRIGONOCEPHALY SYNDROME)

General

Autosomal recessive; consanguinity; early death.

Ocular

Hypertelorism; up-slanted palpebral fissures; strabismus.

Clinical

Polydactyly; unusual facies; cardiac abnormality; cryptorchidism; Omtra-oral anomalies; abnormally modeled ears; cardiac anomalies; neonatal hypotonia; severe mental retardation; short neck with loose skin.

Laboratory

Diagnosis is made by clinical findings.

Treatment

Strabismus: Equalized vision with correct refractive error; surgery may be helpful in patient with diplopia.

Bibliography

1. McKusick VA. Mendelian Inheritance in Man: A Catalog of Human Genes and Genetic Disorders, 12th edition. Baltimore: The Johns Hopkins University Press; 1998.
2. McKusick-Nathans Institute for Genetic Medicine, Johns Hopkins University and National Center for Biotechnology Information, National Library of Medicine. (2007). Online Mendelian Inheritance in Man (OMIM). [online] Available from http://www.ncbi.nlm.nih.gov/omim [Accessed April, 2012].
3. Opitz JM, Johnson RC, McCreadie SR, et al. The C syndrome of multiple congenital anomalies. Birth Defects. 1969;12:161-6.
4. Schaap C, Schrander-Stumpel CT, Fryns JP. Opitz-C syndrome: on the nosology of mental retardation and trigonocephaly. Genet Couns. 1992;3:209-15.
5. Zanini SA, Paglioli Neto E, Viterbo F, et al. Trigonocephaly. J Craniofac Surg. 1992;3:85-9.

222. CAFFEY SYNDROME (CAFFEY-SILVERMAN SYNDROME; INFANTILE CORTICAL HYPEROSTOSIS)

General

Cause unknown, possibly collagen disease or viral infection; prevalent in females; onset in early infancy; sudden onset; benign; self-limited.

Ocular

Periorbital edema and tenderness; transient proptosis; mild conjunctivitis.

Clinical

Tender swelling over regions of cortical hyperostosis (may resemble periostitis); severe anemia; fever; dysphagia; pleurisy.

Laboratory

Radiography is the most valuable diagnostic study in infantile cortical hyperostosis. MRI may also be useful.

Treatment

No specific treatment exists for infantile cortical hyperostosis. The disease is self-limited and usually resolves. Steroids and nonsteroidal anti-inflammatory agents may be useful to reduce symptoms in severe cases.

Additional Resource

1. Novick C (2010). Infantile Cortical Hyperostosis. [online] Available from http://www.emedicine.com/orthoped/TOPIC151.HTM [Accessed April, 2012].

223. CAISSON SYNDROME (BENDS SYNDROME; COMPRESSED-AIR ILLNESS; DIVER'S PALSY)

General

Under high atmospheric pressure (18 lb/in^2 at least) the blood becomes saturated with nitrogen; sudden decompression (e.g. return to normal atmospheric pressure when divers surface too rapidly) causes the nitrogen to bubble out in gas form, with resulting destruction of tissue spaces; symptoms appear usually within 3 hours after decompression.

Ocular

Nystagmus; diplopia; transient blindness; cataract formation with rapidly developing vacuoles and gray opacities; narrowing of the retinal vessels.

Clinical

Severe joint pain; dyspnea with sensation of chest constriction; giddiness; hemiplegia; vertigo; deafness; aphasia; paraplegia; convulsion; pruritus; abdominal pain.

Laboratory

Complete blood count (CBC) and arterial blood gas (ABG) determination.

Treatment

Correct any immediate life-threatening conditions while maintaining adequate oxygenation and perfusion. Patients should be placed on high-flow oxygen and have isotonic fluid infusion to maintain blood pressure and pulse.

Additional Resource

1. Kaplan J (2011). Barotrauma in Emergency Medicine. [online] Available from http://www.emedicine.com/emerg/TOPIC53.HTM [Accessed April, 2012].

224. CALIFORNIA SYNDROME

General

Functional and/or malingering visual complaints in people with psychosocial problems relating to parental divorce, poor school performance and attention-getting behavior; seen in adults as well as children; usually secondary gain motive (e.g. disability benefits, Workmen's Compensation, litigation or income tax).

Ocular

Blurred vision; abnormal vision fields; abnormal color vision; voluntary nystagmus; decreased visual acuity at near or far distance.

Clinical

Hysteria; malingering; social stresses.

Laboratory

Diagnosis is made by clinical findings.

Treatment

Reassurance

Bibliography

1. Keltner JL, May WN, Johnson CA, et al. The California syndrome. Functional visual complaints with potential economic impact. Ophthalmology. 1985;92:427-35.
2. Keltner JL. The California syndrome. A threat to all. Arch Ophthalmol. 1988;106:1053-4.

225. CAMAK SYNDROME (CATARACT-MICROCEPHALY-ARTHROGRYPOSIS-KYPHOSIS SYNDROME)

General

Low birth weight; autosomal recessive.

Ocular

Cataracts at birth or within 3 weeks.

Clinical

Mental retardation; stiffness of joints; microcephaly; bird-like facies; progressive curvature of the spine.

Laboratory

Diagnosis is made by clinical findings.

Treatment

Cataract: Change in glasses can sometimes improve a patient's visual function temporarily; however, the most common treatment is cataract surgery.

Bibliography

1. Lowry RB, MacLean R, McLean DM, et al. Cataracts, microcephaly, kyphosis, and limited joint movement in two siblings: a new syndrome. J Pediatr. 1971;79:282-4.
2. McKusick VA. Mendelian Inheritance in Man: A Catalog of Human Genes and Genetic Disorders, 12th edition. Baltimore: The Johns Hopkins University Press; 1998.
3. McKusick-Nathans Institute for Genetic Medicine, Johns Hopkins University and National Center for Biotechnology Information, National Library of Medicine. (2007). Online Mendelian Inheritance in Man (OMIM). [online] Available from http://www.ncbi.nlm.nih.gov/omim [Accessed April, 2012].

226. CAMFAK SYNDROME (CATARACT-MICROCEPHALY-FAILURE TO THRIVE-KYPHOSCOLIOSIS SYNDROME)

General

Autosomal recessive; there is evidence supporting that it is a neurologic disease characterized by peripheral and central demyelination similar to that seen in Cockayne syndrome.

Ocular

Cataracts

Clinical

Microcephaly; failure to thrive; mental retardation; spasticity; hip dislocation; kyphoscoliosis.

Laboratory

Diagnosis is made by clinical findings.

Treatment

Cataract: Change in glasses can sometimes improve a patient's visual function temporarily; however, the most common treatment is cataract surgery.

Bibliography

1. McKusick VA. Mendelian Inheritance in Man: A Catalog of Human Genes and Genetic Disorders, 12th edition. Baltimore: The Johns Hopkins University Press; 1998.

2. McKusick-Nathans Institute for Genetic Medicine, Johns Hopkins University and National Center for Biotechnology Information, National Library of Medicine. (2007). Online Mendelian Inheritance in Man (OMIM). [online] Available from http://www.ncbi.nlm.nih.gov/omim [Accessed April, 2012].

3. Scott-Emuakpor AB, Heffelfinger J, Higgins JV. A syndrome of microcephaly and cataracts in four siblings. A new genetic syndrome? Am J Dis Child. 1977;131:167-9.

4. Talwar D, Smith SA. CAMFAK syndrome: a demyelinating inherited disease similar to Cockayne syndrome. Am J Med Genet. 1989;34: 194-8.

---

227. CANALIS OPTICUS SYNDROME

General

Loss of vision after blunt trauma to the head (mainly forehead) without direct eye injury; thought to occur because of sudden stretching of the fixed, as well as the movable, portions of the optic nerve during movement of the brain at the time of injury.

Ocular

Spontaneous unilateral or bilateral, reversible or irreversible amaurosis; absent pupil reaction in cases of complete blindness; spontaneous visual recovery has been reported anecdotally.

Clinical

Blunt head injury.

Laboratory

Computed tomography (CT) of optic nerve.

Treatment

Steroids may be helpful.

Bibliography

1. Berlin R. Uber Sehstorungen nach Verletzung durch Stumpfe Gewalt. Klin Monatsbl Augenheilkd. 1878;17.

2. Miller NR. The management of traumatic optic neuropathy. Arch Ophthalmol. 1990;108:1086-7.

3. Seitz R. Canalis opticus syndrome. Ophthalmologica. 1969;158:318-24.

4. Snebold NG. Neuro-ophthalmic manifestations of trauma. In: Albert DM, Jakobiec FA (Eds). Principles and Practice of Ophthalmology. Philadelphia: WB Saunders; 1994.

5. Wolin MJ, Lavin PJ. Spontaneous visual recovery from traumatic optic neuropathy after blunt head injury. Am J Ophthalmol. 1990;109:430-5.

228. CANDIDIASIS

General

Yeast-like opportunistic fungal infection caused by *Candida albicans*.

Ocular

Uveitis; hypopyon; conjunctivitis; keratitis; corneal ulcer; blepharitis; endophthalmitis; dacryocystitis; papillitis; retinal atrophy; Roth spot; vitreous abscess; retrobulbar abscess; retinal detachment; panophthalmitis; chorioretinitis; infectious crystalline keratopathy.

Clinical

C. albicans normally is present as an intestinal saprophyte in 35–75% of the human population; in situations of internal environmental change, however, *Candida* can become pathogenic (e.g. obesity, diabetes mellitus, malignancy and other debilitating conditions).

Laboratory

Common yeast from up to 50% of healthy individuals isolate directly from the eye should be attempted to confirm the presence of organism. Blood agar and Sabouraud's dextrose agar may be used. Polymerase chain reaction (PCR) for species identification.

Treatment

Mucocutaneous infection typically responds to topical therapy. Antifungal therapy should be started immediately after necessary cultures have been obtained from all suspected sites of infection. Infectious disease specialists are typically involved in cases of invasive candidiasis.

Additional Resource

1. Hedayati T (2010). Candidiasis in Emergency Medicine. [online] Available from http://www.emedicine.com/emerg/TOPIC76.HTM [Accessed April, 2012].

229. CANINE TOOTH SYNDROME (CLASS VII SUPERIOR OBLIQUE PALSY)

General

Caused by trauma to the trochlear area, producing a "double Brown syndrome"; secondary to strengthening the superior oblique along with a residual superior oblique palsy, or a combination of local trauma to the trochlea causing restriction to upgaze along with closed head trauma producing a IV nerve palsy.

Ocular

Underaction of the superior oblique and under-action of the inferior oblique on the same side.

Clinical

None

Laboratory

Diagnosis is made by clinical findings.

Treatment

Class I—greatest vertical deviation in field of action of inferior oblique, weaken inferior oblique; Class II—greatest vertical deviation in field of action of the underacting superior oblique-superior oblique strengthening; Class III—equal vertical deviation of inferior oblique and superior oblique either inferior oblique or superior oblique surgery.

Bibliography

1. Ellis FH, Helveston EM. Superior oblique palsy: diagnosis and classification. Int Ophthalmol Clin. 1976;16:127-35.
2. Roy FH, Fraunfelder FW, Fraunfelder FT. Roy and Fraunfelder's Current Ocular Therapy, 6th edition. Philadelphia: WB Saunders; 2008.

230. CAPGRAS SYNDROME (ILLUSION OF DOUBLE SYNDROME; L'ILLUSION DES SOSIES; NONRECOGNITION-MISIDENTIFICATION SYNDROME; PHANTOM DOUBLE SYNDROME)

General

Characterized by misidentification or nonrecognition of a person by the patient who believes that this person appears in double in front of him or her; occurs in paranoid psychosis, and only people familiar or important to the patient appear in double; preponderance in women; agnosia of identification.

Ocular

Illusion of double perception with failure of recognition of a known person.

Clinical

General claims include statements that the person seen is an impostor, although the person is well known to the patient; hallucinations; delusions.

Laboratory

Diagnosis is made by clinical findings.

Treatment

Delusional disorders are difficult to treat for various reasons, including patients' frequent denial that they have any problem, especially of a psychological nature, difficulties in developing a therapeutic alliance, and social/interpersonal conflicts. Careful assessment and diagnosis are crucial to determine an underlying organic illness that warrants specific treatment.

Additional Resource

1. Chopra S (2011). Delusional Disorder. [online] Available from http://www.emedicine.com/med/TOPIC3351.HTM [Accessed April, 2012].

231. CAPSULAR BAG DISTENSION SYNDROME

General

Occurs after phacoemulsification as a result of occlusion of the anterior capsulorhexis opening by the intraocular lens optic.

Ocular

Shallow anterior chamber, pupil peaking, accumulation of turbid fluid in the capsular bag.

Clinical

None

Laboratory

Diagnosis is made by clinical findings.

Treatment

Yttrium-aluminum-garnet (YAG) capsulotomy of posterior capsule.

Bibliography

1. Agrawal S, Agrawal J, Agrawal TP. Incomplete capsular bag distension syndrome after neodymium: YAG capsulotomy. J Cataract Refract Surg. 2006;32:351-2.
2. Davison JA. Capsular bag distension after endophacoemulsification and posterior chamber intraocular lens implantation. J Cataract Refract Surg. 1990;16:99-108.

232. CAPSULAR BLOCK SYNDROME

General

Following cataract surgery.

Ocular

Complete sealing by the anterior capsule opening by the optic and displacement of the posterior capsule far behind the posterior optic surface.

Clinical

None

Laboratory

Diagnosis is made by clinical findings.

Treatment

Yttrium-aluminum-garnet (YAG) capsulotomy of the anterior and posterior capsule.

Bibliography

1. Liu TY, Chou PI. Capsular block syndrome associated with secondary angle-closure glaucoma. J Cataract Refract Surg. 2001;27:1503-5.
2. Nishi O, Nishi K, Takahashi E. Capsular bag distention syndrome noted 5 years after intraocular lens implantation. Am J Ophthalmol. 1998;125: 545-7.
3. Xiao Y, Wang YH, Fu ZY. Capsular block syndrome caused by a reversed-optic intraocular lens. J Cataract Refract Surg. 2004;30:1130-2.

233. CAR SYNDROME (CANCER-ASSOCIATED RETINOPATHY SYNDROME)

General

Rare; antiretinal antibodies in blood of cancer patients experiencing concomitant loss of vision; vision loss may be noted before cancer is diagnosed; mechanisms involved in the vision loss experienced by these patients is not understood, but serologic studies indicate they may include a series of autoimmune reactions directed at specific components of the retina.

Ocular

Vision loss usually progressive; retinal degeneration; retinal hole; abnormal visual fields; loss of color vision; retinal detachment; optic atrophy; ring-like scotoma; night blindness; retinal phlebitis.

Clinical

Carcinoma with or without metastasis to any part of the body.

Laboratory

Diagnosis is made by clinical findings.

Treatment

Treat the antiretinal antibodies.

Bibliography

1. Keltner JL, Roth AM, Chang RS. Photoreceptor degeneration. Possible autoimmune disorder. Arch Ophthalmol. 1983;101:564-9.
2. Ohnishi Y, Ohara S, Sakamoto T, et al. Cancer-associated retinopathy with retinal phlebitis. Br J Ophthalmol. 1993;77:795-8.
3. Thirkill CE, Roth AM, Keltner JL. Cancer-associated retinopathy. Arch Ophthalmol. 1987;105:372-5.
4. Thirkill CE, Tait RC, Tyler NK, et al. The cancer-associated retinopathy antigen is a recoverin-like protein. Invest Ophthalmol Vis Sci. 1992;33: 2768-72.

---

234. CARCINOID SYNDROME

General

Slow-growing neoplasms of enterochromaffin cell; metastatic tumors usually arise from small primary tumors in the ileum.

Ocular

Lacrimation; periorbital edema; choroidal and orbital metastases.

Clinical

Cutaneous flushing; telangiectasia; intestinal hypermotility.

Laboratory

Barium examination, CT, MRI and PET scan.

Treatment

Complete surgical removal of all tumor tissues is the best treatment when feasible because this may result in a complete and permanent cure.

Additional Resource

1. Santacroce L (2012). Malignant Carcinoid Syndrome. [online] Available from http://www.emedicine.com/med/TOPIC2649.HTM [Accessed April, 2012].

---

235. CARDIAC MYXOMAS

General

Myxomas of the heart account for approximately 50% of primary heart tumors; although benign, they can cause serious complications and death by obstruction or embolism; tumor arises from the mural endocardium.

Ocular

Central or branch retinal artery obstruction with ganglion cell edema and a "cherry-red macula"; choroidal and retinal infarct; ischemic optic neuropathy; conjunctival and caruncle pigmentation; eyelid pigmentation; transient loss of vision.

Clinical

Signs and symptoms are a result of emboli that travel to the extremities, brain, liver, spleen, kidney, cerebrum, and, rarely, the coronary arteries.

Laboratory

Echocardiography, CT, MRI and MRA.

Treatment

Myxomas often are asymptomatic, but these tumors can produce symptoms by releasing substances that lead to inflammatory signs, including fever, tachycardia and tachypnea. If myxomas are large, they will cause intracardiac obstruction manifested as dyspnea, syncope or congestive heart. If asymptomatic, treatment depends on the symptom.

Additional Resource

1. Gates J (2011). Cardiac Tumor Imaging. [online] Available from http://www.emedicine.com/radio/TOPIC66.HTM [Accessed April, 2012].

236. CARDIORESPIRATORY OBESITY SYNDROME (PICKWICKIAN SYNDROME)

General

Chronic pulmonary insufficiency caused by extensive obesity.

Ocular

Venous congestion; spontaneous hyphema; chorioretinal venous congestion with retinal hemorrhages and exudates; papilledema; rubeosis iridis (may be bilateral).

Clinical

Pronounced and greatly excessive obesity; headache; dyspnea; drowsiness; cyanosis; heart failure; muscular twitching; disturbed consciousness.

Laboratory

Arterial blood gases, echocardiogram, pulmonary function studies, EKG.

Treatment

Weight loss remains a cornerstone to the treatment. Noninvasive ventilatory support with supplemental oxygen may be necessary.

Additional Resource

1. Cataletto ME (2011). Pediatric Obesity-Hypoventilation Syndrome. [online] Available from http://www.emedicine.com/ped/TOPIC1627.HTM [Accessed April, 2012].

237. CAROTID ARTERY SYNDROME (CAROTID VASCULAR INSUFFICIENCY SYNDROME; OCULAR ISCHEMIC SYNDROME)

General

Causes include microemboli, atherosclerotic plaques, arteritis, arterial compression by cicatricial tissue surrounding the vessel and tumors; male preponderance; onset between the ages of 50 and 70 years.

Ocular

Lacrimation; homolateral transient, painless visual loss; photopsia; hemianopsia; retinal infarcts; cholesterol plaques may be seen in retinal arteries on funduscopic examination; optic atrophy; hypoxic retinopathy; low-tension glaucoma; anterior uveitis; cataract; visual acuity 20/400 or less; iris neovascularization; angle neovascularization; optic disk pale; retinal hemorrhages; Homer syndrome; amaurosis fugax; retinal artery occlusion; ophthalmoparesis; proptosis; chemosis; conjunctival hyperemia; acute orbital infarction.

Clinical

Transient cerebral ischemia with contralateral weakness of arm and leg; hemisensory disturbances; mental confusion and dysphasia; headache; dizziness; epileptiform seizures; carotid dissection.

Laboratory

Erythrocyte sedimentation rate and C-reactive protein levels in patients with suspected GCA. Fluorescein angiography.

Treatment

Panretinal photocoagulation to treat neovascularization of the iris, optic nerve or retina. It was reported to cause regression of neovascularization. Antiplatelet therapy may be useful. Carotid endarterectomy has shown to benefit symptomatic patients.

Additional Resource

1. Leibovitch I (2011). Ocular Ischemic Syndrome. [online] Available from http://www.emedicine.com/oph/TOPIC487.HTM [Accessed April, 2012].

238. CAROTID ARTERY SYNDROME (CAVERNOUS SINUS FISTULA SYNDROME; RED-EYED SHUNT SYNDROME)

General

Seventy-five percent of cases caused by trauma; others occur spontaneously, or are congenital; fistula from carotid artery to cavernous sinus.

Ocular

Progressive, pulsating exophthalmos; distended pulsating superior orbital vein; venous congestion of lids; variable ophthalmoplegia, depending on involvement of cranial nerves III, IV, V and VI; secondary glaucoma; congestion of conjunctiva with chemosis; corneal ulcerations; eversion of the lower lid; loss of corneal sensation; retinal edema; engorgement of retinal veins; papilledema; optic atrophy; ocular bruit that may be subjective and/or objective; diplopia; visual decrease; choroidal folds; dilated superior ophthalmic vein.

Clinical

Severe unilateral headache; buzzing noise.

Laboratory

Orbital ultrasonography, computed tomography, six-vessel cranial digital subtraction angiography-characterization of the arterial supply and venous drainage of fistula.

Treatment

Use of intraocular lowering agent and topical lubrication is the ocular treatment of choice.

Bibliography

1. Dailey EJ, Holloway JA, Murto RE, et al. Evaluation of ocular signs and symptoms in cerebral aneurysms. Arch Ophthalmol. 1964;71:463-74.
2. Duane TD. Clinical Ophthalmology. Philadelphia: JB Lippincott; 1987.
3. Flaharty PM, Lieb WE, Sergott RC, et al. Color Doppler imaging. A new noninvasive technique to diagnose and monitor carotid cavernous sinus fistulas. Arch Ophthalmol. 1991;109:522-6.
4. Roy FH, Fraunfelder FW, Fraunfelder FT. Roy and Fraunfelder's Current Ocular Therapy, 6th edition. Philadelphia: WB Saunders; 2008.
5. Gonshor LG, Kline LB. Choroidal folds and dural cavernous sinus fistula. Arch Ophthalmol. 1991;109:1065-66.
6. Phelps CD, Thompson HS, Ossoinig KC. The diagnosis and prognosis of atypical carotid-cavernous fistula (red-eyed shunt syndrome). Am J Ophthalmol. 1982;93:423-36.
7. Travers B. A case of aneurysm by anastomosis in the orbit, cured by the ligature of the common carotid artery. Med Chir Trans. 1811;2:1-420.1.

239. CARPENTER SYNDROME (ACROCEPHALOPOLYSYNDACTYLY TYPE II)

General

Hereditary; transmitted as an autosomal recessive trait; severe form of Apert syndrome; normal intelligence has been reported with this syndrome; polysyndactyly is not an absolute requirement for this diagnosis.

Ocular

Lateral displacement of inner canthus; epicanthal folds; microcornea; corneal opacities.

Clinical

Acrocephalopolysyndactyly; brachydactyly; peculiar facies; obesity; mental retardation; hypogonadism; generalized aminoaciduria; cryptorchidism; hypogenitalism.

Laboratory

Skull radiography, cranial CT.

Treatment

Carefully monitoring for signs and symptoms of elevated intracranial pressure is important. Surgery typically is indicated for increased intracranial pressure or for cosmetic reasons.

Additional Resource

1. Sheth RD (2010). Pediatric Craniosynostosis. [online] Available from http://www.emedicine.medscape.com/article/1175957-overview [Accessed April, 2012].

240. CAT'S-EYE SYNDROME (PARTIAL TRISOMY G SYNDROME; SCHACHENMANN SYNDROME; SCHMID-FRACCARO SYNDROME)

General

Causative factor is one extra chromosome, a G chromosome, which may be from a 13–15 or 21–22 chromosome; although the ocular findings of the syndrome are similar to the D 13–15 trisomy group, the systemic manifestations usually are less severe; this syndrome is associated with a supernumerary bisatellited marker chromosome which is derived from duplicated regions of 22pter-22q11.2; partial cat's-eye syndrome is characterized by the absence of coloboma.

Ocular

Hypertelorism; microphthalmos; antimongoloid slant of palpebral fissures; strabismus; inferior vertical iris coloboma (cat eye); cataract; choroidal coloboma; epicanthal folds.

Clinical

Anal atresia; preauricular fistulas (bilateral); umbilical hernia; heart anomalies.

Laboratory

Chromosome analysis.

Treatment

Cataract: Change in glasses can sometimes improve a patient's visual function temporarily; however, the most common treatment is cataract surgery.

Strabismus: Equalized vision with correct refractive error; surgery may be helpful in patient with diplopia.

Bibliography

1. Collins JF. Handbook of Clinical Ophthalmology. New York: Masson; 1982.
2. Cory CC, Jamison DL. The cat eye syndrome. Arch Ophthalmol. 1974;92:259-62.
3. Liehr T, Pfeiffer RA, Trautmann U. Typical and partial cat eye syndrome: identification of the marker chromosome by FISH. Clin Genet. 1992;42:91-6.
4. Mears AJ, Duncan AM, Budarf ML, et al. Molecular characterization of the marker chromosome associated with cat eye syndrome. Am J Hum Genet. 1994;55:134-42.
5. Petersen RA. Schmid-Fraccaro syndrome ("cat's eye" syndrome). Arch Ophthalmol. 1973;90:287-91.
6. Schachenmann G, Schmid W, Fraccaro M, et al. Chromosomes in coloboma and anal atresia. Lancet. 1965;2:290.

241. CATARACT AND CONGENITAL ICHTHYOSIS

General

Autosomal recessive; rare.

Ocular

Cortical cataract.

Clinical

Ichthyosis

Laboratory

Diagnosis is made by clinical findings.

Treatment

Cataract: Change in glasses can sometimes improve a patient's visual function temporarily; however, the most common treatment is cataract surgery.

Bibliography

1. McKusick VA. Mendelian Inheritance in Man: A Catalog of Human Genes and Genetic Disorders, 12th edition. Baltimore: The Johns Hopkins University Press; 1998.
2. McKusick-Nathans Institute for Genetic Medicine, Johns Hopkins University and National Center for Biotechnology Information, National Library of Medicine. (2007). Online Mendelian Inheritance in Man (OMIM). [online] Available from http://www.ncbi.nlm.nih.gov/omim [Accessed April, 2012].
3. Pinkerton OD. Cataract associated with congenital ichthyosis. Arch Ophthalmol. 1958;60:393-6.

242. CATARACT, ANTERIOR POLAR

General

Autosomal dominant; imperfect separation of lens from surface ectoderm during the fifth week of embryologic development; abnormal mass in region of anterior pole and incomplete resorption of blood vessels and mesoderm at anterior pole of embryonic lens; they can be associated with chromosomal abnormalities including 3, 18 chromosomal translocation.

Ocular

Small opacities on anterior surface of lens; microphthalmia; cataracts usually do not interfere with vision; corneal astigmatism.

Clinical

None

Laboratory

Diagnosis is made by clinical findings.

Treatment

Cataract surgery if vision decreases.

Bibliography

1. Bouzas AG. Anterior polar congenital cataract and corneal astigmatism. J Pediatr Ophthalmol Strabismus. 1992;29:210-2.
2. McKusick VA. Mendelian Inheritance in Man: A Catalog of Human Genes and Genetic Disorders, 12th edition. Baltimore: The Johns Hopkins University Press; 1998.
3. McKusick-Nathans Institute for Genetic Medicine, Johns Hopkins University and National Center for Biotechnology Information, National Library of Medicine. (2007). Online Mendelian Inheritance in Man (OMIM). [online] Available from http://www.ncbi.nlm.nih.gov/omim/[Accessed April, 2012].

4. Moross T, Vaithilingam SS, Styles S, et al. Autosomal dominant anterior polar cataracts associated with a familial 2;14 translocation. J Med Genet. 1984;21:52-3.

5. Rubin SE, Nelson LB, Pletcher BA. Anterior polar cataract in two sisters with an unbalanced 3;18 chromosomal translocation. Am J Ophthalmol. 1994;117:512-5.

243. CATARACT, CONGENITAL OR JUVENILE (CATARACT, HUTTERITE TYPE, JUVENILE)

General

Autosomal recessive; seen most frequently in people of Japanese origin; autosomal dominant inheritance also has been reported.

Ocular

Retinitis pigmentosa; Usher syndrome (retinitis pigmentosa and congenital deafness); congenital cataract of the "i" phenotype; microphthalmos; keratoconus.

Clinical

Congenital deafness; galactokinase deficiency; epimerase deficiency.

Laboratory

Diagnosis is made by clinical findings.

Treatment

Cataract: Change in glasses can sometimes improve a patient's visual function temporarily; however, the most common treatment is cataract surgery.

Retinitis pigmentosa: Vitamin A 15,000 IU/day is thought to slow the decline of retinal function, dark sunglasses for outdoor use, surgery for cataract, genetic counseling.

Bibliography

1. McKusick VA. Mendelian Inheritance in Man: A Catalog of Human Genes and Genetic Disorders, 12th edition. Baltimore: The Johns Hopkins University Press; 1998.
2. McKusick-Nathans Institute for Genetic Medicine, Johns Hopkins University and National Center for Biotechnology Information, National Library of Medicine. (2007). Online Mendelian Inheritance in Man (OMIM). [online] Available from http://www.ncbi.nlm.nih.gov/omim [Accessed April, 2012].
3. Shokeir MH, Lowry RB. Juvenile cataract in Hutterites. Am J Med Genet. 1985;22:495-500.

244. CATARACT, CONGENITAL TOTAL WITH POSTERIOR SUTURAL OPACITIES

General

Sex-linked; initial lens changes occur in both men and women with continuation of process in men; women show progression at much later age; it has been suggested that several X-linked cataract syndromes are due to deletions of different sizes in the X chromosome.

Ocular

Y-shaped sutural cataracts; congenital cataracts; nuclear cataract; cortical cataract; posterior subcapsular cataract; asymptomatic posterior Y-sutural cataracts; severe visual impairment; bilateral pendular nystagmus; bilateral microcornea; exotropia; keratoconus.

Clinical

Mental retardation.

Laboratory

Diagnosis is made by clinical findings.

Treatment

Change in glasses can sometimes improve a patient's visual function temporarily; however, the most common treatment is cataract surgery.

Bibliography

1. Crews SJ, Bundey SE. Is there an X-linked form of congenital cataracts? Clin Genet. 1982;21:351-3.
2. McKusick VA. Mendelian Inheritance in Man: A Catalog of Human Genes and Genetic Disorders, 12th edition. Baltimore: The Johns Hopkins University Press; 1998.
3. McKusick-Nathans Institute for Genetic Medicine, Johns Hopkins University and National Center for Biotechnology Information, National Library of Medicine. (2007). Online Mendelian Inheritance in Man (OMIM). [online] Available from http://www.ncbi.nlm.nih.gov/omim [Accessed April, 2012].
4. Waarburg M. X-linked cataract and X-linked microphthalmos: how many deletion families? [Letter]. Am J Med Genet. 1989;34:451-3.

245. CATARACT, CRYSTALLINE ACULEIFORM OR FROSTED

General

Autosomal dominant.

Ocular

Small crystal-like opacities of lens.

Clinical

None

Laboratory

Diagnosis is made by clinical findings.

Treatment

Cataract surgery if vision decreases.

Bibliography

1. Gifford SR, Puntenney I. Coralliform cataract and a new form of congenital cataract with crystals in the lens. Arch Ophthalmol. 1937;17:885-92.
2. McKusick VA. Mendelian Inheritance in Man: A Catalog of Human Genes and Genetic Disorders, 12th edition. Baltimore: The Johns Hopkins University Press; 1998.
3. McKusick-Nathans Institute for Genetic Medicine, Johns Hopkins University and National Center for Biotechnology Information, National Library of Medicine. (2007). Online Mendelian Inheritance in Man (OMIM). [online] Available from http://www.ncbi.nlm.nih.gov/omim [Accessed April, 2012].

246. CATARACT, CRYSTALLINE CORALLIFORM

General

Autosomal dominant.

Ocular

Cataracts are characterized by fine crystals in the axial region of the lens.

Clinical

None

Laboratory

Diagnosis is made by clinical findings.

Treatment

Cataract surgery if vision decreases.

Bibliography

1. McKusick VA. Mendelian Inheritance in Man: A Catalog of Human Genes and Genetic Disorders, 12th edition. Baltimore: The Johns Hopkins University Press; 1998.

2. McKusick-Nathans Institute for Genetic Medicine, Johns Hopkins University and National Center for Biotechnology Information, National Library of Medicine. (2007). Online Mendelian Inheritance in Man (OMIM). [online] Available from http://www.ncbi.nlm.nih.gov/omim [Accessed April, 2012].

3. Riad M. Congenital familial cataract with cholesterin deposits. Br J Ophthalmol. 1938;22:745-9.

---

247. CATARACT, FLORIFORM

General

Autosomal dominant; rare.

Ocular

Lens opacity takes the form of annular elements, arranged either independently or grouped together like petals of a flower; lenticonus; aniridia.

Clinical

None

Laboratory

Diagnosis is made by clinical findings.

Treatment

Cataract surgery if vision decreases.

Bibliography

1. Doggart JH. Congenital cataract. Trans Ophthalmol Soc UK. 1957;77:31-7.

2. McKusick VA. Mendelian Inheritance in Man: A Catalog of Human Genes and Genetic Disorders, 12th edition. Baltimore: The Johns Hopkins University Press; 1998.

3. McKusick-Nathans Institute for Genetic Medicine, Johns Hopkins University and National Center for Biotechnology Information, National Library of Medicine. (2007). Online Mendelian Inheritance in Man (OMIM). [online] Available from http://www.ncbi.nlm.nih.gov/omim [Accessed April, 2012].

---

248. CATARACT, MEMBRANOUS

General

Autosomal dominant.

Ocular

Total cataract that has undergone regression or resorption.

Clinical

None

Laboratory

Diagnosis is made by clinical findings.

Treatment

Cataract surgery if vision decreases.

Bibliography

1. Gruber M. Ueber Primaere Familaere Linsendys-plasie. Ophthalmologica. 1945;110:60-73.
2. McKusick VA. Mendelian Inheritance in Man: A Catalog of Human Genes and Genetic Disorders, 12th edition. Baltimore: The Johns Hopkins University Press; 1998.
3. McKusick-Nathans Institute for Genetic Medicine, Johns Hopkins University and National Center for Biotechnology Information, National Library of Medicine. (2007). Online Mendelian Inheritance in Man (OMIM). [online] Available from http://www.ncbi.nlm.nih.gov/omim [Accessed April, 2012].

249. CATARACT, MICROCORNEA SYNDROME

General

Autosomal dominant; prominent in Sicilian families.

Ocular

Cataracts; microcornea; myopia.

Clinical

None

Laboratory

Diagnosis is made by clinical findings.

Treatment

Cataract surgery if vision decreases.

Bibliography

1. McKusick VA. Mendelian Inheritance in Man: A Catalog of Human Genes and Genetic Disorders, 12th edition. Baltimore: The Johns Hopkins University Press; 1998.
2. McKusick-Nathans Institute for Genetic Medicine, Johns Hopkins University and National Center for Biotechnology Information, National Library of Medicine. (2007). Online Mendelian Inheritance in Man (OMIM). [online] Available from http://www.ncbi.nlm.nih.gov/omim [Accessed April, 2012].
3. Mellica F, Li Volti S, Tomarchio S, et al. Autosomal dominant cataract and microcornea associated with myopia in a Sicilian family. Clin Genet. 1985;28:42-6.
4. Polomeno RC, Cummings C. Autosomal dominant cataracts and microcornea. Can J Ophthalmol. 1979;14:227-9.
5. Salmon JF, Wallis CE, Murray AD. Variable expressivity of autosomal dominant microcornea with cataract. Arch Ophthalmol. 1988;106:505-10.

250. CATARACT, MICROPHTHALMIA AND NYSTAGMUS

General

Autosomal recessive.

Ocular

Miosis; cataract; nystagmus; microphthalmia.

Clinical

None

Laboratory

Diagnosis is made by clinical findings.

Treatment

Cataract surgery if vision decreases.

Bibliography

1. McKusick VA. Mendelian Inheritance in Man: A Catalog of Human Genes and Genetic Disorders, 12th edition. Baltimore: The Johns Hopkins University Press; 1998.
2. McKusick-Nathans Institute for Genetic Medicine, Johns Hopkins University and National Center for Biotechnology Information, National Library of Medicine. (2007). [online] Available from http://www.ncbi.nlm.nih.gov/omim [Accessed April, 2012].
3. Temtamy SA, Shalash BA. Genetic heterogeneity of the syndrome: microphthalmia with congenital cataract. Birth Defects Orig Artic Ser. 1974;10:292-3.
4. Zeiter HJ. Congenital microphthalmos. A pedigree of four affected siblings and an additional report of fortyfour sporadic cases. Am J Ophthalmol. 1963;55:910-22.

---

251. CATARACT, NUCLEAR (CATARACT; COPPOCK CATARACT; DISCOID)

General

Autosomal dominant; epidemiologic evidence suggests that a single major gene can account for the correlation among siblings of nuclear sclerosis.

Ocular

Congenital zonular cataract; total nuclear cataract; fetal nucleus with scattered fine diffuse cortical opacities and incomplete cortical riders.

Clinical

None

Laboratory

Diagnosis is made by clinical findings.

Treatment

Cataract surgery if vision decreases.

Bibliography

1. Harman NB. Congenital cataract: a pedigree of five generations. Trans Ophthalmol Soc UK. 1909;29:101-8.
2. Heiba JM, Elston RC, Klein BE, et al. Genetic etiology of nuclear cataract: evidence for a major gene. Am J Med Genet. 1993;47:1208-14.
3. Lee JB, Benedict WL. Hereditary nuclear cataract. Arch Ophthalmol. 1950;44:643-50.
4. McKusick VA. Mendelian Inheritance in Man: A Catalog of Human Genes and Genetic Disorders, 12th edition. Baltimore: The Johns Hopkins University Press; 1998.

---

252. CATARACT, NUCLEAR DIFFUSE NONPROGRESSIVE

General

Autosomal dominant; nonprogressive.

Ocular

Opacity of fetal nucleus resembles senile nuclear sclerosis.

Clinical

None

Laboratory

Diagnosis is made by clinical findings.

Treatment

Cataract surgery if vision decreases.

Bibliography

1. McKusick VA. Mendelian Inheritance in Man: A Catalog of Human Genes and Genetic Disorders, 12th edition. Baltimore: The Johns Hopkins University Press; 1998.
2. McKusick-Nathans Institute for Genetic Medicine, Johns Hopkins University and National Center for Biotechnology Information, National Library of Medicine. (2007). Online Mendelian Inheritance in Man (OMIM). [online] Available from http://www.ncbi.nlm.nih.gov/omim [Accessed April, 2012].

---

253. CATARACT, POSTERIOR POLAR

General

Autosomal dominant; onset in childhood; progressive.

Ocular

Congenital posterior polar opacity; scattered cortical opacities; choroideremia; myopia.

Clinical

None

Laboratory

Diagnosis is made by clinical findings.

Treatment

Cataract surgery if vision decreases.

Bibliography

1. McKusick VA. Mendelian Inheritance in Man: A Catalog of Human Genes and Genetic Disorders, 12th edition. Baltimore: The Johns Hopkins University Press; 1998.
2. McKusick-Nathans Institute for Genetic Medicine, Johns Hopkins University and National Center for Biotechnology Information, National Library of Medicine. (2007). Online Mendelian Inheritance in Man (OMIM). [online] Available from http://www.ncbi.nlm.nih.gov/omim [Accessed April, 2012].
3. Binkhorst PG, Valk LE. A case of familial dwarfism, with choroideremia, myopia, posterior polar cataract, and zonular cataract. Ophthalmologica. 1956;132:299.

---

254. CEBOCEPHALIA

General

Term derived from *Cebus* monkey-like head, defective nose and eyes close together.

Ocular

Hypotelorism; mongoloid obliquity.

Clinical

Flat, incomplete nose; full cheeks; medial nostril; no palate or cleft lips.

Laboratory

None

Treatment

None

Bibliography

1. Cohen MM. Holoprosencephaly revisited. Am J Dis Child. 1974;127:597.
2. Magalini SI, Scrascia E. Dictionary of Medical Syndromes, 2nd edition. Philadelphia: JB Lippincott; 1981.

255. CENTRAL NERVOUS SYSTEM DEFICIENCY SYNDROME (GARLAND SYNDROME; SPILLAN-SCOTT SYNDROME)

General

Cause unknown; found in prisoners who had long been on a deficient diet; no improvement after normal diet resumed.

Ocular

Greatly reduced vision, particularly near vision, increasing over weeks or months but rarely progressing to complete blindness; relative or absolute central or paracentral scotomata; bitemporal pallor of the disks; optic neuropathy.

Clinical

Incomplete bilateral deafness, never proceeding to complete deafness; tinnitus; numbness and tingling in the legs, rarely in the hands; unsteadiness of gait; abnormal tendon reflexes (both hyperactive or absent); peripheral neuropathy.

Laboratory

None

Treatment

Multivitamins

Bibliography

1. Garland HG. A central nervous deficiency syndrome. Proc Roy Soc Med. 1946;39:178-80.
2. Geeraets WJ. Ocular Syndromes, 3rd edition. Philadelphia: Lea & Febiger; 1976.
3. Tucker K, Hedges TR. Food shortages and an epidemic of optic and peripheral neuropathy in Cuba. Nutr Rev. 1993;51:349-57.
4. Wilkinson PB, King A. Amblyopia due to vitamin deficiency. Lancet. 1944;1:528-31.

256. CENTRAL OR BRANCH RETINAL ARTERY OCCLUSION

General

Present with profound monocular vision loss. In branch occlusion the visual loss is partial with a scotoma or visual field loss.

Clinical

None

Ocular

Vision loss, macular edema, macular ischemia, vitreous hemorrhage, traction detachment, rubeosis irides.

Laboratory

Complete blood count, ESR, fasting blood sugar, cholesterol, triglyceride and lipid panels, coagulopathy screen and blood cultures, carotid Doppler ultrasound, ERG, ECG and echocardiogram to identify the cause. OCT to identify area of occlusion.

Treatment

Acetazolamide intravenously, distal ocular massage, hyperbaric oxygen, grid laser photocoagulation for macular edema, vitrectomy without shealthotomy.

Bibliography

1. Campochiaro PA, Heier JS, Feiner L, et al. Ranibizumab for macular edema following branch retinal vein occlusion. Ophthalmology. 2010;117:1102-12.
2. Rogers SL, McIntosh RL, Lim L, et al. Natural history of branch retinal vein occlusion: an evidence based systematic review. Ophthalmology. 2010;117:1094-101.

Additional Resource

1. Graham RH (2012). Central Retinal Artery Occlusion. [online] Available from http://www.emedicine.com/oph/TOPIC387.HTM [Accessed April, 2012].

257. CENTRAL SEROUS CHORIORETINOPATHY

General

Disorder of the central macula.

Clinical

None

Ocular

Decreased visual acuity, metamorphopsia, miscropsia, central color vision deficiency, central scotoma.

Laboratory

Fluorscein angiopathy for "expansile dot" pattern, a "smokestack" pattern or diffuse hyperfluorescence.

Treatment

Observation in most cases. Thermal or photodynamic therapy is necessary in some cases.

Additional Resource

1. Oh KT (2011). Central Serous Chorioretinopathy. [online] Available from http://www.emedicine.com/oph/TOPIC689.HTM [Accessed April, 2012].

258. CENTRAL STERILE CORNEAL ULCERATION

General

Either infectious or sterile, this inflammatory condition is associated with the disruption of the epithelial layer involving the stroma.

Clinical

Herpes simplex virus, herpes zoster virus, Sjögren syndrome, facial palsy, vitamin A deficiency, Wegener granulomatosis, rheumatoid arthritis.

Ocular

Corneal scarring, neovascularization, blindness and corneal perforation. Herpes, contact lens use, lagophthalmos, sicca.

Treatment

It is important to first exclude infectious etiologies. Antibiotics, PF artificial tears, for chemical burs prednisone is useful, oral tetracycline can be use in combination of topical tetracycline.

Laboratory

Corneal smears and cultures, corneal scraping, complete workup to rule out infectious or systemic inflammatory disease.

Additional Resource

1. Farooqui SZ (2011). Central Sterile Corneal Ulceration. [online] Available from http://www.emedicine.medscape.com/article/1196936-overview [Accessed April, 2012].

259. CEREBELLAR ATAXIA, CATARACT, DEAFNESS, AND DEMENTIA OR PSYCHOSIS (HEREDOPATHIA OPHTHALMO-OTO-ENCEPHALICA)

General

Autosomal dominant.

Ocular

Posterior polar cataracts.

Clinical

Tremor; paranoid psychosis; dementia; deafness.

Laboratory

None

Treatment

Cataract surgery if vision decreases.

Bibliography

1. McKusick VA. Mendelian Inheritance in Man: A Catalog of Human Genes and Genetic Disorders, 12th edition. Baltimore: The Johns Hopkins University Press; 1998.
2. McKusick-Nathans Institute for Genetic Medicine, Johns Hopkins University and National Center for Biotechnology Information, National Library of Medicine. (2007). Online Mendelian Inheritance in Man (OMIM). [online] Available from http://www.ncbi.nlm.nih.gov/omim [Accessed April, 2012].
3. Stromgren E. Heredopathia ophthalmo-oto-encephalica. Neurogenetic directory, part 1. Handbook Clin Neurol. 1981;42:150-2.

260. CEREBELLAR ATAXIA, INFANTILE, WITH PROGRESSIVE EXTERNAL OPHTHALMOPLEGIA

General

Autosomal recessive; neurologic lesion.

Ocular

Paralysis of all extraocular muscles; ptosis; retinal degeneration; blindness.

Clinical

Spinocerebellar degeneration; ataxia.

Laboratory

None

Treatment

None

Bibliography

1. Jampel RS, Okazaki H, Bernstein H. Ophthalmoplegia and retinal degeneration associated with spinocerebellar ataxia. Arch Ophthalmol. 1961;66:247-59.
2. McKusick VA. Mendelian Inheritance in Man: A Catalog of Human Genes and Genetic Disorders, 12th edition. Baltimore: The Johns Hopkins University Press; 1998.
3. McKusick-Nathans Institute for Genetic Medicine, Johns Hopkins University and National Center for Biotechnology Information, National Library of Medicine. (2007). [online] Available from http://www.ncbi.nlm.nih.gov/omim [Accessed April, 2012].

261. CEREBELLAR DEGENERATION WITH SLOW MOVEMENTS

General

Autosomal dominant; described only in Indian families; associated with spinocerebellar degeneration and abnormal eye movements.

Ocular

Paramedian pontine reticular formation (horizontal gaze center); absent rapid movements of both eyes and abnormally slow movements.

Clinical

Brainstem lesion of paramedian pontine reticular formation; progressive mental deterioration.

Laboratory

Computed tomography (CT) and MRI.

Treatment

None

Additional Resource

1. Rauschkolb PK (2012). Striatonigral Degeneration. [online] Available from http://www.emedicine.com/neuro/TOPIC354.HTM [Accessed April, 2012].

262. CEREBRAL AUTOSOMAL DOMINANT ARTERIOPATHY

General

Automal dominant, generalized nonatherosclerotic nonamyloid arteriopathy.

Ocular

Scotoma with migraine, cataract, iris atrophy, retinal microinfarction.

Clinical

Recurrent stroke, cognitive decline, subcortical vascular dementia.

Laboratory

Diagnosis is made by clinical observation.

Treatment

Change in glasses can sometimes improve a patient's visual function temporarily; however, the most common treatment is cataract surgery.

Additional Resource

1. Alagiakrishnan K (2012). Vascular Dementia. [online] Available from http://www.emedicine.com/med/TOPIC3150.HTM [Accessed April, 2012].

263. CEREBRAL CHOLESTERINOSIS
(CEREBROTENDINOUS XANTHOMATOSIS; CTX)

General

Autosomal recessive; lipid storage disorder characterized by progressive neurologic dysfunction; large amounts of cholestanol and cholesterol in every tissue in body, particularly in brain and lungs.

Ocular

Cataracts; juvenile cataracts.

Clinical

Cerebellar ataxia; systemic spinal cord involvement; atherosclerosis; mental retardation; unsteady gait; liver damage; jaundice; chronic diarrhea.

Laboratory

Lipid levels.

Treatment

Change in glasses can sometimes improve a patient's visual function temporarily; however, the most common treatment is cataract surgery.

Bibliography

1. Berginer VM, Salen G, Shefer S. Long-term treatment of cerebrotendinous xanthomatosis with chenodeoxycholic acid. N Engl J Med. 1984; 311:1649-52.

2. Cruysberg JR, Wevers RA, Tolboom JJ. Juvenile cataract associated with chronic diarrhea in pediatric cerebrotendinous xanthomatosis. Am J Ophthalmol. 1991;112:606-7.

3. Katz DA, Scheinberg L, Horoupian DS, et al. Peripheral neuropathy in cerebrotendinous xanthomatosis. Arch Neurol. 1985;42:1008-10.

---

264. CEREBRAL PALSY

General

Group of diverse nonprogressive syndromes resulting from injury to the motor centers of the brain; lesions may occur prenatally, in infancy, or in childhood up to age 5 years or more; constitutes the most common cause of permanent physical handicap in children.

Ocular

Strabismus; ptosis; congenital cataract; optic nerve atrophy; papilledema; iris coloboma; nystagmus; uveitis; paresis of extraocular muscles; blepharospasm; leukoma.

Clinical

Systemic abnormalities, such as mental retardation, seizures, microcephalus, hydrocephalus, speech delays, and behavioral or emotional disturbances; motor defect; central visual impairment due to cerebral cortex and white matter malformation.

Laboratory

Diagnosis is made by clinical findings.

Treatment

Multiple medical complications require orthopedic, neurologists and rehabilitation medicine specialists.

Additional Resource

1. Abdel-Hamid HZ (2011). Cerebral Palsy. [online] Available from http://www.emedicine.com/neuro/TOPIC533.HTM [Accessed April, 2012].

---

265. CEREBRO-OCULO-FACIO-SKELETAL SYNDROME (COFS SYNDROME)

General

Inherited as autosomal recessive disorder; death within the first 3 years of life; feeding difficulties secondary to incoordination of the swallowing mechanism.

Ocular

Microphthalmia; blepharophimosis; cataracts.

Clinical

Microcephaly; hypotonia; prominent nasal root; large ear pinnae; flexion contractures at elbows and knees; camptodactylia; osteoporosis; kyphosis; scoliosis; congenital muscular dystrophy.

Laboratory

Diagnosis is made by clinical findings.

Treatment

Change in glasses can sometimes improve a patient's visual function temporarily; however, the most common treatment is cataract surgery.

Bibliography

1. Geeraets WJ. Ocular Syndromes, 3rd edition. Philadelphia: Lea & Febiger; 1976.
2. Gershoni-Baruch R, Ludatscher RM, Lichtig C, et al. Cerebro-oculo-facio-skeletal syndrome: further delineation. Am J Med Genet. 1991;41:74-7.
3. Lowry RB, MacLean R, McLean DM, et al. Cataracts, microcephaly, kyphosis, and limited joint movement in two siblings: a new syndrome. J Pediatr. 1971;79:282-4.
4. McKusick VA. Mendelian Inheritance in Man: A Catalog of Human Genes and Genetic Disorders 12th edition. Baltimore: The Johns Hopkins University Press; 1998.
5. McKusick-Nathans Institute for Genetic Medicine, Johns Hopkins University and National Center for Biotechnology Information, National Library of Medicine. (2007). Online Mendelian Inheritance in Man (OMIM). [online] Available from http://www.ncbi.nlm.nih.gov/omim [Accessed April, 2012].
6. Pena SD, Shokeir MH. Autosomal recessive cerebro-oculo-facio-skeletal (COFS) syndrome. Clin Genet. 1974;5:285-93.

266. CEREBROFACIAL-RENO-ARTHRO-SYNDACTYLIA SYNDROME

General

Cause familial?

Ocular

Trichiasis; slanted and asymmetrical size of lid fissure; blepharitis; contraction of visual fields; peripheral pigmentary anomalies of the retina.

Clinical

Mild oligophrenia; small head for body size; slight facial asymmetry; webbed digits; atrophic unilateral sternocleidomastoid muscle; spontaneous shoulder dislocation; small kidneys with renal dysplasia; chronic interstitial nephritis.

Laboratory

Diagnosis is made by clinical findings.

Treatment

Trichiasis: Epilation, argon laser ablation, cryosurgery, radio surgery and full-thickness wedge resection or eyelid margin rotation procedures are all possible therapies.

Blepharitis: Oral tetracyclines, omega-3 fatty acids, flax seed oil or fish oil. Ocular therapy includes eyelid scrubs, warm compresses, bacitracin ointment to lid margins, topical cyclosporine A and preservative-free lubricants.

Bibliography

1. Geeraets WJ. Ocular Syndromes, 3rd edition. Philadelphia: Lea & Febiger; 1976.
2. Greig DM. Hypertelorism: a hitherto undifferentiated congenital craniofacial deformity. Edinburgh Med J. 1924;31:560.
3. Hanley FJ, Floyd CE, Parker D. Congenital partial hemihypertrophy of the face. J Oral Surg. 1968;26:136-41.

267. CEREBRORETINAL VASCULOPATHY

General

Autosomal dominant; frontoparietal lobe pseudotumor and retinal capillary abnormalities; neuropathologic findings are largely confined to the white matter.

Ocular

Capillary obliteration; retinal telangiectasia; glaucoma; cystoid degeneration; branch retinal vein occlusion; infectious retinitis; reduction in central visual acuity; progressive retinal ischemia.

Clinical

Jacksonian and grand mal seizures; headache; loss of memory; slow speech; cytomegalic virus septicemia; perivascular inflammation; hepatic fibrosis; intracranial mass lesion; systemic collagen vascular disease; systemic lupus erythematosus; central nervous system disease.

Laboratory

Computed tomography (CT) and MRI to identify size and location of pseudotumor.

Treatment

Glaucoma: Its medication should be the first plan of action. If medication is unsuccessful, a filtering surgical procedure with or without antimetabolites may be beneficial.

Retinal vein occlusion: Intraocular pressure lowering medications, carbogen therapy, hyperbaric oxygen. Vitrectomy may be necessary.

Bibliography

1. Grand MG, Kaine J, Fulling K, et al. Cerebroretinal vasculopathy. A new hereditary syndrome. Ophthalmology. 1988;95:649-59.
2. Jabs DA, Fine SL, Hochberg MC, et al. Severe retinal vaso-occlusive disease in systemic lupus erythematosus. Arch Ophthalmol. 1986;104: 558-63.
3. Rizzo J. The retina. In: Lessel S, van Dalen JTW (Eds). Current Neuro-Ophthalmology, 3rd edition. St. Louis.

268. CEROID LIPOFUSCINOSES

General

Ceroid lipofuscinoses are disorders characterized by the accumulation of fluorescent lipopigments in a number of body tissues; included in this group are several diseases that were once considered variants of Tay-Sachs disease but are now classified separately; ceroid lipofuscinoses may be divided into infantile, late infantile (Bielschowsky-Jansky), juvenile (Spielmeyer-Vogt), adult (Kufs) and atypical forms (see Dollinger-Bielschowsky Syndrome; Kufs Disease; Infantile Neuronal Ceroid Lipofuscinosis; Batten-Mayou syndrome).

Ocular

Tapetoretinal degeneration; pigmentary macular changes.

Clinical

Seizures; ataxia; dementia; cerebellar and extrapyramidal signs; "release" hallucinations.

Laboratory

Enzyme levels, MRI, positron emission tomography.

Treatment

No specific treatment is available for these diseases.

Additional Resource

1. Chang CH (2009). Neuronal Ceroid Lipofuscinoses. [online] Available from http://www.emedicine.com/neuro/TOPIC498.HTM [Accessed April, 2012].

269. CESTAN-CHENAIS SYNDROME [CESTAN (1) SYNDROME]

General

Combination of Babinski-Nageotte and Avellis syndromes; lesion in the lateral portion of medulla oblongata.

Ocular

Enophthalmos; ptosis; nystagmus; miosis.

Clinical

Pharyngolaryngeal or glossopharyngeal paralysis; cerebellar hemiataxia; disturbance of sensibility; contralateral side of lesion.

Laboratory

Computed tomography (CT), MRI, transcranial Doppler, ECG.

Treatment

Rehabilitation services have been shown to play a critical role in recovery. Physical, occupational and speech therapy consultations are necessary.

Additional Resource

1. Kaye V (2011). Vertebrobasilar Stroke Overview of Vertebrobasilar Stroke. [online] Available from http://www.emedicine.medscape.com/article/323409-overview [Accessed April, 2012].

270. CHALAZION

General

Common inflammatory lesion of the eyelid; obstruction of the meibomian gland with the accumulation of sebaceous material; most frequently seen in individuals between 30 and 50 years of age.

Clinical

Acne, seborrhea, rosacea.

Ocular

Eyelid swelling; eyelid nodule; injection of the conjunctiva; altered visual acuity; lid tenderness.

Laboratory

Diagnosis is made by clinical findings. Recurrent symptoms may require fine needle aspiration to exclude malignancy and viral or bacterial cultures.

Treatment

Warm compresses; topical or systemic antibiotics; steroid injections; surgical drainage.

Additional Resource

1. Fansler JL (2010). Chalazion in Emergency Medicine. [online] Available from http://www.emedicine.medscape.com/article/797763-overview [Accessed April, 2012].

271. CHARCOT-MARIE-TOOTH DISEASE (PROGRESSIVE PERONEAL MUSCULAR ATROPHY; PROGRESSIVE NEURITIC MUSCULAR ATROPHY)

General

Dominant inheritance; onset between 5 and 15 years of age; rare disease; demonstrates autosomal dominant as well as recessive and X-linked recessive inheritance.

Ocular

Nystagmus; vision reduced if associated with optic nerve involvement; primary optic atrophy (rare).

Clinical

Positive familial history; atrophy of small muscles of hands and feet, slowly progressing to distal and then proximal arm and leg; fibrillary muscle twitchings (fasciculations) are common; cramps are common.

Laboratory

Nerve biopsies show evidence of a hypertrophic demyelinating neuropathy, with chronic remyelination and loss of myelinated fibers.

Treatment

Physical therapy is often required to prevent and treat joint deformities. Nonsteroidal anti-inflammatory drugs (NSAIDs) may also be useful.

Additional Resource

1. Parsons TC (2011). Charcot-Marie-Tooth and Other Hereditary Motor and Sensory Neuropathies. [online] Available from http://www.emedicine com/neuro/TOPIC468.HTM [Accessed April, 2012].

272. CHARCOT-WILBRAND SYNDROME

General

Lesion of artery of angular gyrus of dominant side; lesion can be bilateral; alexia.

Ocular

Visual agnosia; loss of ability to revisualize images; prosopagnosia.

Clinical

Occlusion of a portion of the posterior cerebral artery.

Laboratory

Diagnosis is made by clinical findings.

Treatment

None

Bibliography

1. Charcot JM. Sur un Cas de Cecile Verbale. Oeuvres Completes de Charcot. Paris: Delahaye Lecrosnier; 1887.
2. Feinberg TE, Schindler RJ, Ochoa E, et al. Associative visual agnosia and alexia without prosopagnosia. Cortex. 1994;30:395-411.
3. Magalini SI, Scrascia E. Dictionary of Medical Syndromes, 2nd edition. Philadelphia: JB Lippincott; 1981.
4. Rentschler I, Treutwein B, Landis T. Dissociation of local and global processing in visual agnosia. Vision Res. 1994;34:963-71.
5. Shelton PA, Bowers D, Duara R, et al. Apperceptive visual agnosia: a case study. Brain Cogn. 1994;25:1-23.

273. CHARGE ASSOCIATION (ATRESIA; COLOBOMA; EAR MALFORMATION ASSOCIATION; GENITAL HYPOPLASIA; HEART DISEASE; MULTIPLE CONGENITAL ANOMALIES SYNDROME; RETARDED GROWTH)

General

Syndrome consisting of four of six major manifestations of ocular coloboma, heart disease, atresia, retarded growth and development, genital hypoplasia and ear malformations with or without hearing loss.

Ocular

Blepharoptosis; iris coloboma; optic nerve coloboma; macular hypoplasia; lacrimal canalicular atresia; nasolacrimal duct obstruction.

Clinical

Microcephaly; brachycephaly; malformed ear; bilateral finger contractures; heart disease; genital hypoplasia; heart disease; choanal atresia; retarded growth; hearing loss; facial nerve palsies; mental retardation.

Laboratory

CHD7 mutation analysis is diagnostic in 58–71% of individuals who meet the clinical criteria, head CT and MRI, cranial ultrasound.

Treatment

Secure airway, stabilize the patient, exclude major life-threatening congenital anomalies, and transfer the individual with CHARGE syndrome to a specialist center with pediatric otolaryngologist and other subspecialty services.

Additional Resource

1. Tegay DH (2012). CHARGE Syndrome. [online] Available from http://www.emedicine.com/ped/TOPIC367.HTM [Accessed April, 2012].

274. CHARLIN SYNDROME (NASAL NERVE SYNDROME; NASOCILIARIS NERVE SYNDROME; NASOCILIARY SYNDROME)

General

Neuritis of the nasal branch of the trigeminal nerve; three typical spots of pain according to the nerve distribution: (1) above and outside the nose; (2) above the inner canthus and (3) inferior angle of the medial tarsal ligament (see Sluder Syndrome).

Ocular

Severe ocular and orbital pain, mainly upper nasal-orbital angle; slight inflammatory swelling of upper lid (occasional); photophobia; ciliary and conjunctival injection; pseudopurulent conjunctivitis; anterior uveitis; iritis; hypopyon; keratitis; corneal ulcers.

Clinical

Rhinorrhea; rhinitis always on same side of the ocular involvement; severe pain of ala nasi.

Laboratory

Diagnosis is made by clinical findings.

Treatment

Uveitis: Topical steroids and cycloplegic medication should be the initial treatment of choice. Oral steroids if not responsive to topical steroids, immunosuppressants if bilateral disease that does not respond to oral steroids, periocular steroids for unilateral or posterior uveitis. Vitrectomy can be used for severe vitreous opacification. Cryotherapy and laser photocoagulation may be used for localized pars plana exudates.

Corneal ulcer: Corneal cultures may be taken and treatment initiated. Treatment includes a broad spectrum of antibiotics and cycloplegic drops.

Bibliography

1. Charlin C. Le Syndrome du Nerf Nasal. Ann Ocul. 1931;168:86.
2. Ferrannini G. Charlin's syndrome. Ann Ophthalmol Clin Ocul. 1969;95:807-11.
3. Pau H. Differential Diagnosis of Eye Diseases. New York: Thieme; 1987.

275. CHEDIAK-HIGASHI SYNDROME (ANOMALOUS LEUKOCYTIC INCLUSIONS WITH CONSTITUTIONAL STIGMATA)

General

Occurs in albinoid siblings born of consanguineous parents; tyrosinase-positive type of oculocutaneous albinism associated with a fetal reticuloendothelial incompetence.

Ocular

Decreased iris pigmentation; photophobia; narrowness and decreased number of vessels in retina; decreased pigmentation of choroid elevated disk; papilledema; infiltration of immature leukocytes in the uvea, retina and optic nerve; nystagmus; ocular motor palsies; optic disk edema; oculocutaneous albinism.

Clinical

Anemia; neutropenia; thrombocytopenia; recurrent infections; hepatosplenomegaly; lymphadenopathy; oculocutaneous albinism; hyperpigmentation of sun-exposed areas.

Laboratory

Diagnosis is made by recognition of the characteristic giant granules in neutrophils, eosinophils and granulocytes by using light microscopy in a routine blood smear.

Treatment

Bone marrow transplantation from a sibling is the therapy of choice and should be performed early.

Additional Resource

1. Nowicki RJ (2011). Chediak-Higashi Syndrome. [online] Available from http://www.emedicine.com/derm/TOPIC704.HTM [Accessed April, 2012].

276. CHERRY-RED SPOT MYOCLONUS SYNDROME (TYPE I SIALIDOSIS)

General

Morphologic changes in storage process in lysosomes of retinal ganglion cells, neurons of mesenteric plexus, hepatocytes, and Kupffer cells.

Ocular

Cherry-red spot of macula; horizontal nystagmus; white dot and flake lens changes; decreased visual acuity and gray perimacular halo.

Clinical

Development of a slowly progressive neurologic illness whose most crippling symptoms are myoclonus, seizures, decreased muscle tone, speech disorder and hyperactive reflexes.

Laboratory

Diagnosis is made by demonstrating a deficiency of alpha-N-acetyl neuraminidase activity, which can be measured in amniocytes, leukocytes and cultured fibroblasts.

Treatment

Options remain limited and are directed at supportive care and symptomatic relief.

Additional Resource

1. Roth KS (2010). Sialidosis (Mucolipidosis I). [online] Available from http://www.emedicine.com/ped/TOPIC2093.HTM [Accessed April, 2012].

277. CHICKENPOX (VARICELLA)

General

Acute exanthematous disease; highly contagious; children between the ages of 2 and 8 years.

Ocular

Conjunctival ulcer; corneal ulcer; descemetocele; corneal opacity; keratitis; paresis of third, fourth and sixth nerves; optic neuritis; papilledema; retinitis; hemorrhagic retinopathy; uveitis; cataract; paralytic mydriasis; phthisis bulbi; unifocal choroiditis; dendritic keratitis; acute retinal necrosis [in a patient with acquired immunodeficiency syndrome (AIDS)]; disciform keratitis.

Clinical

Fever; malaise; rash; pruritus.

Laboratory

Diagnosis is made by clinical findings.

Treatment

Isolation oral antihistamines, such as diphenhydramine and hydroxyzine, are used for severe pruritus and acetaminophen is recommended for use for the reduction of fever.

Additional Resource

1. Bechtel KA (2011). Pediatric Chickenpox. [online] Available from http://www.emedicine.com/emerg/TOPIC367.HTM [Accessed April, 2012].

278. CHIKUNGUNYA FEVER

General

Debilitating viral infection spread by the bite of the infected *Aedes* mosquito and is now thought to have mutated enabling it to be transmitted by *A. albopictus*. The disease was first isolated in Tanzania but not outbreaks have occurred in Africa, Asia, India, Vietnam, Myanmar and Indonesia.

Clinical

Arthritis resulting in a stooped posture, fever, headache, fatigue, nausea, vomiting, renal failure, muscle pain, rash and joint pain.

Ocular

Iridocyclitis, viral retinitis, vitreitis, retinal hemorrhage, conjunctivitis and episcleritis.

Laboratory

Specific diagnosis is based on viral isolation or the demonstration of seroconversion, i.e. the presence of specific immunoglobulin M (IgM) antibody or a fourfold increase in the antibody titer.

Treatment

Antiviral therapy may be useful. Acyclovir intravenously or orally is the drug of choice.

Additional Resource

1. Saemi AM (2010). Dermatologic Manifestations of Viral Hemorrhagic Fevers. [online] Available from http://www.emedicine.com/derm/TOPIC880. HTM [Accessed April, 2012].

279. CHLAMYDIA (INCLUSION CONJUNCTIVITIS; PARATRACHOMA)

General

Organism that infects the epithelium of mucoid surfaces; sexually transmitted; major cause of nongonococcal urethritis in men and cervicitis in women; major cause of neonatal ophthalmia; *Chlamydia trachomatis* is an intracellular bacterium lacking respiratory enzymes that has an affinity for mucosal epithelium; serotypes A through C have been epidemiologically associated with trachoma; serotypes E through K have been associated with genital infection and keratoconjunctivitis in sexually active adults and neonates; other serotypes have been associated with lymphogranuloma venereum and Reiter syndrome.

Ocular

Follicular conjunctivitis; corneal opacities; keratitis; corneal ulcer; lid edema; uveitis.

Clinical

Pneumonia; gastrointestinal disturbances; genital discharge.

Laboratory

Giemsa stain, cell culture-time intensive, direct fluorescent monoclonal antibiotics to stain smears.

Treatment

Three to six weeks of oral tetracycline (500 mg qid), oral doxycycline (100 mg bid) or oral erythromycin stearate (500 mg qid). Simultaneous treatment of all sexual partners is important to prevent reinfection.

Additional Resource

1. Bashour M (2010). Chlamydia. [online] Available from http://www.emedicine.com/oph/TOPIC494. HTM [Accessed April, 2012].

280. CHLOROQUINE/HYDROXYCHLOROQUINE TOXICITY (BULL'S EYE MACULOPATHY)

General

Toxicity is caused by use of chloroquine or hydroxychloroquine incidence increased with both the dose and the duration of treatment.

Clinical

Malaria; lupus; rheumatoid arthritis; nausea; rash; sensitivity to ultraviolet light; vertigo; muscle weakness; cranial nerve palsies.

Ocular

Corneal deposits; white flake-like lens opacity; scotoma; stippling of macular pigmentation; concentric zone of hypopigmentation of the retina; generalized hypopigmentation; bone spicule formation; vascular attenuation; optic disk pallor.

Laboratory

Fluorescein angiography; Amsler grid; perimetry; retinal exam and photography; color vision; photostress testing; and electrophysiologic studies are useful. A yearly visual field examination is useful to detect charges from hydroxychloroquine. A small case series study revealed evidence of retinal toxicity that included difficulty with reading, variation in fundus findings from normal to bull's eye maculopathy, ERG findings of reduced rod and cone function and abnormal visual fields. Cessation of the study drug did not result in sustained improved visual function. Chloroquine and hydroxychloroquine are associated with substantial retinal toxicities that require diligent monitoring and management.

Treatment

Withdrawal of the medication; ammonium chloride systemically made necessary if severe toxic symptoms occur.

Bibliography

1. Michaelides M, Stover NB, Francis PJ, et al. Retinal toxicity associated with hydroxychloroquine and chloroquine. Arch Ophthalmol. 2011;129;30-9.

Additional Resource

1. Roque MR (2011). Chloroquine/Hydroxychloroquine Toxicity. [online] Available from http://www.emedicine.medscape.com/article/1229016-overview [Accessed April, 2012].

---

281. CHOLERA

General

Acute illness that results from colonization of small bowel by *Vibrio cholerae*; rare cases of *V. cholerae* meningitis have been reported, some associated with bacteremia.

Ocular

Hyperemia of lids and conjunctivae; subconjunctival hemorrhages; madarosis of lids; xerosis of conjunctiva; lagophthalmos; keratomalacia; retinal ischemia; cataract.

Clinical

Diarrhea; shock; vomiting; muscle cramps; cyanosis; scaphoid abdomen; thready pulse; tachycardia; hypotension; tachypnea; acute tubular necrosis; metabolic acidosis; death.

Laboratory

Diagnosis may be confirmed by identification of *V. cholerae* in the stool.

Treatment

The primary goal of therapy is to replenish fluid losses caused by diarrhea and vomiting.

Additional Resource

1. Thaker VV (2011). Cholera. [online] Available from http://www.emedicine.com/med/TOPIC351.HTM [Accessed April, 2012].

282. CHOLESTASIS WITH GALLSTONE, ATAXIA, AND VISUAL DISTURBANCES

General

Autosomal recessive; not clear if distinct from Byler disease or another form of intrahepatic cholestasis; retinal neurologic features may be secondary to nutritional abnormalities.

Ocular

Retinal lesions; optic atrophy; ptosis.

Clinical

Congenital cholestasis; gallstone; cerebellar ataxia; jaundice; hepatitis; pruritus.

Laboratory

Serum bilirubin levels are elevated, ultrasonography of liver and bile ducts, abdominal CT.

Treatment

Cholestasis often does not respond to medical therapy. Treatment of fat malabsorption principally involves dietary substitution.

Additional Resource

1. Nazer H (2010). Cholestasis. [online] Available from http://www.emedicine.com/ped/TOPIC383. HTM [Accessed April, 2012].

283. CHOREA (ACUTE CHOREA; HUNTINGTON HEREDITARY CHOREA ST. VITUS DANCE; SYDENHAM CHOREA)

General

Mendelian dominant trait.

Ocular

Lid retraction; spasmodic closures; apraxia of lid opening; disoriented ocular movements; anisocoria; mydriasis; hippus.

Clinical

Involuntary purposeless movements; emotional ability; muscle weakness.

Laboratory

Diagnosis of the primary choreatic conditions is based on history and clinical findings.

Treatment

The most widely used agents in the treatment of chorea are the neuroleptics. The basis of their mechanism of action is thought to be related to blocking of dopamine receptors.

Additional Resource

1. Vertrees SM (2012). Chorea in Adults. [online] Available from http://www.emedicine.com/ neuro/TOPIC62.HTM [Accessed April, 2012].

284. CHOROIDAL DETACHMENT (CILIOCHOROIDAL DETACHMENT)

General

Separation of the choroid and sclera is created by a fluid accumulation between the two layers.

Clinical

Sturge Weber syndrome, Vogt-Koyanagi-Harada syndrome.

Ocular

Scleritis, choriditis, orbital pseudotumor.

Laboratory

Diagnosis is made by clinical findings.

Treatment

Topical use of cycloplegic/mydriatic drops in addition to topical steroids when necessary.

Additional Resource

1. Traverso CE (2010). Choroidal Detachment. [online] Available from http://www.emedicine.com/oph/TOPIC63.HTM [Accessed April, 2012].

---

285. CHOROIDAL RUPTURES

General

Tearing of Bruch's membrane and the closely associated choriocapillaris and retinal pigment epithelium after contusive ocular injury.

Clinical

None

Ocular

Subfoveal hemorrhage, pigmentary changes in the macula, angle recession.

Laboratory

Diagnosis is made by clinical findings.

Treatment

There is no treatment for choroidal rupture; however, careful examinations are important to exclude other ocular complications.

Additional Resource

1. Wu L (2012). Choroidal Rupture. [online] Available from http://www.emedicine.com/oph/TOPIC533.HTM [Accessed April, 2012].

---

286. CHOROIDEREMIA (CHOROIDAL SCLEROSIS; PROGRESSIVE; TAPETOCHOROIDAL DYSTROPHY)

General

Sex-linked; onset at early age; progressive; primary degeneration may be of the retina, retinal pigment epithelium or choriocapillaris; pigment stippling or granularity also evident in female carriers who possess normal and abnormal cells, through Barr body inactivation of one X chromosome.

Ocular

Reduction of central vision; constriction of visual fields; night blindness; choroidal and retinal atrophy.

Clinical

None

Laboratory

Diagnosis is made by clinical findings.

Treatment

Therapies are limited. Physicians should emphasize the therapies that are available to help patients. Perhaps, most importantly, it is essential to help patients maximize the vision they do have with refraction and low-vision evaluation. Vitamin A/beta-carotene may or may not be useful.

Additional Resource

1. Telander DG (2012). Retinitis Pigmentosa. [online] Available from http://www.emedicine.com/oph/TOPIC704.HTM [Accessed April, 2012].

287. CHOROIDORETINAL DEGENERATION WITH RETINAL REFLEX IN HETEROZYGOUS WOMEN

General

Sex-linked; choroidoretinal degeneration differentiated by presence in heterozygous women of a tapetal-like retinal reflex; there is probably more than one X-linked locus leading to a retinitis pigmentosa type of picture.

Ocular

Retinitis pigmentosa; golden-hued, patchy appearance around macula.

Clinical

None

Laboratory

Diagnosis is made by clinical findings.

Treatment

Retinitis pigmentosa: Vitamin A 15,000 IU/day is thought to slow the decline of retinal function, dark sunglasses for outdoor use, surgery for cataract, genetic counseling.

Bibliography

1. McKusick VA. Mendelian Inheritance in Man: A Catalog of Human Genes and Genetic Disorders, 12th edition. Baltimore: The Johns Hopkins University Press; 1998.
2. McKusick-Nathans Institute for Genetic Medicine, Johns Hopkins University and National Center for Biotechnology Information, National Library of Medicine. (2007). Online Mendelian Inheritance in Man (OMIM). [online] Available from http://www.ncbi.nlm.nih.gov/omim [Accessed April, 2012].
3. Musarella MA, Anson-Cartwright L, Leal SM, et al. Multipoint linkage analysis and heterogeneity testing in 20 X-linked retinitis pigmentosa families. Genomics. 1990;8:286-96.
4. Nussbaum RL, Lewis RA, Lesko JG, et al. Mapping X-linked ophthalmic diseases: II. Linkage relationship of X-linked retinitis pigmentosa to X chromosomal short arm markers. Hum Genet. 1985;70:45-50.

288. CHOROIDORETINAL DYSTROPHY

General

Sex-linked; similar to retinitis pigmentosa with absence of annular scotoma and little vascular change.

Ocular

Early poor central vision; retinitis pigmentosa; night blindness.

Clinical

None

Laboratory

Diagnosis is made by clinical findings.

Treatment

Retinitis pigmentosa: Vitamin A 15,000 IU/day is thought to slow the decline of retinal function,

dark sunglasses for outdoor use, surgery for cataract, genetic counseling.

Bibliography

1. Hoare GW. Choroidoretinal dystrophy. Br J Ophthalmol. 1965;49:449-51.
2. McKusick VA. Mendelian Inheritance in Man: A Catalog of Human Genes and Genetic Disorders, 12th edition. Baltimore: The Johns Hopkins University Press; 1998.

289. CHROMOSOME 11 LONG-ARM DELETION SYNDROME

General

Patients with deletion of the long arm of chromosome 11 exhibit a distinctive countenance; female preponderance.

Ocular

Colobomas of the choroid, retina and iris; retinal reduplication; retinal dysplasia; epicanthus; blepharoptosis; abnormal slanting of the interpalpebral fissures; bilateral uveal colobomas; hypertelorism; avascular retina (bilateral); abnormal pattern of retinal vessels.

Clinical

Keeled forehead; small carp-shaped mouth; low-set ears; highly arched palate; long upper lip with absent philtrum; short neck; widely spaced nipples; flexion contractures of the knees and elbows;

hypoplastic nails; broad thumbs with low insertion; deeply pigmented skin on buttocks, lower back, and abdomen and in inguinal regions, axillas, and clavicular areas; congenital heart disease.

Laboratory

Diagnosis is made by clinical findings.

Treatment

Ocular/None.

Bibliography

1. Ferry AP, Marchevsky A, Strauss L. Ocular abnormalities in deletion of the long arm of chromosome 11. Ann Ophthalmol. 1981;13:1373-7.
2. Uto H, Shigeto M, Tanaka H, et al. A case of 11q-syndrome associated with abnormalities of the retinal vessels. Ophthalmologica. 1994;208:233-6.

290. CHROMOSOME 13q PARTIAL DELETION (LONG-ARM SYNDROME; 13q SYNDROME)

General

No hereditary factor.

Ocular

Microphthalmos; antimongoloid slant of lid fissures; bilateral epicanthus; esotropia; cataract; choroidal coloboma; ptosis; retinoblastoma.

Clinical

Genital malformations; meningocele; short neck; small mouth; mental and physical retardation; small head; short stature; broad nasal bridge; simian crease; microcephaly; high nasal bridge; thumb hypoplasia.

Laboratory

The red blood cells are usually normochromic normocytic. An elevated white blood cell count (> 12,000/μL) occurs in approximately 60% of patients.

Treatment

Phlebotomy is the mainstay of therapy for this disease. The object is to remove excess cellular elements, mainly red blood cells, to improve the circulation of blood by lowering the blood viscosity.

Additional Resource

1. Besa EC (2012). Polycythemia Vera. [online] Available from http://www.emedicine.medscape.com/article/205114-overview [Accessed April, 2012].

---

291. CHROMOSOME 18 PARTIAL DELETION (LONG-ARM) SYNDROME [MONOSOMY 18 PARTIAL (LONG-ARM) SYNDROME; DE GROUCHY SYNDROME]

General

Deletion of approximately one half of the long arm of chromosome 18.

Ocular

Hypertelorism; epicanthal folds; narrow palpebral fissure; nystagmus (horizontal); strabismus; myopia; astigmatism; glaucoma; oval pupils; microcornea; posterior staphyloma; oblique disk; optic nerve staphyloma; optic nerve atrophy; microphthalmia; corneal opacities; iris hypoplasia; corectopia.

Clinical

Dwarfism; mental retardation; microcephaly; midface dysplasia; prominent antihelix and antitragus; congenital cardiac disease; abnormal, spindle-shaped fingers; genital defects.

Laboratory

Diagnosis is made by clinical findings.

Treatment

Glaucoma: Its medication should be the first plan of action. If medication is unsuccessful, a filtering surgical procedure with or without antimetabolites may be beneficial.

Strabismus: Equalized vision with correct refractive error; surgery may be helpful in patient with diplopia.

Bibliography

1. de Grouchy J, Royer P, Salmon C, et al. Deletion partielle des bras longs du chromosome 18. Pathol Biol (Paris) 1964;12:579-82.
2. Ginsberg J, Perrin EV, Sueoka WT. Ocular manifestations of trisomy 18. Am J Ophthalmol. 1968;66:59-67.
3. Izquierdo NJ, Maumenee IH, Traboulsi EI. Anterior segment malformations in 18q- (de Grouchy) syndrome. Ophthalmic Paediatr Genet. 1993;14:91-4.
4. Levenson JE, Crandall BF, Sparkes RS. Partial deletion syndromes of chromosome 18. Ann Ophthalmol. 1971;3:756-60.

292. CHROMOSOME 18 PARTIAL DELETION (SHORT-ARM) SYNDROME
[MONOSOMY 18 PARTIAL (SHORT-ARM) SYNDROME]

General

Deletion of the short arm of chromosome 18 (note similarity of clinical features to those of the Cri-du-chat syndrome or B1 deletion syndrome) (see Cri-du-Chat Syndrome).

Ocular

Hypertelorism; epicanthal folds; ptosis; mongolian or antimongolian slant; strabismus; eccentric pupil; cataract; corneal opacities; concentric visual field defects.

Clinical

Short stature; mental retardation; low-set ears; dysphagia; moon face; oliguria; arhinencephaly; microcephaly; congenital alopecia; flat bridge of nose; pyramidal tract signs; weakness and focal dystonia of the lower extremities.

Laboratory

Diagnosis is made by clinical findings.

Treatment

Ptosis: If visual acuity is affected most cases require surgical correction, and there are several procedures that may be used including levator resection, repair or advancement and Fasanella-Servat.

Strabismus: Equalized vision with correct refractive error; surgery may be helpful in patient with diplopia.

Bibliography

1. Buhler EM, Buhler UK, Stalder GR. Partial monosomy 18 and anomaly of thyroxine synthesis. Lancet. 1964;1:170.
2. Levenson JE, Crandall BF, Sparkes RS. Partial deletion syndromes of chromosome 18. Ann Ophthalmol. 1971;3:756-60.
3. Yanoff M, Rorke LB, Niederer BS. Ocular and cerebral abnormalities in chromosome 18 deletion defect. Am J Ophthalmol. 1970;70:391-402.

293. CHRONIC EPSTEIN-BARR VIRUS
(CHRONIC INFECTIOUS MONONUCLEOSIS; EPSTEIN-BARR VIRUS, CHRONIC)

General

Onset late adolescence or early adulthood; rare.

Ocular

Bilateral uveitis; cystoid macular edema; papilledema; cataract; keratitis; peripapillary and macular preretinal membranes; vitreitis; lacrimal gland swelling; conjunctivitis; corneal edema; keratoconjunctivitis; follicular conjunctivitis; subepithelial corneal opacities; retinitis; ophthalmoplegia; optic neuritis; endophthalmitis; dacryocystitis; nasolacrimal duct obstruction.

Clinical

Recurrent fever; pharyngitis; lymphadenopathy; fatigue; malaise; weight loss; splenomegaly.

Laboratory

Criteria for laboratory confirmation include lymphocytosis, the presence of at least 10% atypical lymphocytes on peripheral smear, and a positive serologic test result for Epstein-Barr virus.

Treatment

A self-limited illness that does not usually require specific therapy. If splenic rupture is an acute abdominal emergency that usually requires surgical intervention.

Additional Resource

1. Bennett NJ (2010). Pediatric Mononucleosis and Epstein-Barr Virus Infection. [online] Available from http://www.emedicine.com/ped/TOPIC705.HTM [Accessed April, 2012].

---

294. CHRONIC GRANULOMATOUS DISEASE OF CHILDHOOD

General

Genetically determined metabolic defect manifested by inability of the leukocytes to operate the hexose monophosphate shunt during phagocytosis.

Ocular

Conjunctivitis; keratitis; destructive chorioretinal lesions.

Clinical

Eczematous dermatitis; microabscesses of the skin, lymph nodes and viscera.

Laboratory

The standard is the NBT test.

Treatment

Antimicrobial prophylaxis, early and aggressive treatment of infections, and IFN-gamma are the cornerstones of current therapy.

Additional Resource

1. Wolfe LC (2010). Pediatric Chronic Granulomatous Disease. [online] Available from http://www.emedicine.com/ped/TOPIC1590.HTM [Accessed April, 2012].

---

295. CHRONIC PROGRESSIVE EXTERNAL OPHTHALMOPLEGIA (CPEO; OPHTHALMOPLEGIA PLUS)

General

A general term covering many conditions; onset at any age; familial history; conditions associated with CPEO include myotonic dystrophy, Kearns-Sayre syndrome and oculopharyngeal dystrophy; disorders that rarely cause external ophthalmoplegia include congenital disorders (abetalipoproteinemia, Refsum disease, extraocular fibrosis syndrome, Möbius syndrome), progressive supranuclear palsy, endocrine exophthalmos, myasthenia gravis and multiple sclerosis; now considered to be a mitochondrial cytopathy with varied clinical presentation; four distinct disorders of ophthalmic importance are: (1) CPEO or Kearns-Sayre syndrome, (2) myoclonus epilepsy with ragged red fibers (MERRF), (3) mitochondrial encephalopathy, lactic acidosis and stroke-like episodes (MELAS) and (4) Leber optic neuropathy.

Ocular

Exposure keratopathy; filamentary keratitis; keratoconjunctivitis sicca; corneal scarring; esotropia; exotropia; gaze paralysis; ptosis; levator paralysis;

cataract; optic atrophy; diplopia; tapetoretinal degeneration; constriction of visual field; retinitis pigmentosa.

Clinical

Weakness; weight loss; myopathic or Hutchinson facies; cardiac abnormalities; central nervous system abnormalities.

Laboratory

No specific test diagnosis on clinical evidence.

Treatment

Ophthalmoplegia: A complex disorder requiring the involvement of physicians from various specialties including neurology, cardiology, ophthalmology and endocrinology.

Additional Resource

1. Roy H (2011). Chronic Progressive External Ophthalmoplegia. [online] Available from http://www.emedicine.com/oph/TOPIC510.HTM [Accessed April, 2012].

296. CHURG-STRAUSS SYNDROME (ALLERGIC GRANULOMATOSIS AND ANGIITIS)

General

Severe multisystem vasculitis.

Ocular

Allergic granulomas in the extravascular tissues are characterized by a central eosinophilic core consisting of necrotic eosinophilic leukocytes and fibrinoid swelling of collagen fibers; uveoscleritis; papilledema; anterior ischemic optic neuropathy; sensory motor neuropathy; reversible monocular blindness; myositis; episcleritis; amaurosis fugax; central branch retinal artery occlusion; retinal vasculitis; retinal hemorrhage; cranial nerve palsies; orbital inflammatory syndrome; corneal ulcer; conjunctival nodules.

Clinical

Bronchial asthma; fever; eosinophilia; necrotizing of small arteries and veins with an infiltration of vessels and perivascular tissues by eosinophils; systemic vasculitis.

Laboratory

Eosinophil count, ESR, testing for rheumatoid factor, CT, MRI.

Treatment

Medical management of cardiovascular, cardiac, renal and gastrointestinal complications falls that requires subspecialty consultation.

Additional Resource

1. Rust RS (2010). Churg-Strauss Disease. [online] Available from http://www.emedicine.com/neuro/TOPIC501.HTM [Accessed April, 2012].

297. CILIARY BODY CONCUSSIONS AND LACERATIONS

General

Trauma which can frequently result in damage to other structures of the eye as well as the ciliary body. Choroid can be separated from the sclera and allow aqueous to drain into the suprachoroidal space.

Ocular

Hypotony, iris atrophy, angle-closure glaucoma, cataract, loss of retinal pigment epithelium, choroidal folds, cystoid macular edema, optic atrophy, phthisis bulbi.

Laboratory

Diagnosis is made by clinical findings.

Treatment

Topical steroids and cyclopentolate, surgery—sodium hyaluronate into the anterior chamber to close the cyclodialysis cleft, argon laser photocoagulation.

Bibliography

1. Roy FH, Fraunfelder FW, Fraunfelder FT. Roy and Fraunfelder's Current Ocular Therapy, 6th edition. Philadelphia: WB Saunders; 2008.

298. CITRULLINEMIA

General

Autosomal recessive; enzyme deficiency called argininosuccinic acid synthetase; mutations causing human citrullinemia are extremely heterogeneous; nonconsanguineous persons studied until 1991 had been found to be compound heterozygotes.

Ocular

Hypotonicity; low intraocular pressure; irregular choroidal and retinal pigment epithelium folding; engorged retinal vessels; pallor of optic disk.

Clinical

Mental retardation; nausea; vomiting; tremors; intermittent hyperammonemia.

Laboratory

Citrulline levels are elevated. Urine amino acid, urine organic acid and urine orotic acid levels should be analyzed.

Treatment

Restrict dietary protein. Emphasize other nonprotein caloric sources to compensate.

Additional Resource

1. Roth KS (2012). Citrullinemia. [online] Available from http://www.emedicine.com/ped/TOPIC406. HTM [Accessed April, 2012].

299. CLAUDE SYNDROME (INFERIOR NUCLEUS RUBER SYNDROME; RUBRO-SPINAL-CEREBELLAR-PEDUNCLE SYNDROME)

General

Paramedian mesencephalic lesion starting in midbrain; often occlusion of terminal branches of the paramedian arteries supplying the inferior portion of the nucleus ruber.

Ocular

Paralysis of ipsilateral oculomotor (III) and trochlear (IV) nerves.

Clinical

May be associated with motor hemiplegia.

Laboratory

Diagnosis is made by clinical findings.

Treatment

Prisms may be useful for small deviations. Botulinum toxin may also be useful. For deviation greater than 15 prism diopters, strabismus surgery may be required.

Bibliography

1. Claude H. Inferior nucleus ruber syndrome. Rev Neurol. 1912;1:311.
2. Cremieux G, Serratrice G. A case of retraction nystagmus (associated with Claude's syndrome). Mars Med. 1972;109:635-7.
3. Gaymard B, Saudeau D, de Toffol B, et al. Two mesencephalic lacunar infarcts presenting as Claude's syndrome and pure motor hemiparesis. Eur Neurol. 1991;31:152-5.
4. Geeraets WJ. Ocular Syndromes, 3rd edition. Philadelphia: Lea & Febiger; 1976.

300. CLIVUS EDGE SYNDROME

General

Elevated intracranial pressure; root of oculomotor nerve pressed against bone as it enters cavernous sinus; includes subdural hematoma, temporal lobe tumor and supraclinoid aneurysm.

Ocular

Brief miosis, then mydriasis and sluggish reaction of pupil; extraocular muscle paresis.

Clinical

None

Laboratory

Computed tomography (CT) and MRI to identify cause of increased intracranial pressure.

Treatment

Strabismus: Equalized vision with correct refractive error; surgery may be helpful in patient with diplopia.

Bibliography

1. Fischer-Brugge E. Anatomische Ursachen Funktionaler Kreislaufstorungen des Gehirns und am N. Oculomotorius Bruns. Beitr Klin Chir. 1951; 181:323-36.
2. Pau H. Differential Diagnosis of Eye Diseases. New York: Thieme; 1987.

301. CLOSTRIDIUM PERFRINGENS

General

Gram-positive rod; most important cause of gas gangrene infection.

Ocular

Hypopyon; gas bubbles in anterior chamber; endophthalmitis; proptosis; glaucoma; coffee-colored discharge; eyelid edema; severe ocular pain; endophthalmitis after penetrating trauma or metastatic.

Clinical

Traumatized ischemic skeletal muscle, abdominal wall or uterus; hemolytic anemia; shock; death.

Laboratory

Enzyme-linked immunosorbent assay (ELISA) of the wound exudate, tissue samples or serum can confirm diagnosis.

Treatment

Antibiotic therapy and hyperbaric oxygen may be useful. In more severe cases fasciotomy, debridement and amputation may be necessary.

Additional Resource

1. Ho H (2011). Gas Gangrene. [online] Available from http://www.emedicine.com/med/TOPIC843. HTM [Accessed April, 2012].

---

302. COARCTATION OF THE AORTA

General

Congenital, local and developmental; occurs in 1 of 2,000; not familial; not predictable by sex.

Ocular

Straightening of the arteriolar tree; arteriovenous crossing defects; focal caliber changes; cotton-wool spots; retinal edema; pronounced corkscrew tortuosity of the arterioles with little other retinal changes in 50% of patients; retinal vascular anomalies secondary to hemodynamic changes.

Clinical

Aorta narrowed to less than 1 cm in the region of the insertion of the ductus arteriosus; dyspnea; headache; epistaxis; palpitations of the heart; thoracic pain; intermittent claudication.

Laboratory

Chest X-ray, EKG, MRI, CT, ECG and cardiac catherization may all be beneficial in determining the diagnosis.

Treatment

Initially cardiac failure or hypertension should be treated to stabilize the patient. The aortic obstruction then should be repaired. The therapy can include surgical and catheter interventional procedures; the latter procedures include balloon angioplasty and bare or covered stents.

Additional Resource

1. Rao PS (2012). Coarctation of the Aorta. [online] Available from http://www.emedicine.com/ped/ TOPIC2504.HTM [Accessed April, 2012].

---

303. COATS DISEASE (LEBER MILIARY ANEURYSM; RETINAL TELANGIECTASIA)

General

Exudative retinitis; rare; more common in males than females; 95% unilateral.

Ocular

Leukocoria; telangiectatic retinal vessels; solid gray-yellow retinal detachment; optic atrophy; vitreous hemorrhage; anterior uveitis; glaucoma; intraocular calcification (rare); fibro-osseous retinal nodules (atypical); hemorrhagic retinal macrocysts; cystoid macular edema.

Clinical

None

Laboratory

Fluorescein angiography demonstrates large aneurismal (light bulb) dilatation of the retinal vessels.

Treatment

Cryotherapy and vitrectomy can be used to obliterate the vascular abnormalities.

Bibliography

1. Cameron JO. Coats' disease and Turner's syndrome. Am J Ophthalmol. 1974;78:852-4.
2. Senft SH, Hidayat AA, Cavender JC. Atypical presentation of Coats disease. Retina. 1994;14:36-8.

304. COCAINE INTOXICATION SYNDROME

General

Neonates born to cocaine-abusing mothers.

Ocular

Dilation and tortuosity of the iris vasculature; use of intranasal cocaine has been associated with optic neuropathy.

Clinical

Signs of withdrawal; jittery; irritable.

Laboratory

Urine, blood, gastric contents may be sent for toxicologic evaluation. Cocaine exhibits first-order kinetics over a wide dose range; therefore, after 5 half-lives (approximately 4 hours), virtually all of the cocaine should have been converted to its metabolites.

Treatment

Patients presenting with cocaine toxicity should receive interventions directed at the unstable condition, including attention ABCs, oxygen, IV and monitoring (cardiac monitoring and pulse oximetry). Consultation with a regional poison control center or a medical toxicologist may be appropriate in complicated cases.

Additional Resource

1. Burnett LB (2010). Cocaine Toxicity in Emergency Medicine. [online] Available from http://www.emedicine.com/emerg/TOPIC102.HTM [Accessed April, 2012].

305. COCCIDIOIDOMYCOSIS (SAN JOAQUIN FEVER; VALLEY FEVER)

General

Caused by a fungus, *Coccidioides immitis.*

Ocular

Conjunctivitis; choroiditis; uveitis; retinal hemorrhages; vitreal opacity; vitreal floaters; episcleritis; hypopyon; granulomatous lesion of optic nerve head; paralysis of VI cranial nerve; secondary glaucoma; papilledema; mutton fat keratitic precipitates; necrotizing granulomatous conjunctivitis; iridocyclitis.

Clinical

Mild respiratory illness; cavity lung lesion.

Laboratory

Routine culture media, IgM antibody for acute, IgG antibody for present or past infection.

Treatment

Systemic fluconazole or amphotericin B are the treatments of choice. Ocular treatment includes topical amphotericin B and use of steroids sparingly.

Additional Resource

1. Hospenthal DR (2011). Coccidioidomycosis. [online] Available from http://www.emedicine. com/ped/TOPIC423.HTM [Accessed April, 2012].

---

306. COCKAYNE SYNDROME (DWARFISM WITH RETINAL ATROPHY AND DEAFNESS; MICKEY MOUSE SYNDROME)

General

Autosomal recessive; onset in the second year of life; wide spectrum of symptoms and severity of the disease suggest that biochemical and genetic heterogeneity exist.

Ocular

Enophthalmos; cataracts; pigmentary degeneration of retina; optic atrophy; band keratopathy; exotropia; nystagmus; absence of foveal reflex; corneal dystrophy; corneal perforation; anhidrosis; exposure keratitis; decreased blinking.

Clinical

Dwarfism (nanism) with disproportionately long limbs, large hands and large feet; kyphosis; deformed limbs; thickened skull; intracranial calcifications; mental retardation; prognathism; deafness (often partial); precociously senile appearance; sensitivity to sunlight, with skin pigmentation and scarring; dental caries.

Laboratory

Brain CT scan may reveal calcifications and cortical atrophy.

Treatment

Photoprotection with sunscreens and clothing are useful. Cochlear implantation can help minimize the effects of auditory impairment.

Additional Resource

1. Imaeda S (2012). Cockayne Syndrome. [online] Available from http://www.emedicine.com/ derm/TOPIC717.HTM [Accessed April, 2012].

---

307. COENUROSIS (TAPEWORM)

General

Rare human infestation of the cystic larval stage of the dog tapeworm; usually infestation in the muscle, subcutaneous tissue, eye, nervous system or brain; three species may be involved: (1) *Multiceps taenia*, (2) *M. serialis* and (3) *M. glomeratus*.

Ocular

Hypopyon; retinal detachment; retinal edema; anterior uveitis; conjunctivitis; proptosis; miosis; vitreal haze; increased intraocular pressure; coenurus cysts of the conjunctiva and iris.

Clinical

Ataxia; headache; loss of weight; somnolence; stiffness of neck and shoulders.

Laboratory

Perianal and stool examinations are useful.

Treatment

Anthelmintic drugs are used to rid the GI tract of worms or systemically to rid the body of the helminth forms that invade organs and tissues.

Additional Resource

1. Irizarry L (2011). Tapeworm Infestation. [online] Available from http://www.emedicine.com/emerg/TOPIC567.HTM [Accessed April, 2012].

308. COFFIN-LOWRY SYNDROME

General

X-linked dominant pattern. Seen in both sexes but more severe in males.

Clinical

Mental retardation; prominent forehead, short nose with wide tip, wide mouth with full lips, short hands with tapered fingers; short stature, microcephaly, kyphoscoliosis loss of ambulation.

Ocular

Telecanthus, antimongoloid palpebral fissure.

Laboratory

Diagnosis is made by clincial findings.

Treatment

None

Bibliography

1. Hunter AG. Coffin-Lowry syndrome: a 20-year follow-up and review of long-term outcomes. Am J Med Genet. 2002;111:345-55.

309. COGAN (1) SYNDROME (NONSYPHILITIC INTERSTITIAL KERATITIS)

General

Cause unknown; perhaps a generalized hypersensitivity reaction; most frequently affects young adults; unclear etiology; several studies suggest an autoimmune-mediated process, possibly a vasculitis.

Ocular

Blepharospasm; lacrimation; congested conjunctival vessels; little or no reaction in anterior chamber but ciliary injection present; interstitial keratitis (unilateral or bilateral); granular-type infiltrates; patchy distribution in deeper stroma; later vascularization; conjunctivitis; corneal opacity; uveitis; nystagmus.

Clinical

Vestibuloauditory symptoms (similar to Ménière syndrome); nausea; vomiting; vertigo; tinnitus (abrupt onset); rapidly progressive deafness; loss of equilibration (see Ménière Syndrome); aortic insufficiency; sensorineural testing; lacunar infarcts.

Laboratory

Leukocytosis in 75%, Neutrophilia in 50%, mild eosinophilia in 17%, relative lymphopenia in 25%, anemia in 33%, thrombocytosis in 30% and erthocyte sedimentation rate of greater than 20 in 75%.

Treatment

Corticosteroids and antibiotics are useful. Corneal transplantation may be necessary for corneal opacity.

Additional Resource

1. Majmudar PA (2011). Interstitial Keratitis Overview of Interstitial Keratitis. [online] Available from http://www.emedicine.com/oph/TOPIC101.HTM [Accessed April, 2012].

---

310. COGAN (2) SYNDROME (OCULOMOTOR APRAXIA SYNDROME; WIEACKER SYNDROME)

General

X-linked; oculomotor apraxia and muscle atrophy; prevalent in males; corpus callosum can be hypoplastic.

Ocular

Rapid and frequent blinking; conjugate palsy; congenital oculomotor apraxia with patient unable to move eyes voluntarily to one side but with otherwise normal ocular movements; patient fixes objects by head tilt and turning, which causes further ocular deviation via the vestibular reflex; compensation for this overshoot is accomplished by some jerky eye movements with final fixation possible and gradual return of the head to the primary position; may be associated with abnormal electroretinographic responses.

Clinical

Slow progression, predominantly distal muscle atrophy; congenital contracture of feet; dyspraxia of face and tongue muscles; mild mental retardation.

Laboratory

Diagnosis is made by clinical findings.

Treatment

None

Bibliography

1. Borchert MS, Sadun AA, Sommers JD, et al. Congenital ocular motor apraxia in twins. Findings with magnetic resonance imaging. J Clin Neuroophthalmol. 1987;7:104-7.
2. Cogan DG. A type of congenital ocular motor apraxia presenting jerky head movements. Trans Am Acad Ophthalmol Otolaryngol. 1952;56:853-62.
3. Magni R, Spadea L, Pece A, et al. Electroretinographic findings in congenital oculomotor apraxia (Cogan's syndrome). Doc Ophthalmol. 1994;86:259-66.
4. Vassella F, Lütschg J, Mumenthaler M. Cogan's congenital ocular motor apraxia in two successive generations. Dev Med Child Neurol. 1972;14:788-96.

311. COGAN-GUERRY SYNDROME (MAP-DOT FINGERPRINT DYSTROPHY; MICROCYSTIC CORNEAL DYSTROPHY)

General

Etiology obscure; condition benign and asymptomatic; females predominantly affected; ultrastructural studies show discontinuous multilaminar thickened basement membrane under abnormal epithelium; the primary defect appears to be synthesis of abnormal basement membrane and adhesion complexes by the dystrophic epithelium.

Ocular

Reduced vision mainly with involvement of center of cornea; very fine wavy lines resembling fingerprints within or very close to corneal epithelium and best seen on biomicroscopy with retroillumination; fine grayish spheres (0.1–0.5 mm diameter) in superficial corneal epithelium; maplike irregular border-lined slightly grayish area.

Clinical

None

Laboratory

Diagnosis is made by clinical findings.

Treatment

Pain suppression with pressure patch and antibiotic ointment, recurrence suppression with Muro drops or ointment, persistent erosion may be helped by mechanical debridement, local cycloplegics and a diamond burr to "polish Bowman's membrane, anterior stromal puncture in resistant erosion and PTK may be useful.

Bibliography

1. Cogan DG, Donaldson DD, Kuwabara T, et al. Microcystic dystrophy of the corneal epithelium. Trans Am Ophthalmol Soc. 1964;62:213-25.
2. Guerry DuP. Fingerprint-like lines in the cornea. Am J Ophthalmol. 1950;33:724-6.
3. Luxenberg MN, Friedland BR, Holder JM. Superficial microcystic corneal dystrophy. Arch Ophthalmol. 1975;93:107-10.
4. Starck T, Hersh PS, Kenyon KR. Corneal dysgeneses, dystrophies and degenerations. In: Albert DM, Jakobiec FA (Eds). Principles and Practice of Ophthalmology. Philadelphia: WB Saunders; 1994. pp. 26-30.

Additional Resource

1. Verdier D (2012). Map-dot-fingerprint Dystrophy. [online] Available from http://www.emedicine.medscape.com/article/1193945-overview [Accessed April, 2012].

312. COHEN SYNDROME (OBESITY-HYPOTONIA SYNDROME)

General

Autosomal recessive transmission, rare, characterized by developmental delay, mental retardation, microcephaly and hypotonia.

Clinical

Thick hair and eyebrows, prominent upper central teeth, neutropenia, obesity, narrow hands and feet, slender fingers.

Ocular

Progressive myopia, retinal dystrophy, optic atrophy, microphthalmia, chorioretinitis, nystagmus and retinal coloboma.

Laboratory

Diagnosis is made by clinical appearance.

Treatment

Treat the individual characteristics.

Bibliography

1. Chandler KE, Kidd A, Al-Gazali L, et al. Diagnostic criteria, clinical characteristics, and natural history of Cohen syndrome. J Med Genet. 2003;40:233-41.
2. Kivitie-Kallio S, Summanen P, Raitta C, et al. Ophthalmologic findings in Cohen syndrome. A long-term follow-up. Ophthalmology. 2000;107: 1737-45.

---

313. COLOBOMA, OCULAR

General

Autosomal recessive; congenital or secondary to faulty closure of embryonic fissure.

Ocular

Optic nerve coloboma; retinochoroidal coloboma; orbital cysts; retinal dysplasia; retinal detachment; iris coloboma.

Clinical

White sponge nevus.

Laboratory

Diagnosis is made by clinical findings.

Treatment

Retinal detachment: Scleral buckle, pneumatic retinopexy and vitrectomy may be used to close all the breaks.

Bibliography

1. Hayasaka S, Furuse N, Noda S, et al. Typical ocular coloboma affects three generations in one family. Ann Ophthalmol. 1992;24:209-12.
2. McKusick VA. Mendelian Inheritance in Man: A Catalog of Human Genes and Genetic Disorders, 12th edition. Baltimore: The Johns Hopkins University Press; 1998.
3. McKusick-Nathans Institute for Genetic Medicine, Johns Hopkins University and National Center for Biotechnology Information, National Library of Medicine. (2007). Online Mendelian Inheritance in Man (OMIM). [online] Available from http://www.ncbi.nlm.nih.gov/omim/ [Accessed April, 2012].
4. Pagon RA, Kalina RE, Lechner DJ. Possible autosomal-recessive ocular coloboma. Am J Med Genet. 1981;9:189-93.
5. Wright S, Levy IS. White sponge naevus and ocular coloboma. Arch Dis Child. 1991;66:514-6.

---

314. COLOBOMA OF MACULA (AGENESIS OF MACULA)

General

Autosomal dominant; can be caused by intrauterine inflammation, birth hemorrhage; infantile inflammation.

Ocular

Defect in central area of fundus; coloboma can be pigmented, nonpigmented, or have abnormal vessels associated or completely absent; visual defect; absolute central scotoma; nystagmus; myopia; destruction of pigment epithelium; microphthalmos; coloboma of optic nerve (rare); keratoconus; paravenous retinochoroidal atrophy.

Clinical

Microencephaly

Laboratory

Diagnosis is made by clinical findings.

Treatment

Keratoconus: Spectacle correction, hard contacts and avoid eye rubbing may be useful. If hydrops occurs discontinue contact lens, use NaCl drops and ointment, patching and short course of steroids. As the disease advances penetrating keratoplasty, deep anterior lamellar keratoplasty, intacs with laser grooves or collagen stabilization of cornea.

Bibliography

1. Chen MS, Yang CH, Huang JS. Bilateral macular coloboma and pigmented paravenous retinochoroidal atrophy. Br J Ophthalmol. 1992;76: 250-1.
2. Duane TD. Clinical Ophthalmology. Philadelphia: JB Lippincott; 1987.
3. McKusick VA. Mendelian Inheritance in Man: A Catalog of Human Genes and Genetic Disorders, 12th edition. Baltimore: The Johns Hopkins University Press; 1998.
4. McKusick-Nathans Institute for Genetic Medicine, Johns Hopkins University and National Center for Biotechnology Information, National Library of Medicine. (2007). Online Mendelian Inheritance in Man (OMIM). [online] Available from http://www.ncbi.nlm.nih.gov/omim [Accessed April, 2012].
5. Ranchod TM, Quiram PA, Hathaway N, et al. Microcornea, posterior megalolenticonus, persistent fetal vasculature, and coloboma: a new syndrome. Ophthalmology. 2010;117:1843-7.

315. COLOBOMA OF MACULA WITH TYPE B BRACHYDACTYLY (APICAL DYSTROPHY)

General

Autosomal dominant; bilateral pigmented macular coloboma and brachydactyly.

Ocular

Myopia; retinal detachment; coloboma of retina, choroid, sclera and macula.

Clinical

Cleft palate; flexion deformity of distal interphalangeal joints of little fingers of hand; retarded growth; delayed sexual maturity; recurrent dis-location of left patella; short feet; coxa valga; genu valgum.

Laboratory

Diagnosis is made by clinical findings.

Treatment

Myopia: Generally treated with glasses, contact lens and refractive surgery.

Retinal detachment: Scleral buckle, pneumatic retinopexy and vitrectomy may be used to close all the breaks.

Bibliography

1. McKusick VA. Mendelian Inheritance in Man: A Catalog of Human Genes and Genetic Disorders, 12th edition. Baltimore: The Johns Hopkins University Press; 1998.
2. McKusick-Nathans Institute for Genetic Medicine, Johns Hopkins University and National Center for Biotechnology Information, National Library of Medicine. (2007). Online Mendelian Inheritance in Man (OMIM). [online] Available from http:// www.ncbi.nlm.nih.gov/omim [Accessed April, 2012].
3. Smith RD, Fineman RM, Sillence DO, et al. Congenital macular colobomas and short-limb skeletal dysplasia. Am J Med Genet. 1980;5:365-71.
4. Sorsby A. Congenital coloboma of the macula: together with an account of the familial occurrence of bilateral macular coloboma in association with apical dystrophy of hands and feet. Br J Ophthalmol. 1935;19:65-90.

316. COLOBOMATOUS, MICROPHTHALMIA AND MICROCORNEA SYNDROME

General

Autosomal dominant pattern of inheritance with complete penetrance.

Ocular

Bilateral infernasal coloboma; axial enlargement; myopia; iridocorneal angle abnormalities; elevated IOP.

Clinical

None

Laboratory

Diagnosis is made by clinical findings.

Treatment

Glaucoma: Its medication should be the first plan of action. If medication is unsuccessful, a filtering surgical procedure with or without antimetabolites may be beneficial.

Bibliography

1. Toker E, Elcioglu N, Ozcan E, et al. Colobomatous macrophthalmia with microcornea syndrome: report of a new pedigree. Am J Med Genet. 2003;121:25-30.

317. COLOR BLINDNESS, BLUE-MONO-CONE MONOCHROMATIC TYPE

General

Sex-linked; progressive.

Ocular

Total to partial color blindness; macular scar; poor central vision; poor color discrimination; infantile nystagmus; nearly normal retinal appearance in most cases; there is evidence showing alterations in the red and green visual pigment gene cluster.

Clinical

None

Laboratory

Color vision tests to identify type.

Treatment

None

Bibliography

1. McKusick VA. Mendelian Inheritance in Man: A Catalog of Human Genes and Genetic Disorders, 12th edition. Baltimore: The Johns Hopkins University Press; 1998.
2. McKusick-Nathans Institute for Genetic Medicine, Johns Hopkins University and National Center for Biotechnology Information, National Library of Medicine. (2007). Online Mendelian Inheritance in Man (OMIM). [online] Available from http://www.ncbi.nlm.nih.gov/omim [Accessed April, 2012].
3. Nathans J, Davenport CM, Maumenee IH, et al. Molecular genetics of human blue cone monochromacy. Science. 1989;245:831-8.
4. Spivey BE. The X-linked recessive inheritance of atypical monochromatism. Arch Ophthalmol. 1965;74:327-33.

---

318. COLOR BLINDNESS, PARTIAL, DEUTAN SERIES (DEUTERANOPIA)

General

Sex-linked; affects males; deuteranopes can have one red pigment gene and one anomalous hybrid red-green gene with a spectral absorbance close to the red pigment gene.

Ocular

Red-green color blindness.

Clinical

None

Laboratory

None

Treatment

None

Bibliography

1. Adam A, Fraser GR. The linkage between protan and deutan loci. Am J Hum Genet. 1970;22:691-3.
2. Boger WP, Petersen RA. Pediatric ophthalmology. Protan and deutan color blindness. In: Pavan-Langston D (Ed). Manual of Ocular Diagnosis and Therapy, 4th edition. Boston: Little, Brown and Company; 1995. pp. 285-6.
3. McKusick VA. Mendelian Inheritance in Man: A Catalog of Human Genes and Genetic Disorders, 12th edition. Baltimore: The Johns Hopkins University Press; 1998.
4. McKusick-Nathans Institute for Genetic Medicine, Johns Hopkins University and National Center for Biotechnology Information, National Library of Medicine. (2007). Online Mendelian Inheritance in Man (OMIM). [online] Available from http://www.ncbi.nlm.nih.gov/omim/ [Accessed April, 2012].
5. Nathans J, Piantanida TP, Eddy RL, et al. Molecular genetics of inherited variation in human color vision. Science. 1986;232:203-10.

---

319. COMEDO CATARACT

General

Etiology unknown; possibly in the group of neurectodermal dysplasia syndromes (phakomatoses).

Ocular

Bilateral cataract, or both unilateral comedo nevus and cataract.

Clinical

Bilateral comedo nevus (dermatosis is character-ized by groups of dilated, keratin-filled follicular spaces).

Laboratory

Diagnosis is made by clinical findings.

Treatment

Cataract surgery if vision decreases.

Bibliography

1. Mutton P, Lewis M, Harley J, et al. Comedo naevus: an unusual association of infantile cataract. Aust Paediatr J. 1975;11:46-8.
2. Popov L, Boianov L. Undescribed congenital cutaneo-ocular syndrome (congenital cataract-comedo syndrome). Surv Med (Sofiia). 1962;13:49-50.
3. Whyte HJ. Unilateral comedo nevus and cataract. Arch Dermatol. 1968;97:533-5.

320. COMPUTER USER SYNDROME

General

Seen in people who use computers extensively.

Ocular

Ocular pain; asthenopia; excyclotorsion; depression of gaze; ocular synkinesis.

Clinical

Hand-wrist pronation; ulnar abduction; headache; fatigue; various types of head and shoulder distress; carpal tunnel syndrome.

Laboratory

Diagnosis is made by clinical findings.

Treatment

Use newer computer keyboards, treat dry eyes, and try various screen backgrounds.

Bibliography

1. Bernbaum MH. Symposium on near point visual stress. Am J Optom Physiol Opt. 1985;62:361-4.
2. Grant AH. The computer users syndrome. J Am Optom Assoc. 1987;58:892-901.
3. Tsubota K, Nakamori K. Dry eyes and video display terminals [Letter]. N Engl J Med. 1993;328:584.

321. CONE DYSFUNCTION SYNDROME (ACHROMATOPSIA)

General

Male-linked recessive inheritance; condition is stagnant and nonprogressive; all modes of inheritance have been reported as well as many sporadic cases.

Ocular

Nystagmus; vision decreased 20/50 to 20/200 or less with no or reduced color vision; color vision might be affected with or without amblyopia; peripheral field loss if rods and cones are involved; photophobia; general fundus lesions, mainly macular involvement with depigmentation and degenerative changes; decreased central vision; difficulty adjusting from light to dark environment.

Clinical

Head movements.

Laboratory

Diagnosis is made by clinical findings.

Treatment

Gabapentin may be beneficial in congenital nystagmus, botulinum toxin has been demonstrated to abolish nystagmus temporarily and sometimes strabismus surgery.

Bibliography

1. Magalini SI, Scrascia E. Dictionary of Medical Syndromes, 2nd edition. Philadelphia: JB Lippincott; 1981.
2. Boger WP, Petersen RA. Achromatopsia. In: Pavan-Langston D (Ed). Manual of Ocular Diagnosis and Therapy, 4th edition. Boston: Little, Brown and Company; 1995. p. 283.

322. CONE-ROD DYSTROPHY (CRD)

General

Autosomal dominant; retinal dystrophy of photoreceptors, characterized by abiotrophic degeneration of rods and cones; onset before age 10 years; it has been suggested that a locus for cone-rod dystrophy may be located in the segment 18q21.1–q21.3 and 19q.

Ocular

Decreased central vision with progressive constriction of peripheral visual fields; degeneration of rods and cones.

Clinical

None

Laboratory

Diagnosis is made by clinical findings.

Treatment

Maximize the vision with refraction and low-vision evaluation and aids.

Additional Resource

1. Telander DG (2012). Retinitis Pigmentosa. [online] Available from http://www.emedicine.com/oph/TOPIC704.HTM [Accessed April, 2012].

323. CATARACT, CONGENITAL OR JUVENILE (CATARACT, HUTTERITE TYPE, JUVENILE)

General

Autosomal recessive; seen most frequently in people of Japanese origin; autosomal dominant inheritance also has been reported.

Ocular

Retinitis pigmentosa; Usher syndrome (retinitis pigmentosa and congenital deafness); congenital cataract of the "i" phenotype; microphthalmos; keratoconus.

Clinical

Congenital deafness; galactokinase deficiency; epimerase deficiency.

Laboratory

Diagnosis is made by clinical findings.

Treatment

Retinitis pigmentosa: Vitamin A 15,000 IU/day is thought to slow the decline of retinal function, dark sunglasses for outdoor use, surgery for cataract, genetic counseling.

Cataract: Change in glasses can sometimes improve a patient's visual function temporarily; however, the most common treatment is cataract surgery.

Bibliography

1. McKusick VA. Mendelian Inheritance in Man: A Catalog of Human Genes and Genetic Disorders, 12th edition. Baltimore: The Johns Hopkins University Press; 1998.

2. McKusick-Nathans Institute for Genetic Medicine, Johns Hopkins University and National Center for Biotechnology Information, National Library of Medicine. (2007). Online Mendelian Inheritance in Man (OMIM). [online] Available from http://www.ncbi.nlm.nih.gov/omim [Accessed April, 2012].

3. Skokeir MH, Lowry RB. Juvenile cataract in Hutterites. Am J Med Genet. 1985;22:495-500.

324. CONGENITAL ANOMALIES OF THE LACRIMAL SYSTEM (ACCESSARY PUNCTUM, CANALICULAR STENOSIS, CONGENITAL NASOLACRIMAL DUCT OBSTRUCTION, DACRYOCYSTITIS, DACRYOCYSTOCELE, PUNCTAL STENOSIS)

General

Common congenital anomalities of lacrimal drainage system.

Clinical

None

Ocular

Tearing, recurrent mucopurulent discharge, reflux of tears and mucopurulent material from the punctum with pressure in the nasolacrimal sac.

Laboratory

Diagnosis is made by clinical findings.

Treatment

Spontaneously resolves during the first year of life if not probing and irrigation of the nasolacrimal duct can be done in an office setting.

Additional Resource

1. Bashour M (2012). Congenital Anomalies of the Nasolacrimal Duct. [online] Available from http://www.emedicine.com/oph/TOPIC592.HTM [Accessed April, 2012].

325. CONGENITAL CATARACT AND HYPERTROPHIC CARDIOMYOPATHY SYNDROME

General

Autosomal recessive; characterized by congenital cataract, hypertrophic cardiomyopathy, mitochondrial myopathy of voluntary muscles and exercise-related lactic acidosis.

Ocular

Cataract; hyperplastic primary vitreous; aniridia; iris colobomas; microphthalmos; nystagmus; strabismus; myopia; keratoconus.

Clinical

Pulmonary stenosis; ventricular septal defects; structurally abnormal mitochondria.

Laboratory

Diagnosis is made by clinical findings.

Treatment

Cataract surgery if vision decreases.

Bibliography

1. Cruysberg JR, Sengers RC, Pinckers A, et al. Features of a syndrome with congenital cataract and hypertrophic cardiomyopathy. Am J Ophthalmol. 1986;102:740-9.
2. McKusick VA. Mendelian Inheritance in Man: A Catalog of Human Genes and Genetic Disorders, 12th edition. Baltimore: The Johns Hopkins University Press; 1998.
3. McKusick-Nathans Institute for Genetic Medicine, Johns Hopkins University and National Center for Biotechnology Information, National Library of Medicine. (2007). Online Mendelian Inheritance in Man (OMIM). [online] Available from http://www.ncbi.nlm.nih.gov/omim [Accessed April, 2012].

326. CONGENITAL CATARACT, MICROCORNEA, ABNORMAL IRIDES, NYSTAGMUS AND CONGENITAL GLAUCOMA SYNDROME

General

Autosomal dominant.

Ocular

Microphakia; cataract with two concentric disks, with the anterior being swollen; microphthalmos; microcornea; nystagmus; congenital glaucoma; honey-colored iris with absence of pattern; peripheral anterior synechiae; pupillary abnormality; corneal edema; posterior synechiae; vitreous hemorrhage; shallow anterior chamber; vitreous loss; corneal staphyloma; keratoconus.

Clinical

High-arched palate; increased webbing of fingers and toes; deafness.

Laboratory

Diagnosis is made by clinical findings.

Treatment

Cataract surgery if vision decreases.

Bibliography

1. Cebon L, West RH. A syndrome involving congenital cataracts of unusual morphology, microcornea, abnormal irides, nystagmus and congenital glaucoma, inherited as an autosomal dominant trait. Aust J Ophthalmol. 1982;10:237-42.
2. Henkind P, Friedman AH. Iridogoniodysgenesis with cataract. Am J Ophthalmol. 1971;72:949-54.

327. CONGENITAL CATARACT WITH OXYCEPHALY (TOWER SKULL SYNDROME)

General

Autosomal dominant; craniostenosis.

Ocular

Congenital cataracts; keratoconus.

Clinical

Large fontanelles; deformed skull; dwarfing; osteopetrosis.

Laboratory

Diagnosis is made by clinical findings.

Treatment

Cataract surgery if vision decreases.

Bibliography

1. McKusick VA. Mendelian Inheritance in Man: A Catalog of Human Genes and Genetic Disorders, 12th edition. Baltimore: The Johns Hopkins University Press; 1998.
2. McKusick-Nathans Institute for Genetic Medicine, Johns Hopkins University and National Center for Biotechnology Information, National Library of Medicine. (2007). Online Mendelian Inheritance in Man (OMIM). [online] Available from http://www.ncbi.nlm.nih.gov/omim [Accessed April, 2012].
3. Roy FH. Ocular Differential Diagnosis, 8th edition. Philadelphia: Lippincott Williams & Wilkins; 2007.

328. CONGENITAL CATARACTS FACIAL DYSMORPHISM NEUROPATHY SYNDROME

General

Autosomal recessive; motor and sensory neuropathy.

Ocular

Congenital cataracts, microcorneas, strabismus, pendular nystagmus, bilateral blepharoptosis.

Clinical

Patients are recognized in infancy by the presence of congenital cataracts and microcorneas; initially, a predominantly motor neuropathy begins in the lower limbs followed by upper limb involvement; severe disability occurs by the third decade; short stature, moderate nonprogressive cognitive deficits, pyramidal signs and mild chorea are characteristic.

Laboratory

Diagnosis is made by clinical findings.

Treatment

Change in glasses can sometimes improve a patient's visual function temporarily; however, the most common treatment is cataract surgery.

Bibliography

1. Mullner-Eidenbock A, Moser E, Klebermass N, et al. Ocular features of the congenital cataracts facial dysmorphism neuropathy syndrome. Ophthalmology. 2004;111:1415-23.
2. Tournev I, Kalaydjieva L, Youl B, et al. Congenital cataracts facial dysmorphism neuropathy syndrome, a novel complex genetic disease in Balkan Gypsies: clinical and electrophysiological observations. Ann Neurol. 1999;45:742-50.

329. CONGENITAL CLOUDING OF THE CORNEA

General

Glaucoma is one common reason for this condition. Other metabolic, genetic, idiopathic and developmental can result in congenital clouding of the cornea.

Clinical

Fryns syndrome, Goldenhar-Gorlin syndrome, birth trauma, Peters anomaly.

Ocular

Sclerocornea, dermoid tumors and congenital endothelial dystrophy. Rare cases include: cornea plana, cornea keloids and congenital hereditary stromal dystrophy.

Laboratory

No laboratory findings for corneal clouding unless is due to mucopolysaccharidoses, in that case, laboratory testing activity in leukocytes may be warranted.

Treatment

Treatment is primary surgical. Patients with bilateral corneal opacity, PK is recommended.

Additional Resource

1. Scheinfeld NS (2011). Congenital Clouding of the Cornea. [online] Available from http://www.emedicine.medscape.com/article/1197148-overview [Accessed April, 2012].

---

330. CONGENITAL DYSLEXIA SYNDROME (ATTENTION DEFICIT DISORDER; CONGENITAL WORD BLINDNESS CONGENITAL WORD BLINDNESS OF HERMANN; DEVELOPMENTAL DYSLEXIA OF CRITCHLEY; DYSLEXIA SYNDROME; MINIMAL BRAIN DYSFUNCTION SYNDROME; PRIMARY DYSLEXIA)

General

Primary reading disability in children with an average or above-average intelligence; male preponderance; dysfunction of the dominating parietotemporal lobe; Levinson postulates a primary cerebellar-vestibular (inner ear) dysfunction underlying this syndrome resulting in a secondary scrambled sensory input and motor output.

Ocular

No obvious connection seems to exist between coordination of ocular functions and dyslexia, although associated ocular findings may exist in reading problems (e.g. abnormal optokinetic nystagmus, metamorphopsia, defective color vision, convergence insufficiency, muscle imbalance, refractive errors); low accommodative converge/accommodation associated with decreased visual acuity and contrast sensitivity.

Clinical

General clumsiness; disorientation (time-space, right-left); behavioral changes; lack of integration of visual and auditory stimuli.

Laboratory

An educational diagnostician, an educator trained as a reading specialist and a school psychologist are the professionals charged with evaluation.

Treatment

No medical care is indicated. Appropriate referrals to a special education (SPED) setting, specialized tutoring setting, or both can prove important for long-term progress.

Additional Resource

1. Crouch ER (2011). Reading Learning Disorder. [online] Available from http://www.emedicine.com/ped/TOPIC2792.HTM [Accessed April, 2012].

331. CONGENITAL EPIBLEPHARON INFERIOR OBLIQUE INSUFFICIENCY SYNDROME

General

Prognosis is good with treatment; present in infancy; inversion of lash line occurs with epiblepharon and is exaggerated by the inferior oblique insufficiency.

Ocular

Narrow interpupillary distance; some ocular prominence; epicanthus; epiblepharon exaggerated in downward gaze; spastic entropion with retroflexion of the eyelashes; epiblepharon becomes less pronounced with growth and development; usually bilateral but in some cases asymmetrical; inferior oblique insufficiency usually unilateral; persistent unilateral keratoconjunctival irritation by the inverted cilia; lacrimation due to conjunctival and corneal irritation.

Clinical

Chubby cheeks (occasionally).

Laboratory

Diagnosis is made by clinical findings.

Treatment

None

Bibliography

1. Duke-Elder S (Ed). System of Ophthalmology. St. Louis: CV Mosby; 1976.
2. Swan KC. The syndrome of congenital epiblepharon and inferior oblique insufficiency. Am J Ophthalmol. 1955;39:130-6.

332. CONGENITAL ESOTROPIA (INFANTILE ESOTROPIA)

General

Inward turning of the eye which is manifested by 6 months of age.

Clinical

None

Ocular

Esotropia, amblyopia, coloboma, hypoplasia, retinoblastoma.

Laboratory

Diagnosis is made by clinical findings.

Treatment

Correct refractive error, amblyopia therapy, medial rectus recession and/or lateral rectus resection in one or both eyes.

Additional Resource

1. Ocampo VVD (2010). Infantile Esotropia. [online] Available from http://www.emedicine.com/oph/TOPIC328.HTM [Accessed April, 2012].

333. CONGENITAL HEART DISEASE

General

Represents a wide variety of cardiac diseases or defects.

Ocular

Dilated, tortuous conjunctival vessels; tortuous retinal vessels; retinal edema; papilledema; retinal arterial macroaneurysm; Duane retraction syndrome; double elevator palsy.

Clinical

Hypoxia; increased cerebrospinal fluid; features vary because of a wide variety of cardiac diseases and defects.

Laboratory

Complete blood count with peripheral smear to look for Howell-Jolly bodies and evidence of impaired splenic function.

Treatment

Anticongestive medication is often required in patients with significant left-to-right shunts. Patients with significant cardiac disease may require staged palliation or definitive repair, whereas patients with biliary atresia may require initial palliative surgery followed by liver transplantation.

Additional Resource

1. http://www.emedicine.medscape.com/article/2035949-overview [Accessed April, 2012].

334. CONGENITAL HEREDITARY RETINOSCHISIS (CHRS; JUVENILE X-LINKED RETINOSCHISIS)

General

X-linked recessive; bilateral; develops early in life but often stabilized toward the end of the second decade; severity varies widely.

Ocular

Bilateral vitreoretinal dystrophy; retinoschisis; vitreous veil; vitreous detachment; vitreous hemorrhage; decreased visual fields; maculopathy; cataract; neovascular glaucoma; vitreoretinopathy; proliferative retinal detachment; Mizuo phenomenon.

Laboratory

Optical coherence tomography (OCT) provides high-resolution cross-sectional images of the macular region indocyanine green (ICG) angiography performed on patients with XJR shows a distinct hyperfluorescence in the macular region that is associated with radial lines of hypofluorescence centered on the foveola in the early phase.

Treatment

No treatment is available to halt the natural progression of schisis formation.

Additional Resource

1. Song MK (2010). Retinoschisis, Juvenile. [online] Available from http://www.emedicine.com/oph/TOPIC639.HTM [Accessed April, 2012].

335. CONGENITAL LUES (CONGENITAL SYPHILIS)

General

Caused by intrauterine transplacental infection of fetus by *Treponema pallidum (see Syphilis)*.

Ocular

Conjunctivitis; keratitis; dacryocystitis; optic nerve atrophy; periostitis; anisocoria; Argyll Robertson pupil; retinal degeneration; nystagmus; gumma of conjunctiva, eyelids and orbit; paresis of extraocular muscles; secondary glaucoma; uveitis; iridoschisis.

Clinical

Cutaneous and mucous membrane lesions; periostitis; anemia; hepatosplenomegaly; ectodermal defects; central nervous system involvement; gummatous lesions.

Laboratory

Fluorescent treponemal antibody absorption (FTA-ABS) and MHA-TP are the standard tests.

All patients with syphilis should also be tested for HIV.

Treatment

Parenteral penicillin is the preferred treatment for all stage of syphilis. The treatment varies from primary and secondary syphilis, late latent syphilis, tertiary syphilis and neurosyphilis. Ocular treatment includes topical steroids and cycloplegics and it can relieve the symptoms of anterior uveitis and interstitial keratitis. Subconjunctival steroids have been used to relieve recurrent anterior segment inflammation. Sever corneal opacification may require keratoplasty. However with recurrent inflammation and graft rejection.

Additional Resource

1. Waseem M (2011). Pediatric Syphilis. [online] Available from http://www.emedicine.com/ped/TOPIC2193.HTM [Accessed April, 2012].

336. CONGENITAL PIT OF OPTIC DISK

General

Single, unilateral and occurs most commonly in the temporal sector of larger than normal disk.

Clinical

None

Ocular

Visual loss due to serous detachment of the macula, visual field defect.

Laboratory

Diagnosis is made by clinical findings.

Treatment

Linear photocoagulation between pit and macula, uncomplicated optic pits require no treatment.

Bibliography

1. Roy FH, Fraunfelder FW, Fraunfelder FT. Roy and Fraunfelder's Current Ocular Therapy, 6th edition. Philadelphia: WB Saunders; 2008.

337. CONGENITAL RETINAL NONATTACHMENT

General

Autosomal dominant or recessive; acquired prenatally or perinatally; retinal dysplasia typical; X-ray irradiation has been reported to cause retinal nonattachment.

Ocular

Vascularized mass behind the lens; malformation of the chamber angle and elongation of the ciliary processes; retinal dysplasia.

Clinical

Severe fragility of the bones.

Laboratory

Diagnosis can usually be made clinically. Ultrasound is a useful when the media is hazy.

Treatment

The medical and surgical treatments of exudative retinal detachments have to be tailored to the underlying condition.

Additional Resource

1. Wu L (2010). Retinal Detachment, Exudative. [online] Available from http://www.emedicine.com/oph/TOPIC407.HTM [Accessed April, 2012].

338. CONGENITAL RETINAL NONATTACHMENT WITH MENTAL RETARDATION, OSTEOPOROSIS AND HYPOTONIA

General

Autosomal recessive; well-demarcated entity; affects both males and females.

Ocular

Retinoblastoma; retina nonattached.

Clinical

Mentally retarded; osteoporosis; hypotonia; ligamentous laxity; dwarfism; microcephaly.

Laboratory

Diagnosis is made by clinical findings.

Treatment

External beam radiation therapy is recommended on patients with significant vitreous seeding. Radioactive isotope plaques and chemotherapy are also an option. Removal of the tumor is the standard management for retinoblastoma.

Bibliography

1. McKusick VA. Mendelian Inheritance in Man: A Catalog of Human Genes and Genetic Disorders, 12th edition. Baltimore: The Johns Hopkins University Press; 1998.
2. McKusick-Nathans Institute for Genetic Medicine, Johns Hopkins University and National Center for Biotechnology Information, National Library of Medicine. (2007). Online Mendelian Inheritance in Man (OMIM). [online] Available from http://www.ncbi.nlm.nih.gov/omim [Accessed April, 2012].
3. Warburg M. Heterogeneity of congenital retinal non-attachment, falciform folds and retinal dysplasia. A guide to genetic counselling. Hum Hered. 1976;26:137-48.

339. CONGENITAL SPHEROCYTIC ANEMIA (CONGENITAL HEMOLYTIC JAUNDICE; HEREDITARY SPHEROCYTOSIS)

General

Hereditary deficiency of erythrocyte glucose-6-phosphate after exposure to certain drugs, chemicals and foods such as fava beans.

Ocular

Congenital cataract; ring-shaped pigmentary deposits of cornea; tortuosity of retinal vessels; mongoloid palpebral aperture; microphthalmos.

Clinical

Leukemia; anemia.

Laboratory

The most sensitive test is the incubated osmotic fragility test performed after incubating RBCs for 18–24 hours under sterile conditions.

Treatment

The treatment involves presplenectomy care, splenectomy and postsplenectomy complications.

Additional Resource

1. Gonzalez G (2012). Hereditary Spherocytosis. [online] Available from http://www.emedicine. com/med/TOPIC2147.HTM [Accessed April, 2012].

340. CONGENITAL VERTICAL RETRACTION SYNDROME

General

Congenital

Ocular

Aberrant regeneration of the oculomotor nerve; concurrent protective eyelid closure; congenital alterations in the extraocular muscle, its insertion, and its peripheral innervation; nystagmus retractorius; surgical or traumatic rearrangement of orbital structures may account for retraction.

Clinical

None

Laboratory

Diagnosis is made by clinical findings.

Treatment

None

Bibliography

1. Khodadoust AA, von Noorden GK. Bilateral vertical retraction syndrome. A family study. Arch Ophthalmol. 1967;78:606-12.
2. Osher RH, Schatz NJ, Duane TD. Acquired orbital retraction syndrome. Arch Ophthalmol. 1980;98:1798-802.
3. Pesando P, Nuzzi G, Maraini G. Vertical retraction syndrome. Ophthalmologica. 1978;177:254-9.

341. CONGENITAL FIBROSIS OF THE EXTRAOCULAR MUSCLES

General

Familial congenital; autosomal dominant or recessive.

Clinical

None

Ocular

Large angle exotropia; bilateral hypotropia; bilateral ptosis; sluggish pupil; almost complete ophthalmoplegia; refractive error and amblyopia.

Laboratory

Venous blood sampling for genetic analysis.

Treatment

Genetic counseling, correction of refractive error, amblyopia therapy and traditional surgical treatment for exotropia and ptosis.

Bibliography

1. Khan AO, Khalil DS, Al Sharif LJ, et al. Germline mosaicism for KIF21A mutation (p.R954L) mimicking recessive inheritance for congenital fibrosis of the extraocular muscles. Ophthalmology. 2010;117:154-8.
2. Demer JL, Clark RA, Engle EC. Magnetic resonance imaging evidence for widespread orbital dysinnervation in congenital fibrosis of extraocular muscles due to mutations in KIF21A. Invest Ophthalmol Vis Sci. 2005;46:530-9.
3. Roy FH, Fraunfelder FW, Fraunfelder FT. Roy and Fraunfelder's Current Ocular Therapy, 6th edition. Philadelphia: WB Saunders; 2008.

342. CONJUNCTIVAL MELANOTIC LESIONS (BLUE NEVUS, COMPOUND NEVUS, CONGENITAL MELANOCYTOSIS, CONJUNCTIVAL MELANOMA, CONJUNCTIVAL MALIGNANT MELANOMA, CONJUNCTIVAL MELANOSIS, CONJUNCTIVAL NEVUS, CONJUNCTIVAL JUNCTIONAL NEVUS, EPITHELIAL NELANOSIS, MALIGNANT MELANOMA, MELANOSIS OCULI, PRIMARY ACQUIRED MELANOSIS, RACIAL MELANOSIS, SUBEPITHELIAL MELANOCYTOSIS, SUBEPITHELIAL NEVUS)

General

Conjunctival lesions may be melanocytic or nonmelanocytic.

Clinical

None

Ocular

Conjunctival lesion.

Laboratory

Photographic documentation, biopsy of the lesion.

Treatment

Complete excision, with tumor-free margins of primary acquired melanosis with atypical. Cryotherapy, radiotherapy, topical mitomycin C or CO_2 laser are useful adjunctive therapies.

Additional Resource

1. Roque MR (2011). Conjunctival Melanoma. [online] Available from http://www.emedicine.com/oph/TOPIC110.HTM [Accessed April, 2012].

343. CONJUNCTIVITIS, LIGNEOUS

General

Autosomal recessive; palpebral conjunctiva becomes the site of dense woody membrane that has global shape; associated with systemic use of tranexamic acid.

Ocular

Corneal scarring; dense membrane of the conjunctiva; may occur as a complication following strabismus surgery.

Clinical

None

Laboratory

Diagnosis is made by clinical findings.

Treatment

Surgical excision of conjunctiva membrane followed by cautery, cryoplexy and grafting of conjunctiva or sclera.

Bibliography

1. Bierly JR, Blandford DL, Weeks JA, et al. Ligneous conjunctivitis as a complication following strabismus surgery. J Pediatr Ophthalmol Strabismus. 1994;31:99-103.
2. Diamond JP, Chandna A, Williams C, et al. Tranexamic acid-associated ligneous conjunctivitis with gingival and peritoneal lesions. Br J Ophthalmol. 1991;75:753-4.
3. McKusick VA. Mendelian Inheritance in Man: A Catalog of Human Genes and Genetic Disorders, 12th edition. Baltimore: The Johns Hopkins University Press; 1998.
4. McKusick-Nathans Institute for Genetic Medicine, Johns Hopkins University and National Center for Biotechnology Information, National Library of Medicine. (2007). Online Mendelian Inheritance in Man (OMIM). [online] Available from http://www.ncbi.nlm.nih.gov/omim [Accessed April, 2012].
5. Pavan-Langston D. Cornea and external disease. Ligneous conjunctivitis. In: Pavan-Langston D (Ed). Manual of Ocular Diagnosis and Therapy, 4th edition. Boston: Little, Brown and Company; 1995. p. 103.

344. CONJUNCTIVITIS, VIRAL

General

Characterized commonly by an acute follicular conjunctival reaction and preauricular adenopathy. Adenovirus is the most common cause but can be result of herpes simplex, molluscum, vaccina, HIV and others. Generally self-limited and benign but tends to follow a longer course than bacterial. May last 2–4 weeks.

Clinical

Herpes simplex virus, varicella-zoster virus, picornavirus, poxvirus and human immunodeficiencey virus. Rarely: Epstein-Barr virus, paramyxovirus, rubella and HIV.

Ocular

Foreign body sensation, tearing, itching, photophobia, redness HSV keratoconjunctivitis, VSV keratoconjunctivitis, ocular chlamydia, vernal keratoconjunctivitis, blepharoconjunctivitis, epithelial keratitis.

Laboratory

Diagnosis is made by clinical findings. If inflammation is severe or chronic culture and smear for viral identity should be considered.

Treatment

No evidence exists that demonstrates efficacy of antiviral agents. It is recommended for patients to use cold compresses and artificial tears, for comfort. Topical steroids may be used when subepithelial infiltrates impair vision.

Additional Resource

1. Scott IU (2011). Viral Conjunctivitis. [online] Available from http://www.emedicine.medscape.com/article/1191370-diagnosis [Accessed April, 2012].

345. CONJUNCTIVOCHALASIS (CCH)

General

Relaxation of conjunctiva; redundant loose nonedematous inferior bulbar conjunctiva; associated with disruption of the tear meniscus; causative agent not yet determined but may be associated with age-related elastotic degeneration and chronic inflammation.

Ocular

Dry eye; punctal occlusion; delayed tear clearance; age-related elastotic degeneration; chronic inflammation; epiphora.

Laboratory

Diagnosis is determined by clinical observation.

Treatment

High frequency radiowave electrosurgery has proven to be beneficial.

Bibliography

1. Youm DJ, Kim JM, Choi CY. Simple surgical approach with high-frequency radio-wave electrosurgery for conjunctivochalasis. Ophthalmology. 2010;117:2129-33.

346. CONRADI SYNDROME (CALCINOSIS UNIVERSALIS; CHONDRODYSPLASIA PUNCTATA; CHONDRODYSTROPHIA FOETALIS HYPOPLASTICA; CONGENITAL CALCIFYING CHONDRODYSTROPHY; CONRADI-HÜNERMANN SYNDROME; DYSPLASIA EPIPHYSEALIS CONGENITA; MULTIPLE EPIPHYSEAL DYSPLASIA CONGENITA; STIPPLED EPIPHYSES SYNDROME)

General

Autosomal recessive; manifestations within the first 6 months of life; epiphyseal stippling present at birth; perinatal manifestations include disorganization of the spine, premature echogenicity of femoral epiphyses and frontal bossing with depressed nasal bridge.

Ocular

Hypertelorism; heterochromia iridis (rare); bilateral total congenital cataract appearing at or shortly after birth; primary optic atrophy (rare); bilateral corneal punctate erosions.

Clinical

Short limbs (mainly proximal part) resulting in "short-limbed dwarfism"; deformities of hip, knee and elbow joints by contraction and immobility, and possible transformation of muscles into fibrous tissue as a result; congenital heart defect with calcium deposits in the cardiac valves; skin anomalies (dyskeratosis); mental retardation.

Laboratory

Diagnosis is made by clinical findings.

Treatment

Cataract: Change in glasses can sometimes improve a patient's visual function temporarily; however, the most common treatment is cataract surgery.

Corneal erosion: The goal of therapy is regenerating or repairing the epithelial basement membrane to restore the adhesion between the epithelium and the anterior stroma; topical lubrication therapy, bandage soft contact lenses, debridement of the epithelium and basement membrane or anterior stromal micropuncture may be useful.

Bibliography

1. Bellson FA. Optic nerve hypoplasia in chondrodysplasia punctata. J Pediatr Ophthalmol. 1977;14:144-7.
2. Conradi E. Vorzeitiges Auftreten von Knochenund Eigenartigen Verkalkungskernen bei Chondrodystrophia Fotalis Hypoplastica. Histologische un Rontgenuntersuchungen. Jahrb Kinderhk. 1914; 80:86.
3. Happle R. Cataracts as a marker of genetic heterogeneity in chondrodysplasia punctata. Clin Genet. 1981;19:64-6.
4. Massey JY, Roy FH. Ocular manifestations of Conradi disease. Arch Ophthalmol. 1974;92:524-6.
5. Pryde PG, Bawle E, Brandt F, et al. Prenatal diagnosis of nonrhizomelic chondrodysplasia punctata (Conradi-Hunermann syndrome). Am J Med Genet. 1993;47:426-31.
6. Spierer A, Neumann D. Corneal changes in chondrodysplasia punctata syndrome. Ann Ophthalmol. 1993;25:356-8.

347. CONTACT DERMATITIS (DERMATITIS VENENATA)

General

Reaction of skin due to contact with foreign material; inflammatory disorder of the skin that may result from immunologic hypersensitivity (allergic contact dermatitis) or cutaneous injury not involving immunologic mechanisms (irritant contact dermatitis) from offending topical agents.

Ocular

Keratoconjunctivitis; chemosis; leukoma; corneal ulcer; pruritus of lids.

Clinical

Dermatitis; itching; erythema; vesiculation; edema with weeping and crusting.

Laboratory

Diagnosis is made by clinical findings.

Treatment

Adequate hygiene and avoidance of the contactant may be helpful. Many cases of localized mild contact dermatitis respond well to cool compresses and adequate wound care. Antibiotic therapy may be necessary for secondary infection. Low-strength topical steroids, such as hydrocortisone, may be effective in decreasing inflammation and symptoms associated with very mild contact dermatitis. Systemic steroids are the mainstay of therapy in acute episodes of severe extensive allergic contact dermatitis.

Additional Resource

1. Elston DM (2011). Pediatric Contact Dermatitis. [online] Available from http://www.emedicine.com/ped/TOPIC2569.HTM [Accessed April, 2012].

348. CONVERGENCE INSUFFICIENCY SYNDROME (ASTHENOVERGENCE OF STUTTERHEIM)

General

An exodeviation that is greater at near distances than at far ones; inadequate accommodative and fusional convergence impulses; prevalence is generally considered to be low in children under age 10 years and higher in females.

Ocular

Burning, itching, blurred vision; diplopia; difficulty in following moving objects; astigmatism; decreased visual acuity; exotropia; hypermetropia; orthotropia.

Clinical

Headache; associated with thyroid eye disease.

Laboratory

Diagnosis is made by clinical findings.

Treatment

Orthoptics, nearpoint of convergent exercises, base out prisms and base in prism for near only.

Bibliography

1. Burke JP, Shipman TC, Watts MT. Convergence insufficiency in thyroid eye disease. J Pediatr Ophthalmol Strabismus. 1993;30:127-9.
2. Roy FH, Fraunfelder FW, Fraunfelder FT. Roy and Fraunfelder's Current Ocular Therapy, 6th edition. Philadelphia: WB Saunders; 2008.
3. Harley RD (Ed). Pediatric Ophthalmology, 4th edition. Philadelphia: WB Saunders; 1998.
4. Norm MS. Convergence insufficiency: incidence in ophthalmic practice. Results of orthoptic treatment. Acta Ophthalmol. 1966;44:132-8.

---

349. COOLEY ANEMIA (THALASSEMIA; THALASSEMIA MAJOR; THALASSEMIA MINOR)

General

Autosomal dominant in synthesis of the alpha or beta chain of hemoglobin; most prevalent in Mediterranean and Oriental populations.

Ocular

Retinal hemorrhages; angioid streaks; macular vascular abnormalities; pigmented chorioretinal scars (black sunbursts); occlusion of peripheral retinal arteries; vitreous hemorrhages.

Clinical

Hemolytic anemia; hypochromic anemia.

Laboratory

Blood-hypochromic, microcystic anemia.

Treatment

The goals of medical therapy are correction of anemia, suppression of erythropoiesis and inhibition of increased GI iron.

Additional Resource

1. Takeshita K (2011). Beta Thalassemia. [online] Available from http://www.emedicine.com/med/TOPIC438.HTM [Accessed April, 2012].

---

350. CORNEA PLANA

General

Autosomal dominant; may be inherited as autosomal dominant or recessive.

Ocular

Hyperopia; hazy corneal limbus; opacities in corneal parenchyma and marked arcus; posterior embryotoxon; iris and lens abnormalities.

Clinical

Associated with epidermolysis bullosa dystrophica.

Laboratory

Diagnosis is made by clinical findings.

Treatment

Medical treatment includes the use of hyperosmotic drops, nonsteroidal and steroid eye drops. Corneal transplant may be necessary.

Bibliography

1. Duane TD. Clinical Ophthalmology. Philadelphia: JB Lippincott; 1987.
2. Hemady RK, Blum S, Sylvia BM. Duplication of the lens, hourglass cornea, and cornea plana. Arch Ophthalmol. 1993;111:303.
3. McKusick VA. Mendelian Inheritance in Man: A Catalog of Human Genes and Genetic Disorders, 12th edition. Baltimore: The Johns Hopkins University Press; 1998.
4. McKusick-Nathans Institute for Genetic Medicine, Johns Hopkins University and National Center for Biotechnology Information, National Library of Medicine. (2007). Online Mendelian Inheritance in Man (OMIM). [online] Available from http://www.ncbi.nlm.nih.gov/omim/ [Accessed April, 2012].
5. Sharkey JA, Kervick GN, Jackson AJ, et al. Cornea plana and sclerocornea in association with recessive epidermolysis bullosa dystrophica. Case report. Cornea. 1992;11:83-5.

351. CORNEAL ABRASIONS, CONTUSIONS, LACERATIONS AND PERFORATIONS

General

Loss of corneal epithelium from direct or indirect injury.

Clinical

None

Ocular

Photophobia, tearing, eye pain, foreign body sensation, corneal abrasion, laceration or perforation.

Laboratory

Diagnosis is made by clinical findings.

Treatment

Topical antibiotic and cycloplegic agents, pain medication, pressure patching and bandage contact lens.

Additional Resources

1. Verma A (2011). Corneal Abrasion. [online] Available from http://www.emedicine.com/oph/TOPIC247.HTM [Accessed April, 2012].
2. Giri G (2012). Corneoscleral Laceration. [online] Available from http://www.emedicine.com/oph/TOPIC108.HTM [Accessed April, 2012].

352. CORNEAL AND CONJUNCTIVAL CALCIFICATIONS

General

Eye calcium may occur as isolated conditions or in association with a variety of disease entities.

Clinical

None

Ocular

Calcific band keratopathy, calcium deposits of conjunctiva, chronic uveitis causes deposits, ocular trauma.

Laboratory

Diagnosis is made by clinical findings.

Treatment

Symptomatic treatment includes chelation of calcium salt deposit with EDTA.

Additional Resource

1. Taravella M (2011). Band Keratopathy. [online] Available from http://www.emedicine.medscape.com/article/1194813-overview [Accessed April, 2012].

353. CORNEAL CRYSTALS, MYOPATHY AND NEPHROPATHY

General

Etiology unknown; may represent an atypical variant of myotonic dystrophy.

Ocular

Retinal pigment epithelial mottling; nystagmus; deep corneal crystals; conjunctival crystals.

Clinical

Weakness and atrophy of pharyngeal, facial and intrinsic hand muscles; decreased hearing; hypertension; chronic renal disease with decreased glomerular filtration and proteinuria; asymmetrical smile; diminished gag reflex; chronic serous otitis media.

Laboratory

Diagnosis is made by clinical findings.

Treatment

PTK can be used to treat subepithelial crystals and penetrating keratoplasty may be necessary.

Bibliography

1. Arnold RW, Stickler GB, Bourne WM, et al. Corneal crystals, myopathy and nephropathy: a new syndrome? J Pediatr Ophthalmol Strabismus. 1987;24:151-5.
2. Reiss GR, Campbell RJ, Bourne WM. Infectious crystalline keratopathy. Surv Ophthalmol. 1986;31: 69-72.

354. CORNEAL DYSTROPHY, GRANULAR TYPE (GROENOUW TYPE I CORNEAL DYSTROPHY)

General

Autosomal dominant; hyaline degeneration with absence of acid mucopolysaccharide deposition; autosomal dominant with complete penetrance; evidence links it with chromosome 5q; Avellino dystrophy is a variant of granular corneal dystrophy with lattice changes.

Ocular

Grayish-white granules in a disk-shaped area of central cornea; hyaline material separates epithelium from Bowman's membrane; keratoconus.

Clinical

None

Laboratory

Diagnosis is made by clinical findings.

Treatment

If recurrent corneal erosions occur despite medical therapy, then excimer laser phototherapeutic keratectomy (PTK) may be considered. If deep opacities are causing significant visual symptoms, PK or DALK may be required.

Additional Resource

1. Afshari N (2010). Granular Dystrophy. [online] Available from http://www.emedicine.com/oph/TOPIC92.HTM [Accessed April, 2012].

---

355. CORNEAL DYSTROPHY, HEREDITARY POLYMORPHOUS POSTERIOR (PCD)

General

Autosomal dominant.

Ocular

Clouding of posterior cornea; reduced number of endothelial cells; thickening and opacities of Descemet's membrane; associated with keratoconus; iridocorneal adhesions; glassy membranes; pupillary ectropion (rare).

Clinical

None

Laboratory

Diagnosis is made by clinical findings.

Treatment

Keratoconus: Spectaclce correction, hard contacts and avoid eye rubbing may be useful. If hydrops occurs discontinue contact lens, use NaC1 drops and ointment, and short-term steroids may be beneficial. As the disease advances penetrating keratoplasty, deep anterior lamellar keratoplasty, intacs with laser grooves or collagen stabilization may be necessary.

Bibliography

1. Driver PJ, Reed JW, Davis RM. Familial cases of keratoconus associated with posterior polymorphous dystrophy. Am J Ophthalmol. 1994;118: 256-7.
2. Laganowski HC, Sherrard ES, Muir MG, et al. Distinguishing features of the iridocorneal endothelial syndrome and posterior polymorphous dystrophy: value of endothelial specular microscopy. Br J Ophthalmol. 1991;75:212-6.
3. McKusick VA. Mendelian Inheritance in Man: A Catalog of Human Genes and Genetic Disorders, 12th edition. Baltimore: The Johns Hopkins University Press; 1998.
4. McKusick-Nathans Institute for Genetic Medicine, Johns Hopkins University and National Center for Biotechnology Information, National Library of Medicine. (2007). Online Mendelian Inheritance in Man (OMIM). [online] Available from http://www.ncbi.nlm.nih.gov/omim [Accessed April, 2012].
5. Rodrigues MM, Sun T, Krachmer J, et al. Posterior polymorphous corneal dystrophy: recent developments. Birth Defects Orig Artic Ser. 1982;18: 479-91.
6. Sekundo W, Lee WR, Kirkness CM, et al. An ultrastructural investigation of an early manifestation of the posterior polymorphous dystrophy of the cornea. Ophthalmology. 1994;101:1422-31.

356. CORNEAL DYSTROPHY, LATTICE TYPE (BIBER-HAAB-DIMMER DYSTROPHY; LATTICE CORNEAL DYSTROPHY, LCD; LATTICE DYSTROPHY TYPE I)

General

Autosomal dominant; progression to severe visual impairment by fifth or sixth decade.

Ocular

Grayish lines between the centers of cornea and periphery; rounded dots scattered over the cornea; elongated deposits that form reticular pattern in corneal stoma; keratoconus.

Clinical

Secondary form of inherited localized amyloidosis inherited as an autosomal dominant trait with low penetrance.

Laboratory

Diagnosis is made by clinical findings.

Treatment

Excessive corneal erosions can be treated with PTK. If the visual acuity drops and the opacities are deep, a lamellar or full-thickness corneal transplant can be performed. Although the success rate for a corneal transplant is very high, lattice deposits can recur. DALK may also be an option.

Additional Resource

1. Afshari N (2010). Lattice Dystrophy. [online] Available from http://www.emedicine.com/oph/TOPIC93.HTM [Accessed April, 2012].

357. CORNEAL DYSTROPHY, MACULAR TYPE (GROENOUW TYPE II CORNEAL DYSTROPHY)

General

Autosomal recessive; onset in the first decade, between 5 and 9 years of age; progressive; acid mucopolysaccharides found in corneal fibroblasts; it has been suggested that the defect may not be limited to the cornea.

Ocular

Minute gray, punctate opacities; reduced corneal sensitivity; photophobia; foreign body sensations; recurrent corneal erosions; keratoconus.

Clinical

Defect in metabolism of glycoprotein processing.

Laboratory

Diagnosis is made by clinical findings.

Treatment

Once the acute episode of recurrent corneal erosion resolves, preventive treatment may include sodium chloride 5% drops or artificial tear lubricating drops during the day and sodium chloride 5% ointment or lubricating ointment at bedtime. Excessive corneal erosions or a mild visual decrease can be treated with excimer laser PTK. If visual acuity drops and the opacities are deep, lamellar or full-thickness corneal transplantation can be performed.

Additional Resource

1. Afshari N (2010). Macular Dystrophy. [online] Available from http://www.emedicine.com/oph/TOPIC94.HTM [Accessed April, 2012].

358. CORNEAL DYSTROPHY, MEESMANN EPITHELIAL (MEESMANN EPITHELIAL DYSTROPHY OF CORNEA)

General

Autosomal dominant; rare; onset in the first year of life; possible that a disturbance of the cytoplasmic ground substance results in cellular homogenization with cyst formation.

Ocular

Myriads of fine punctate opacities in epithelium and Bowman's membrane of cornea; thickening of the epithelial basement membrane of cornea; keratoconus.

Clinical

None

Laboratory

Diagnosis is made by clinical findings.

Treatment

Usually not treatment. Bandage contact lens can be used to reduce discomfort and reduce visual loss.

Bibliography

1. Tremblay M, Dubé I. Meesmann's corneal dystrophy: ultrastructural features. Can J Ophthalmol. 1982;17:24-8.
2. Fine BS, Yanoff M, Pitts E, et al. Meesmann's epithelial dystrophy of cornea. Am J Ophthalmol. 1977;83:633-42.
3. McKusick VA. Mendelian Inheritance in Man: A Catalog of Human Genes and Genetic Disorders, 12th edition. Baltimore: The Johns Hopkins University Press; 1998.
4. McKusick-Nathans Institute for Genetic Medicine, Johns Hopkins University and National Center for Biotechnology Information, National Library of Medicine. (2007). Online Mendelian Inheritance in Man (OMIM). [online] Available from http://www.ncbi.nlm.nih.gov/omim [Accessed April, 2012].

359. CORNEAL ECTASIA

General

Thining of the cornea, usually inferior, most frequently following refractive surgery such as LASIK or PRK.

Clinical

None

Ocular

Irregular astigmatism, decreased visual acuity, keratoconus, thin corneal bed.

Laboratory

Corneal topography, videokeratography.

Treatment

Rigid gas permeable contact lens may be useful. Intacs or corneal collagen cross-linking may be beneficial. Penetrating keratopathy or DSEK may be necessary.

Bibliography

1. Duffey RJ, Hardten DR, Lindstrom RL, et al. Ectasia after refractive surgery. Ophthalmology. 2008;115:1849-50.

2. Reznik J, Salz JJ, Klimava A. Development of unilateral corneal ectasia after PRK with ipsilateral preoperative forme fruste keratoconus. J Refract Surg. 2008;24:843-7.
3. Raecker ME, Erie JC, Patel SV, et al. Long-term keratometric changes after penetrating keratoplasty for keratoconus and Fuchs endothelial dystrophy. Trans Am Ophthalmol Soc. 2008;106:187-93.

360. CORNEAL EDEMA (BULLOUS KERATOPATHY, EPITHELIAL EDEMA, STROMAL EDEMA)

General

Corneal edema may be caused by endothelial dysfunction, corneal hypoxia and elevated intraocular pressure (IOP).

Clinical

None

Ocular

Swelling of cornea, loss of vision, pain.

Laboratory

Diagnosis is made by clinical findings.

Treatment

Control IOP, hypertonic salt solution or ointment, soft contact lens, anterior stromal puncture or conjunctival flap, phototherapeutic keratectomy (PTK), hairdryer held at arm's length and posterior lamellar keratoplasty.

Additional Resource

1. Taravella M (2012). Postoperative Corneal Edema. [online] Available from http://www.emedicine.com/oph/TOPIC64.HTM [Accessed April, 2012].

361. CORNEAL FOREIGN BODY

General

Foreign body lodged in the corneal epithelium usually metal, glass or organic material; may be superficial or embedded. Seen in males more frequently than females, secondary to their activities.

Clinical

None

Ocular

Pain, photophobia, tearing, conjunctival and ciliary injection; epithelial defect; corneal edema; rust ring with metallic injury.

Laboratory

Slit lamp examination; Seidel test; and if intraocular involvement is suspected B-scan, orbital CT scan and ultrasound biomicroscopy.

Treatment

Removal with a sterile spud or needle under topical anestheia; if a rust ring remains a rust ring drill may be used. The patient is treated with antibiotics, cycloplegics and a pressure patch or bandage contact lens.

Additional Resource

1. Bashour M (2010). Corneal Foreign Body Treatment & Management. [online] Available from http://www.emedicine.medscape.com/article/1195581-treatment [Accessed April, 2012].

362. CORNEAL GRAFT REJECTION OR FAILURE

General

Five-year failure rate for grafts is approximately 35% most are do to rejection; immunologic response of the host to the donor corneal tissue; more frequent in individuals under the age of 60.

Clinical

None

Ocular

Decreased visual acuity, redness, irritation, photophobia; epithelial, stromal and endothelial edema.

Laboratory

Diagnosis is made by clinical findings.

Treatment

Topical corticosteroids are used aggressively; subconjunctival injections of corticosteroids; systemic corticosteroids. Intraocular pressure must be monitored and if the pressure becomes elevated glaucoma medication will be necessary.

Additional Resource

1. Jacobs J (2010). Corneal Graft Rejection. [online] Available from http://www.emedicine.medscape. com/article/1193505-overview [Accessed April, 2012].

363. CORNEAL HYPESTHESIA, FAMILIAL

General

Autosomal dominant; decreased corneal sensation, reflex tearing, blinking and foreign body sensation.

Ocular

Punctate epithelial erosions; corneal edema; neurotrophic keratitis; corneal ulcers; poor blinking; decreased tearing; decreased corneal sensation.

Clinical

Trigeminal anesthesia; hypoplastic trigeminal nerves and gasserian ganglia.

Laboratory

Diagnosis is made by clinical findings.

Treatment

Stage 1: Punctate keratopathy—treated with intermittent patching. Oral tetracyclines and discontinuing contact lens may be helpful.

Stage 2: Epithelial detachment—atropine, Blenderm or temporary tarsorrhaphy. Inject botulism toxin into the levator palpebrae superioris.
Stage 3: Closure of lid—atropine, botulism toxin, local antibiotics and systemic antibiotics. Permanent tarsorrhaphy.

Bibliography

1. McKusick VA. Mendelian Inheritance in Man: A Catalog of Human Genes and Genetic Disorders, 12th edition. Baltimore: The Johns Hopkins University Press; 1998.
2. McKusick-Nathans Institute for Genetic Medicine, Johns Hopkins University and National Center for Biotechnology Information, National Library of Medicine. (2007). Online Mendelian Inheritance in Man (OMIM). [online] Available from http://www.ncbi.nlm.nih.gov/omim [Accessed April, 2012].
3. Purcell JJ, Krachmer JH. Familial corneal hypesthesia. Arch Ophthalmol. 1979;97:872-4.

364. CORNEAL MELT POSTOPERATIVE

General

Corneal melt may be associated with infectious, inflammatory or trophic causes. Two of the most common causes of corneal melt are: (1) herpes simplex virus and (2) retained lenticular material.

Ocular

Postoperative corneal melt can occur with almost all ocular operations. Some of the major surgeries include: pterygium surgery, refractive surgery, epikeratophakia, keratomileusis, keratoplasty, glaucoma surgeries, trabeculectomy, vitreous surgery, cataract surgery and rectus muscle surgery (rare).

Clinical

Sjögren syndrome; rheumatoid arthritis; lupus.

Laboratory

Diagnosis is made by clinical findings.

Treatment

Frequent lubrication with drops and ointment and closely monitored for the development of hypopyon which would indicate bacterial, viral or fungal infection. If infection should develop topical, systemic and intraocular antibiotics may be necessary. If corneal continues to thin, corneal gluing may be necessary. Causative factor, such as rheumatoid arthritis or lupus, should be identified and treated.

Additional Resource

1. Verma A (2011). Postoperative Corneal Melt. [online] Available from http://www.emedicine.medscape.com/article/1193347-overview [Accessed April, 2012].

365. CORNEAL MUCOUS PLAQUES

General

Abnormal collections of a mixture of mucus, epithelial cells and proteinaceous and lipoidal material adhering to cornea.

Clinical

None

Ocular

Corneal mucous plaque.

Laboratory

Diagnosis is made by clinical findings.

Treatment

Lubricants for dry eyes, cyclosporine A, steroids and nonsteroidal anti-inflammatory agents may also be necessary.

Additional Resource

1. Graham RH (2012). Corneal Mucous Plaques. [online] Available from http://www.emedicine.com/oph/TOPIC682.HTM [Accessed April, 2012].

366. CORNEAL NEOVASCULARIZATION

General

Pathologic state in which new blood vessels extending in the corneal stroma from trauma, inflammation, infection, toxic insults, and underlying inherited corneal dystrophy or degeneration.

Clinical

None

Ocular

Vessel ingrowth into the cornea, ocular irritation.

Laboratory

Diagnosis is made by clinical findings.

Treatment

Observation, eliminate cause, topical steroid drops, reduce time individual uses contact lens, corneal laser photocoagulation.

Additional Resource

1. Weissman BA (2011). Neovascularization, Corneal, CL-Related. [online] Available from http://www.emedicine.com/oph/TOPIC466.HTM [Accessed April, 2012].

367. CORNEAL SNOWFLAKE DYSTROPHY

General

Autosomal dominant; prevalence of green irides.

Ocular

Star-shaped chromatophore-like cells attached to anterior lens capsule; Bitot spots; white flecks on endothelium and Descemet's membrane.

Clinical

Lactose intolerance; malabsorption of fat; vitamin A deficiency; dry skin; nevi; freckles.

Laboratory

Diagnosis is made by clinical findings.

Treatment

Sodium chloride drops or ointment.

Bibliography

1. Meretoja J. Inherited corneal snowflake dystrophy with oculocutaneous pigmentation disturbances and other symptoms. Ophthalmologica (Basel). 1985;191:197-205.
2. Meretoja J. Inherited syndrome with corneal snowflake dystrophy, oculocutaneous pigmentary disturbances, pseudoexfoliation and malabsorption. Ophthalmic Res. 1987;19:245-54.

368. CORNEAL ULCER (BACTERIAL CORNEAL ULCERS, BACTERIAL KERATITIS)

General

Rapid progression with corneal destruction within 48 hours. Predisposing factors include contact lens wearers, trauma, contaminated ocular medications.

Clinical

None

Ocular

Corneal ulceration, stromal abscess formation and anterior segment inflammation.

Laboratory

Chocolate agar plate, Gram stain, blood agar plate, brain-heart infusion broth, meat-glucose broth, Giemsa stain, Sabouraud's dextrose agar (fungus).

Treatment

Fluoroquinoline

Additional Resource

1. Murillo-Lopez FH (2011). Bacterial Keratitis. [online] Available from http://www.emedicine.com/oph/TOPIC98.HTM [Accessed April, 2012].

369. CORNEAL ULCERATION AND ULCERATIVE KERATITIS

General

Although corneal ulcers may at times be sterile, most are infectious. Bacterial ulcers occur generally after trauma to the epithelium, thereby providing an entry to bacteria. Ulcerative keratitis is a complication of rheumatoid arthritis that can lead to corneal destruction and loss of vision.

Clinical

Rheumatoid arthritis, herpes simplex, varicella-zoster viruses.

Ocular

Corneal melt, corneal scarring and vision loss.

Laboratory

Corneal scraping to identify the underlying organism, rheumatoid arthritis evaluation.

Treatment

Corneal cultures may be taken and treatment initiated. Treatment includes a broad spectrum of antibiotics and cycloplegic drops.

Additional Resource

1. Mills TJ (2011). Corneal Ulceration and Ulcerative Keratitis in Emergency Medicine. [online] Available from http://www.emedicine.medscape.com/article/798100-overview [Accessed April, 2012].

370. CORNEO-DERMATO-OSSEOUS SYNDROME (CDO SYNDROME; CORNEAL DYSTROPHY, EPITHELIAL WITH SKIN AND SKELETAL CHANGES)

General

Autosomal dominant; similar lesions of palms, soles and cornea occur in Richner-Hanhart syndrome.

Ocular

Epithelial and stromal corneal changes; photophobia; keratoconus.

Clinical

Palmoplantar hyperkeratosis; brachydactyly, short stature; premature birth; soft teeth.

Laboratory

Diagnosis is made by clinical findings.

Treatment

Usually not treatment.

Keratoconus: Spectacle correction, hard contacts and avoid eye rubbing may be useful. If hydrops occurs discontinue contact lens, use NaCl drops and ointment, patching and short course of steroids. As the disease advances penetrating keratoplasty, deep anterior lamellar keratoplasty, intacs with laser grooves or collagen stabilization of cornea.

Bibliography

1. McKusick VA. Mendelian Inheritance in Man: A Catalog of Human Genes and Genetic Disorders, 12th edition. Baltimore: The Johns Hopkins University Press; 1998.
2. McKusick-Nathans Institute for Genetic Medicine, Johns Hopkins University and National Center for Biotechnology Information, National Library of Medicine. (2007). Online Mendelian Inheritance in Man (OMIM). [online] Available from http://www.ncbi.nlm.nih.gov/omim [Accessed April, 2012].
3. Stern JK, Lubinsky MS, Durrie DS, et al. Corneal changes, hyperkeratosis, short stature, brachydactyly, and premature birth: a new autosomal dominant syndrome. Am J Med Genet. 1984;18:67-77.

371. CORTICOSTEROID INDUCED GLAUCOMA

General

Oral, inhaled, topical and periocular corticosteroids can cause elevated IOP.

Clinical

None

Ocular

Open-angle glaucoma secondary to the use of corticosteroids.

Laboratory

Diagnosis is made by clinical findings.

Treatment

Discontinue the use of steroids if possible, use antiglaucoma agents, filter surgery may be effective.

Additional Resource

1. Rhee DJ (2012). Drug-Induced Glaucoma. [online] Available from http://www.emedicine.com/oph/TOPIC124.HTM [Accessed April, 2012].

372. COSTEN SYNDROME (TEMPOROMANDIBULAR JOINT SYNDROME)

General

Dental malocclusion; overaction of jaw joint followed by the development of a loose joint due to absorption of the meniscus, condyles and bone.

Ocular

Headaches; facial pain.

Clinical

Severe neuralgia; "full" ear sensation with reduced hearing; tinnitus; dizziness; associated with vertigo.

Laboratory

X-ray of the TMJ joint.

Treatment

Consult dental specialist.

Bibliography

1. Chole RA, Parker WS. Tinnitus and vertigo in patients with temporomandibular disorder. Arch Otolaryngology Head Neck Surg. 1992;118:817-21.
2. Costen JB. A syndrome of ear and sinus symptoms dependent upon disturbed function of the temporomandibular joint. 1934. Ann Otol Rhinol Laryngol. 1997;106:805-19.
3. Freese AS. Costen's syndrome: a reinterpretation. AMA Arch Otolaryngol. 1959;70:309-14.

373. COWDEN DISEASE (MULTIPLE HAMARTOMA SYNDROME)

General

Autosomal dominant; *PTEN* gene; tumor suppressor gene.

Ocular

Cataract; angoid streaks; myopia; multiple trichilemmomas of eyelids.

Clinical

Malignancies of breast, thyroid, ovary, uterus, colon or bladder; seizures; tremor; mental retardation; cerebellar gangliocytoma.

Laboratory

Monitor patients closely using appropriate laboratory procedures. Annual or biannual mammograms, chest radiograph thyroid scans, MRI if CNS symptoms are present, barium swallow and ultrasound of the testes are all useful if the prompt symptoms are present.

Treatment

Consult specialists as determined necessary by laboratory tests and physical examination.

Additional Resource

1. Adkisson K (2010). Cowden Disease (Multiple Hamartoma Syndrome). [online] Available from http://www.emedicine.com/derm/TOPIC86.HTM [Accessed April, 2012].

374. CRANIAL NERVES, CONGENITAL PARESIS

General

Autosomal recessive; damage to peripheral nerve and brainstem.

Ocular

Paralysis of pupillary sphincter; oculomotor synkinesis; ptosis; exotropia; hypotropia; amblyopia; diplopia.

Clinical

Vascular lesion from damage to peripheral nerve and brainstem; generalized developmental delay; seizures; facial paralysis; malformed external ears; abnormalities of motor system of arms and legs.

Laboratory

Diagnosis is made by clinical findings.

Treatment

Ptosis: If visual acuity is affected most cases require surgical correction, and there are several procedures that may be used including levator resection, repair or advancement and Fasanella-Servat.

Strabismus: Equalized vision with correct refractive error; surgery may be helpful in patient with diplopia.

Bibliography

1. Balkan R, Hoyt CS. Associated neurologic abnormalities in congenital third nerve palsies. Am J Ophthalmol. 1984;97:315-9.
2. McKusick VA. Mendelian Inheritance in Man: A Catalog of Human Genes and Genetic Disorders, 12th edition. Baltimore: The Johns Hopkins University Press; 1998.
3. McKusick-Nathans Institute for Genetic Medicine, Johns Hopkins University and National Center for Biotechnology Information, National Library of Medicine. (2007). Online Mendelian Inheritance in Man (OMIM). [online] Available from http://www.ncbi.nlm.nih.gov/omim [Accessed April, 2012].

---

375. CRANIAL NERVES, RECURRENT PARESIS

General

Autosomal recessive; rare, recurrent episodes of Bell palsy and external ophthalmoplegia; lack of iridoplegia distinguishes it from aneurysm.

Ocular

External ophthalmoplegia; III nerve palsy.

Clinical

Bell palsy; diabetes; polycythemia.

Laboratory

Check for diabetes and polycythemia.

Treatment

Prisms may be useful for small deviations. Botulinum toxin may also be useful. For deviation greater than 15 prism diopters, strabismus surgery may be required.

Bibliography

1. Currie S. Familial oculomotor palsy with Bell's palsy. Brain. 1970;93:193-8.
2. McKusick VA. Mendelian Inheritance in Man: A Catalog of Human Genes and Genetic Disorders, 12th edition. Baltimore: The Johns Hopkins University Press; 1998.
3. McKusick-Nathans Institute for Genetic Medicine, Johns Hopkins University and National Center for Biotechnology Information, National Library of Medicine. (2007). Online Mendelian Inheritance in Man (OMIM). [online] Available from http://www.ncbi.nlm.nih.gov/omim [Accessed April, 2012].

376. CRANIO-ORO-DIGITAL SYNDROME (FACIO-PALATO-OSSEOUS SYNDROME; FPO; OTOPALATODIGITAL SYNDROME; OPD II SYNDROME)

General

Sex-linked; can occur as a sporadic condition.

Ocular

Downward-slanting palpebral fissures (antimongoloid obliquity).

Clinical

Microcephaly; small mouth; midface hypoplasia; cleft palate; flexed, overlapping fingers with syndactyly of digits 3 and 4; syndactyly of toes 2 and 5; bifid uvula; slight deviation of the terminal phalanges of the third fingers; radial deviation of the terminal phalanx of the right fourth finger; short first toe and long second toe; short first metacarpal; extra bone in the capitate-hamate complex; small thorax; bowed limbs with absent fibula; mild frontal bossing; conductive hearing impairment; flat facies; broad nasal base; wavy irregular clavicles and ribs; widely spaced eyes; prominent forehead.

Laboratory

Diagnosis is made by clinical findings.

Treatment

Ocular/None.

Additional Resource

1. Patel PK (2012). Orthognathic Surgery. [online] Available from http://www.emedicine.com/plastic/TOPIC177.HTM [Accessed April, 2012].

377. CRANIOCERVICAL SYNDROME (WHIPLASH INJURY)

General

Disturbed accommodation is due to a central lesion rather than a peripheral lesion of the ciliary muscle; Horner syndrome observed where a palsy of the cervical sympathetics occurs (see Horner Syndrome).

Ocular

General ocular pain; enophthalmos; mild ptosis; reduced ability to accommodate; disturbance in ocular movements; primarily those extraocular muscles innervated by the oculomotor nerve are involved; convergence insufficiency; nystagmus (gaze direction and vestibular, central, peripheral and mixed type); vestibular impairment in more than 50% of cases; asthenopia; fogging; double vision; miosis; mydriasis; retinal arteriolar pressure may show changes in systolic and diastolic pressure and be more pronounced than changes in the brachial blood pressure; decreased stereoacuity; vitreous detachment.

Clinical

Headache; vertigo; dizziness; neck and back pain.

Laboratory

Radiographs in the neutral, flexed and extended positions, should be obtained and the degree of movement measured.

Treatment

Physical therapy, cervical fusion should be considered with great caution and only after aggressive nonsurgical care has failed, intra-articular facet joint injections and medial branch blocks.

Additional Resource

1. Windsor RE (2012). Cervical Facet Syndrome. [online] Available from http://www.emedicine.com/sports/TOPIC20.HTM [Accessed April, 2012].

378. CRANIOCLEIDODYSOSTOSIS SYNDROME (CLEIDOCRANIAL DYSOSTOSIS SYNDROME; HULKCRANTZ ANOSTEOPLASIA; MARIE-SAINTON SYNDROME; MUTATIONAL DYSOSTOSIS SYNDROME; SCHEUTHAURER SYNDROME)

General

Autosomal dominant; hypoplastic dysostosis of the skull; shows brachycephaly or platycephaly.

Ocular

Proptosis (unilateral); prominent orbital ridges; greater vertical diameter of the orbit compared with horizontal diameter; hypertelorism; anti-mongoloid palpebral fissure.

Clinical

Saddle nose; prominent forehead (frontal bossing); hypoplasia of facial bones and clavicles; high arched palate and protruding jaw; oligodontia; pathologic fractures; hyperlaxia of joints; kyphoscoliosis and spina bifida; scoliosis; hemiplegia; spastic paraplegia; mental deficiency; psychosis; incomplete closure of fontanelles; dwarfism; epilepsy; hypoplasia/aplasia of nasal bones; high and narrow orbital opening; absent or diminished paranasal sinuses; small sella; skeletal immaturity due to defect in bone remodeling.

Laboratory

Diagnosis is made by clinical findings.

Treatment

Ocular lubricants are beneficial for control of the corneal exposure.

Bibliography

1. Gorlin RJ, Cervenka J. Syndrome of facial clefting. Scand J Plast Reconstr Surg. 1974;8:13-25.
2. Jensen BL. Cleidocranial dysplasia: craniofacial morphology in adult patients. J Craniofac Genet Dev Biol. 1994;14:163-76.
3. Marie P, Sainton P. Sur la Dysostose Cleido-Cranienne Hereditaire. Bull Soc Med Hop Paris. 1898;15:436.
4. McKusick VA. Mendelian Inheritance in Man: A Catalog of Human Genes and Genetic Disorders, 12th edition. Baltimore: The Johns Hopkins University Press; 1998.
5. McKusick-Nathans Institute for Genetic Medicine, Johns Hopkins University and National Center for Biotechnology Information, National Library of Medicine. (2007). Online Mendelian Inheritance in Man (OMIM). [online] Available from http://www.ncbi.nlm.nih.gov/omim [Accessed April, 2012].

379. CRANIOFACIAL, DEAFNESS, HAND SYNDROME

General

Autosomal dominant.

Ocular

Hypertelorism

Clinical

Flat facial profile; hypoplastic nose with slitlike nares; hearing loss; ulnar deviation of hands.

Laboratory

Diagnosis is made by clinical findings.

Treatment

None

Bibliography

1. McKusick VA. Mendelian Inheritance in Man: A Catalog of Human Genes and Genetic Disorders, 12th edition. Baltimore: The Johns Hopkins University Press; 1998.
2. McKusick-Nathans Institute for Genetic Medicine, Johns Hopkins University and National Center for Biotechnology Information, National Library of Medicine. (2007). Online Mendelian Inheritance in Man (OMIM). [online] Available from http://www.ncbi.nlm.nih.gov/omim [Accessed April, 2012].
3. Sommer A, Young-Wee T, Frye T. Previously undescribed syndrome of craniofacial, hand anomalies, and sensorineural deafness. Am J Med Genet. 1983;15:71-7.

380. CRANIOFRONTONASAL DYSPLASIA

General

Sex-linked; unexplained higher prevalence in females.

Ocular

Down-slanting palpebral fissures; hypertelorism.

Clinical

Coronal synostosis; brachycephaly; clefting of the nasal tip; joint anomalies; longitudinally grooved fingernails; other digital anomalies.

Laboratory

Skull X-ray, ultrasound and CT are useful.

Treatment

Ocular/None.

Additional Resource

1. Podda S (2011). Craniosynostosis Management. [online] Available from http://www.emedicine.com/plastic/TOPIC534.HTM [Accessed April, 2012].

381. CRANIOMETAPHYSEAL DYSPLASIA SYNDROME (BAKWIN-KRIDA SYNDROME; FAMILIAL METAPHYSEAL DYSPLASIA; LEONTIASIS OSSEA; PYLE SYNDROME)

General

Autosomal recessive; absorption of secondary spongiosa is lacking, with resulting long-bone deformities.

Ocular

Hypertelorism

Clinical

Splaying of metaphyseal ends of long bones; thick and dense base of bony skull; absent air filling of mastoid process and paranasal sinuses; late dentition; deafness; progressive headache; vomiting; low intelligence; prominent glabella and zygomatic arch; genu valgus deformity.

Laboratory

Diagnosis is made by clinical findings.

Treatment

Ocular/None.

Additional Resource

1. Tewfik TL (2011). Manifestations of Craniofacial Syndromes. [online] Available from http://www.emedicine.com/ent/TOPIC319.HTM [Accessed April, 2012].

---

382. CRANIOPHARYNGIOMA

General

Benign congenital tumors arising from epithelial remnants of Rathke pouch; most common nonglial intracranial tumors in childhood; second most common sellar-parasellar tumor primarily in children or young adults; 35% of cases occur in patients over age 40 years.

Ocular

Paresis of third or sixth nerve; optic nerve atrophy; optic neuritis; papilledema; dilation of pupil; diplopia; hemianopsia; nystagmus; scotoma; visual field defects; visual loss.

Clinical

Hydrocephalus; infantilism; diabetes insipidus; abnormal sexual development; headache; acute aseptic meningitis.

Laboratory

Cranial CT and MRI are the current imaging standard.

Treatment

Although controversial, aggressive surgical treatment to attempt gross total resection is sometimes considered. Second option is planned limited surgery followed by radiotherapy.

Additional Resource

1. Bobustuc GC (2012). Craniopharyngioma. [online] Available from http://www.emedicine.com/neuro/TOPIC584.HTM [Accessed April, 2012].

---

383. CRANIOSTENOSIS

General

Skull deformity caused by premature fusion of cranial sutures.

Ocular

Optic atrophy; exophthalmos; strabismus; papilledema; nystagmus; ocular colobomas; swollen optic nerves; dissociated eye movements; ptosis; anisometropia; corneal exposure; amblyopia.

Clinical

Elevated cerebrospinal fluid; abnormal development of the skull.

Laboratory

Skull, spine and hand radiography are usually necessary to confirm the diagnosis.

Treatment

Neurosurgical procedure is recommended in cases of intracranial hypertension leading to further optic atrophy.

Additional Resource

1. Chen H (2011). Genetics of Crouzon Syndrome. [online] Available from http://www.emedicine.com/ped/TOPIC511.HTM [Accessed April, 2012].

384. CRANIOSYNOSTOSIS-MENTAL RETARDATION-CLEFTING SYNDROME

General

Autosomal recessive.

Ocular

Choroidal coloboma.

Clinical

Craniosynostosis; mental retardation; seizures; dysplastic kidneys; bat ears; cleft lip and palate; beaked nose; small posterior fontanelle.

Laboratory

Serial radiographs, CT, MRI.

Treatment

Surgical treatment involves cranial expansion procedures.

Additional Resource

1. Jane JA (2010). Surgery for Craniosynostosis. [online] Available from http://www.emedicine.com/med/TOPIC2897.HTM [Accessed April, 2012].

385. CRANIOTELENCEPHALIC DYSPLASIA

General

Autosomal recessive.

Ocular

Optic nerve hypoplasia.

Clinical

Frontal bone protrusion; encephalocele; craniosynostosis; developmental retardation; agenesis of the corpus callosum; lissencephaly; arhinencephaly.

Laboratory

Diagnosis is made by clinical findings.

Treatment

Ocular/None.

Bibliography

1. Hughes HE, Harwood-Nash DC, Becker LE. Craniotelencephalic dysplasia in sisters: further delineation of a possible syndrome. Am J Med Genet. 1983;14:557-65.
2. McKusick VA. Mendelian Inheritance in Man: A Catalog of Human Genes and Genetic Disorders, 12th edition. Baltimore: The Johns Hopkins University Press; 1998.
3. McKusick-Nathans Institute for Genetic Medicine, Johns Hopkins University and National Center for Biotechnology Information, National Library of Medicine. (2007). Online Mendelian Inheritance in Man (OMIM). [online] Available from http://www.ncbi.nlm.nih.gov/omim [Accessed April, 2012].

386. CRETINISM (HYPOTHYROID GOITER; HYPOTHYROIDISM; JUVENILE HYPOTHYROIDISM; MYXEDEMA)

General

Deficient thyroid function.

Ocular

Blepharitis; ptosis; enophthalmos; temporal madarosis; decreased tear secretion; glaucoma;

proptosis; optic atrophy; optic neuritis; blue dot cataract; conjunctivitis; scleritis; optic disk hemorrhage and arcuate scotoma associated with glaucoma.

Clinical

Myxedema; larynx and tongue swollen; hoarse speech; dry, yellowish skin; slow pulse; mental retardation; infertility; pericardial effusion; cardiac enlargement; physical development retarded.

Laboratory

Diagnosis is made by clinical findings.

Treatment

Blepharitis: Oral tetracyclines, omega-3 fatty acids, flax seed oil or fish oil. Ocular therapy includes eyelid scrubs, warm compresses, bacitracin ointment to lid margins, topical cyclosporine A and preservative-free lubricants.

Ptosis: If visual acuity is affected most cases require surgical correction, and there are several procedures that may be used including levator resection, repair or advancement and Fasanella-Servat.

Glaucoma: Its medication should be the first plan of action. If medication is unsuccessful, a filtering surgical procedure with or without antimetabolites may be beneficial.

Cataract: Change in glasses can sometimes improve a patient's visual function temporarily; however, the most common treatment is cataract surgery.

Bibliography

1. Lin HC, Kang JH, Jiang YD, et al. Hypothyroidism and the risk of developing open angle glaucoma. Ophthalmology. 2010;117:1960-6.

Additional Resource

1. Postellon DC (2011). Congenital Hypothyroidism. [online] Available from http://www.emedicine.com/ped/TOPIC501.HTM [Accessed April, 2012].

---

387. CREUTZFELDT-JAKOB SYNDROME (CORTICOSTRIATOSPINAL DEGENERATION; DISSEMINATED ENCEPHALOPATHY; HEIDENHAIM SYNDROME; PRESENILE DEMENTIA WITH SPASTIC PARALYSIS; PRESENILE DEMENTIA-CORTICAL DEGENERATION SYNDROME; SPASTIC PSEUDOSCLEROSIS)

General

Heredofamilial occurrence; caused by degenerative changes in cerebral cortex, basal ganglion and spinal cord; disease is progressive; begins in middle or later age; occurs in both sexes.

Ocular

Cortical blindness; myoclonic conjugate eye movements; paralysis of seventh nerve; ptosis; dyschromatopsia; homonymous hemianopsia; nystagmus; slow vertical saccades; mild demyelination of the optic nerve.

Clinical

Mental deterioration; psychosis; stupor; weakness and stiffness of extremities; slow development of pyramidal signs; loss of reflexes; tremor, rigidity; dysarthria; aphasia; ataxia; myoclonus; convulsive seizures; cerebellar ataxia decerebrate posture.

Laboratory

Diagnosis is based on clinical and biological tests.

Treatment

There is no effective therapy but discontinuing medications that cause confusion and possibly psychiatric care may be beneficial.

Additional Resource

1. Thomas FP (2010). Variant Creutzfeldt-Jakob Disease and Bovine Spongiform Encephalopathy. [online] Available from http://www.emedicine.com/neuro/TOPIC725.HTM [Accessed April, 2012].

388. CRI-DU-CHAT SYNDROME (BI DELETION SYNDROME; CAT-CRY (5p-) SYNDROME; CRYING CAT SYNDROME; LEJEUNE SYNDROME)

General

Short arm deletion of a no. 5 chromosome (5p-); increased inheritance risk; 13% have one parent with balanced translocation; female preponderance (2:1) (see Wolf Syndrome).

Ocular

Hypertelorism; epicanthal folds; antimongoloid slanting of palpebral fissures; strabismus; increased tortuosity of retinal vessels.

Clinical

High-pitched, plaintive cry by an infant (reminiscent of a crying cat); mental retardation; broad nasal root; micrognathia or retrognathia; low-set ears; simian crease; congenital heart defect; small larynx and epiglottis.

Laboratory

Conventional cytogenetic studies, skeletal radiography, MRI, echocardiography.

Treatment

No treatment exists for the underlying disorder. Correction of congenital heart defects may be indicated.

Additional Resource

1. Chen H (2011). Cri-du-chat Syndrome. [online] Available from http://www.emedicine.com/ped/TOPIC504.HTM [Accessed April, 2012].

389. CRISWICK-SCHEPENS SYNDROME (FAMILIAL EXUDATIVE VITREORETINOPATHY)

General

Familial exudative vitreoretinopathy, similar to retrolental fibroplasia; bilateral; slowly progressive; full-term babies; no oxygen therapy; autosomal dominant; may be inherited as X-linked or autosomal dominant condition.

Ocular

Posterior vitreous detachment of organized membranes of vitreous; snowflake-like opacities of vitreous; heterotropia of macula; subretinal exudates; retinal detachment; degenerative retinal changes; retinal hemorrhage; retinal folds; enophthalmos; phthisis; intraretinal exudate; vitreous hemorrhage; amblyopia; falciform retinal fold.

Clinical

Normal general development; normal birth weight.

Laboratory

Fluorescein angiography especially temporal periphery.

Treatment

Retinal detachment: Scleral buckle, pneumatic retinopexy and vitrectomy may be used to close all the breaks.

Vitreous hemorrhage: If possible the source of the bleeding needs to be isolated and treated with laser. Vitrectomy may be necessary.

Bibliography

1. Brockhurst RJ, Okamura ID, Schepens CL. Uveitis. I. Gonioscopy. Am J Ophthalmol. 1956;42:545-54.
2. Criswick VG, Schepens CL. Familial exudative vitreoretinopathy. Am J Ophthalmol. 1969;68:578-94.
3. Ebert EM, Mukai S. Familial exudative vitreoretinopathy. Int Ophthalmol Clin. 1993;33:237-47.
4. Fullwood P, Jones J, Bundey S, et al. X-linked exudative vitreoretinopathy: clinical features and genetic linkage analysis. Br J Ophthalmol. 1993;77: 168-70.
5. Nicholson DH, Galvis V. Criswick-Schepens syndrome (familial exudative vitreoretinopathy). Study of a Colombian kindred. Arch Ophthalmol. 1984;102:1519-22.
6. Plager DA, Orgel IK, Ellis FD, et al. X-linked recessive familial exudative vitreoretinopathy. Am J Ophthalmol. 1992;114:145-8.
7. van Nouhuys CE. Signs, complications, and platelet aggregation in familial exudative vitreoretinopathy. Am J Ophthalmol. 1991;111:34-41.

---

390. CROHN DISEASE (GRANULOMATOUS ILEOCOLITIS)

General

Autoimmune or hypersensitivity inflammatory change; slight prevalence in males; Jewish people most frequently affected; onset at any age; more severe in young people; remission; relapses.

Ocular

Recurrent conjunctivitis; marginal corneal ulcers; keratitis; blepharitis; dry eye; scleritis; episcleritis; iris atrophy; uveitis; pupil immobility and dilatation; macular edema; macular hemorrhages; extraocular muscles palsy; vitreal haze; retinal vasculitis; subconjunctival nodules; conjunctival ulcer; pannus; acute dacryoadenitis; orbital pseudotumor.

Clinical

Inflammatory bowel disease; abdominal distention; tenderness of abdomen; mass in right lower quadrant of abdomen; diarrhea; abdominal cramps; bloating; flatulence; weight loss; nervousness; tension; depression; pyoderma gangrenosum.

Laboratory

Test result positive for ASCA and negative for p-ANCA antigen suggests the presence of Crohn disease. CT, MRI, barium contrast studies, colonoscopy and upper endoscopy may also be useful.

Treatment

Treat diarrhea, antibiotic and anti-inflammatory drugs, antimetabolites, antitumor necrosis factor antibody, immunosuppressive agents, surgical correction for fibrostenotic obstruction may be necessary.

Additional Resource

1. Rangasamy P (2011). Crohn Disease. [online] Available from http://www.emedicine.com/med/TOPIC477.HTM [Accessed April, 2012].

391. CROME SYNDROME

General

Fatal; death usually at 4–8 months; autosomal recessive.

Ocular

Congenital cataracts.

Clinical

Epileptic seizures; mental retardation; small stature; renal tubular necrosis; encephalopathy.

Laboratory

Diagnosis is made by clinical findings.

Treatment

Cataract: Change in glasses can sometimes improve a patient's visual function temporarily; however, the most common treatment is cataract surgery.

Bibliography

1. Crome L, Duckett S, Franklin AW. Congenital cataracts, renal tubular necrosis and encephalopathy in two sisters. Arch Dis Child. 1963;38: 505-15.
2. McKusick VA. Mendelian Inheritance in Man: A Catalog of Human Genes and Genetic Disorders, 12th edition. Baltimore: The Johns Hopkins University Press; 1998.
3. McKusick-Nathans Institute for Genetic Medicine, Johns Hopkins University and National Center for Biotechnology Information, National Library of Medicine. (2007). Online Mendelian Inheritance in Man (OMIM). [online] Available from http://www.ncbi.nlm.nih.gov/omim [Accessed April, 2012].

392. CRONKHITE-CANADA SYNDROME

General

Hypoproteinemia; hypocalcemia.

Ocular

Nuclear and posterior subcapsular cataract.

Clinical

Gastrointestinal polyposis; hyperpigmentation of skin; hair loss; nail atrophy.

Laboratory

Universal finding is hamartomatous polyps throughout the GI tract without typically involving the esophagus and this can be determined by upper GI, colonoscopy and diagnostic endoscopy.

Treatment

Therapy is supportive which includes fluid and electrolyte replacement and maintenance of macronutrient and micronutrient requirements. Antibiotics are given orally to treat small-bowel overgrowth or parenterally to treat systemic infections. Corticosteroids are frequently used for advanced stages. Anabolic steroids are used as a last resort.

Additional Resource

1. Rabinowitz SS (2010). Pediatric Cronkhite-Canada Syndrome. [online] Available from http://www.emedicine.com/ped/TOPIC508.HTM [Accessed April, 2012].

393. CROUZON SYNDROME (CRANIOFACIAL DYSOSTOSIS; DYSOSTOSIS CRANIOFACIALIS; HEREDITARY CRANIOFACIAL DYSOSTOSIS; OXYCEPHALY; MÖBIUS-CROUZON SYNDROME; PARROT-HEAD SYNDROME)

General

Autosomal dominant; manifestations present at birth.

Ocular

Bilateral exophthalmos; hypertelorism (wide interpupillary distance); obliquity of palpebral fissures with outer canthus slanting downward; nystagmus; exotropia; upper field defects due to pressure upon the optic nerve on its lower part; bluish sclera; exposure keratitis in extreme exophthalmos; cataract; papilledema; secondary optic atrophy; corneal dystrophy; ptosis; strabismus; keratoconus.

Clinical

Prognathism; maxillary hypoplasia with short upper lip; synostosis of coronal and lambda sutures; parrot-beaked nose (psittachosrhina); widening temporal fossae; headache.

Laboratory

Skull, spine and hand radiography are usually necessary to confirm the diagnosis.

Treatment

Neurosurgical procedure is recommended in cases of intracranial hypertension leading to further optic atrophy.

Additional Resource

1. Chen H (2011). Genetics of Crouzon Syndrome. [online] Available from http://www.emedicine.com/ped/TOPIC511.HTM [Accessed April, 2012].

394. CROWDED DISK SYNDROME (BILATERAL CHOROIDAL FOLDS AND OPTIC NEUROPATHY)

Ocular

Bilateral choroidal folds; optic disk congestion; optic atrophy; hyperopia; shortened axial length.

Clinical

Elevated intracranial ruled out.

Laboratory

Fluorescein angiogram, CT or MRI when orbital tumor or inflammation suspected, ultrasonography when posterior scleritis is suspected.

Treatment

Reversal of underlying cause is the therapy of choice.

Additional Resources

1. Younge BR (2012). Anterior Ischemic Optic Neuropathy. [online] Available from http://www.emedicine.com/oph/TOPIC161.HTM [Accessed April, 2012].
2. Kim JW (2011). Compressive Optic Neuropathy. [online] Available from http://www.emedicine.com/oph/TOPIC167.HTM [Accessed April, 2012].

395. CRST SYNDROME (CALCINOSIS, RAYNAUD PHENOMENON, SCLERODACTYLY, AND TELANGIECTASIA; THIBIERGE-WEISSENBACH SYNDROME)

General

Scleroderma variant; possible autosomal dominant transmission; resembles Rendu-Osler-Weber disease; well-established association with primary biliary cirrhosis; prevalent in females; average age of onset is 45 years; reported only in whites.

Ocular

Conjunctival hyperemia; keratitis; profuse tear lysozyme; gritty, burning sensations; bilateral optic neuropathy.

Clinical

Dermal and subcutaneous calcinosis; Raynaud phenomenon; sclerodactyly; telangiectasia; calcinosis cutis; multiple intracranial aneurysms.

Laboratory

Early rise in ANA levels, particularly of the immunoglobulin G3 subclass, CT, barium studies.

Treatment

This syndrome involves both physical and psychological consequences, so a holistic approach to patient care should be taken. An evaluation of organ involvement, patient education regarding the clinical course, patient and family support, and treatment based on disease severity and organ involvement are necessary.

Additional Resource

1. Yoon JC (2012). CREST Syndrome. [online] Available from http://www.emedicine.com/derm/TOPIC88.HTM [Accessed April, 2012].

---

396. CRYOGLOBULINEMIA

General

Hematologic disorder in which a group of proteins precipitate from serum on exposure to cold but redissolve when warmed. Frequently occurs in diseases of reticuloendothelial systems, multiple myeloma and Hodgkin disease.

Ocular

Congestive retinopathy; vitreous hemorrhage; retinal detachment; rubeosis iridis; neovascular glaucoma; optic disk edema; conjunctival vascular congestion.

Clinical

Widespread intravascular coagulation in small vessels throughout body.

Laboratory

Evaluation for serum cryoglobulins, CT, chest X-ray, angiography.

Treatment

The goal of therapy is to treat underlying conditions, as well as to limit the precipitant cryoglobulin and the resultant inflammatory effects. CT, chest X-ray, angiography and nonsteroidal anti-inflammatory agents are useful. Plasmaphersis may be necessary in severe cases.

Additional Resource

1. Tritsch AM (2012). Cryoglobulinemia. [online] Available from http://www.emedicine.com/med/TOPIC480.HTM [Accessed April, 2012].

397. CRYPTOCOCCOSIS (TORULOSIS)

General

A pulmonary infection caused by *Cryptococcus neoformans*, a saprophyte found in weathered pigeon droppings, soil, and unpasteurized cow's milk; infection acquired through respiratory system and usually manifests as meningoencephalitis; higher incidence in patients with AIDS.

Ocular

Blurred or poor vision; diplopia; uveitis; papilledema; retinal detachment; retinal hemorrhage and exudates; secondary glaucoma; vitreous reaction; retinitis; proptosis; a mass over the optic nerve head; disease process can be bilateral or unilateral; cranial nerve VI (abducens) palsy; visual loss; conjunctivitis.

Clinical

Severe headache; dizziness; ataxia; vomiting; tinnitus; memory disturbances; jacksonian convulsions; fever usually is absent; occurs frequently in patients with leukemia or lymphoma.

Laboratory

The diagnosis is based on skin biopsy findings evaluated after fungal staining and culture.

Treatment

The goal of pharmacotherapy is either to terminate the infection when possible or to control the infection and to reduce morbidity when cure is not possible.

Additional Resource

1. King JW (2011). Cryptococcosis. [online] Available from http://www.emedicine.com/med/TOPIC482.HTM [Accessed April, 2012].

398. CRYPTOPHTHALMIA SYNDROME (CRYPTOPHTHALMOS SYNDACTYLY SYNDROME; FRASER SYNDROME)

General

Autosomal recessive.

Ocular

Microphthalmia; epibulbar dermoid; cryptophthalmos; enophthalmia; eyebrows partially or completely missing; skin from forehead completely covers one or both eyes, but the globes can be palpated beneath the skin; in unilateral cases, the fellow eye may present lid coloboma; buphthalmos; conjunctival sac partially or totally obliterated; absence of trabeculae, Schlemm canal and ciliary muscles; cornea is differentiated from the sclera; lens anomalies from complete absence to hypoplasia, dislocation and calcification.

Clinical

Syndactyly (finger, toes) (about 40%); coloboma of alae nasi and nostrils; urogenital abnormalities, including pseudohermaphroditism and renal hypoplasia; abnormal, bizarre hairline; narrow external auditory meatus and malformation of ossicles; cleft lip and palate may occur; atresia or hypoplasia of larynx in some cases; hoarse voice; dysplastic pinna; meatal stenosis; glottic web and subglottic stenosis.

Laboratory

Computed tomography (CT) and MRI.

Treatment

Ocular/None.

Additional Resource

1. Mamalis N (2010). Anophthalmos. [online] Available from http://www.emedicine.com/oph/TOPIC572. HTM [Accessed April, 2012].

399. CURLY HAIR-ANKYLOBLEPHARON-NAIL DYSPLASIA SYNDROME (CHANDS)

General

Autosomal recessive with pseudodominance.

Ocular

Congenital ankyloblepharon (fused eyelids).

Clinical

Curly hair; hypoplastic nails.

Laboratory

Diagnosis is made by clinical findings.

Treatment

Ankyloblepharon: Fine bands can sometimes be broken with the muscle hook or by forcibly separating the lids. This can be done in the office on small infants. More severe congenital ankyloblepharon requires surgery to separate and reconstruct the lid margins. Young children require general anesthesia.

Bibliography

1. Baughman FA. CHANDS: the curly hair-ankyloblepharon-nail dysplasia syndrome. Birth Defects Orig Artic Ser. 1971;7:100-2.

400. CURTIUS SYNDROME (ECTODERMAL DYSPLASIA WITH OCULAR MALFORMATIONS)

General

Ectodermal dysplasia of the skin with ocular involvement; occasional combinations such as hypoplasia of nails and hair, and malformation of cheeks, temples and breasts.

Ocular

Hypertelorism; sparse eyelashes (hypotrichosis); nystagmus; decreased tear secretion; congenital cataract; tapetoretinal degeneration; coloboma.

Clinical

Hidrotic ectodermal dysplasia; ichthyosis vulgaris; acrofacial syndactylic dysostosis; hypodontia.

Laboratory

Diagnosis is made by clinical findings.

Treatment

The care of affected patients depends on which ectodermal structures are involved.

Additional Resource

1. Shah KN (2012). Ectodermal Dysplasia. [online] Available from http://www.emedicine.com/derm/ TOPIC114.HTM [Accessed April, 2012].

401. CUSHING (1) SYNDROME (ADRENOCORTICAL SYNDROME; HYPERADRENALISM SYNDROME; PITUITARY BASOPHILISM; SUPRARENAL SYNDROME)

General

Excessive secretion of adrenal cortical hormones due to primary or secondary adrenal hyperplasia or induced by adrenal or extra-adrenal neoplastic tissue; common in females of childbearing age.

Ocular

Proptosis (rare); ocular muscle palsies; uncharacteristic visual field changes (not necessarily resembling bitemporal hemianopsia); optic nerve and/or chiasmal compression either unilateral or bilateral; posterior subcapsular cataract; central serous retinopathy; Lisch nodules.

Clinical

Hirsutism; obesity; "buffalo hump"; hypertension; diabetes; skin pigmentation; osteoporosis; abdominal striae; polycythemia and lymphopenia; weakness; nervousness; irritability; dysmenorrhea.

Laboratory

Diagnosis identifying the overproduction of cortisol and can be seen in inappropriately high serum or urine cortisol levels. This can be tested in urinary free cortisol level, low-dose dexamethasone suppression test, evening serum and salivary cortisol level, and dexamethasone-corticotropin releasing hormone test.

Treatment

Therapy should reduce the cortisol secretion to normal to reduce the risk of comorbidities associated with hypercortisolism. A tumor should be removed if possible. The treatment of choice for endogenous Cushing syndrome is surgical resection of the causative tumor. The primary therapy for Cushing disease is transsphenoidal surgery, and the primary therapy for adrenal tumors is adrenalectomy.

Additional Resource

1. http://www.emedicine.medscape.com/ article/117365-overview [Accessed April, 2012].

402. CUSHING (2) SYNDROME (ACOUSTIC NEUROMA SYNDROME; ANGLE TUMOR SYNDROME; CEREBELLOPONTINE ANGLE SYNDROME; PONTOCEREBELLAR ANGLE TUMOR SYNDROME)

General

Tumor involving cranial nerves V (trigeminal), VI (abducens), VII (facial), and VIII (vestibulocochlear) and brainstem; occurs between the ages of 30 and 45 years.

Ocular

Paresis orbicularis muscle (VII); paresis external rectus muscle (VI); mixed nystagmus with head tilt; palsies of extraocular muscles are accounted for by increased intracranial pressure if the aqueduct of Sylvius is closed by the growing tumor; decreased corneal reflex V (homolateral and early sign); bilateral papilledema (increased intracranial pressure).

Clinical

Deafness (homolateral); labyrinth function disturbed or lost; tinnitus; hyperesthesia of the face; homolateral facial nerve paresis (total paralysis rare); hoarseness; difficulties in swallowing; uni-lateral limb ataxia; gait ataxia; nuchal headache; emesis; facial pain, numbness and paresis; progressive unilateral hearing loss.

Laboratory

The diagnostic test for acoustic tumors is gadolinium-enhanced MRI.

Treatment

Surgical excision of the tumor, arresting tumor growth using stereotactic radiation therapy, careful serial observation.

Additional Resource

1. Kutz JW (2011). Acoustic Neuroma. [online] Available from http://www.emedicine.com/ent/TOPIC239.HTM [Accessed April, 2012].

403. CUSHING (3) SYNDROME (CHIASMAL SYNDROME)

General

Suprasellar meningioma, aneurysm in the anterior part of the circle of Willis and craniopharyngioma are the three most common lesions; usually occurs in adult patients.

Ocular

Bitemporal hemianopsia (progressive); in early stages, optic disk may appear normal or only slightly pale; later, sharp, border-lined white optic disk.

Clinical

Craniopharyngiomas; pituitary adenoma; aneurysm; chiasmal glioma; nasopharyngeal carcinoma; germinoma; glioma; choristoma; chordoma; hemangioma; leukemia; lymphoma; metastatic tumor; arteriovenous malformation; sarcoidosis; pituitary abscess; sphenoid sinus mucocele; arachnoid cyst.

Laboratory

Visual fields and ophthalmologic evaluation are critical in defining the presence of a chiasmal syndrome; neuroimaging is also useful.

Treatment

Dopamine receptor agonists, somatostatin analogs can be helpful, transsphenoidal surgery may be necessary.

Additional Resource

1. Kattah JC (2011). Pituitary Tumors. [online] Available from http://www.emedicine.com/neuro/TOPIC312.HTM [Accessed April, 2012].

404. CUTIS MARMORATA SYNDROME (MARBLE SKIN SYNDROME)

General

Prominent in children; etiology unknown; possibly a mild form of livedo reticularis; in severe cases, vessel dilation and skin changes may be permanent; occurs with exposure to cold and subsides in a warm environment; extremities and pectoral region most frequently affected.

Ocular

Congenital glaucoma; corneal and scleral thinning; staphyloma; sclerotic appearance to trabecular meshwork; corneal edema; cataracts; optic nerve atrophy; heterochromia iridium; iris anterior layer dysplasia; intraoperative suprachoroidal hemorrhage (rare).

Clinical

Bluish-red mottling of skin; spasmodic narrowing of arterioles with dilation of vessels; ulceration and scaling of skin; congenital hypothyroidism.

Laboratory

Diagnosis is made by clinical findings.

Treatment

No treatment is needed unless associated anomalies such as glaucoma, hypospadias, syndactyly, multicystic renal disease, cardiac malformation and limb asymmetry require treatment.

Additional Resource

1. Schwartz RA (2011). Cutis Marmorata Telangiectatica Congenita. [online] Available from http://www.emedicine.com/derm/TOPIC793.HTM [Accessed April, 2012].

---

405. CYSTIC FIBROSIS SYNDROME (FIBROCYSTIC DISEASE OF PANCREAS)

General

Autosomal recessive; Caucasians; lungs, pancreas and salivary glands are mainly involved.

Ocular

Ischemic retinopathy is caused by carbon dioxide retention and chronic respiratory insufficiency; vein congestion and capillary dilation around the optic nerve; retinal hemorrhages; macular degeneration; papilledema; optic atrophy; xerosis of conjunctiva; optic neuritis; abnormal pupillary responses; decreased contrast sensitivity.

Clinical

Failure to gain weight properly; recurrent pulmonary infections; salty skin; pancreatic insufficiency with malabsorption; abdominal cramps; diarrhea; increased appetite; dyspnea; chronic cough; production of viscous tenacious sputum; fever; retarded growth; delayed puberty; distended abdomen; hyperresonant chest; depressed diaphragm; clubbing of fingers.

Laboratory

The diagnosis is based pulmonary and/or gastrointestinal tract manifestations, a family history, and positive results on sweat test.

Treatment

Because of the complex and multisystemic involvement the need for care by specialists, treatment and follow-up care at specialty centers with multidisciplinary care teams is recommended.

Additional Resource

1. Sharma GD (2012). Cystic Fibrosis. [online] Available from http://www.emedicine.com/ped/TOPIC535.HTM [Accessed April, 2012].

---

406. CYSTICERCOSIS

General

Caused by *Taenia solium*.

Ocular

Tenonitis; endophthalmitis; optic atrophy; papilledema; retinal detachment; retinal hemorrhages and exudates; vitreal hemorrhages; hypopyon; uveitis; paresis of extraocular muscles; periretinal proliferation; cysts may be present almost anywhere in or around the eye; orbital lesion; extraocular myositis; subretinal cysticercosis; acute preseptal cellulitis.

Clinical

Dead larvae may cause muscle pain; weakness; fever; eosinophilia; calcification of tissues.

Laboratory

The enzyme immunotransfer blot assay for the detection of serum and CSF antibodies to *T. solium* is the antibody test of choice. Diagnosis of neurocysticercosis is primarily based on CT scanning or MRI results.

Treatment

Medical treatment depends on the location of the cysts and the symptoms. Live parenchymal cysts can be treated with either albendazole or praziquantel, but corticosteroids and antiseizure medications are often required in addition. Cases that do not respond to medical therapy, shunt placement, removal of large solitary cysts for decompression, and the removal of mobile cysts that cause ventricular obstruction should be considered.

Additional Resource

1. Ghadishah D (2012). Pediatric Cysticercosis. [online] Available from http://www.emedicine. com/ped/TOPIC537.HTM [Accessed April, 2012].

407. CYSTICERCOSIS (TAENIA SAGINATA AND TAENIA SOLIUM)

General

Infestation by humans of cysticercus cellulosae, the larva from *Taenia solium* or the pork tapeworm.

Clinical

Brain lesions.

Ocular

Intraocular and orbital/adnexal cysticercosis; subretinal cysticerosis; orbital myocysticercosis, subconjunctival cysticercus, retinal detachment; proliferative vitreoretinopathy.

Laboratory

Fecal sample and perianal swabbing. Radiologic exam of limbs and skull may show calcified cysts. CT and MRI of brain for other lesions.

Treatment

Paraziquantel or albendazole are drugs of choice.

Bibliography

1. Roy FH, Fraunfelder FW, Fraunfelder FT. Roy and Fraunfelder's Current Ocular Therapy, 6th edition. Philadelphia: WB Saunders; 2008.

408. CYSTINURIA

General

Caused by abnormal protein metabolism; recessive or incomplete recessive.

Ocular

Pigmentary retinopathy; gyrate atrophy.

Clinical

Impaired intestinal absorption and renal tubular reabsorption of cystine, lysine, arginine and ornithine lead to excretion of these dibasic amino acids into urine; associated with renal dwarfism, pyramidal and extrapyramidal symptoms, and deaf mutism.

Laboratory

Urinalysis, 24-hour urinalysis, sodium cyanide-nitroprusside test, renal function, CT, renal ultrasound.

Treatment

Hyperdiuresis, alkalinization, chelating agents, lithotripsy, nephrolithotomy, nephrostomy.

Additional Resource

1. Biyani CS (2012). Cystinuria. [online] Available from http://www.emedicine.com/med/TOPIC498. HTM [Accessed April, 2012].

---

409. CYSTOID MACULAR EDEMA

General

Common cause of decrease central vision, resulting from fluid accumulation in intraretinal spaces in the macular region.

Clinical

Concomitant hypertension, arteriosclerosis.

Ocular

Central vision loss.

Laboratory

Diagnosis is made by clinical findings.

Treatment

Antiprostaglandin agents, steroids, nonsteroidal anti-inflammatory drops.

Additional Resource

1. Telander DG (2010). Macular Edema, Pseudophakic (Irvine-Gass). [online] Available from http://www.emedicine.com/oph/TOPIC400. HTM [Accessed April, 2012].

---

410. CYTOMEGALIC INCLUSION DISEASE (CONGENITAL CYTOMEGALIC INCLUSION DISEASE; CYTOMEGALOVIRUS)

General

Cytomegalovirus passes transplacentally from an asymptomatic mother to fetus.

Ocular

Uveitis; cataract; optic atrophy; inclusion bodies in the aqueous humor; severe conjunctivitis; corneal opacities; microphthalmos; strabismus; dacryoadenitis; chorioretinitis; cytomegalovirus retinitis (most common cause of acquired viral retinitis, primarily because of the AIDS virus); glaucoma.

Clinical

Cerebral calcifications; microcephaly; mental retardation; inclusion bodies in the urine; spastic diplegia; seizures; cerebellar hypoplasia; intraventricular hemorrhage; hydrocephalus.

Laboratory

Antigen testing, qualitative and quantitative polymerase chain reaction, shell vial assay.

Treatment

Ganciclovir, foscarnet, acyclovir and cidofovir.

Additional Resource

1. Akhter K (2011). Cytomegalovirus. [online] Available from http://www.emedicine.com/med/TOPIC504.HTM [Accessed April, 2012].

411. CYTOMEGALOVIRUS RETINITIS

General

Ubiquitous DNA virus that infects the majority of adults and generally only an issue in immunocompromised individuals such as with AIDS, transplant and those immunosuppressive medication.

Clinical

AIDS, transplantation patients; myalgia, cervical lymphadenopathy; hepatitis.

Ocular

Decreased visual acuity; blindness; retinitis; retinal detachment; retinal breaks; necrotic retina.

Laboratory

Lab testing to determine the cause; ultrasound to evaluate for retinal detachment; dilated fundus exam.

Treatment

Intravitreal ganciclovir implant or injection may be used; retinal detachment surgery may be necessary.

Additional Resource

1. Altaweel M (2010). CMV Retinitis. [online] Available from http://www.emedicine.medscape.com/article/1227228-overview [Accessed April, 2012].

412. DACRYOADENITIS

General

Acute or chronic inflammatory enlargement of lacrimal gland is usually/generally caused by a virus; however, IgG4 systemic disease has also been linked as a cause.

Clinical

Sarcoid, Sjögren syndrome Graves' disease, lupus, Wegener granulamatosis, benign lymphoepithelial lesions.

Ocular

Orbital pain, edema of upper lid, S-shaped upper lid.

Laboratory

Computed tomography (CT)—enlarged gland.

Treatment

Determine the cause and treat, systemic steroids or antibiotics, lavage the conjunctival sac if discharge is present, ocular therapy with tear substitutes, incision of lacrimal palpebral lobe if involved.

Additional Resource

1. Singh GJ (2011). Dacryoadenitis. [online] Available from http://www.emedicine.com/oph/TOPIC594.HTM [Accessed April, 2012].

413. DACRYOCYSTITIS AND DACRYOLITH

General

Inflammation in the lacrimal sac resulting from stairs of tears in lacrimal drainage system and secondary infection by bacteria or fungus. Dacryolith is concretion of material in canaliculi or lacrimal sac.

Clinical

None

Ocular

Redness and tenderness of medial area.

Laboratory

Diagnosis is made by clinical findings.

Treatment

Warm compresses and topical antibiotics, pressure over the sac to express material into conjunctiva, topical nystatin, external dacryocystorhinostomy.

Additional Resource

1. Gilliland GD (2012). Dacryocystitis. [online] Available from http://www.emedicine.com/oph/TOPIC708.HTM [Accessed April, 2012].

414. DANBOLT-CLOSS SYNDROME
(ACRODERMATITIS ENTEROPATHICA; BRANDT SYNDROME)

General

Etiology unknown; autosomal recessive; occurs in both sexes with onset in early infancy; characterized by intermittent simultaneous occurrence of diarrhea and dermatitis with failure to thrive.

Ocular

Loss of eyebrows; blepharitis; ectropion; loss of eyelashes; photophobia; conjunctivitis; scattered superficial corneal opacities; keratitis; lacrimal punctal stenosis; corneal superficial punctate lesions, nebulous subepithelial opacities and linear epithelial erosions.

Clinical

Symmetrical skin eruptions on hands, feet, elbows, knees and buttocks usually dry up to an erythematosquamous type; glossitis and stomatitis; alopecia; paronychia with nail dystrophy; gastrointestinal disturbances; diarrhea (intermittent).

Laboratory

Determining hair, urine and parotid saliva zinc levels as well as serum alkaline phosphatase activity (which lowers later in the disease) may be helpful.

Treatment

Oral zinc supplementation per day for life.

Additional Resource

1. Dela Rosa KM (2011). Acrodermatitis Enteropathica. [online] Available from http://www.emedicine.com/derm/TOPIC5.HTM [Accessed April, 2012].

415. DANDY-WALKER SYNDROME (ATRESIA OF THE FORAMEN OF MAGENDIE)

General

Manifested in infants; malformation and stenosis of the foramina of Luschka and Magendie; dilation of fourth ventricle.

Ocular

Ptosis; sixth nerve paralysis; papilledema.

Clinical

Hydrocephalus (varies in severity) with enlargement of the skull and thinning of the bone predominantly in occipital region; loss of tendon reflexes; basilar impression; scoliosis; hydromelia.

Laboratory

Computed tomography (CT), MRI, ultrasound, angiography.

Treatment

Shunt to treat associated hydrocephalus.

Additional Resource

1. Incesu L (2011). Imaging in Dandy-Walker Malformation. [online] Available from http://www.emedicine.com/radio/TOPIC206.HTM [Accessed April, 2012].

416. DARIER-WHITE SYNDROME (DYSKERATOSIS FOLLICULARIS SYNDROME; KERATOSIS FOLLICULARIS; PSOROSPERMOSIS)

General

Unknown etiology; defect in the synthesis, organization, and maturation of tonofilament-desmosome complex; irregular dominant inheritance; both sexes equally affected, with onset in childhood; chronic but relatively benign and more aggravated in the summer.

Ocular

Conjunctival keratosis; bilateral corneal sub-epithelial infiltrations and sometimes corneal ulceration; cataract formation (rare).

Clinical

Confluent flesh-colored keratotic papules on head, neck, back, abdomen and groin; small stature; mild mental retardation; hair loss; genital hypoplasia; oral-mucosal lesions; hypertrophic flexural involvement; acral signs.

Laboratory

The *ATP2A2* gene sequencing and skin biopsy can be used to confirm the diagnosis.

Treatment

Systemic antibiotics, acyclovir, contraceptives, retinoids. Topical emollients, retinoids and 5-fluorouracil. Dermabrasion.

Additional Resource

1. Kwok PY (2010). Keratosis Follicularis (Darier Disease). [online] Available from http://www.emedicine.com/derm/TOPIC209.HTM [Accessed April, 2012].

417. DAWSON DISEASE (DAWSON ENCEPHALITIS; INCLUSION-BODY ENCEPHALITIS; SUBACUTE SCLEROSING PANENCEPHALITIS)

General

Sclerosing panencephalitis classified as a degenerative, progressive neurologic disorder caused by a measles virus infection of the central nervous system.

Ocular

Nystagmus; ptosis; papilledema; optic neuritis; macular pigmentation and degeneration; focal retinitis; ocular motor palsies; optic atrophy; preretinal vitreous membrane; exophthalmos; visual agnosia; chorioretinitis; retinal vasculitis; macular chorioretinitis.

Clinical

Chronic inflammation of brain with neuronal degeneration; gliosis; eosinophilic inclusion bodies in brain tissue; decline in intellect; behavioral changes; slurred speech; drooling; motor abnormalities; disorientation; seizures; death.

Laboratory

Refer to neurologist.

Treatment

Ptosis: If visual acuity is affected most cases require surgical correction, and there are several procedures that may be used including levator resection, repair or advancement and Fasanella-Servat.

Optic neuritis: Intravenous steroids may be used with optic neuritis or ischemic neuropathy. Stem cell treatment may be the future treatment of choice.

Bibliography

1. Fenichel GM. Subacute sclerosing panencephalitis. In: Fenichel GM (Ed). Clinical Pediatric Neurology, 2nd edition. Philadelphia: WB Saunders; 1993. p. 137.
2. Gravina RF, Nakanishi AS, Faden A. Subacute sclerosing panencephalitis. Am J Ophthalmol. 1978;86:106-9.
3. Johnston HM, Wise GA, Henry JG. Visual deterioration as presentation of subacute sclerosing panencephalitis. Arch Dis Child. 1980;55: 899-901.
4. Kovacs B, Vastag O. Fluoroangiographic picture of the acute stage of the retinal lesion in subacute sclerosing panencephalitis. Ophthalmologica. 1978;177:264-9.
5. Meyer E, Majlin M, Zonis S. Subacute sclerosing panencephalitis: clinicopathological study of the eyes. J Pediatr Ophthalmol Strabismus. 1978;15:19-23.
6. Miller JR, Jubelt B. Viral infections. In: Rowland LP (Ed). Merritt's Textbook of Neurology, 9th edition. Baltimore: Williams & Wilkins; 1995. pp. 164-5.
7. Miller NR: Walsh & Hoyt's Clinical Neuro-Ophthalmology 6th ed. Lippincott, Williams and Wilkins, Baltimore: 2004.
8. Salmon JF, Pan EL, Murray AD. Visual loss with dancing extremities and mental disturbances. Surv Ophthalmol. 1991;35:299-306.
9. Takayama S, Iwasaki Y, Yamanouchi H, et al. Characteristic clinical features in a case of fulminant subacute sclerosing panencephalitis. Brain Dev. 1994;16:132-5.
10. Vignaendra V, Lim CL, Chen ST. Subacute sclerosing panencephalitis with unusual ocular movements: polygraphic studies. Neurology. 1978;28:1052-6.
11. Zagami AS, Lethlean AK. Chorioretinitis as a possible very early manifestation of subacute sclerosing panencephalitis. Aust N Z J Med. 1991; 21:350-2.

418. DE LANGE SYNDROME (I) (BRACHMANN-DE LANGE SYNDROME; CONGENITAL MUSCULAR HYPERTROPHY CEREBRAL SYNDROME)

General

Etiology not known; autosomal recessive inheritance.

Ocular

Antimongoloid slant of palpebral fissures; mild exophthalmos; hypertrichosis of eyebrows; long eyelashes; telecanthus; ptosis; blepharophimosis; nystagmus on lateral gaze; constant coarse nystagmus; strabismus; alternating exotropia; high myopia; anisocoria; chronic conjunctivitis; blue sclera; pallor of optic disk.

Clinical

Mental retardation; growth retardation; extrapyramidal motor disturbances; multiple skeletal abnormalities with congenital muscular hypertrophy; long philtrum; thin lips; crescent-shaped mouth.

Laboratory

Molecular diagnosis with screening of the NIPBL gene, X-ray, ultrasonography, echocardiography.

Treatment

Early intervention for feeding problems, hearing and visual impairment, congenital heart disease, and urinary system abnormalities and psychomotor delay.

Additional Resource

1. Tekin M (2011). Cornelia De Lange Syndrome. [online] Available from http://www.emedicine. com/ped/TOPIC482.HTM [Accessed April, 2012].

419. DE MORSIER SYNDROME (SEPTO-OPTIC DYSPLASIA)

General

Absence of the septum pellucidum; agenesis of corpus callosum; enlargement of ventricles; infundibulum primary site of structural derangement in patients with optic nerve hypoplasia.

Ocular

Optic disk hypoplasia; bitemporal hemianopia; poor vision; nystagmus, hyperplastic primary vitreous.

Clinical

Growth retardation; pituitary insufficiency; diabetes insipidus; normal cognitive development; intact neurologic status; normal language development; late appropriate behavior; abnormal early poor motor coordination; subtle visual alterational problems; association between optic nerve hypoplasia and cerebral hemispheric abnormalities, especially schizencephaly, due to migration anomalies.

Laboratory

Computed tomography (CT) and MRI of head.

Treatment

Vitrectomy may be necessary.

Bibliography

1. Brodsky MC, Glasier CM. Optic nerve hypoplasia. Clinical significance of associated central nervous system abnormalities on magnetic resonance imaging. Arch Ophthalmol. 1993;11:66-74.

2. de Morsier G. Median craniocephalic dysraphia and olfactogenital dysplasia. World Neurol. 1962; 3:485-506.
3. Rush JA, Bajandas FJ. Septo-optic dysplasia (de Morsier syndrome). Am J Ophthalmol. 1978;86: 202-5.

4. Williams J, Brodsky MC, Griebel M, et al. Septo-optic dysplasia: the clinical insignificance of an absent septum pellucidum. Dev Med Child Neurol. 1993;35:490-501.

420. DE BARSY SYNDROME

General

Rare progeroid syndrome associated with characteristic ocular, facial, skeletal, dermatologic and neurologic abnormalities.

Ocular

Congenital corneal opacification (loss of Bowman's layer); cataracts.

Clinical

Short stature, pectus excavatum, skeletal dysplasia with short legs, multiple joint dislocations, especially involving the hands; skin redundancy (as seen in cutis laxa); midface hypoplasia; thin transparent skin with prominent superficial veins; frontal bossing and aged, progeroid facies; early death; hypotonia; mental retardation; brisk deep tendon reflexes.

Laboratory

None

Treatment

Corneal opacification: Check for elevated intraocular pressure. Medical treatment includes the use of hyperosmotic drops, nonsteroidal and steroid eye drops. Corneal transplant may be necessary.

Cataract: Change in glasses can sometimes improve a patient's visual function temporarily; however, the most common treatment is cataract surgery.

Bibliography

1. Aldave AJ, Eagle RC, Streeten BW, et al. Congenital corneal opacification in De Barsy syndrome. Arch Ophthalmol. 2001;119:285-8.
2. Bartsocas CS, Dimitriou J, Kavadias A, et al. De Barsy syndrome. Prog Clin Biol Res. 1982;104: 157-60.
3. De Barsy AM, Moens E, Dierckx L. Dwarfism, oligophrenia and degeneration of the elastic tissue in skin and cornea. A new syndrome? Helv Paediatr Acta. 1968;23:305-13.

421. DEERFLY FEVER (DEERFLY TULAREMIA; FRANCIS DISEASE; RABBIT FEVER; TULAREMIA)

General

Acute infectious disease caused by *Francisella (Pasteurella) tularensis.*

Ocular

Chemosis; conjunctivitis; corneal ulcer; endophthalmitis; dacryocystitis; optic atrophy; iris prolapse; chalazion; corneal opacity; pannus.

Clinical

Local ulcerative lesion; suppuration of regional lymph nodes; fever; prostration; myalgia; severe headache; pneumonia.

Laboratory

Diagnosis is usually based on serology results. Tularemia tube agglutination testing is the most commonly used serological test.

Treatment

Systemic antibiotics.

Additional Resource

1. Cleveland KO (2012). Tularemia. [online] Available from http://www.emedicine.com/med/TOPIC2326. HTM [Accessed April, 2012].

422. DEGOS SYNDROME (CUTANEOINTESTINAL SYNDROME; DEGOS-DELORT-TRICOT SYNDROME; KOHLMEIER-DEGOS SYNDROME; MALIGNANT ATROPHIC PAPULOSIS)

General

Rare cutaneovisceral disease; male preponderance; death occurs within a few months after diffuse eruption of skin lesions; multiple cerebral infarcts and/or thrombosis of small arteries; lymphocytic-mediated necrotizing vasculitis with mucin deposits in the dermis.

Ocular

Atrophic skin of eyelids; intermittent diplopia; conjunctiva may be atrophic; telangiectasias of conjunctiva with microaneurysms; peripheral choroiditis; papilledema has occurred with progressive central nervous system involvement; necrotic papules of lids, bulbar conjunctivae and episcleral tissues.

Clinical

Porcelain-white skin lesions (asymptomatic and diffuse); anorexia and/or weight loss; gastrointestinal involvement; peritonitis; intermittent paresthesias with early central nervous system involvement; signs of progressive cerebral and cerebellar atrophy; peripheral telangiectatic rim.

Laboratory

Magnetic resonance imaging, cerebral angiogram, EEG, CT and endoscopy of gastrointestinal tract.

Treatment

Antiplatelet drugs may reduce the number of new lesions in some patients with only skin involvement. Surgical intervention may be necessary with gastrointestinal bleeding.

Additional Resource

1. Scheinfeld NS (2011). Degos Disease. [online] Available from http://www.emedicine.com/derm/TOPIC931.HTM [Accessed April, 2012].

423. DEJEAN SYNDROME (ORBITAL FLOOR SYNDROME)

General

Usually secondary to a traumatic lesion involving the floor of the orbit.

Ocular

Enophthalmos; exophthalmos; lid hematoma; diplopia due to displacement of the globe or restricted function of the inferior rectus and/or inferior oblique muscles; orbital emphysema.

Clinical

Severe pain in superior maxillary region; numbness in area of first and second branches of trigeminal nerve; nausea and vomiting.

Laboratory

Computed tomography (CT) and MRI of orbit.

Treatment

Repair orbital floor fracture.

Bibliography

1. Roy FH. Ocular Syndromes and Systemic Diseases, 4th edition. Philadelphia: Lippincott Williams & Wilkins; 2007.

424. DEJERINE-KLUMPKE SYNDROME (KLUMPKE PARALYSIS; KLUMPKE SYNDROME; LOWER RADICULAR SYNDROME)

General

Lesion involving the inferior roots of the brachial plexus with nerves derived from the eighth cervical and first thoracic root.

Ocular

Enophthalmos; ptosis; narrowed palpebral fissure; miosis.

Clinical

Paralysis and atrophy of the small muscles of forearm and hand (flexor carpi ulnaris, flexor digitorum, interossei, thenar, hypothenar); decreased sensation or increased sensibility on the inner side of the forearm.

Laboratory

Neurologic evaluation, CT, MRI.

Treatment

Primary exploration and repair of brachial plexus. Secondary deformities may require surgical intervention and therapy.

Additional Resource

1. Bienstock A (2011). Brachial Plexus Hand Surgery. [online] Available from http://www.emedicine.com/plastic/TOPIC450.HTM [Accessed April, 2012].

425. DEJERINE-ROUSSY SYNDROME (DEJERINE-ROUSSY SYNDROME; POSTERIOR THALAMIC SYNDROME; RETROLENTICULAR SYNDROME; THALAMIC HYPERESTHETIC ANESTHESIA SYNDROME; THALAMIC SYNDROME)

General

Posterior thalamic lesion.

Ocular

Hemianopsia when the thalamogeniculate artery is thrombosed near its origin from the posterior cerebral artery, because there is involvement of the medial aspect of the lateral geniculate body; if the posterior cerebral artery is thrombosed, complete hemianopsia with macular sparing results; clinical transient acute esotropia; possible association between thalamic lesions and mononuclear supranuclear palsy; unilateral blepharospasm.

Clinical

Sensory disturbances: contralateral; hemiataxia: contralateral; hemiplegia (transient): contralateral; choreoathetoid movements: contralateral; spontaneous pain: contralateral.

Laboratory

Computed tomography (CT) scan and MRI of head.

Treatment

Consult neurosurgeon.

Bibliography

1. Barroso L, Hoyt WF. Episodic exotropia from lateral rectus neuromyotonia-appearance and remission after radiation therapy for a thalamic glioma. J Pediatr Ophthalmol Strabismus. 1993;30:56-7.
2. Dejerine J, Roussy G. Le Syndrome Thalamique. Rev Neurol. 1906;14:521-32.
3. Kulisevsky J, Avila A, Roig C, et al. Unilateral blepharospasm stemming from a thalamomesen-cephalic lesion. Mov Disord. 1993;8:239-40.
4. Miller NR: Walsh & Hoyt's Clinical Neuro-Ophthalmology 6th ed. Lippincott, Williams and Wilkins, Baltimore: 2004.
5. Scoditti U, Colonna F, Bettoni L, et al. Acute esotropia from small thalamic hemorrhage. Acta Neurol Belg. 1993;93:290-4.

426. DELETION OF CHROMOSOME 12q 15-q23

General

Interstitial deletion of chromosome 12; autosomal dominant or autosomal recessive.

Ocular

Corneal plana.

Clinical

Deletion of the *KERA* gene.

Laboratory

Chromsome studies.

Treatment

None

Bibliography

1. Tocyap ML, Azar N, Chen T, et al. Clinical and molecular characterization of a patient with an interstitial deletion of chromosome 12q15-q23 and peripheral corneal abnormalities. Am J Ophthalmol. 2006;141:566-7.

427. DEMODICOSIS

General

Demodex folliculorum and *Demodex brevis* infestation; exact role in causing blepharitis is unclear; most patients are asymptomatic.

Ocular

Blepharitis; follicular distention and hyperplasia; lid hyperemia; lid hyperkeratinization; madarosis; meibomian gland destruction; mite colonies of eyelashes and eyebrows.

Clinical

Pruritus.

Laboratory

Presence of parasites on epilated eyelashes.

Treatment

Brushed vigorously across the external lid margin, following 0.5% proparacaine instillation. Five minutes later, a solution of 70% alcohol is applied in a similar manner. This regimen is reported to successfully reduce both the symptoms and the observed number of mites by the end of 3 weekly visits. Ether and alcohol should be used with caution, and corneal contact should be prevented. Home regimen includes scrubbing the eyelids twice daily with baby shampoo diluted with water to yield a 50% dilution and applying an antibiotic ointment at night until resolution of symptoms. Discard makeup, clean sheets, check household members and pets.

Bibliography

1. Li J, O'Reilly N, Sheha H, et al. Correleation between ocular demodex infestation and serum immunoreactivity to bacillus proteins in patients with facial rosacea. Ophthalmology. 2010;117:870-7.

Additional Resource

1. Roque MR (2011). Demodicosis. [online] Available from http://www.emedicine.com/oph/TOPIC517. HTM [Accessed April, 2012].

428. DENGUE FEVER

General

Endemic over the tropics and subtropics; caused by four distinct serogroups of dengue viruses, types 1,2,3 and 4, group B arboviruses; transmitted solely by mosquitoes of the genus *Aedes*.

Ocular

Lid edema; conjunctivitis; ocular and retrobulbar pain accentuated by ocular movement; dacryoadenitis; keratitis; corneal ulcer; iritis; retinal or vitreous hemorrhages; ocular motor paresis; optic atrophy.

Clinical

Hemorrhagic fever, severe headache; backache; joint pain; rigors; insomnia; anorexia; loss of taste; epistaxis; rashes; maculopapular rash; myalgia; human infection with four serotypes of Dengue virus causing two diseases: (1) classic Dengue fever and (2) Dengue hemorrhagic fever (50% mortality).

Laboratory

Basic metabolic panel, liver function test (LFT), coagulation studies, chest X-ray, serial ultrasonography.

Treatment

A self-limited illness, and only supportive care is required. Acetaminophen may be used to treat patients with symptomatic fever. Dengue hemorrhagic fever warrant closer observation. Rehydration with intravenous fluids, plasma expander, transfusion and shock therapy may be necessary.

Additional Resource

1. Shepherd SM (2012). Dengue. [online] Available from http://www.emedicine.com/med/TOPIC528. HTM [Accessed April, 2012].

---

429. DENTAL-OCULAR-CUTANEOUS SYNDROME

General

Abnormal tooth roots; distinctive features separate this syndrome from oculodentodigital or faciodentodigital syndromes.

Ocular

Entropion lower eyelids; glaucoma (juvenile type).

Clinical

Unusual upper lip with lack of "cupid's bow" and thickening and widening of the philtrum; syndactyly; cutaneous hyperpigmentation overlying the interphalangeal joints; clinodactyly; single conical roots in all primary teeth and permanent first molars; scant body hair; horizontal ridging of fingernails.

Laboratory

X-rays.

Treatment

Entropion: Topical antibiotics and lubricants, temporary sutures to evert the eyelid, lateral cantholysis with subconjunctival incision just inferior to the tarsus. Inferior retractors are isolated and reattached to anteroinferior portion of tarsus with multiple interrupted sutures.

Glaucoma: Its medication should be the first plan of action. If medication is unsuccessful, a filtering surgical procedure with or without antimetabolites may be beneficial.

Bibliography

1. Ackerman JL, Ackerman AL, Ackerman AB. A new dental, ocular and cutaneous syndrome. Int J Dermatol. 1973;12:285-9.

---

430. DERMATITIS HERPETIFORMIS (DUHRING-BROCQ DISEASE)

General

Malignant; atypical; does not respond well to sulfone or sulfapyridine therapy; uncommon; autoimmune blistering dermatosis; pruritic eruption involving the scalp, buttocks, lower back and extensor surface of arms; autoantibody is generally of immunoglobulin A class causing deposition at the dermal-epidermal junction.

Ocular

Bullae of conjunctiva, skin and mucous membranes; blisters are intraepithelial (acantholysis) and usually do not leave scars; epithelium desquamates in patches; corneal and conjunctival vascularization; symblepharon; cataract.

Clinical

Vesicles; erythema; pruritus; burning; eruption classically involves extensor surface of the knees, elbows, buttocks, sacrum, scapula and scalp.

Laboratory

Diagnosis is made by clinical findings and skin biopsy.

Treatment

Dapsone and sulfapyridine are the primary medications used for therapy. Avoidance of gluten is also helpful.

Additional Resource

1. Miller JL (2011). Dermatitis Herpetiformis. [online] Available from http://www.emedicine. com/derm/TOPIC95.HTM [Accessed April, 2012].

---

431. DERMATOCHALASIS

General

Redundant and lax eyelid skin and muscle commonly seen in the elderly; loss of elastic tissue and weakening of connective tissue is the causative factor; most frequent in the upper lid but can be seen in lower lid.

Clinical

Renal failure, trauma, cutis laxa, Ehlers-Danlos syndrome, amyloidosis, xanthelasma, thyroid abnormalities and genetics predipose individuals.

Ocular

Visual field loss, blepharitis, entropion, ectropion and trichiasis.

Laboratory

Diagnosis is made by clinical findings. Visual field testing can document field loss.

Treatment

Blepharoplasty is the treatment of choice. Lid hygiene and topical antibiotic may be necessary for blepharitis.

Additional Resource

1. Gilliland GD (2012). Dermatochalasis. [online] Available from http://www.emedicine.medscape. com/article/1212294-overview [Accessed April, 2012].

---

432. DERMATOPHYTOSIS (EPIDERMOMYCOSIS; EPIDERMOPHYTOSIS; RUBROPHYTIA; TINEA; TRICHOPHYTOSIS)

General

Superficial infection of the skin; ringworm fungi; most frequently seen in children during hot, humid weather.

Ocular

Conjunctivitis; corneal ulcer; madarosis; scaly rash; folliculitis; blepharitis; lid edema.

Clinical

Scalp, facial and lid ringworm lesions.

Laboratory

Rapid identification on polymerase chain reaction. Septate hyphae branches on 20% potassium hydroxide stain.

Treatment

Topical treatment involves antifungal cream. Systemic treatment involves use of ketoconazole for 2–4 weeks.

Additional Resource

1. Kao GF (2011). Tinea Capitis. [online] Available from http://www.emedicine.com/derm/TOPIC420. HTM [Accessed April, 2012].

433. DERMOID (DERMOID CHORISTOMA; DERMOID CYST; DERMOLIPOMA; LIPODERMOID)

General

Benign tumors composed of epidermal tissue, dermal adnexal structures, skin appendages, hair follicles, sebaceous gland and sweat glands; slowly growing.

Ocular

Dermoid of conjunctiva, cornea and lids; keratitis; extraocular muscle paralysis; exophthalmos; astigmatism; visual loss; orbital lesions causing diplopia and proptosis; may be connected with the lacrimal canaliculum.

Clinical

Subcutaneous dermoids of the skin; aplasia cutis congenita possibly associated with strabismus has been reported.

Laboratory

Radiographs of the orbit reveal the deeper orbital cysts; CT is commonly used to image orbital cysts; MRI of dermoid cyst is especially valuable in deeper orbital lesions.

Treatment

Surgery for function or cosmesis.

Additional Resource

1. Schwartz RA (2012). Dermoid Cyst. [online] Available from http://www.emedicine.com/derm/ TOPIC686.HTM [Accessed April, 2012].

434. DERMOID, ORBITAL

General

Choristomas, tumors that originate from aberrant primordial tissue; may displace structures in the orbit, especially the globe. If the displacement is great, interference with vision by compression of the optic nerve.

Ocular

Mass in the orbital area; decreased visual acuity, color vision and brightness perception; afferent pupillary defect; optic nerve compression.

Laboratory

Radiography, CT, MRI and ultrasound can be used to diagnosis.

Treatment

No treatment is generally required unless there is optic nerve compression or for cosmetic problems. If surgery is required the location of the cyst helps to determine the appropriate type of orbitotomy.

Additional Resource

1. Cooper T (Ted) (2010). Dermoid, Orbital. [online] Available from http://www.emedicine.medscape. com/article/1218740-overview [Accessed April, 2012].

---

435. DESCEMET'S MEMBRANE FOLDS

General

Descemet's membrane is positioned between the stroma and the endothelial cell layer. Any condition that may cause inflammation to the cornea or the anterior chamber can result in Descemet's membrane folds.

Clinical

Diagnosis is made by clinical findings.

Ocular

Corneal edema and anterior chamber inflamm- ation. Ocular infections, inflammation after sur- gery, retained lens fragments, retina detachment, endophthalmitis, trauma or injury, such as blunt trauma or chemical injury.

Laboratory

B-scan if the view of the posterior pole is obscured, gonioscopy may be performed to reveal lens fragments in the anterior chamber.

Treatment

Treat inflammation using steroidal, nonsteroidal and osmotic agents. Surgical care via penetrating keratoplasty is available.

Additional Resource

1. Graham RH (2012). Descemet Membrane Folds. [online] Available from http://www.emedicine. medscape.com/article/1196103-overview [Accessed April, 2012].

---

436. DESERT LUNG AND CATARACT SYNDROME

General

Nonoccupational pneumoconiosis; common in desert areas; excessive exposure to atmospheric dust; inhalant of fine, sandy dust.

Ocular

Cataracts (posterior subcapsular most prevalent); corneal opacities.

Clinical

Miliary infiltrates; thickening of bronchial walls; mild restrictive changes with pulmonary function.

Laboratory

Chest X-ray, ultrasound, CT and bronchoscopy.

Treatment

Maintenance of airways and clearance of secretions with tracheal suctioning, oxygen supplementation, antibiotics.

Additional Resource

1. Ocampo VVD (2012). Senile Cataract. [online] Available from http://www.emedicine.com/oph/ TOPIC49.HTM [Accessed April, 2012].

437. DETACHMENT OF DESCEMET'S MEMBRANE

General

Complication of intraocular surgery.

Clinical

None

Ocular

Detachment of Descemet's membrane.

Laboratory

Diagnosis is made by clinical findings.

Treatment

Unscroll surgically, full-thickness suturing may be necessary.

Bibliography

1. Roy FH, Fraunfelder FW, Fraunfelder FT. Roy and Fraunfelder's Current Ocular Therapy, 6th edition. Philadelphia: WB Saunders; 2008.

438. DEVIC SYNDROME (NEUROMYELITIS OPTICA; OPHTHALMOENCEPHALOMYELOPATHY; OPTIC MYELITIS)

General

Etiology unknown; frequent between the ages of 20 and 50 years; mortality rate up to 50%; associated with chickenpox.

Ocular

Ptosis is rare; ocular muscle palsy (rare); abducens and oculomotor palsy; paralysis of conjugate gaze; blindness; onset usually very sudden in one eye, followed soon by blindness in the other eye; miosis; bilateral optic neuritis (unilateral involvement is rare); optic atrophy; pupillary dysfunction.

Clinical

Prodromal signs: headache; sore throat; fever and malaise; ascending myelitis with resulting pain, which may be severe; numbness; weakness; paralysis.

Laboratory

Diagnosis is made by clinical findings.

Treatment

Steroids orally or intravenously may be useful.

Additional Resource

1. Schatz MP (2011). Childhood Optic Neuritis. [online] Available from http://www.emedicine.com/oph/TOPIC343.HTM [Accessed April, 2012].

439. DIABETES MELLITUS

General

Complex disorder of carbohydrate, lipid and protein metabolism characterized by hyper-glycemia and a relative or total lack of insulin. Development is influenced by both genetic and environmental factors. Most commonly occurs in middle or late life (Type II) and is seen most commonly in the obese. Diabetes can occur in the first or second decade of life (Type I) and usually involves the lack of insulin production by the pancreas and the need for insulin therapy.

Clinical

Atherosclerosis, nephropathy, neuropathy, polyuria, polydipsia, polyphagia, obesity, elevated plasma glucose and elevated A1C.

Ocular

Diabetic retinopathy, vitreous hemorrhage, macular edema, cataract, glaucoma, asteroid hyalosis, extraocular muscle paralysis, rubeosis iridis, corneal hypesthesia, optic nerve atrophy, papillopathy.

Laboratory

Diagnosis is made by fasting plasma glucose of greater than 126 mg/dL and 2-hour post-glucose load (75 g) plasma glucose of greater than 200 mg/dL and confirmed by repeat test.

Treatment

Goals include elimination of symptoms, by reduction of blood sugar and blood pressure. Smoking cessation, aspirin therapy, weight loss, exercise, diabetic diet as well as oral medication and/or insulin are all used in the treatment of diabetes. Diabetic retinopathy is most successfully treated with retinal photocoagulation. Pars plana vitrectomy is sometimes necessary to remove vitreous hemorrhage. Other ocular problems are caused by diabetes, such as cataracts and glaucoma, and are treated in traditional methods.

Bibliography

1. Ostri C, Lund-Andersen H, Sander B, et al. Bilateral diabetic papillopathy and metabolic control. Ophthalmology. 2010;117:2214-7.

Additional Resource

1. Khardori R (2012). Type 2 Diabetes Mellitus. [online] Available from http://www.emedicine. medscape.com/article/117853-overview [Accessed April, 2012].

---

440. DIABETIC MACULAR EDEMA

General

Diabetes is a major medical problem that is growing in numbers. Seen most commonly in Western countries in individuals that consume more calories than they use each day. Caused by the pancreas not making or not making enough insulin.

Clinical

Renal, neuropathic and cardiovasuclar disease, polyuria, polydipsia, polyphagia and weight loss.

Ocular

Cataracts, glaucoma, corneal abnormalities, iris neovascularization, macular edema, microaneurysms, retinal hemorrhage, cotton-wool spots changes in refractive error.

Laboratory

Fasting glucose and A1C, fluorescein angiography and optical coherence tomography (OCT), color stereo fundus photographs.

Treatment

Glucose control with diet, exercise and medication, lowering blood pressure and lipid levels, laser photocoagulation, intravitreal triamcinolone acetonide and anti VEGT agents. Pars plana vitrectomy may also be necessary.

Bibliography

1. Murakami T, Nishijima K, Sakamoto A, et al. Foveal cystoid spaces are associated with enlarged foveal avascular zone and microaneurysms in diabetic macular edema. Ophthalmology. 2011;118:359-67.

Additional Resource

1. Mavrikakis E (2011). Macular Edema in Diabetes. [online] Available from http://www.emedicine. medscape.com/article/1224138-overview [Acessed April, 2012].

441. DIABETIC RETINOPATHY, BACKGROUND

General

Diabetes is a major medical problem that is growing in numbers. Seen most commonly in Western countries in individuals that consume more calories than they use each day. Caused by the pancreas not making or not making enough insulin.

Clinical

Renal, neuropathic and cardiovasuclar disease, polyuria, polydipsia, polyphagia and weight loss.

Ocular

Cataracts, glaucoma, corneal abnormalities, iris neovascularization, macular edema, microaneurysms, retinal hemorrhage, cotton-wool spots changes in refractive error.

Laboratory

Fasting glucose and A1C, fluorescein angiography and optical coherence tomography (OCT).

Treatment

Glucose control with diet, exercise and medication, daily dose of aspirin (650 mg), laser photocoagulation, Avastin and Lucentis is also being used off label.

Additional Resource

1. Bhavsar AR (2011). Diabetic Retinopathy. [online] Available from http://www.emedicine.medscape. com/article/1225122-overview [Accessed April, 2012].

442. DIABETIC RETINOPATHY, PROLIFERATIVE

General

Diabetes is a major medical problem that is growing in numbers. Seen most commonly in Western countries in individuals that consume more calories than they use each day. Caused by the pancreas not making or not making enough insulin.

Clinical

Renal, neuropathic and cardiovascular disease, polyuria, polydipsia, polyphagia and weight loss.

Ocular

Cataracts, glaucoma, corneal abnormalities, iris neovascularization, macular edema, microaneurysms, retinal hemorrhage, cotton-wool spots changes in refractive error.

Laboratory

Fasting glucose and A1C, fluorescein angiography and optical coherence tomography (OCT). B-scan may be necessary to evaluate the retina if vitreous hemorrhage is present.

Treatment

Glucose control with diet, exercise and medication, daily dose of aspirin (650 mg), laser photocoagulation, intravitreal injections of triamcinolone, Avastin and Lucentis can be used. The use of Avastin and Lucentis is off label. Vitrectomy and cryotherapy may also be necessary.

Additional Resource

1. Bhavsar AR (2011). Diabetic Retinopathy. [online] Available from http://www.emedicine.medscape.com/article/1225210-overview [Accessed April, 2012].

443. DIALINAS-AMALRIC SYNDROME (AMALRIC-DIALINAS SYNDROME; DEAF MUTISM-RETINAL DEGENERATION SYNDROME)

General

Retinal pigmentary disturbances and deafness as outstanding findings but without severe general systemic disorders as seen in the syndromes of Hallgren, Cockayne, Alport, Laurence-Moon-Bardet-Biedl (see Hallgren Syndrome; Cockayne Syndrome; Alport Syndrome; Laurence-Moon-Bardet-Biedl Syndrome).

Ocular

No night blindness but heterochromia iridis; atypical retinitis pigmentosa with small, scattered, fine-pigmented deposits in the macular region with some accumulations and accompanied by small white and yellow spots.

Clinical

Deaf mutism.

Laboratory

None/Ocular.

Treatment

Retinitis pigmentosa: Vitamin A 15,000 IU/day is thought to slow the decline of retinal function, dark sunglasses for outdoor use, surgery for cataract, genetic counseling.

Bibliography

1. Amalric P. Nouveau Type de Degenerescence Tapeto-Retienne au Cours de la Surdumutite. Bull Soc Ophthalmol Fr. 1960;196:211.
2. Charamis J et al. Deaf-mutism and ophthalmic lesions. J Pediatr Ophthalmol. 1968;5:230.
3. Dialinas NP. Les Alterations Oculaires chez les Sourds-Muets. Genet Hum. 1959;8:225.
4. Geeraets WJ. Ocular Syndromes, 3rd edition. Philadelphia: Lea & Febiger; 1976.

444. DIAMOND BLACKFAN SYNDROME

General

Rare, congenital hematologic disorder characterized by isolated erythroid hypoplasia (hypoplastic anemia).

Ocular

Strabismus, hypertelorism, microphthalmos and infantile glaucoma.

Clinical

May have musculoskeletal abnormalities.

Laboratory

Hemoglobin studies, imaging studies may be helpful in revealing occult malformations.

Treatment

Packed red cell transfusions may be necessary.

Additional Resource

1. Huang LH (2009). Transient Erythroblastopenia of Childhood. [online] Available from http://www.emedicine.medscape.com/article/959644-overview [Accessed April, 2012].

445. DIENCEPHALIC SYNDROME (ANTERIOR DIENCEPHALIC AUTONOMIC EPILEPSY SYNDROME; AUTONOMIC EPILEPSY SYNDROME; DIENCEPHALIC EPILEPSY SYNDROME; PENFIELD SYNDROME)

General

Occurs in males at ages 6–7 years; caused by hypothalamic dysfunction and a localized epileptic stimulus originating in the dorsal nucleus of the thalamus.

Ocular

Proptosis (occasionally); excessive lacrimation; pupillary abnormalities.

Clinical

Abdominal pain; headache; irritability; rapid pulse; elevated blood pressure; salivation; hiccup; chills; dyspnea (Cheyne-Stokes); seizures (possible); sudden onset of vasodilation of the skin (cervical sympathetic).

Laboratory

Brain MRI, head CT, EEG.

Treatment

Anticonvulsant medication.

Additional Resource

1. Nouri S (2011). Epilepsy and the Autonomic Nervous System. [online] Available from http://www.emedicine.com/neuro/TOPIC658.HTM [Accessed April, 2012].

446. DIFFUSE KERATOSES SYNDROME

General

Ophthalmic complications and manifestations following a group of dermatologic conditions for which the etiology is unknown, including scleroderma, CRST syndrome, Rendu-Osler-Weber syndrome, progressive systemic sclerosis with calcinosis, Spanlang-Tappeiner syndrome and Savin syndrome (see Rendu-Osler-Weber Syndrome; Progressive Systemic Sclerosis; Spanlang-Tappeiner Syndrome; Savin Syndrome; CRST Syndrome; Scleroderma).

Ocular

Dermatologic and cicatricial skin changes; hydrophthalmos; corneal changes with nodular thickening in the stroma, which worsen in fall and improve during spring (particularly Savin syndrome); retinal phlebitis.

Clinical

Ichthyosis (usually congenital); microcephalus (CRST); facial dermatoses; deafness; urticarial (allergic) manifestations; subcutaneous calcinous plaques, mainly on hands; sclerodactyly.

Laboratory

Consult internist.

Treatment

Corneal clouding: Check for elevated intraocular pressure. Medical treatment includes the use of hyperosmotic drops, nonsteroidal and steroid eye drops. Corneal transplant may be necessary.

Additional Resource

1. Lee RA (2011). Keratosis Palmaris et Plantaris. [online] Available from http://www.emedicine. com/derm/TOPIC589.HTM [Accessed April, 2012].

---

447. DIFFUSE UNILATERAL SUBACUTE NEURORETINITIS SYNDROME (DUSN; UNILATERAL WIPEOUT SYNDROME; WIPEOUT SYNDROME)

General

Caused by a nematode that is not *Toxocara canis*, i.e. at least two nematodes of different sizes; usually occurs in children or young adults; nematode may remain viable in eye for 3 years or longer.

Ocular

Vitreitis; papillitis; gray-white lesions of retina; optic atrophy; retinal vessel narrowing; diffuse pigment epithelial degeneration; endophthalmitis; nematode in fundus; the pathognomonic finding in DUSN is the presence of a motile intraocular nematode.

Clinical

Weight loss; lack of appetite; cough; fever; pulmonary infiltration; hepatomegaly; leukocytosis; persistent eosinophilia.

Laboratory

Electroretinopathy, enzyme-linked immunosorbent assays for individual nematode species.

Treatment

Direct laser photocoagulation of the nematode is the treatment of choice for DUSN, surgical transvitreal removal of the nematode may be indicated in selected cases.

Additional Resource

1. Kooragayala LM (2011). Diffuse Unilateral Subacute Neuroretinitis. [online] Available from http://www.emedicine.com/oph/TOPIC684.HTM [Accessed April, 2012].

---

448. DIMMER SYNDROME (KERATITIS NUMMULARIS)

General

Onset after minor ocular trauma.

Ocular

Photophobia; ocular pain; excessive lacrimation; discoid infiltration of superficial layers of cornea without adjacent conjunctivitis.

Laboratory

None

Treatment

Keratitis: Local treatment is use for prevention and reduction of corneal damage. Systemic therapy is used for controlling the underlying disease. Tissue adhesives may be necessary for impending perforation. Keratectomy, conjunctival resection, amniotic membrane transplatation and keratoplasty may necessary.

Bibliography

1. Dimmer F. Weber Eine der Keratitis Nurmnularis. Mahestehende Hirnhutentzuendung Augenheilkd. 1905;13:621-35.
2. Magalini SI, Scrascia E. Dictionary of Medical Syndromes, 2nd edition. Philadelphia: JB Lippincott; 1981.

---

449. DIPHTHERIA

General

Acute infectious disease caused by *Corynebacterium diphtheriae*; severity is dependent upon the amount of exotoxin absorbed prior to initiation of specific therapy.

Ocular

Conjunctivitis; xerophthalmia; keratitis; corneal ulcer; blepharitis; cellulitis of lid; meibomianitis; ptosis; dacryocystitis; cataract; central retinal artery occlusion; optic neuritis; accommodative spasm or paralysis; convergence paralysis; divergence paralysis; paralysis of third, fourth or sixth nerve; paralysis of accommodation (in children); ocular motor nerve paresis; choroiditis; cranial neuropathies involving the V (trigeminal), X (vagus) and XII (hypoglossal) cranial nerves; myocarditis.

Clinical

Local inflammatory lesion, with effect on heart, kidneys and nervous system.

Laboratory

Gram-positive rods commonly affect children younger than 10 years.

Treatment

Systemic treatment involves use of diphtheria antitoxin and antibiotics. Ocular treatment includes diphtheria antitoxin and high titer Y-globulin preparation. Topical penicillin G ointment helps to eradicate the bacilli.

Additional Resource

1. Demirci CS (2011). Pediatric Diphtheria. [online] Available from http://www.emedicine.com/ped/TOPIC596.HTM [Accessed April, 2012].

---

450. DIPLOPIA

General

Double vision; first manifestation of many systemic disorders, especially muscular or neurologic processes; can be binocular or monocular.

Clinical

Blunt head trauma; Marfan syndrome; myasthenia gravis; following refractive surgery; thyroid disease; tumor of orbit or cranial nerve pathway; increased intracranial pressure; aneurysm; carotid cavernous fistula.

Ocular

Distortion of images; corneal distortion or scarring; openings of the iris; cataract; subluxation of natural or pseudophakic lens; vitreous abnormalities; strabismus; abnormal head position; refractive abnormalities.

Laboratory

Careful history and extraocular muscle evaluation; CT or MRI to rule out systemic disease; tensilon test to exclude myasthenia gravis.

Treatment

Patching, stick on occlusive lenses and fresnel prisms; occasionally strabismus surgery, transposition surgery, Knapp superior oblique surgery and chemodenervation is necessary. Treatment of the causative disease.

Additional Resource

1. Wessels IF (2011). Diplopia. [online] Available from http://www.emedicine.medscape.com article/1214490-overview#IntroductionPathophysi ology [Accessed April, 2012].

451. DIROFILARIASIS

General

Caused by the parasitic nematode of the genus *Dirofilaria*.

Ocular

Chemosis; tenonitis; proptosis; granuloma of conjunctiva, eyelid, orbit and sclera; periocular soft tissue mass.

Clinical

Pulmonary symptoms; coughing; cardiac infection; "coin" lesions in the lung; pruritus, most commonly in subepithelial tissues of eyelids, fingers, cheeks, breast, abdomen and conjunctivae (rarely); allergic reactions; hemoptysis.

Laboratory

Dirofilariae serology, chest X-ray, CT, MRI, ultrasound of abdomen, bronchoscopy and lung biopsy.

Treatment

Surgical excision of lesions and affected areas is the treatment of choice for patients with human dirofilariasis.

Additional Resource

1. Klotchko A (2010). Dirofilariasis. [online] Available from http://www.emedicine.com/med/ TOPIC3446.HTM [Accessed April, 2012].

452. DISLOCATION OF INTRAOCULAR LENS

General

Following cataract surgery or YAG posterior capsulotomy. Intraocular lens (IOL) malpositions range from decentration to luxation into the posterior segment. Subluxated IOLs involve such extreme decentration that the IOL optic covers only a small fraction of the pupillary space. Luxation involves total dislocation of the IOL into the posterior segment. Causes include improper fixation, trauma, internal forces such as scarring, anterior synechiae and capsular contraction pseudoexofoliation syndrome.

Clinical

Facial trauma.

Ocular

Pseudoexofoliation; decreased vision, edge glare, diplopia streaks of light; haloes; photobia; ghost images; aphakia; retinal detchment; cystoid macular edema; vitreous hemorrhage; irregular pupil; corneal decompensation; torn zonules.

Laboratory

Generally diagnosis is made by clinical observation. If vitreous hemorrhage or severe corneal edema is present B-scan ultrasonic imaging may be necessary to determine the position of the IOL.

Treatment

In the absence of symptoms, observation is the necessary treatment. IOL repositioning with or without a McCannel suture; IOL exchange and IOL explantation are all surgical procedures used in the more severe, symptomatic cases.

Additional Resource

1. Wu L (2011). Intraocular Lens Dislocation. [online] Available from http://www.emedicine.medscape.com/article/1211310-overview [Accessed April, 2012].

---

453. DISLOCATION OF THE LENS

General

Ectopia lentis, occurs when the lens is not in its normal position.

Clinical

Marfan syndrome, Weill-Marchesani syndrome, sulfite oxidase deficiency.

Laboratory

Diagnosis is made by clinical findings.

Treatment

Careful phacoemulsification, topical steroids to control ocular inflammation.

Additional Resource

1. Eifrig CW (2011). Ectopia Lentis. [online] Available from http://www.emedicine.com/oph/TOPIC55.HTM [Accessed April, 2012].

---

454. DISSEMINATED INTRAVASCULAR COAGULATION

General

Intravascular coagulation in small vessels throughout the body.

Ocular

Serous retinal detachment; choroidal, retinal, and vitreous hemorrhage and hyphema; recurrent choroidal hemorrhagic detachment.

Clinical

Hypocoagulable, hemorrhagic state.

Laboratory

Imaging studies are useful only to detect an underlying etiology; the diagnosis is made by combining the clinical impression and laboratory abnormalities.

Treatment

Treat underlying disease, platelet and plasma transfusion, anticoagulant therapy.

Additional Resource

1. Levi MM (2011). Disseminated Intravascular Coagulation. [online] Available from http://www.emedicine.com/med/TOPIC577.HTM [Accessed April, 2012].

455. DISSEMINATED LUPUS ERYTHEMATOSUS (KAPOSI-LIBMAN-SACKS SYNDROME, LUPUS ERYTHEMATOSUS; SYSTEMIC LUPUS ERYTHEMATOSUS, SLE)

General

Possible etiology includes viral infections and genetic predisposition; immunologic abnormalities.

Ocular

Keratitis; keratoconjunctivitis sicca; corneal ulcer; optic nerve atrophy; optic neuritis; papilledema; arteritis; central retinal vein occlusion; retinal detachment; microaneurysm; scleritis; uveitis; ptosis; conjunctivitis; paralysis of third nerve; homonymous hemianopsia; multifocal microinfarcts; mydriasis; nystagmus; proptosis; orbital myositis; pseudoretinitis pigmentosa; photophobia.

Clinical

Polyarthritis; morning stiffness; fever; malaise; fatigue; polyserositis; renal disease; central nervous system disease; anemia; leukopenia; maculopapular rash in a "butterfly" distribution over malar region; alopecia.

Laboratory

Antibodies to double-stranded DNA or the SM antigen or a false-positive serology test for syphilis; positive antinuclear antibody test that is caused by a medication.

Treatment

Fever, rash, musculoskeletal and serositis manifestations respond to hydroxychloroquine and NSAIDs. Low-to-moderate dose steroids are necessary for acute flares. CNS involvement and renal disease constitute more serious disease and often require high-dose steroids and other immunosuppression agents. Diffuse proliferative lupus nephritis has been treated with cyclophosphamide induction therapy.

Additional Resource

1. Bartels CM (2012). Systemic Lupus Erythematosus (SLE). [online] Available from http://www.emedicine.com/med/TOPIC2228.HTM [Accessed April, 2012].

456. DISSOCIATED VERTICAL DEVIATION (DISSOCIATED STRABISMUS COMPLEX, ALTERNATING SURSUMDUCTION, DISSOCIATED VERTICAL DIVERGENCE, DOUBLE-DISSOCIATED HYPERTROPIA, OCCLUSION HYPERTROPIA, DISSOCIATED TORSIONAL DEVIATION, DISSOCIATED HORIZONTAL DEVIATION)

General

Ocular misalignment with elevation, abduction and excyclotorsion, usually bilateral and almost always associated with infantile strabismus.

Clinical

None

Ocular

Head tilt, inferior oblique overaction, latent nystagmus, amblyopia, esotropia, exotropia.

Laboratory

Diagnosis is made by clinical findings.

Treatment

Superior muscle rectus recession is the most common therapy.

Bibliography

1. Roy FH, Fraunfelder FW, Fraunfelder FT. Roy and Fraunfelder's Current Ocular Therapy, 6th edition. Philadelphia: WB Saunders; 2008.

457. DISTICHIASIS (DISTICHIASIS WITH CONGENITAL ANOMALIES OF THE HEART AND PERIPHERAL VASCULATURE)

General

Autosomal dominant.

Ocular

Double rows of eyelashes; congenital ectropion; absence of meibomian glands; replacement of dense collagenous tissue of the tarsal plates by loose areolar tissue.

Clinical

Congenital heart defects; ventricular septal defects; stress-induced asystole; visible varicosities; chronic venous disease of the legs; sinus bradycardia.

Laboratory

Diagnosis is made by clinical findings.

Treatment

Symptomatic-therapeutic contact lenses as well as lubricating drops and ointments. Epilation with electrolysis cryosurgery, double freeze-thaw down to -20°F, lid splitting procedure.

Additional Resource

1. Rostami S (2011). Distichiasis. [online] Available from http://www.emedicine.com/oph/TOPIC603.HTM [Accessed April, 2012].

458. DIVERTICULOSIS OF BOWEL, HERNIA, RETINAL DETACHMENT

General

Autosomal recessive.

Ocular

Severe myopia; esotropia; retinal detachment.

Clinical

Femoral or inguinal hernias; diverticula of bowel or bladder.

Laboratory

Diagnosis is made by clinical findings.

Treatment

Esotropia: Equalized vision with correct refractive error; surgery may be helpful in patient with diplopia.

Retinal detachment: Scleral buckle, pneumatic retinopexy and vitrectomy may be used to close all the breaks.

Bibliography

1. Clunie GJ, Mason JM. Visceral diverticula and the Marfan syndrome. Br J Surg. 1962:50:51-2.
2. McKusick VA. Mendelian Inheritance in Man: A Catalog of Human Genes and Genetic Disorders, 12th edition. Baltimore: The Johns Hopkins University Press; 1998.
3. McKusick-Nathans Institute for Genetic Medicine, Johns Hopkins University and National Center for Biotechnology Information, National Library of Medicine. (2007). Online Mendelian Inheritance in Man (OMIM). [online] Available from http://www.ncbi.nlm.nih.gov/omim [Accessed April, 2012].

459. DOLLINGER-BIELSCHOWSKY SYNDROME [BIELSCHOWSKY-JANSKY DISEASE; INFANTILE AMAUROTIC FAMILIAL IDIOCY (LATE); INFANTILE GANGLIOSIDE LIPIDOSIS (LATE); JANSKY-BIELSCHOWSKY SYNDROME]

General

Late infantile form of neuronal ceroid lipofuscinosis; onset between the ages of 2 and 5 years; autosomal recessive; other neuronal ceroid lipofuscinoses include infantile (Santavuori-Haltia), juvenile (Spiel-Meyer-Sjögren) and adult (Kufs-Hallervorden).

Ocular

Optic nerve atrophy; macular pigmentation.

Clinical

Cerebroretinal degeneration; cerebellar ataxia; defective hearing; convulsions; spasticity; contractures; progressive mental deterioration.

Laboratory

Diagnosis is made by clinical findings.

Treatment

No treatment available for optic nerve atrophy. Intravenous steroids may be used with optic neuritis or ischemic neuropathy. Stem cell treatment may be the future treatment of choice.

Bibliography

1. Bateman JB, Philippart M. Ocular features of the Hagberg-Santavuori syndrome. Am J Ophthalmol. 1986;102:262-71.

2. Bielschowsky M. Uber Spatintatile Familiare Amaurotische Idiotie Mit Klein Hirn-symptomen. Dtsch Z Nervenh. 1914;50:7-29.
3. Brod RD, Packer AJ, Van Dyk HJ. Diagnosis of neuronal ceroid lipofuscinosis by ultrastructural examination of peripheral blood lymphocytes. Arch Ophthalmol. 1987;105:1388-93.
4. Dollinger A. Zur Klinik der Infantiler Form der Familioren Amaurotischen Idiotie (Tay-Sachs).

Einige neue Symptome. Ein Beitrag zu den von Magnus beschrie-benen Tonischer. Hals-und Labyrinth Reflex. Z Kinderh. 1919;22:167-94.
5. Goebel HH, Zeman W, Damaske E. An ultrastructural study of the retina in the Jansky-Bielschowsky type of neuronal ceroid-lipofuscinosis. Am J Ophthalmol. 1977;83:70-9.

460. DOMINANT OPTIC ATROPHY SYNDROME (DEAFNESS, DOMINANT OPTIC ATROPHY, DYSTAXIA AND MYOPATHY, OPHTHALMOPLEGIA, PTOSIS)

General

Autosomal dominant disorder; ptosis, ophthalmoplegia, dystaxia and nonspecific myopathy occur in midlife; optic atrophy and hearing loss occur in early life; autosomal dominant inheritance.

Ocular

Ptosis; ophthalmoplegia; progressive optic atrophy; abnormal electroretinography; diplopia; ocular myopathy; nystagmus; focal temporal excavation of optic disk; dyschromatopsia (blue-yellow); myopia; temporal pallor of the optic nerve.

Clinical

Sensorineural hearing loss; myopathy; dystaxia.

Laboratory

Diagnosis is made by clinical findings.

Treatment

Oral steroids and sometimes intravenous steroids are necessary.

Bibliography

1. Del Porto G, Vingolo EM, Steindl K, et al. Clinical heterogeneity of dominant optic atrophy: the contribution of visual function investigations to diagnosis. Graefes Arch Clin Exp Ophthalmol. 1994;232:717-27.
2. Eliott D, Traboulsi EI, Maumenee IH. Visual prognosis in autosomal dominant optic atrophy (Kjer type). Am J Ophthalmol. 1993;115:360-7.
3. Grehn F, Kommerell G, Ropers HH, et al. Dominant optic atrophy with sensorineural hearing loss. Ophthalmic Paediatr Genet. 1982;1:77-88.
4. Treft RL, Sanborn GE, Carey J, et al. Dominant optic atrophy, deafness, ptosis, ophthalmoplegia, dystaxia, and myopathy. A new syndrome. Ophthalmology. 1984;91:908-15.

461. DONOHUE SYNDROME (LEPRECHAUNISM)

General

Etiology unknown; possibly autosomal recessive; prevalent in females; present at birth; possible correlation between Donohue syndrome and insulin receptor gene defects.

Ocular

Hypertelorism

Clinical

Failure to thrive; mental retardation; sexual precocity; hirsutism; broad nose; hypertrophic nipples; hypertrophy of external genitals; intra-uterine growth retardation; extreme insulin resistance hyperkeratosis; precocious tooth eruption.

Laboratory

Fasting blood glucose and lipid profile, creatinine evaluation, and urinalysis for protein, X-ray, MRI.

Treatment

Biguanides and thiazolidinediones have been used in the treatment of the insulin-resistant state.

Bibliography

1. Donohue WL, Clark DR, Edwards HE, et al. Dysendocrinism. J Pediatr. 1948;32:739-48.
2. Krook A, Brueton L, O'Rahilly S. Homozygous nonsense mutation in the insulin receptor gene in infant with leprechaunism. Lancet. 1993;342: 277-8.

---

462. DORSAL MIDBRAIN SYNDROME

General

Caused by lesions of the posterior commissure located in the dorsal midbrain, pineal tumors, shunt malfunction or hydrocephalus; less common causes include midbrain hemorrhage or infection, hypoxia, multiple sclerosis, trauma, lipid storage disease, Wilson disease, Whipple disease, syphilis and tuberculosis.

Ocular

Loss of upward gaze; lid retraction; light-near dissociation; impaired convergence and divergence; convergence-retraction nystagmus.

Clinical

Patients tend to adopt abnormal head postures to fixate or maintain binocularity.

Laboratory

High-resolution MRI with gadolinium.

Treatment

Radiotherapy, chemotherapy, stereotactic radiation, stereotactic biopsy and open recession.

Bibliography

1. Kawasaki A, Miller NR, Kardon R. Pupillographic investigation of the relative afferent pupillary defect associated with a midbrain lesion. Ophthalmology. 2010;117:175-7.

Additional Resource

1. Bruce JN (2011). Pineal Tumors. [online] Available from http://www.emedicine.com/med/TOPIC2911.HTM [Accessed April, 2012].

---

463. DOUBLE WHAMMY SYNDROME (VOLUNTARY PROPULSION OF THE EYES)

General

Ability to displace the globe forward actively while retracting the upper and lower lids behind the equator of the eyeball.

Ocular

Voluntary dislocation of either eye separately or of both simultaneously.

Laboratory

Diagnosis is made by clinical findings.

Treatment

Dry eye treatment.

Bibliography

1. Friedenwald H. Luxation and avulsion of eyeball during birth. Am J Ophthalmol. 1918;1:9.
2. Walsh TJ, Gilman M. Voluntary propulsion of the eyes. Am J Ophthalmol. 1969;67:583.

464. DOWN SYNDROME (MONGOLISM; MONGOLOID IDIOCY; TRISOMY G; TRISOMY 21 SYNDROME)

General

Trisomy of chromosome 21.

Ocular

Hypertelorism; epicanthus; blepharitis; ectropion; nystagmus; esotropia; high myopia (30%); hyperopia; color blindness; yellow spots on the iris; hypoplasia of the iris; blepharoconjunctivitis; lens opacities (50%); keratoconus (may be acute); corneal hydrops; corneal ectasia; corneal edema; leukoma; lateral displacement of canaliculi and puncta; megaloblepharon; euryblepharon; decreased accommodation; Leber congenital amaurosis.

Clinical

Mental retardation; skeletal abnormalities; overextension of joints; deformed and low-set ears; short fifth finger; transverse palmar crease; fissured tongue; heart anomalies.

Laboratory

Aminocentesis during 2nd trimester to check mothers who have low alpha-fetoprotein serum values, prenatal echography, craniofacial X-ray to check features and echocardiography.

Treatment

Primary care provider should coordinate the multisystemic evaluation. Awareness of systemic and ocular findings is essential for managing patients.

Additional Resource

1. Izquierdo NJ (2011). Ophthalmologic Manifestations of Down Syndrome. [online] Available from http://www.emedicine.com/oph/TOPIC522.HTM [Accessed April, 2012].

465. DOYNE HONEYCOMB CHOROIDITIS (DOMINANT ORBRUCH MEMBRANE DRUSEN; HOLTHOUSE-BATTEN SUPERFICIAL CHOROIDITIS; HUTCHINSON-TAYS CENTRAL GUTTATE CHOROIDITIS; MALATTIA-LEVENTINESE SYNDROME)

General

Autosomal dominant; represents early manifestation of senile macular degeneration; both sexes affected; onset in advanced age; patients present with drusen at an early age (second to third year of life) with near-normal visual acuity in childhood.

Ocular

Drusen with multiple yellow lesions becoming calcified and presenting crystalline appearance.

Clinical

None

Laboratory

Diagnosis is made by clinical findings.

Treatment

Vitamins, antioxidants, cessation of smoking and proper control of hypertension. There is evidence that patients with early or moderate dry macular degeneration should consume adequate quantities of antioxidants, including vitamin A, vitamin E, zinc and lutein. Prevention is the best treatment in this case because no satisfactory method exists.

Additional Resource

1. Maturi RK (2011). Nonexudative ARMD. [online] Available from http://www.emedicine.com/oph/TOPIC383.HTM [Accessed April, 2012].

---

466. DRACONTIASIS (DRACUNCULIASIS; DRACUNCULOSIS; GUINEA WORM INFECTION)

General

Caused by *Dracunculus medinensis*; affects connective and subcutaneous tissues.

Ocular

Conjunctivitis; proptosis; nematode present in the conjunctiva, eyelid, globe and orbit.

Clinical

Itching; urticaria; small blisters; tetany; septicemia; arthritis; paraplegia; constrictive pericarditis; urogenital involvement.

Laboratory

Complete blood count with differential, serum immunoglobulin levels.

Treatment

The most common practice to treat dracunculiasis still involves wrapping the worm around a stick. Metronidazole or thiabendazole (in adults) is usually adjunctive to stick therapy.

Additional Resource

1. Dhawan VK (2011). Dracunculiasis. [online] Available from http://www.emedicine.com/ped/TOPIC616.HTM [Accessed April, 2012].

---

467. DRAGGED-FOVEA DIPLOPIA SYNDROME

General

Binocular double vision with macular conditions such as epiretinal membrane, choroidal neovascular membranes, localized retinal detachment or paramacular scars dragging the fovea.

Ocular

Maculopathy; metamorphopsia; vascular wrinkling; central diplopia in the presence of peripheral fusion.

Clinical

Lights on-off test with 20/70 to 20/100 is diagnostic.

Laboratory

Diagnosis is made by clinical findings.

Treatment

Patching is often required, Fresnel prisms, Hummelsheim surgery with permanent paralysis of the lateral rectus muscle.

Additional Resource

1. Wessels IF (2011). Diplopia. [online] Available from http://www.emedicine.com/oph/TOPIC191.HTM [Accessed April, 2012].

468. DRUG INDUCED OPTIC ATROPHY

General

Selective symmetric involvement of maculopapillary axons, ganglion cells or both. Toxic optic neuropathies seem to be directly related to the dosage and duration of treatment.

Clinical

Renal or hepatic failure, diabetes, arteriosclerosis, dietary deficiencies.

Ocular

Central vision loss, cecocentral scotoma, visual field constriction, fluctuating hemianopsia defects.

Laboratory

Diagnosis is made by clinical findings.

Treatment

Discontinuation of suspected drug at first sign of optic atrophy.

Additional Resource

1. Zafar A (2011). Toxic/Nutritional Optic Neuropathy. [online] Available from http://www.emedicine.com/oph/TOPIC750.HTM [Accessed April, 2012].

469. DRUMMOND SYNDROME (BLUE DIAPER SYNDROME; IDIOPATHIC HYPERCALCEMIA)

General

Autosomal recessive; manifests itself in infancy; defective intestinal transport of tryptophan, which oxidizes to indigo blue and stains the diaper blue.

Ocular

Sclerosis of optic foramina (occasionally); prominent epicanthal folds; nystagmus; strabismus; peripheral retinal atrophy; papilledema; optic atrophy; microcornea; hypoplasia of the optic nerve; abnormal eye movements.

Clinical

Dwarfism; osteosclerosis; craniostenosis; depressed bridge of nose; "elfin-like" face; mental retardation; anorexia; vomiting; constipation.

Laboratory

Measurement of serum phosphate, alkaline phosphatase, serum chloride, serum bicarbonate and urinary calcium.

Treatment

Treatment depends on the severity of symptoms and the underlying cause.

Additional Resource

1. Agraharkar M (2010). Hypercalcemia. [online] Available from http://www.emedicine.com/med/TOPIC1068.HTM [Accessed April, 2012].

470. DRY EYE SYNDROME

General

Multifactorial disease of the tears and the ocular surface that results in symptoms of discomfort, visual disturbance, and tear film instability with potential damage to the ocular surface increased osmolarity of the tear film and inflammation of the ocular surface. Most common cause is aqueous tear deficiency. Keratoconjunctivitis sicca which is an ocular surface disorder may also be a cause. Associated with connective tissue disease such as rheumatoid arthritis and systemic sclerosis; postmenopausal women; pregnant women; and individuals taking oral contraceptives and hormone replacement.

Clinical

Rheumatoid arthritis; systemic sclerosis; menopause; pregnancy, prostate disease.

Ocular

Foreign body sensation; burning; itching; photophobic; blurred vision; excessive tearing; irregular corneal surface; decreased tear break up time; punctate epithelial keratopathy; debri in the tear film; corneal ulcer.

Laboratory

Diagnosis is generally made by clinical observation; careful history; tear break-up test; schirmer test, and the use of rose bengal and fluorescein to check for staining is useful. Additional testing can be used to determine the tear components. These include conjunctival biopsy, tear function index, tear ferning test, impression cytology and meibometry.

Treatment

Environmental and dietary modifcations; elimination of systemic medications if possible; artificial tears, gels and ointments; anti-inflammatory agents such as topical corticosteroids, cyclosporine A and omega-3 fatty acids; and tetracyclines for meibomianitis. Punctal plugs; moisture chamber spectacles and autologous serum tears may be necessary if the symptoms persist. Sometimes systemic anti-inflammatory agents, tarsorrhaphy, mucous membrane grafting; amniotic membrane transplantation and salivary gland duct transposition may be necessary in the worst cases.

Additional Resource

1. Foster CS (2012). Dry Eye Syndrome. [online] Available from http://www.emedicine.medscape.com/article/1210417-overview [Accessed April, 2012].

471. DUANE SYNDROME (RETRACTION SYNDROME; STILLING SYNDROME; TURK-STILLING SYNDROME)

General

Autosomal dominant; more frequent in females; manifestations in infancy; was thought to be secondary to fibrosis of the lateral rectus muscle or abnormal check ligaments; now established to be due to congenital aberrant innervation affecting III and VII cranial nerves.

Ocular

Narrowing of palpebral fissure on adduction, widening on abduction; primary global retraction; deficiency of medial and lateral recti motility; limitation of abduction in affected eye usually is complete; retraction of the globe with attempted adduction varies from 1 to 10 mm; convergence insufficiency; heterochromia irides; left eye is more frequently involved.

Clinical

Associated Klippel-Feil syndrome; malformation of face, ears and teeth.

Laboratory

Diagnosis is made by clinical findings.

Treatment

Indications for surgery include anomalous head position, strabismus in primary gaze, significant upshot or downshoot in adduction and cosmetically significant palpebral fissure. Type 1 DRS (absent abduction, esotropia in primary position and head turn toward the affected side to fuse) medial recuts recession of the affected eye, DRS with exotropia—recess lateral rectus of involved side. Retraction of the globe—recess medial and lateral rectus of involved eye. Upshoots and downshoots—recess the lateral rectus.

Additional Resource

1. Verma A (2011). Duane Syndrome. [online] Available from http://www.emedicine.com/oph/TOPIC326.HTM [Accessed April, 2012].

---

472. DUBIN-JOHNSON SYNDROME (CHRONIC IDIOPATHIC JAUNDICE; ROTOR SYNDROME)

General

Onset in infancy, but may be present at birth; autosomal dominant; liver cells are unable to excrete conjugated bilirubin; manifestations similar to Rotor syndrome, except that in the latter there is no melanin pigment present in the liver cells.

Ocular

Jaundice of sclera and conjunctiva in infancy.

Clinical

Abdominal pain right hypochondrium; nausea; vomiting; diarrhea; anorexia; weakness; hepatomegaly.

Laboratory

Urinary excretion of coproporphyrin is altered, cholescintigraphy, hepatic biopsy.

Treatment

Treatment is generally not required.

Additional Resource

1. Rabinowitz SS (2010). Pediatric Dubin-Johnson Syndrome. [online] Available from http://www.emedicine.com/ped/TOPIC621.HTM [Accessed April, 2012].

---

473. DUBOWITZ SYNDROME (DWARFISM-ECZEMA-PECULIAR FACIES)

General

Affects both sexes; congenital; may be autosomal recessive inheritance.

Ocular

Hypertelorism; lateral telecanthus; palpebral ptosis; short palpebral tissues.

Clinical

Eczema; sparse hair; cleft palate; hypospadia; microcephaly; low birth weight; mild mental retardation; characteristic face; short stature; spontaneous keloids; intrauterine growth retardation.

Laboratory

Bone marrow biopsy, quantitative hemoglobin electrophoresis, cytogenetic studies, human leukocyte antigen.

Treatment

Management involves supportive care that includes transfusion, treatment of infections, and a search for an allogeneic stem cell donor.

Additional Resource

1. Dixon N (2011). Pediatric Myelodysplasia. [online] Available from http://www.emedicine.medscape.com/article/956631-overview [Accessed April, 2012].

---

474. DUCK-BILL LIPS AND PTOSIS

General

Autosomal dominant.

Ocular

Ptosis; strabismus; hypertelorism.

Clinical

Short philtrum; duck-bill lips; low-set ears; broad forehead; slightly anteverted nose and flat nasal bridge; slightly wide-spaced teeth and high-arched palate; slightly receding chin; slightly wide-set nipples; two phalanges in both fifth fingers; impaired speech.

Laboratory

Diagnosis is made by clinical findings.

Treatment

Observation in mild cases with no abnormal head position or amblyopia. More severe cases may require levator muscle resection, frontalis suspension procedure, Fasanella-Servat procedure, Müller's muscle-conjunctival resection.

Additional Resource

1. Suh DW (2012). Congenital Ptosis. [online] Available from http://www.emedicine.com/oph/TOPIC345.HTM [Accessed April, 2012].

---

475. DUPLICATION 14q SYNDROME

General

Chromosomal 14q duplication syndrome.

Ocular

Hypertelorism; sparse eyelashes and eyebrows; slanted palpebral fissures; ocular colobomata.

Clinical

Postnatal growth retardation; mental retardation; hypotonia; microcephaly; nasal dysmorphism; tented lip; micrognathia; posteriorly rotated ears; minor skeletal anomalies.

Laboratory

Diagnosis is made by clinical findings.

Treatment

None/Ocular.

Bibliography

1. Onwochei BC, Simon JW, Bateman JB, et al. Ocular colobomata. Surv Ophthalmol. 2000;45:175-94.

2. Sklower SL, Jenkins EC, Nolin SL, et al. Distal duplication 14q: report of three cases and further delineation of the syndrome. Hum Genet. 1984;68:159-64.

476. DYSCHONDROPLASIA SYNDROME (ENCHONDROMATOSIS; OLLIER SYNDROME)

General

Chondrodysplasia in which ossification in the epiphyseal region is delayed or absent, with resulting continuation of excessive hypertrophic cartilage formation; dyschondroplasia associated with hemangiomas is referred to as Maffucci syndrome (see Maffucci Syndrome).

Ocular

Narrowing of the optic foramen and supraorbital fissure; ophthalmoplegia; optic atrophy; retinal pigmentation.

Clinical

Joint deformities with functional disturbances; coxa vara or valga; scoliosis; facial asymmetry; unilateral bone involvement with resulting shortening of the extremity; intracranial gliomas; intracavernous chondrosarcoma; clival chondroma.

Laboratory

Cytogenetics, radiographs of the skull, spine and extremities, computed tomography (CT) and magnetic resonance imaging (MRI).

Treatment

Somatotropin (recombinant human growth hormone) is the treatment of choice.

Additional Resource

1. Parikh S (2012). Achondroplasia. [online] Available from http://www.emedicine.com/orthoped/TOPIC4.HTM [Accessed April, 2012].

477. EALES DISEASE (PERIPHLEBITIS)

General

Common; young adults.

Ocular

Sheathing of peripheral veins; hemorrhage in new vessels and later retinal detachment; retinal vascular tortuosity; microaneurysms of retina; postneovascularization of vitreous; internuclear ophthalmoplegia.

Clinical

Epilepsy and hemiplegia have been reported; chronic encephalitis; ulcerative colitis; central nervous infarction.

Laboratory

Fluorescein angiography and tuberculosis screening test.

Treatment

Thyroid extract, osteogenic hormones, androgenic hormones and systemic steroids. The antioxidant vitamins A, C and E have been suggested as a possible therapy because antioxidizing enzymes are deficient in the vitreous samples.

Additional Resource

1. Roth DB (2010). Eales Disease. [online] Available from http://www.emedicine.com/oph/TOPIC637. HTM [Accessed April, 2012].

---

478. EAST-WEST SYNDROME

General

Caused when an intraocular lens is placed so that the edge of the optic, a positioning hole and the components of the loop-optic junction are well within the papillary aperture.

Ocular

Glare; halos; monocular diplopia; irregular pupil.

Clinical

None

Laboratory

Diagnosis is made by clinical findings.

Treatment

Reposition the dislocated intraocular lens (IOL) or suture the dislocated IOL sometimes the IOL will need to be exchanged or removed.

Additional Resource

1. Wu L (2011). Intraocular Lens Dislocation. [online] Available from http://www.emedicine.com/oph/ TOPIC392.HTM [Accessed April, 2012].

---

479. EATON-LAMBERT SYNDROME (MYASTHENIC SYNDROME; MYOCLONIC SYNDROME; OCULAR MYOCLONUS SYNDROME)

General

Males; over 40 years of age; intrathoracic tumor; myasthenia-like condition less likely to have ocular manifestations; positive association with small cell cancer of the lung; underlying autoimmune basis.

Ocular

Decreased amplitude of version in all directions of gaze; ocular myoclonus; corneal abrasion; decreased corneal sensitivity; conjunctival injection; miotic pupil.

Clinical

Weakness; fatigue; peripheral paresthesia; dryness of mouth.

Laboratory

Magnetic resonance imaging (MRI) or computed tomography (CT) of the chest.

Treatment

Search for and treat the underlying malignancy.

Additional Resource

1. Stickler DE (2011). Lambert-Eaton Myasthenic Syndrome (LEMS). [online] Available from http:// www.emedicine.com/neuro/TOPIC181.HTM [Accessed April, 2012].

480. ECLAMPSIA AND PREECLAMPSIA (PREECLAMPSIA; TOXEMIA OF PREGNANCY)

General

Disorders of cells in glomeruli of kidneys that occur during gestation or shortly after delivery.

Ocular

Cortical blindness; nystagmus; mydriasis; absolute pupillary paralysis; ptosis; choroidal detachment; retinal detachment; cotton-wool exudates; optic atrophy; retinal hemorrhages; petechial hemorrhages and focal edema in the occipital cortex.

Clinical

Hypertension; edema; proteinuria; convulsions; coma; death; cardiac failure; weight gain.

Laboratory

Computed tomography of head, MRI, cerebral angiography, laboratory studies—complete blood cell count, platelet count, 24-hour urine for protein/creatinine, electrolytes, liver function tests, aspartate aminotransferase, uric acid, serum glucose.

Treatment

Eclamptic convulsions are life-threatening emergencies and require the proper treatment to decrease maternal morbidity and mortality, Deliver immediately by cesarean delivery, depending on the maternal and fetal condition.

Additional Resource

1. Ross MG (2011). Eclampsia. [online] Available from http://www.emedicine.com/med/TOPIC633. HTM [Accessed April, 2012].

481. ECTOPIA LENTIS WITH ECTOPIA OF PUPIL (ECTOPIA LENTIS ET PUPILLAE)

General

Autosomal recessive.

Ocular

Lens and pupil displaced in opposite directions; bilateral cataracts; acute intermittent intraocular pressure crises; persistent pupillary membrane; poor pupillary dilation.

Clinical

None

Laboratory

Perform appropriate diagnostic and laboratory evaluation—cardiac evaluation for Marfan syndrome, check serum and urine levels of homocysteine or methionine for homocystinuria.

Treatment

Repair of an impending dissecting aortic aneurysm, treatment of glaucoma, lensectomy.

Additional Resource

1. Eifrig CW (2011). Ectopia Lentis. [online] Available from http://www.emedicine.com/oph/TOPIC55. HTM [Accessed April, 2012].

482. ECTRODACTYLY, ECTODERMAL DYSPLASIA, CLEFTING SYNDROME (EEC SYNDROME)

General

Autosomal dominant; low penetrance; variable expressivity.

Ocular

Dacryocystitis; photophobia; corneal ulceration; blepharophimosis; atresia or absence of lacrimal puncta; strabismus; decreased visual acuity.

Clinical

Cleft lip; cleft palate; abnormalities of the urinary tract, hands, feet, and nail hypoplasia, granulomatous perlèche; scalp dermatitis.

Laboratory

X-ray films of hands and feet to demonstrate specific skeletal deformities, renal ultrasonography, sweat pore counts.

Treatment

Therapy depends on which ectodermal structures are involved.

Additional Resource

1. Shah KN (2012). Ectodermal Dysplasia. [online] Available from http://www.emedicine.com/derm/TOPIC114.HTM [Accessed April, 2012].

483. ECTROPION

General

Outward turning of eyelid which can be congenital or acquired.

Clinical

Facial abnormalities.

Ocular

Eyelid turning outward, exposure keratopathy, ocular irritation or infection.

Laboratory

Diagnosis is made by clinical findings.

Treatment

Topical ocular lubricants. Congenital-full thickness skin graft with canthal tendon tightening. Involutional-tighten lid by resecting full thickness wedge-medial spindle procedure for punctal eversion. Paralytic may require a fascia lata sling procedure if does not resolve in 3–6 months.

Additional Resource

1. Ing E (2012). Ectropion. [online] Available from http://www.emedicine.com/oph/TOPIC211.HTM [Accessed April, 2012].

484. EHLERS-DANLOS SYNDROME (CUTIS HYPERELASTICA; CUTIS LAXA; FIBRODYSPLASIA ELASTICA GENERALISATA; INDIAN RUBBER MAN SYNDROME; MEEKEREN-EHLERS-DANLOS SYNDROME)

General

Present at birth; autosomal dominant; two groups: (1) cutaneous and (2) articular; syndrome is one of three primary disorders of elastic tissue (other two are pseudoxanthoma elasticum (Grönblad-Strandberg syndrome) and senile elastosis); inherited disorder of collagen biosynthesis.

Ocular

Hyperelasticity of palpebral skin; easy eversion of upper lid; ptosis; epicanthal folds; hypotony of extraocular muscles; strabismus; microcornea; thinning of cornea with keratoconus; thinning of sclera (blue sclera); subluxation of lens; angioid streaks; chorioretinal hemorrhages; retinitis proliferans with secondary detachment; macular degeneration; myopia; ruptured globe after minor trauma; limbus-to-limbus corneal thinning; acute hydrops; cornea plana; keratoglobus.

Clinical

Cutaneous manifestations include thin, atrophic, fragile skin, cutaneous hyperelasticity and pseudomolluscoid tumors; articular manifestations include excessive articular laxity and luxations; hypermobile joints.

Laboratory

Biochemical studies can detect alterations in collagen molecules in cultured skin fibroblasts. Molecular (DNA-based) testing is available. Diagnosis may be by urinary analyte assay, and clinical examination is the most common.

Treatment

Ascorbic acid therapy, in the event of skin lacerations seriously consider alternatives to sutures, including adhesive strips and wound glues, monitor for cardiac conditions and scolosis.

Additional Resource

1. Steiner RD (2011). Genetics of Ehlers-Danlos Syndrome. [online] Available from http://www. emedicine.com/ped/TOPIC654.HTM [Accessed April, 2012].

---

485. ELDRIDGE SYNDROME

General

Autosomal recessive inheritance; also may involve an enzyme deficiency.

Ocular

Myopia, onset between the ages of 4 and 6 years; increased retinal translucency; temporal crescents; mild electroretinographic abnormalities.

Clinical

Severe myopia; sensorineural hearing loss; low intelligence; mild renal disease.

Laboratory

Diagnosis is made by clinical findings.

Treatment

None/Ocular.

Bibliography

1. Eldridge R, Berlin CI, Money JW, et al. Cochlear deafness, myopia and intellectual impairment in an Amish family. Arch Otolaryngol. 1968;88:49-54.
2. Ohlsson L. Congenital renal disease, deafness and myopia in one family. Acta Med Scand. 1963; 174:77-84.

486. ELECTRICAL INJURY

General

Electric current passes through the body; voltage ranging from 100 to 200 million volts may cause electrical burns.

Ocular

Choroidal atrophy; corneal perforation; necrosis of cornea or lids; blepharospasm; anterior or posterior subcapsular cataracts and vacuoles; optic neuritis; optic nerve atrophy; retinal edema; retinal hemorrhage; pigmentary degeneration; retinal holes; anterior uveitis; hyphema; hypotony; glaucoma; night blindness; nystagmus; paralysis of extraocular muscles; visual field defects; dilation of retinal veins.

Clinical

Skin burns; injury to cardiovascular, central nervous and musculoskeletal systems; tissue necrosis; vascular injury.

Laboratory

Diagnosis is made from clinical findings.

Treatment

Basics of supportive care, and appropriate advanced cardiac life support measures should be administered. Limb-saving measures, such as escharotomy and fasciotomy, may be needed to restore tissue perfusion.

Additional Resource

1. Cushing TA (2010). Electrical Injuries in Emergency Medicine. [online] Available from http://www. emedicine.com/derm/TOPIC859.HTM [Accessed April, 2012].

487. ELLIS-VAN CREVELD SYNDROME (CHONDROECTODERMAL DYSPLASIA)

General

Autosomal recessive inheritance; occurs in the Amish; associated with de novo chromosomal abnormality: deletion of 12 (p11.21p12.2).

Ocular

Esotropia; iris coloboma; congenital cataract.

Clinical

Bilateral polydactyly; short and plump limbs; genu valgum; talipes (equinovarus, calcaneovalgus); thoracic constriction; fusion of middle part of upper lip to maxillary gingival margin; dental anomalies: number, shape, spacing; congenital heart defect in about 50% of patients; dystrophic fingernails; genital anomalies; mild mental retardation; short stature; hypoplastic hair and skin; oligodontia; small thoracic cage; hypoplastic pelvis; cone-shaped epiphyses of hands.

Laboratory

Diagnosis is made by clinical findings.

Treatment

Esotropia: Equalized vision with correct refractive error; surgery may be helpful in patient with diplopia.

Retinal detachment: Scleral buckle, pneumatic retinopexy and vitrectomy may be used to close all the breaks.

Additional Resource

1. Chen H (2011). Ellis-van Creveld Syndrome. [online] Available from http://www.emedicine.com/ped/TOPIC660.HTM [Accessed April, 2012].

488. ELSCHNIG SYNDROME (ELSCHNIG SYNDROME II)

General

Present from birth; etiology unknown.

Ocular

Elongation of lid fissure with downward displacement of the lateral angle; ectropion of lower lid.

Clinical

Cleft lip and palate may occur.

Laboratory

Diagnosis is made by clinical findings.

Treatment

Ectropion: Topical ocular lubricants. Congenital-full thickness skin graft with canthal tendon tightening. Involutional-tighten lid by resecting full thickness wedge-medial spindle procedure for punctal eversion. Paralytic may require a fascia lata sling procedure if does not resolve in 3–6 months.

Bibliography

1. Elschnig A. Zur Kenntnis der Anomalien der Lidspalten Form. Klin Monatsbl Augenheilkd. 1912;17-30.
2. Magalini SI, Scrascia E. Dictionary of Medical Syndromes, 2nd edition. Philadelphia: JB Lippincott; 1981. p. 253.
3. Pau H. Differential Diagnosis of Eye Diseases. New York: Thieme; 1987.

489. ELSCHNIG SYNDROME I (MEIBOMIAN CONJUNCTIVITIS)

General

Chronic inflammations; characteristic foamy secretion; benign.

Ocular

Conjunctivitis; foamy secretion; ocular irritation; photophobia; minimal visual impairment.

Clinical

Hyperplasia of tarsal glands.

Laboratory

Diagnosis is made by clinical findings.

Treatment

Symptomatic control may include cold compresses and artificial tears; nonsteroidal and occasionally steroidal drops to relieve itching.

Bibliography

1. Elschnig A. Belt ray Artiologie und Therapie der chronischen Conjunctivitis. Dtsch Med Wochenschr. 1908;34:1133-5.
2. Magalini SI, Scrascia E. Dictionary of Medical Syndromes, 2nd edition. Philadelphia: JB Lippincott; 1981.

490. EMPTY SELLA SYNDROME

General

Further progression of ocular findings and symptoms after treatment of pituitary tumors.

Ocular

Reduced visual acuity and possible blindness; hemianopsia; quadranopsia; irregular field defects; central scotoma; pale optic disks; central retinal vein occlusion.

Clinical

Acromegalic features and other general systemic manifestations depend on the type of the primary tumor the patient had and are not part of the "empty sella syndrome" that is responsible for progression of ocular pathologic condition.

Laboratory

Laboratory and radiographic tests are necessary to confirm the diagnosis. ACTH deficiency in the morning during its highest circadian levels suggests a pituitary/hypothalamic etiology. The corticotropin stimulation test, which evaluates the hypothalamic-pituitary-adrenal axis, is a superior tool in distinguishing hypopituitarism from primary adrenal insufficiency.

Treatment

The treatment of patients with hypopituitarism is often complex because of multiple endocrine deficiencies and consequent abnormalities that require close specific laboratory testing and monitoring during treatment. Interventions including sodium replacement, glucose replacement, bradycardia treatment, steroid administration and fluid resuscitation may be necessary.

Bibliography

1. Dahlstrom R, Acers TE. Chiasmatic arachnoiditis and empty sella: report and discussion of a case. Ann Ophthalmol. 1975;7:73-6.
2. Pollock SC, Bromberg BS. Visual loss in a patient with primary empty sella. Arch Ophthalmol. 1987;105:1487-8.

491. ENCEPHALITIS, ACUTE

General

In approximately 0.1–0.2% of patients having rubeola (measles), an acute encephalitis is seen within 1 week after the onset of the rash; a case of immunosuppressive encephalitis can present with focal seizures leading to progressive obtundation.

Ocular

Papillitis; optic atrophy; ocular motor palsies; nystagmus; optic neuritis or neuroretinitis.

Clinical

Rise in temperature; drowsiness; irritability; meningismus; vomiting and headache; stupor; convulsions; coma.

Laboratory

Perform head CT, with or without contrast agent, before LP to search for evidence of elevated intracerebral pressure MRI is useful; viral serology.

Treatment

Evaluate and treat for shock or hypotension, treat systemic complications, acyclovir.

Additional Resource

1. Howes DS (2012). Encephalitis. [online] Available from http://www.emedicine.com/emerg/TOPIC163.HTM [Accessed April, 2012].

492. ENDOCARDITIS

General

Common in people with arteriosclerosis; subacute form leads to pyemia; bacterial endocarditis without heart murmur seen in intravenous drug users.

Ocular

Retinal hemorrhages; conjunctival petechiae; choroiditis; Roth spots; spastic mydriasis; optic neuritis; central retinal artery occlusion; choroidal abscess, subretinal neovascularization.

Clinical

Heart murmur; fever; intracranial aneurysm; cerebral hemorrhage; subarachnoid hemorrhage.

Laboratory

Electrocardiogram (ECG or EKG), chest X-ray, ventilation/perfusion and CT.

Treatment

Stabilize the patient with acute disease and cardiovascular instability, empiric antibiotic therapy, suspected infectious endocarditis should be admitted to the hospital for IV antibiotics while blood cultures are pending.

Additional Resource

1. Brusch JL (2011). Infective Endocarditis. [online] Available from http://www.emedicine.com/emerg/TOPIC164.HTM [Accessed April, 2012].

493. ENGELMANN SYNDROME [CAMURATI-ENGELMANN DISEASE; HEREDITARY MULTIPLE DIAPHYSEAL SCLEROSIS; JUVENILE PAGET DISEASE; MULTIPLEX INFANTILIS; OSTEOPATHIA HYPEROSTOTICA (SCLEROTICANS) DIAPHYSEAL DYSPLASIA]

General

Etiology unknown; progressive resorption and deposits of bone with thickening of periosteum and changes of cortex as evident by diagnostic X-ray studies in the intermediate portion of the long bones.

Ocular

Exophthalmos; hypertelorism (secondary); ptosis; lagophthalmos; lateral rectus palsy; convergence insufficiency; epiphora; cataract; tortuous retinal vessels; papilledema; optic atrophy.

Clinical

Pain in extremities; poorly developed musculature; waddling gait; delayed ambulation; scaly skin; delayed dentition; deafness; hypogonadism; pain in both legs; aching in the forearms; episodic temporofrontal and occipital headache.

Laboratory

Diagnosis is made by clinical findings.

Treatment

Exophthalmos: Reversing the problem, which is causing the exophthalmos, is the treatment of choice and will minimize the ocular complications. Ocular lubricants are beneficial for control of the corneal exposure.

Ptosis: If visual acuity is affected most cases require surgical correction, and there are several procedures that may be used including levator resection, repair or advancement and Fasanella-Servat.

Cataract: Change in glasses can sometimes improve a patient's visual function temporarily; however, the most common treatment is cataract surgery.

Papilledema: Underlying cause should be determined and treated. Systemic acetazolamide is the medical therapy of choice.

Bibliography

1. Brodrick JD. Luxation of the globe in Engelmann's disease. Am J Ophthalmol. 1977;83:870-3.
2. De Vits A, Keymeulen B, Bossuyt A, et al. Progressive diaphyseal dysplasia (Camurati-Engelmann's disease). Improvement of clinical signs and of bone scintigraphy during pregnancy. Clin Nucl Med. 1994;19:104-7.
3. Engelmann G. Ein Fall von Osteopathia Hyperostotica (Scleroticans) Infantilis. Fortschr Geb Roentgen Strahl. 1929;39:1101.
4. Morse PH, Walsh FB, McCormick JR. Ocular findings in hereditary diaphyseal dysplasia (Engelmann's disease). Am J Ophthalmol. 1969;68:100-4.
5. Roy FH, Fraunfelder FW, Fraunfelder FT. Roy and Fraunfelder's Current Ocular Therapy, 6th edition. Philadelphia: WB Saunders; 2008.

494. ENTEROBIASIS (OXYURIASIS; PINWORM; SEATWORM)

General

Intestinal infection caused by *Enterobius vermicularis*; worm's head attached to cecal mucosa, appendix or parts of bowel; worms travel anal canal and deposit eggs on perianal skin; eggs infective for 10–20 days; airborne transmission; common in children; extraintestinal pinworm infection has been reported.

Ocular

Palpebral edema; blepharitis; keratoconjunctivitis; macular edema.

Clinical

Pruritus; eczema; pyogenic infection; vaginal discharge; chronic granulomatous salpingitis; endometritis.

Laboratory

Wide (2 inches) transparent tape is pressed against the perineum at night or in the morning before the patient bathes to capture eggs. Three such specimens are usually consecutively collected. Diagnosis is made by identifying eggs under the low power lens of microscope. Dilute sodium hydroxide or toluene should be added to the slide.

Treatment

Mebendazole or albendazole are recommended as first-line treatment of pinworms, simultaneously treating all household members may be reasonable.

Additional Resource

1. Wolfram W (2011). Enterobiasis. [online] Available from http://www.emedicine.com/ped/TOPIC684.HTM [Accessed April, 2012].

495. ENTROPION

General

Inversion of eyelid can be classified as congenital, cicatricial, spastic and involutional.

Clinical

None

Ocular

Inversion of either the upper or lower eyelid, ocular irritation, corneal scarring and corneal staining.

Laboratory

Diagnosis is made by clinical findings.

Treatment

Topical antibiotics and lubricants, temporary sutures to event the eyelid, lateral cantholysis with subconjunctival incision just inferior to the tarsus. Inferior retractors are isolated and reattached to anteroinferior portion of tarsus with multiple interrupted sutures.

Bibliography

1. Kakizaki H, Selva D, Leibovitch I. Cilial entropion: surgical outcome with a new modification of the Hotz procedure. Ophthalmology. 2009;116:2224-9.

Additional Resource

1. DeBacker C (2011). Entropion. [online] Available from http://www.emedicine.com/oph/TOPIC212. HTM [Accessed April, 2012].

496. EPIBLEPHARON

General

Autosomal dominant; occurs predominantly in Chinese individuals.

Ocular

Epicanthus; epiblepharon of the upper and lower lids.

Clinical

None

Laboratory

Diagnosis is made by clinical findings.

Treatment

Epicanthus: Skin resection such as Verwey's Y to V operation, double Z-plasty, Mustard's technique or five-flap procedure works.

Bibliography

1. Hu DN. Ophthalmic genetics in China. Ophthalmic Paediatr Genet. 1983;2:39-45.

497. EPICANTHUS

General

Autosomal dominant.

Ocular

Epicanthus; epiblepharon of the upper and lower lids; ptosis.

Clinical

None

Laboratory

Diagnosis is made by clinical findings.

Treatment

Epicanthus tarsalis, palpebralis and supraculiarus will decrease with age. Skin resection such as Verwey's Y to V operation, double Z-plasty, Mustard's technique or five-flap procedure works.

Bibliography

1. Hu DN. Ophthalmic genetics in China. Ophthalmic Paediatr Genet. 1983;2:39-45.

498. EPIDEMIC KERATOCONJUNCTIVITIS

General

Highly communicable; adenovirus types 8 and 19; usually bilateral; epidemic keratoconjunctivitis has been reported worldwide associated with 11 virus serotypes, with serotypes 8, 11 and 19 being the most common responsible ones.

Ocular

Follicular or membranous conjunctivitis; chemosis; subconjunctival hemorrhages; corneal opacity; punctate epithelial keratitis; corneal ulcer; blepharospasm; lid edema; serous discharge; uveitis; epiphora.

Clinical

Submaxillary and cervical lymphadenopathy.

Laboratory

Viral insolation on cell culture from conjunctival scrapings.

Treatment

No effective topical or systemic treatment available. Topical steroids may be used if epithelial keratitis occurs.

Additional Resource

1. Bawazeer A (2011). Epidemic Keratoconjunctivitis. [online] Available from http://www.emedicine.com/oph/TOPIC677.HTM [Accessed April, 2012].

499. EPIDERMAL NEVUS SYNDROME (ICHTHYOSIS HYSTRIX)

General

One or a combination of the following epidermal nevi described as nevus unius lateris, ichthyosis hystrix, linear nevus sebaceous or congenital acanthosis nigricans; autosomal dominant.

Ocular

Blepharoptosis and fibroma on bulbar conjunctiva; antimongoloid eyelid fissures; eyelid colobomata; horizontal and rotary nystagmus; esotropia; conjunctival tumors; corneal opacities; corectopia and colobomata of the iris.

Clinical

Somatic anomalies involving the skeletal and central nervous system; anomalies of bone formation; atrophy; ankylosis; vitamin D-resistant rickets; bone cysts; mental retardation; cortical atrophy; hydrocephalus; focal and grand mal epilepsy; cerebrovascular tumors; cortical blindness.

Laboratory

Histologic examination, EEG, MRI.

Treatment

Vitamin D analogs may work by inhibiting epidermal proliferation, promoting keratinocyte differentiation, and/or exerting immunosuppressive effects on lymphoid cells.

Additional Resource

1. Schwartz RA (2012). Epidermal Nevus Syndrome. [online] Available from http://www.emedicine.com/derm/TOPIC732.HTM [Accessed April, 2012].

500. EPILEPSY, LIGHT-SENSITIVE

General

Autosomal dominant.

Ocular

Photic stimulation of 15–30 flashes per second, inducing epileptic seizure.

Clinical

Spastic paraparesis; mental retardation; light sensitivity.

Laboratory

Electroencephalography (EEG), clinical history.

Treatment

Both ethosuximide and valproate suppress absence seizures in more than 80% of patients.

Additional Resource

1. Kaddurah AK (2011). Benign Childhood Epilepsy. [online] Available from http://www.emedicine.com/neuro/TOPIC641.HTM [Accessed April, 2012].

501. EPIMACULAR PROLIFERATION (MACULAR PUCKER)

General

Condition in which the macular region is destroyed by the contraction of a fibrocellular epiretinal membrane that has grown across the inner retinal surface.

Clinical

None

Laboratory

Optical coherence tomography (OCT) demonstrates extent of epiretinal membrane, fluorescein angiography.

Treatment

Three port pars plana vitrectomy.

Additional Resource

1. Oh KT (2012). Epimacular Membrane. [online] Available from http://www.emedicine.com/oph/TOPIC396.HTM [Accessed April, 2012].

502. EPIPHORIA

General

Hypersecretion or failure of the lacrimal excretory system to function.

Clinical

Nasal pathology.

Ocular

Epiphoria, corneal foreign body, trichiasis, corneal ulcer, entropion, ectropion or lid retraction.

Laboratory

Diagnosis is made by clinical findings.

Treatment

Treat the underlying cause, massage the tear sac and antibiotics, conjunctival dacryocystorhinostomy with Jones tube.

Bibliography

1. Roy FH, Fraunfelder FW, Fraunfelder FT. Roy and Fraunfelder's Current Ocular Therapy, 6th edition. Philadelphia: WB Saunders; 2008.

503. EPIPHYSEAL DYSPLASIA, MICROCEPHALY, AND NYSTAGMUS

General

Autosomal recessive.

Ocular

Nystagmus; retinitis pigmentosa.

Clinical

Epiphyseal dysplasia; microcephaly; short stature.

Laboratory

Diagnosis is made by clinical findings.

Treatment

Retinitis pigmentosa: Vitamin A 15,000 IU/day is thought to slow the decline of retinal function, dark sunglasses for outdoor use, surgery for cataract, genetic counseling.

Additional Resource

1. Parikh S (2012). Diastrophic Dysplasia. [online] Available from http://www.emedicine.com/orthoped/TOPIC632.HTM [Accessed April, 2012].

504. EPIPHYSEAL DYSPLASIA OF FEMORAL HEADS, MYOPIA, AND DEAFNESS

General

Autosomal recessive.

Ocular

Severe myopia.

Clinical

Femoral epiphyseal dysplasia; deafness.

Laboratory

Diagnosis is made by clinical findings.

Treatment

Myopia: Generally treated with glasses, contact lens and refractive surgery.

Additional Resource

1. Parikh S (2012). Diastrophic Dysplasia. [online] Available from http://www.emedicine.medscape.com/article/1257787-overview [Accessed April, 2012].

505. EPISCLERITIS

General

Benign, recurrent, self-limiting inflammation of the highly vascularized episclera which is closely attached to the underlying sclera and the mobile Tenon's capsule.

Clinical

Episcleritis may be the first sign of a systemic connective tissue disorder.

Ocular

Pain, redness and swelling around the eyes.

Laboratory

Diagnosis is made by clinical findings.

Treatment

Topical prednisolone, artificial tears and cold compresses.

Additional Resources

1. Roy H (2012). Episcleritis. [online] Available from http://www.emedicine.com/oph/TOPIC641.HTM [Accessed April, 2012].
2. de la Maza MS (2010). Scleritis. [online] Available from http://www.emedicine.com/oph/TOPIC642. HTM [Accessed April, 2012].

---

506. EPISKOPI BLINDNESS

General

Sex-linked; confined to male members of Greek Cypriot family group, most of whom live in Episkopi.

Ocular

Microphthalmia; corneal opacities; transverse corneal band; iritis; cataract; retrolental opacities; retinitis pigmentosa; Leber optic atrophy; amaurosis.

Clinical

None

Laboratory

Diagnosis is made by clinical findings.

Treatment

Cataract: Change in glasses can sometimes improve a patient's visual function temporarily; however, the most common treatment is cataract surgery.

Retinitis pigmentosa: Vitamin A 15,000 IU/day is thought to slow the decline of retinal function, dark sunglasses for outdoor use, surgery for cataract, genetic counseling.

Iritis: Oral steroids if not responsive to topical steroids, immunosuppressants if bilateral disease that does not respond to oral steroids, periocular steroids for unilateral or posterior uveitis. Vitrectomy can be used for severe vitreous opacification. Cryotherapy and laser photocoagulation may be used for localized pars plana exudates.

Bibliography

1. Roy FH. Ocular Differential Diagnosis, 8th edition. Philadelphia: Lippincott Williams & Wilkins; 2007.
2. Taylor PJ, Coates T, Newhouse ML. Episkopi blindness: hereditary blindness in a Greek Cypriot family. Br J Ophthalmol. 1959;43:340-4.

507. EPITHELIAL EROSION SYNDROME (FRANCESCHETTI DYSTROPHY; KAUFMAN SYNDROME; METAHERPETIC KERATITIS; POST-TRAUMATIC KERATITIS)

General

Most likely caused by herpes simplex virus; previous corneal trauma or autosomal dominant.

Ocular

Recurrent erosions of the corneal epithelium, usually seen within weeks or months after herpes simplex infection of the cornea; "loose" epithelium is removed from the underlying Bowman's membrane mechanically by lid blinking; defects are irregular in shape and stain positively with fluorescein dye; underlying corneal stroma usually shows some edema; pain upon opening eyes in morning.

Clinical

Mild fever; occasionally herpetic skin lesions.

Laboratory

Diagnosis is made by clinical findings.

Treatment

Corneal erosion: The goal of therapy is regenerating or repairing the epithelial basement membrane to restore the adhesion between the epithelium and the anterior stroma; topical lubrication therapy, bandage soft contact lenses, debridement of the epithelium and basement membrane or anterior stromal micropuncture may be useful.

Additional Resource

1. Verma A (2012). Recurrent Corneal Erosion. [online] Available from http://www.emedicine.com/oph/TOPIC113.HTM [Accessed April, 2012].

508. EPITHELIAL INGROWTH (EPITHELIAL DOWNGROWTH)

General

Epithelial ingrowth in a sheet-like fashion which is a rare complication of ocular trauma or anterior segment surgery.

Clinical

None

Ocular

Hypotony, prolonged inflammation.

Laboratory

Diagnosis is made from clinical findings.

Treatment

Excision of epithelial sheets has been reported with variable success. A corneoscleral graft is necessary following this procedure.

Bibliography

1. Roy FH, Fraunfelder FW, Fraunfelder FT. Roy and Fraunfelder's Current Ocular Therapy, 6th edition. Philadelphia: WB Saunders; 2008.

509. ERB-GOLDFLAM SYNDROME (ERB II SYNDROME; HOPPE-GOLDFLAM DISEASE; PSEUDOPARALYTIC SYNDROME; MYASTHENIA GRAVIS)

General

Occurs at any age; more frequent between the ages of 20 and 40 years; more females affected than males; progressive; spontaneous; symptoms improve or resolve with rest in early stages of disease (see Myasthenia Gravis, Neonatal or Infantile); caused by autoantibodies against the acetylcholine receptor at the neuromuscular junction, leading to abnormal fatigability and weakness of skeletal muscle.

Ocular

Transient diplopia; ptosis of upper eyelids.

Clinical

Excessive fatigability of musculature; symptoms appear and increase as day progresses; expressionless face; sagging jaw; difficulty in chewing and talking; nasal regurgitation.

Laboratory

"Ice test" crushed ice in surgical glove over ptotic eyelid for 2 minutes and watch for brief-elevation of eyelid; Tensilon test and Prostigmin test may result in elevation of ptotic eyelid or improved strabismus in individuals with myasthemia gravis.

Treatment

Adrenal corticosteroids are frequently used. In some cases mycophenolate, mofetil, cyclosporine and cyclophosphamide may be useful. Patching one eye or using prisms may be helpful.

Bibliography

1. Erb W. Zur Casuistick der Bulbaren La hmungen. Arch Psychiatr Vervenkr. 1879;9:325-50.
2. Goldflam S. Vebereinen Scheinbar Keilbaren Bulbarparalytischem Symptom Complex mit Betheiligung der Extremitaten. Dtsch Z Nerven. 1983;4:312-52.
3. Kim JH, Hwang JM, Hwang YS, et al. Childhood ocular myasthenia gravis. Ophthalmology. 2003; 110:1458-62.
4. Roy FH, Fraunfelder FW, Fraunfelder FT. Roy and Fraunfelder's Current Ocular Therapy, 6th edition. Philadelphia: WB Saunders; 2008.
5. Sommer N, Melms A, Weller M, et al. Ocular myasthenia gravis. A critical review of clinical and pathophysiological aspects. Doc Ophthalmol. 1993;84:309-33.

510. EROSION SYNDROME

General

Caused by imperfect adherence of corneal epithelium due to abnormalities in basement membrane; abnormalities may be inherent, induced by trauma, or both; disease is not vision threatening.

Ocular

Disabling episodes of pain; stabbing pain in the eye like that from a foreign body, most frequent on awakening; lesser forms of irritation; blurring of vision; drying associated with a stinging in the eyes; irregular astigmatism; corneal findings include anterior membrane dystrophies (epithelial and subepithelial dot, map or fingerprint-type changes).

Clinical

None

Laboratory

Diagnosis is made by clinical findings.

Treatment

Corneal erosion: The goal of therapy is regenerating or repairing the epithelial basement membrane to restore the adhesion between the epithelium and the anterior stroma; topical lubrication therapy, bandage soft contact lenses, debridement of the epithelium and basement membrane or anterior stromal micropuncture may be useful.

Additional Resource

1. Verma A (2012). Recurrent Corneal Erosion. [online] Available from http://www.emedicine.com/oph/TOPIC113.HTM [Accessed April, 2012].

---

511. ERYTHEMA NODOSUM (DERMATITIS CONTUSIFORMIS)

General

Young females; hypersensitive reaction secondary to viral, bacterial and fungal infections; duration 2–4 weeks; recurrences possible.

Ocular

Subcutaneous nodules involving lids; keratitis; uveitis.

Clinical

Painful nodules on surface of thighs, arms and face; fever; malaise; red lesions that progress to bruise-like and disappear in a few days to 3 weeks; cervical lymphadenopathy; exquisitely tender, erythematous nodules distributed symmetrically on the extensor surfaces of the lower extremities.

Laboratory

Throat culture as part of the initial workup to exclude group A beta-hemolytic streptococcal infection. Erythrocyte sedimentation rates are often very high. Antistreptolysin titer is elevated in some patients with streptococcal disease, but normal values do not exclude streptococcal infection. Evaluate titer levels during the initial workup, since streptococcal disease is a common cause of erythema nodosum (EN). Order stool examination, since along with the appropriate history of gastrointestinal complaints, a stool examination can exclude infection by Yersinia, Salmonella and Campylobacter organisms. Order blood cultures according to preliminary indications and findings.

Treatment

Self-limited disease and requires only symptomatic relief using nonsteroidal anti-inflammatory drugs (NSAIDs), cool wet compresses, elevation and bed rest.

Additional Resource

1. Hebel JL (2010). Erythema Nodosum. [online] Available from http://www.emedicine.com/derm/TOPIC138.HTM [Accessed April, 2012].

---

512. ESCHERICHIA COLI

General

Gram-negative rod is found in the gastrointestinal tract; urinary tract is the usual portal of entry.

Ocular

Uveitis; hyphema; hypopyon; gas bubbles in anterior chamber; purulent conjunctivitis; keratitis; corneal edema; panophthalmitis; endo-phthalmitis; glaucoma.

Clinical

Diarrhea; gastroenteritis; dehydration.

Laboratory

Anaerobic Gram-negative rod.

Treatment

Antibiotic therapy should start with ampicillin until sensitivity reports return.

Additional Resource

1. Suh DW (2012). Ophthalmologic Manifestations of Escherichia Coli. [online] Available from http://www.emedicine.com/oph/TOPIC496.HTM [Accessed April, 2012].

---

513. ESOTROPIA: HIGH ACCOMMODATIVE CONVERGENCE TO ACCOMMODATION RATIO

General

The ratio of accommodative convergence (AC) to accommodation (A) (AC/A) is measure of responsiveness of convergence for each diopter of accommodation, onset is from age 1 to 7.

Clinical

None

Ocular

Esotropia, accommodation is greater at near than distance.

Laboratory

Diagnosis is made by clinical findings.

Treatment

Goal—achievement of alignment distance and near by use of single vision lens—full prescription.

Additional Resource

1. Noyes C (2012). Esotropia with High AC/A Ratio. [online] Available from http://www.emedicine.com/oph/TOPIC557.HTM [Accessed April, 2012].

---

514. ESPILDORA-LUQUE SYNDROME (OPHTHALMIC SYLVIAN SYNDROME)

General

Embolism of the ophthalmic artery with refectory spasm of the middle cerebral artery.

Ocular

Unilateral blindness (caused by ophthalmic artery embolism).

Clinical

Temporary hemiplegia contralateral side of amaurosis (caused by reflex spasm of the middle cerebral artery).

Laboratory

Diagnosis is made by clinical findings.

Treatment

Lowering of intraocular pressure with oral and topical medications, carbogen therapy and hyperbaric oxygen may be useful.

Bibliography

1. Espildora-Luque C. Ophthalmic sylvian syndrome. Arch Oft Hisp Am. 1934;34:616.
2. Geeraets WJ. Ocular Syndromes, 3rd edition. Philadelphia: Lea & Febiger; 1976.

515. ETHAN SYNDROME, PRIMARY

General

Congenital, esotropia, head turn and nystagmus coexistent with nystagmus compensation and nystagmus blockage syndrome (see Nystagmus Compensation Syndrome; Nystagmus Blockage Syndrome).

Ocular

Esotropia; esophoria; nystagmus; amblyopia; orthophoria.

Clinical

Head turn and chin elevation to compensate for nystagmus.

Laboratory

Diagnosis is made by clinical findings.

Treatment

Strabismus surgery is used in patients with certain forms of nystagmus with varying degrees of success.

Additional Resources

1. Ocampo VVD (2010). Infantile Esotropia. [online] Available from http://www.emedicine.com/oph/TOPIC328.HTM [Accessed April, 2012].
2. Curtis T (2010). Nystagmus, Congenital. [online] Available from http://www.emedicine.com/oph/TOPIC688.HTM [Accessed April, 2012].

516. ETHAN SYNDROME, SECONDARY

General

Classic nystagmus blockage syndrome, but after strabismus surgery development of head turn with straight eyes and appearance of nystagmus compensation syndrome (see Nystagmus Blockage Syndrome; Nystagmus Compensation Syndrome).

Ocular

Esotropia; nystagmus; orthophoria; amblyopia; nystagmus increased in abduction.

Clinical

Abnormal head position.

Laboratory

Diagnosis is made by clinical findings.

Treatment

Strabismus surgery is used in patients with certain forms of nystagmus with varying degrees.

Additional Resources

1. Ocampo VVD (2010). Infantile Esotropia. [online] Available from http://www.emedicine.com/oph/TOPIC328.HTM [Accessed April, 2012].
2. Curtis T (2010). Nystagmus, Congenital. [online] Available from http://www.emedicine.com/oph/TOPIC688.HTM [Accessed April, 2012].

517. EWING SARCOMA (EWING SYNDROME)

General

Highly metastatic round cell tumor of bone; most commonly involves long or trunk bones; metastasizes at high rate; usually occurs between the ages of 10 and 25 years; seen more frequently in males than in females.

Ocular

Exophthalmos; orbital hemorrhages; orbital necrosis; commonly found as the second malignancy in patients with hereditary retinoblastoma.

Clinical

Lytic bone destruction; pain; edema; slight fever.

Laboratory

Histologic testing requires fresh tissue. Biopsy site to be in area of radiation.

Treatment

Tumor spread must be recognized, and methods such as PET scanning with FDG and/or bone scanning can help in detecting metastases.

Additional Resource

1. Strauss LG (2011). Ewing Sarcoma Imaging. [online] Available from http://www.emedicine.com/radio/TOPIC275.HTM [Accessed April, 2012].

---

518. EXFOLIATION SYNDROME (CAPSULAR EXFOLIATION SYNDROME)

General

Only in men older than 60 years.

Ocular

Iridodonesis; rubeosis iridis; cataract; phacodonesis; dislocated lens; corneal dystrophy; choroidal sclerosis; primary optic atrophy; lens capsule exfoliation; lower endothelial cell density.

Clinical

None

Laboratory

Diagnosis is made by clinical findings.

Treatment

Aggressive open-angle glaucoma therapy with topical agents is the initial treatment. Laser trabeculatomy and filtering surgery may be necessary.

Additional Resource

1. Pons ME (2011). Pseudoexfoliation Glaucoma. [online] Available from http://www.emedicine.com/oph/TOPIC140.HTM [Accessed April, 2012].

---

519. EXOPHTHALMOS (PROPTOSIS)

General

Abnormal protrusion of the eyeball. Etiology is varied and can include inflammatory, vascular or infections. Thyroid disease is the most frequent cause for both unilateral or bilateral exophthalmos.

Clinical

Thyroid disease, lymphoma, cavernous hemangiomas, leukemia, sinsus disease.

Ocular

Proptosis, orbital cellulitis, orbital emphysema, lid retraction, punctate keratopathy, corneal ulcer, corneal perforation, diplopia.

Laboratory

Thyroid function studies, CT, MRI, ocular ultrasonography can all be used to determine the cause.

Treatment

Reversing the problem, which is causing the exophthalmos, is the treatment of choice and will minimize the ocular complications. Ocular lubricants are beneficial for control of the corneal exposure.

Additional Resource

1. Mercandetti M (2010). Exophthalmos. [online] Available from http://www.emedicine.com/oph/TOPIC616.HTM [Accessed April, 2012].

520. EXTERNAL ORBITAL FRACTURES

General

External fracture of the orbit results in direct disjunction of any portion of the orbital rim usually with bony orbital wall involvement.

Clinical

Tripod fractures of the zygoma, naso-orbital ethnoid fractures.

Laboratory

Computed tomography (CT) and ultrasound.

Treatment

Surgery is indicated when bone displacement causes cosmetic or functional defects.

Additional Resource

1. Seiff S (2012). Zygomatic Orbital Fracture. [online] Available from http://www.emedicine.com/oph/TOPIC231.HTM [Accessed April, 2012].

521. EXTRAOCULAR MUSCLE LACERATIONS

General

Rare without damage to globe, eyelid and adjacent structures.

Clinical

None

Ocular

Laceration of extraocular muscles most frequently the lateral or medial muscle.

Laboratory

Diagnosis is made by clinical findings and history.

Treatment

Reattachment of lacerated ends of muscle or tendon immediately after trauma.

Bibliography

1. Roy FH, Fraunfelder FW, Fraunfelder FT. Roy and Fraunfelder's Current Ocular Therapy, 6th edition. Philadelphia: WB Saunders; 2008.

522. EXTREME HYDROCEPHALUS SYNDROME (CHONDRODYSTROPHICUS CONGENITA; CLOVERLEAF SKULL SYNDROME; HYDROCEPHALUS; KLEEBLATTSCHÄDEL SYNDROME)

General

Secondary obstruction of cerebrospinal fluid circulation is caused by some primary disease such as maternal rubella, Rh incompatibility or hydramnion; Arnold-Chiari syndrome has similar associated findings; almost all affected children are born dead.

Ocular

Exophthalmos with downward placement and downward rotation of the globes; propulsion of globes; upper lid retraction and lower lids covering almost half of the downwardly rotated cornea; nystagmus; strabismus; exposure keratitis; optic nerve atrophy.

Clinical

Extreme hydrocephalus; low-set ears; thin and spastic extremities with digital anomalies; convulsions; spina bifida.

Laboratory

Computed tomography, MRI, ultrasound through the anterior fontanelle.

Treatment

Surgical treatment is the preferred therapeutic option and shunts are performed in the majority of patients.

Additional Resource

1. Espay AJ (2010). Hydrocephalus. [online] Available from http://www.emedicine.com/neuro/TOPIC161.HTM [Accessed April, 2012].

523. EYEBROW WHORL

General

Autosomal dominant.

Ocular

Whorl in the hair of the eyebrow; myopia; telecanthus; hypertelorism.

Clinical

Deafness, proteinuria.

Laboratory

Diagnosis is made by clinical findings.

Treatment

None/Ocular.

Bibliography

1. McKusick VA. Mendelian Inheritance in Man: A Catalog of Human Genes and Genetic Disorders, 12th edition. Baltimore: The Johns Hopkins University Press; 1998.

524. EYELID CONTUSIONS, LACERATIONS, AND AVUSIONS

General

Trauma to the eyelid, blowout fracture.

Clinical

None

Ocular

Eyelid contusion, laceration or avulsion.

Laboratory

Computed tomography (CT) scan for orbital fracture, MRI for soft tissue contrast.

Treatment

Oral and topical antibiotics, debridement of wound, repair of laceration with sutures, repair of canalicular injury. Laceration of canthus may require an oculoplastic surgeon.

Additional Resource

1. Ing E (2010). Eyelid Laceration. [online] Available from http://www.emedicine.com/oph/TOPIC219. HTM [Accessed April, 2012].

---

525. FABRY DISEASE (ANGIOKERATOMA CORPORIS DIFFUSUM SYNDROME; DIFFUSE ANGIOKERATOSIS; FABRY-ANDERSON SYNDROME; GLYCOSPHINGOLIPID LIPIDOSIS; GLYCOSPHINGOLIPIDOSIS)

General

Lipoid storage disorder; X-linked recessive inheritance; lack of alpha-galactosidase A enzyme.

Ocular

Swelling of eyelids; varicosities of palpebral and bulbar conjunctiva; corneal dystrophy; corneal opacities; increased tortuosity of retinal vessels and aneurismal dilatations; cornea verticillata; cataract; central retinal artery occlusion; internuclear paralysis of extraocular muscles; papilledema; tortuosity and caliber irregularity of conjunctival vessels; characteristic cream-colored whorl-like opacity in deep part of corneal epithelium; posterior cataract; occasional edema of optic disk and retina.

Clinical

Angiokeratoma of the skin with small, grouped papular lesions mainly over the scrotum, thighs, buttocks, sacral area, umbilical area and lips; elevated blood pressure; disturbance in sweat secretion; pain in arms and legs; enlarged heart; albuminuria.

Laboratory

Reduced alpha-galactosidase A level in plasma; elevated trihexosyl ceramide levels in urine and plasma.

Treatment

Primarily surgical and is usually a corneal transplant. After surgery, treatment of amblyopia and optical therapy can be helpful.

Additional Resource

1. Banikazemi M (2012). Genetics of Fabry Disease. [online] Available from http://www.emedicine. com/ped/TOPIC2888.HTM [Accessed April, 2012].

526. FACIAL MOVEMENT DISORDERS (BENIGN ESSENTIAL BLEPHAROSPASM, HEMIFACIAL SPASM)

General

Bilateral-blepharospasm and unilateral-hemifacial spasm; can be associated with Parkinson disease.

Clinical

Spasms of the face.

Ocular

Forceful closure of one or both eyelids.

Laboratory

Diagnosis is made by clinical findings.

Treatment

Artane by mouth or botulinum toxin injections may be useful. Surgically—resect of the obicularis oculi muscles or decompression of the facial nerve may be necessary.

Additional Resource

1. Graham RH (2011). Benign Essential Blepharospasm. [online] Available from http://www.emedicine.com/oph/TOPIC202.HTM [Accessed April, 2012].

527. FACIO-OCULO-ACOUSTICO-RENAL SYNDROME

General

Autosomal recessive.

Ocular

Congenital myopia; undeveloped filtration angle; persistent pupillary remnant membrane; hypertelorism; dysplasia carthonum; antimongoloid obliquity of palpebral fissure.

Clinical

Large head; sensorineural hearing loss; proteinuria; epiphyseal dysplasia of the femoral heads.

Laboratory

Diagnosis is made by clinical findings.

Treatment

Trial topical medical therapy. If IOPs are uncontrolled—iridectomy, goniotomy, trabeculectomy, filtration surgery or cyclodestructive may be necessary.

Bibliography

1. Holmes Lb, Schepens CL. Syndrome of ocular and facial anomalies, telecanthus, and deafness. J Pediatr. 1972;81:552-5.

2. Murdoch JL, Mengel MC. An unusual eye-ear syndrome with renal abnormality. Birth Defects Orig Artic Ser. 1971;7:136.

528. FACIO-SCAPULO-HUMERAL MUSCULAR DYSTROPHY (FSH MUSCULAR DYSTROPHY)

General

Autosomal dominant disorder; onset varies from infancy to old age; severity varies from scarcely detectable to incapacitating; recessive inheritance has been reported.

Ocular

Retinal telangiectasis; macular lesion; macular edema; retinal sea fans.

Clinical

Deafness; wasting of shoulder girdle, upper deltoid, pectoralis, biceps and triceps; difficulty whistling, drinking through straws and playing wind instruments; foot dragging; mental retardation.

Laboratory

Diagnosis is made by clinical findings.

Treatment

Macular edema: Uses of corticosteroids, carbonic anhydrase inhibitors and NSAIDs are the mainstay of treatment. If traditional therapy is not effective, intraocular injections of Avastin may be helpful. In cases that have vitreous strand tugging against the macula, pars plana vitrectomy may be necessary.

Bibliography

1. Brouwer OF, Padberg GW, Ruys CJ, et al. Hearing loss in facioscapulohumeral muscular dystrophy. Neurology. 1991;41:1878-81.
2. McKusick VA. Mendelian Inheritance in Man: A Catalog of Human Genes and Genetic Disorders, 12th edition. Baltimore: The johns Hopkins University Press; 1998.

529. FALCIFORM DETACHMENT

General

Autosomal dominant or recessive; preperinatally acquired; characterized by ocular signs only; falciform detachment and congenital total detachment may alternate in affected siblings; falciform detachment and folds; retina projects as a wedge-shaped fold from the posterior pole of eye into the vitreous, occasionally as far anterior as the lens; less typical fold flattens and tapers out in the midperiphery of the retina.

Ocular

Falciform folds; retinal detachment; retrolental fibroplasia.

Clinical

None

Laboratory

Diagnosis is made by clinical findings.

Treatment

Encircling buckle, gas injection, vitrectomy and peeling the tractional (falciform) fold.

Bibliography

1. McKusick VA. Mendelian Inheritance in Man: A Catalog of Human Genes and Genetic Disorders, 12th edition. Baltimore: The Johns Hopkins University Press; 1998.

530. FALCIFORM DETACHMENT WITH MICROPHTHALMIA AND MICROCEPHALY

General

Rare; both sexes affected; etiology unknown.

Ocular

Microphthalmia; congenital cataract; corneal opacities; falciform folds; glaucoma; buphthalmos; congenital detachment of retina; vitreous hemorrhages; persistent hyperplastic primary vitreous; retinal neovascularization; retinal dysplasia.

Clinical

Microcephaly; vestigial cerebellum; cleft palate; micrognathia; hydrocephalus.

Laboratory

Diagnosis is made by clinical findings.

Treatment

Referral to retinal specialist.

Bibliography

1. Geeraets WJ. Ocular Syndromes, 3rd edition. Philadelphia: Lea & Febiger; 1976.

531. FALCIFORM FOLDS WITH OBESITY, NONTOXIC GOITER, HYPOGENITALISM, AND CRYPTORCHIDISM

General

Etiology unknown; isolated rare cases.

Ocular

Falciform folds; vitreous opacity.

Clinical

Obesity; nontoxic goiter; hypogenitalism; cryptorchidism.

Laboratory

Diagnosis is made by clinical findings.

Treatment

Referral to retinal specialist.

Bibliography

1. Geeraets WJ. Ocular Syndromes, 3rd edition. Philadelphia: Lea & Febiger; 1976.

532. FAMILIAL EXUDATIVE VITREORETINOPATHY

General

Herditary abnormality characterized by abnormal vascularization of the peripheral retina which may appear similar to retinopathy of prematurity.

Clinical

Norrie disease gene mutation.

Laboratory

Fluorescein angiography especially temporal periphery.

Treatment

Ablation of the peripheral avascular zone, sclera buckling, vitrectomy or both.

Bibliography

1. Roy FH, Fraunfelder FW, Fraunfelder FT. Roy and Fraunfelder's Current Ocular Therapy, 6th edition. Philadelphia: WB Saunders; 2008.

---

533. FAMILIAL HYPOGONADISM SYNDROME

General

Defect in testosterone biosynthesis.

Ocular

Progressive visual loss to complete blindness beginning shortly after birth; cataract; retinal degeneration.

Clinical

Partial deafness (neural type); obesity; shortness of stature; normal virilization.

Laboratory

Determine FSH, LH, prolactin and testosterone levels and obtain thyroid function test results. Examination of seminal fluid, karyotyping and testicular biopsy may be helpful. If gonadotropin levels are elevated, measure antiovarian antibody levels in females.

Treatment

Hormonal replacement therapy, replacement of sex steroids, nonfunctioning testicular tissue should undergo orchiectomy and replacement with prostheses.

Additional Resource

1. Kemp S (2010). Hypogonadism. [online] Available from http://www.emedicine.com/ped/TOPIC1118. HTM [Accessed April, 2012].

---

534. FAMILIAL JUVENILE NEPHRONOPHTHISIS (MEDULLARY CYSTIC DISEASE)

General

Number of closely related renal disorders are associated with tapetoretinal degeneration; cause unknown.

Ocular

Retinitis pigmentosa; night blindness; progressive constriction of peripheral fields; retinal arterioles narrowed; yellow pigment deposits present throughout retina; macular degeneration.

Clinical

Renal disorders; polydipsia; polyuria.

Laboratory

The urine has elevated sodium levels and low specific gravity with minimal proteinuria and normal sediment. Renal tubular acidosis may result in alkalotic urine and systemic acidosis. Intravenous pyelography (IVP), sonography, CT and MRI may be useful.

Treatment

Increase fluid intake, prevent and treat infection.

Additional Resource

1. Frye TP (2010). Cystic Diseases of the Kidney. [online] Available from http://www.emedicine.com/med/TOPIC3189.HTM [Accessed April, 2012].

535. FAMILIAL MEDITERRANEAN FEVER

General

Recessive inherited polyserositis; progressive, fatal complications are renal failure and amyloidosis.

Ocular

Episcleritis; uveitis; colloid bodies; optic neuritis.

Clinical

Peritonitis; pleuritis; arthritis; fever; skin rash; renal failure; amyloidosis; recurrent attacks of fever and polyserositis of unknown origin.

Laboratory

Synovial fluid is inflammatory, with cell counts high.

Treatment

Colchicine therapy daily is the treatment of choice.

Additional Resource

1. Meyerhoff JO (2012). Familial Mediterranean Fever. [online] Available from http://www.emedicine.com/med/TOPIC1410.HTM [Accessed April, 2012].

536. FANCONI SYNDROME (AMINO DIABETES; DE TONI-FANCONI SYNDROME; HYPOCHLOREMIC-GLYCOSURIC OSTEONEPHROPATHY SYNDROME; TONI FANCONI SYNDROME)

General

Autosomal recessive inheritance; hematologic manifestations mainly in young patients; in adults, the syndrome resembles Milkman syndrome with disorder of calcium and phosphorus metabolism; chronic organic acidosis in Fanconi syndrome due to an inborn error of protein metabolism.

Ocular

Massive retinal hemorrhage may be present secondary to blood dyscrasia; bilateral anterior uveitis.

Clinical

Ecchymoses and mucous membrane hemorrhages; skin hyperpigmentation; osteomalacia; pseudo fractures; deformities of radius and absence of thumbs; hypophosphatemia.

Laboratory

Diagnosis is made by clinical findings.

Treatment

Treat the underlying cause as quickly as possible, vitrectomy.

Bibliography

1. Fanconi G, Turler U. Kogenitale Kleinhirnatrophie mit Supranuklearen Storungen der Motilitat der Augenmuskein. Helv Paediatr Acta. 1951;6:475-83.
2. Geeraets WJ. Ocular Syndromes, 3rd edition. Philadelphia: Lea & Febiger; 1976.
3. Tsilou ET, Giri N, Weinstein S, et al. Ocular and orbital manifestations of the inherited bone marrow failure syndromes: Fanconi anemia and dyskeratosis congenita. Ophthalmology. 2010;117: 615-22.

537. FANCONI-TURLER SYNDROME (ATAXIC DIPLEGIA; FAMILIAL ATAXIC DIPLEGIA)

General

Aberration of the III cranial nerve (supranuclear type); ataxic diplegia is cerebellar ataxia with spastic pareses mainly of lower extremities; affects both sexes; onset at birth.

Ocular

Nystagmus; uncoordinated eye movements; dysmetria.

Clinical

Cerebellar ataxia; mental deficiency; spastic pareses.

Laboratory

Diagnosis is made by clinical findings.

Treatment

Nystagmus: See-saw nystagmus—visual field to consider neoplastic or vascular etiologies. Upbeat nystagmus—may indicate multiple sclerosis, cerebellar degeneration, tumors or infarcts. Treatment is directed toward identification and resolution of underlying cause. Downbeat nystagmus—affects the cerebellum or craniocervical junction including Arnold-Chiari malformation, multiple sclerosis, trauma, tumor, infarction and many toxic metabolic entities. MRI may indicate a surgically correctable lesion. Periodic alternating nystagmus is continuous horizontal nystagmus from stroke, tumor, multiple sclerosis, trauma, infection and drug intoxication. Can occur from cataract, vitreous hemorrhage or optic atrophy.

Bibliography

1. Fanconi G, Turler U. Kongenitale Kleinhimatrophie mit Supranuklearen Storungen der Motilitat der Augenrnuskeln. Helv Paediatr Acta. 1951;6: 475-83.
2. Geeraets WJ. Ocular Syndromes, 3rd edition. Philadelphia: Lea & Febiger; 1976.
3. Pfeiffer RA, Palm D, Jünemann G, et al. Nosology of congenital non-progressive cerebellar ataxia. Report on six cases in three families. Neuropediatrie. 1974;5:91-102.

538. FARBER SYNDROME (DISSEMINATED LIPOGRANULOMATOSIS; FARBER LIPOGRANULOMATOSIS)

General

Autosomal recessive inheritance; onset shortly after birth; rare; ceramidase deficiency.

Ocular

Parafoveal edema with mild cherry-red spot; grayness of the macula; diffuse fine pigmentary changes in the fundus.

Clinical

Progressive hoarseness; swelling of extremities; nodular and granulomatous infiltrations of periarticular and subcutaneous tissue; mild lymphadenopathy; fever attacks; dysphonia and dyspnea; irritability; ceramidase deficiency associated with storage of ceramide in body tissues.

Laboratory

Diagnosis is made by clinical findings.

Treatment

Identify and treat the cause. Cherry-red spot— options remain limited and are directed at supportive care and symptomatic relief.

Bibliography

1. Cogan DG, Kuwabara T, Moser H, et al. Retinopathy in a case of Farber's lipogranulomatosis. Arch Ophthalmol. 1966;75:752-7.
2. Collins JF. Handbook of Clinical Ophthalmology. New York: Masson; 1982.
3. Farber S, Cohen J, Uzman LL. Lipogranulomatosis: a new lipo-glycoprotein storage disease. J Mt Sinai Hosp N Y. 1957; 24:816-37.
4. Smith LH. Inherited metabolic disease with pediatric ocular manifestations. In: Albert DM, Jakobiec FA (Eds). Principles and Practice of Ophthalmology. Philadelphia: WB Saunders; 1994. p. 2778.

---

539. FAT ADHERENCE SYNDROME

General

Presence of a scar or adhesion that originates in extraconal fat and extends through Tenon's capsule to attach to the muscle insertion or sclera; seen following retinal surgery.

Ocular

Persistent acquired restrictive strabismus after retinal surgery; diplopia.

Clinical

None

Laboratory

Diagnosis is made by clinical findings.

Treatment

Consult with strabismologist.

Bibliography

1. Mets MB, Wendell ME, Gieser RG. Ocular deviation after retinal detachment surgery. Am J Ophthalmol. 1985;99:667-72.
2. Parks MM. Causes of the adhesive syndrome. Symposium on Strabismus; Transactions of the New Orleans Academy of Ophthalmology. St. Louis: CV Mosby; 1978. pp. 269-79.
3. Wright KW. The fat adherence syndrome and strabismus after retina surgery. Ophthalmology. 1986;93:411-5.

---

540. FAVRE-RACOUCHOT SYNDROME (NODULAR ELASTOIDOSIS)

General

Reaction to sun; permanent, slowly progressing condition; occurs in people chronically exposed to sun; usually apparent in the fourth or fifth decade.

Ocular

Yellowish thickening of skin, with comedones and follicular cysts in and around orbit.

Clinical

Elastotic degeneration of skin; raised yellow patches and numerous comedones; orifices enlarged; citrine skin; cutis rhomboidalis nuchae; elastoma Dubreuilh.

Laboratory

Diagnosis is made by clinical findings.

Treatment

Consult dermatologist.

Additional Resource

1. Feinstein RP (2011). Favre-Racouchot Syndrome (Nodular Elastosis With Cysts and Comedones). [online] Available from http://www.emedicine.com/derm/TOPIC151.HTM [Accessed April, 2012].

---

541. FEER SYNDROME (ACRODYNIA; INFANTILE ACRODYNIA PINK DISEASE; SWIFT-FEER SYNDROME)

General

Etiology unknown, possibly allergic reaction to mercury or infection; onset in early childhood; both sexes equally affected.

Ocular

Proptosis; lacrimation; pronounced photophobia; severe conjunctival itching; conjunctival injection with occasional marked signs of inflammation; severe keratitis; mild optic neuritis; mydriasis.

Clinical

Restlessness; irritability; continuous profuse sweating; muscle hypotony; tachycardia; exanthema of palms and soles with exfoliation of large skin flaps; stomatitis; sleeplessness; cyanosis of fingers, toes and nose; loss of teeth; rectal prolapse; muscle hypotonia; hypertension; hypertrichosis; gangrene of fingers.

Laboratory

Evidence of excess mercury in the urine of affected persons has been noted. A 24-hour urine collection is recommended. Blood evaluation is valuable to determine acute intoxication.

Treatment

Removal of the inciting agent is the goal of treatment. Peritoneal dialysis and plasma exchange may also be of benefit. Tolazoline (priscoline) has been shown to offer symptomatic relief from sympathetic overactivity. Antibiotics are necessary when massive hyperhidrosis.

Additional Resource

1. Padlewska KK (2012). Acrodynia. [online] Available from http://www.emedicine.com/derm/TOPIC592.HTM [Accessed April, 2012].

---

542. FELTY SYNDROME (CHAUFFARD-STILL SYNDROME; PRIMARY SPLENIC NEUTROPENIA WITH ARTHRITIS; RHEUMATOID ARTHRITIS WITH HYPERSPLENISM; STILL-CHAUFFARD SYNDROME; UVEITIS-RHEUMATOID ARTHRITIS SYNDROME)

General

Etiology not fully understood, possibly infection or allergy; onset in middle-aged patients or children; prognosis poor; collagen disorder; occasionally can occur without articular disease.

Ocular

Decreased tear formation; scleromalacia perforans; keratoconjunctivitis; chronic anterior uveitis; scleritis; vitreous opacities; macular edema; choroidal inflammation; papillitis; keratitic precipitates; band-shaped keratopathy.

Clinical

Rheumatoid arthritis; splenomegaly; leukopenia; anemia (mild); oral lesion with ulcers and atrophy.

Laboratory

Complete blood count with differential, CT, erythrocyte sedimentation rate (ESR) and serum immunoglobulin levels invariably are elevated.

Treatment

Control the underlying rheumatoid arthritis (RA), with immunosuppressive therapy for RA often improves granulocytopenia and splenomegaly.

Additional Resource

1. Keating RM (2011). Felty Syndrome. [online] Available from http://www.emedicine.com/med/TOPIC782.HTM [Accessed April, 2012].

543. FETAL ALCOHOL SYNDROME

General

Dysgenesis in children born to alcoholic mothers; both sexes affected; onset from birth.

Ocular

Antimongoloid slant of lid fissures; lateral displacement of inner canthi; ptosis; epicanthi; strabismus; myopia; optic nerve hypoplasia; diffuse corneal clouding; iridocorneal abnormalities with central corneal edema; lens opacification; motility disorders.

Clinical

Growth retardation; delayed development (physical and intellectual); maxillary hypoplasia; micrognathia; large, low-set ears; abnormal motor function; irritability; microcephaly; cerebral nervous system dysfunctions; abnormal philtrum; flattened nasal bridge; cardiovascular defects; thin upper lip.

Laboratory

If suspected, consult a subspecialist (e.g. geneticist, developmentalist) to confirm the diagnosis.

Treatment

Treat for associated birth defects and intervention for potential cognitive and behavioral abnormalities. Vitrectomy may be necessary.

Additional Resource

1. Vaux KK (2010). Fetal Alcohol Syndrome. [online] Available from http://www.emedicine.com/ped/TOPIC767.HTM [Accessed April, 2012].

544. FETAL ANTICONVULSANT SYNDROME

General

Congenital after maternal ingestion of sodium valproate, carbamazepine and phenytoin.

Ocular

Myopia; astigmatism; strabismus; anisometropia; optic nerve hypoplasia.

Clinical

Craniofacial dysmorphisms vary with type of abnormality.

Laboratory

If suspected, consult a subspecialist (e.g. geneticist, developmentalist) to confirm the diagnosis.

Treatment

Treat for associated birth defects and intervention for potential cognitive and behavioral abnormalities.

Additional Resource

1. Jain VD (2011). Psychosocial and Environmental Pregnancy Risks. [online] Available from http://www.emedicine.com/med/TOPIC3237.HTM [Accessed April, 2012].

545. FETAL HYDANTOIN SYNDROME

General

Syndrome due to an epoxide hydrolase 1, microsomal, arene oxide detoxification defect.

Ocular

Nystagmus

Clinical

In vitro testing for the defect correlates most highly with congenital heart disease, cleft lip/palate, microcephaly, and major genitourinary, eye and limb defects; hypersensitivity to phenytoin has occurred.

Laboratory

If suspected, consult a subspecialist (e.g. geneticist, developmentalist) to confirm the diagnosis.

Treatment

Treat for associated birth defects and intervention for potential cognitive and behavioral abnormalities.

Bibliography

1. Buehler BA, Delimont D, van Waes M, et al. Prenatal prediction of risk of the fetal hydantoin syndrome. N Engl J Med. 1990;322:1567-72.
2. Gennis MA, Vemuri R, Burns EA, et al. Familial occurrence of hypersensitivity to phenytoin. Am J Med. 1991;91:631-4.
3. McKusick VA. Mendelian Inheritance in Man: A Catalog of Human Genes and Genetic Disorders, 12th edition. Baltimore: The Johns Hopkins University Press; 1998.

546. FIBRINOID SYNDROME

General

From 2 to 14 days postvitrectomy, white-gray criss-cross layers of fibrin appear on the surface of the retina and immediately behind the plane of the iris; occurs only in patients with diabetes mellitus and usually in those requiring insulin; seen more frequently in people who have been diabetic for 15 years or more.

Ocular

Fibrin material interlaced on the surface of the retina and behind the iris; retinal detachment; neovascular glaucoma; rubeosis irides.

Clinical

Diabetes mellitus.

Laboratory

Diagnosis is made by clinical findings.

Treatment

Although prognosis is poor, lensectomy (in phakic eyes), excision of the posterior hyaloid face and vitreous base dissection, extensive pan-retinal photocoagulation (to induce regression of or prevent anterior hyaloidal fibrovascular proliferation) and silicone oil infusion can be useful.

Bibliography

1. Ho T, Smiddy WE, Flynn HW. Vitrectomy in the management of diabetic eye disease. Surv Ophthalmol. 1992;37:190-202.
2. Schepens CL. Clinical and research aspects of subtotal open-sky vitrectomy. XXXVII Edward Jackson Memorial Lecture. Am J Ophthalmol. 1981;91:143-71.
3. Sebestyen JG. Fibrinoid syndrome: a severe complication of vitrectomy surgery in diabetics. Ann Ophthalmol. 1982;14:853-6.

547. FIBROSARCOMA

General

Malignant tumor of fibrous connective tissue; most commonly seen in persons 30–70 years old; frequent metastases to lung; true fibrosarcoma has a tendency to occur in children (better prognosis); most fibrosarcomas now would be classified as malignant fibrous histiocytomas.

Ocular

Paralysis of extraocular muscles; proptosis; orbital edema; erosion of orbital bony walls; increased intraorbital pressure; metastases to choroid/orbit.

Clinical

Tumors of mesenchymal soft tissues of the extre-mities, especially in the knee region; progressive pain; edema; tumors of the sinuses; tumors of the lungs.

Laboratory

Neuroimaging with CT and MRI are no diagnostic. Excisional or incisional biopsy is diagnostic.

Treatment

Surgical resection with a cuff of normal tissue and reconstruction of the subsequent defect are necessary. Radiation treatment and chemotherapy may also be necessary.

Additional Resource

1. Dickey ID (2010). Fibrosarcoma. [online] Available from http://www.emedicine.com/orthoped/TOPIC599.HTM [Accessed April, 2012].

548. FILAMENTARY KERATITIS

General

Etiology unknown.

Clinical

None

Ocular

Fine filaments develop on front surface of cornea. Move with lid movement.

Laboratory

Diagnosis is made by clinical findings.

Treatment

Debridement of filaments with forceps or cotton-tipped applicator, sodium chloride drops and ointment, soft contact lens and punctal occlusion.

Bibliography

1. Roy FH, Fraunfelder FW, Fraunfelder FT. Roy and Fraunfelder's Current Ocular Therapy, 6th edition. Philadelphia: WB Saunders; 2008.

549. FILTERING BLEBS AND ASSOCIATED PROBLEMS

General

Elevation of conjunctiva and Tenon's capsule from anterior chamber fistula is caused by antimetabolite/antifibrotic usage, trabeculectomy, bleb leaks or overfiltering blebs.

Clinical

None

Ocular

Overfiltering blebs, overhanging blebs and bleb dysesthesia. Complications include hypotony, flat anterior chamber, corneal edema, choroidal effusion, enophthalmitis, dellen, uncontrolled glaucoma, astigmatism, cataract and suprachoroidal hemorrhage.

Laboratory

Diagnosis is made by clinical findings and Seidel test.

Treatment

Conservative treatment includes pressure patching, large diameter bandage contact lens. Cryotherapy, laser thermotherapy and autologous blood injection, cyanoacrylate to dry conjunctiva to close leaking bleb and compression sutures may be used if conservative therapy does not resolve the problem.

Additional Resource

1. Traverso CE (2010). Filtering Bleb Complications. [online] Available from http://www.emedicine.com/oph/TOPIC541.HTM [Accessed April, 2012].

550. FISH-EYE DISEASE (CORNEAL OPACITIES-DYSLIPOPROTEINEMIA)

General

Etiology unknown; rare; described in Swedish family; currently considered a unique dyslipoproteinemia.

Ocular

Visual impairment; marked corneal opacities.

Clinical

Very-low-density triglycerides and cholesterol raised.

Laboratory

Diagnosis is made by clinical findings.

Treatment

Primarily surgical; after surgery, treatment of amblyopia and optical therapy can be helpful.

Bibliography

1. Carlson LA, Philipson B. Fish-eye disease. A new familial condition with massive corneal opacities and dyslipoproteinaemia. Lancet. 1979;2:922-4.
2. Koster H, Savoldelli M, Dumon MF, et al. A fish-eye disease-like familial condition with massive corneal clouding and dyslipoproteinemia. Report of clinical, histologic, electron microscopic, and biochemical features. Cornea. 1992;11:452-64.
3. Magalini SI, Scrascia E. Dictionary of Medical Syndromes, 2nd edition. Philadelphia: JB Lippincott; 1981.

551. FISH ODOR SYNDROME (TRIMETHYLAMINURIA)

General

Metabolic syndrome characterized by a strong body odor of rotting fish; trimethylamine levels elevated; it appears that the enzyme flavin-containing monooxygenase is defective in this disorder; possibly autosomal recessive pattern of inheritance.

Ocular

Hypertelorism, cortical blindness.

Clinical

Hydrocephalus; mental retardation; unusual facies; short stature; skeletal abnormalities; cryptorchidism; hyperextensible skin.

Laboratory

Specific testing of urine or sweat may be indicated to detect the aberrant amino acid product.

Treatment

None/Ocular.

Bibliography

1. Chen H, Aiello F. Trimethylaminuria in a girl with Prader-Willi syndrome and del(15)(q11q13). Am J Med Genet. 1993;45:335-9.
2. Humbert JA, Hammond KB, Hathaway WE. Trimethylaminuria: the fish-odour syndrome. Lancet. 1970;2:770-1.
3. Shelley ED, Shelley WB. The fish odor syndrome. Trimethylaminuria. JAMA. 1984;251:253-5.

552. FISHER SYNDROME (MILLER-FISHER SYNDROME; OPHTHALMOPLEGIA ATAXIA AREFLEXIA SYNDROME)

General

Acute idiopathic polyneuritis; prognosis good; complete recovery over several weeks (see Variant of Guillain-Barré Syndrome).

Ocular

Moderate ptosis; complete external and almost complete internal ophthalmoplegia; diplopia; sluggish pupil reaction to light; may present without total ophthalmoplegia.

Clinical

Dizziness; severe ataxia; loss of tendon reflexes; chest pains; difficulties in chewing; diminished or absent sense of vibration; upper respiratory tract infection preceding this syndrome.

Laboratory

Diagnosis usually is made on clinical grounds. Laboratory studies are useful to rule out other diagnoses.

Treatment

Monitored closely for changes in blood pressure, heart rate and other arrhythmias. Temporary pacing may be required for patients with second-degree and third-degree heart block.

Bibliography

1. Fisher M. An unusual variant of acute idiopathic polyneuritis (syndrome of ophthalmoplegia, ataxia and areflexia). N Engl J Med. 1956;255:57-65.
2. Igarashi Y, Takeda M, Maekawa H, et al. Fisher's syndrome without total ophthalmoplegia. Ophthalmologica. 1992;205:163-7.
3. Swick HM. Pseudointernuclear ophthalmoplegia in acute idiopathic polyneuritis (Fisher's syndrome). Am J Ophthalmol. 1974;77:725-8.

553. FLECK RETINA OF KANDORI SYNDROME (KANDORI SYNDROME)

General

Possibly hereditary; onset young age; focal disturbance of the retinal pigment epithelium (RPE); affects both sexes; toxic causes also considered.

Ocular

Relatively large, irregular, yellowish flecks, sharply border-lined without pigmentation underneath retinal vessels and usually in the midperiphery; poor dark adaptation; normal photopic electroretinographic response; delay in generation of the scotopic response.

Clinical

None

Laboratory

Diagnosis is made by clinical findings.

Treatment

None/Ocular.

Bibliography

1. Bullock JD, Albert DM. Flecked retina. Appearance secondary to oxalate crystals from methoxyflurane anesthesia. Arch Ophthalmol. 1975;93:26-31.
2. Carr RE. Abnormalities of cone and rod function. In: Ryan SJ (Ed). Retina, 2nd edition. St. Louis: Mosby; 1994. pp. 512-3.
3. Kandori F, Kurimoto S, Fukunaga K, et al. Studies on fluorescein fundus photography in cases of "fleck retina with congenital nonprogressive nightblindness. Nihon Ganka Gakkai Zasshi. 1968; 72:1253-9.

554. FLOPPY EYELID SYNDROME

General

Origin unknown; more common in males; overweight; X chromosome-linked inheritance pattern or possible hormonal influence; has been postulated that the degenerative changes in the tarsus may result from the combination of local pressure-induced lid ischemia and systemic hypoventilation.

Ocular

Easily everted, floppy upper eyelid and papillary conjunctivitis of the upper palpebral conjunctiva; upper eyelid everts during sleep, resulting in irritation, papillary conjunctivitis and conjunctival keratinization; most distinct feature is rubbery, malleable upper tarsus; keratoconus; punctate keratopathy; blepharoptosis; lash ptosis.

Clinical

Obesity; sleep apnea.

Laboratory

Conjunctival scrapings reveal keratinized epithelial cells. Bacterial cultures are important.

Treatment

Full-thickness upper and lower eyelid resection.

Bibliography

1. Ezra DG, Beaconsfield M, Sira M, et al. Long-term outcomes of surgical approaches to the treatment of floppy eyelid syndrome. Ophthalmology. 2010; 117:839-46.
2. Ezra DG, Beaconsfield M, Sira M, et al. The associations of floppy eyelid syndrome: a case control study. Ophthalmology. 2010;117:831-8.

Additional Resource

1. Blaydon SM (2011). Floppy Eyelid Syndrome. [online] Available from http://www.emedicine.com/oph/TOPIC605.HTM [Accessed April, 2012].

---

555. FLOPPY IRIS SYNDROME

General

Flomax (tamsulosin) is causative agent during cataract. Flomax is commonly prescribed for benign prostate hypertrophy.

Ocular

Floppy iris.

Clinical

Benign prostate hypertrophy; noted during cataract surgery.

Laboratory

Diagnosis is made by clinical findings.

Treatment

Stop tamsulosin at least 3 days before cataract surgery.

Bibliography

1. Chang DF, Campbell JR. Intraoperative floppy iris syndrome associated with tamsulosin. J Cataract Refract Surg. 2005;31:664-73.
2. Gurbaxani A, Packard R. Intracameral phenylephrine to prevent floppy iris syndrome during cataract surgery in patients on tamsulosin. Eye (Lond). 2007;21:331-2.
3. Schlötzer-Schrehardt U, Stojkovic M, Hofmann-Rummelt C, et al. The pathogenesis of floppy eyelid syndrome. Ophthalmology. 2005;112:694-704.

---

556. FLYNN-AIRD SYNDROME

General

It may be basic hereditary enzyme deficiency, probably autosomal dominant; no sex predilection apparent.

Ocular

Severe myopia; bilateral cataracts; retinitis pigmentosa; total blindness; onset of visual difficulties in the first or second decade of life.

Clinical

Hearing loss; joint stiffness; muscular wasting; kyphoscoliosis.

Laboratory

Computed tomography (CT) and MRI.

Treatment

Assistive listening devices and personal systems.

Bibliography

1. Flynn P, Aird RB. A neuroectodermal syndrome of dominant inheritance. J Neurol Sci. 1965;2:161-82.

2. McKusick VA. Mendelian Inheritance in Man: A Catalog of Human Genes and Genetic Disorders, 12th edition. Baltimore: The Johns Hopkins University Press; 1998.

3. McKusick-Nathans Institute for Genetic Medicine, Johns Hopkins University and National Center for Biotechnology Information, National Library of Medicine. (2007). Online Mendelian Inheritance in Man (OMIM). [online] Available from http://www.ncbi.nlm.nih.gov/omim/ [Accessed April, 2012].

4. Regenbogen LS, Coscas GJ. Oculo-auditory Syndromes. New York: Masson; 1985. pp. 99-103.

557. FOIX SYNDROME (CAVERNOUS SINUS-NASOPHARYNGEAL TUMOR SYNDROME; CAVERNOUS SINUS THROMBOSIS; CAVERNOUS SINUS NEURALGIA SYNDROME; CAVERNOUS SINUS SYNDROME; GODTFREDSEN SYNDROME; HYPOPHYSEAL-SPHENOIDAL SYNDROME)

General

Causes include tumor of lateral sinus wall or sphenoid bone, intracranial aneurysm, cavernous and lateral sinus thrombosis, or lesions; multiple myeloma; may result from infarctions or cancer or be idiopathic.

Ocular

Proptosis; severe ocular and periorbital pain; lid edema; paresis or paralysis of cranial nerves III, IV, V and VI; corneal anesthesia; optic atrophy.

Clinical

Postauricular edema; trigeminal neuralgia; deviation of the tongue toward paralyzed side; patients usually have prominent manifestations of sepsis and paranasal sinus; local skin infections are the most common cause.

Laboratory

Computed tomography (CT) and MRI.

Treatment

Radiotherapy, anticoagulation and high-dose antibiotic therapy.

Additional Resource

1. Kattah JC (2012). Cavernous Sinus Syndromes. [online] Available from http://www.emedicine.com/neuro/TOPIC572.HTM [Accessed April, 2012].

558. FOLLING SYNDROME (IKIOTIA PHENYLKETONURIA SYNDROME; PHENYLKETONURIA; PHENYLPYRUVIC OLIGOPHRENIA)

General

Rare; autosomal recessive; phenylalanine cannot be converted to tyrosine; poor prognosis without early diet therapy; both sexes affected.

Ocular

Blue sclera; severe photophobia; corneal opacities; cataracts (controversial); partial ocular albinism; macular atrophy.

Clinical

Phenylketonuria (PKU); oligophrenia; partial albinism; muscle hypertonicity; hyper-reflexia of tendons; epilepsy; microcephaly; mousy odor of habitus; fair skin.

Laboratory

Newborn screening, low-grade elevations of phenylalanine may require repeat screening. More significant elevations may require definitive testing and/or referral to a metabolic treatment facility experienced with phenylketonuria.

Treatment

Most patients are treated in a specialty metabolic clinic, usually under the auspices of a genetics or pediatric endocrinology clinic. Treatment consists of dietary restriction of phenylalanine with tyrosine supplementation.

Additional Resource

1. Steiner RD (2011). Phenylketonuria. [online] Available from http://www.emedicine.com/ped/TOPIC1787.HTM [Accessed April, 2012].

559. FOOT-IN-THE-WOUND SYNDROME

General

Occurs when the anterior chamber intraocular lens haptic is within the wound.

Ocular

Haptic in the wound.

Clinical

None

Laboratory

Diagnosis is made by clinical findings.

Treatment

Reposition intraocular lens.

Bibliography

1. Hessburg PC. Complications noted in PMMA IOL haptics: fracture, pupillary capture named problems. Ophthal Times. August 21, 1983.

560. FORAMEN LACERUM SYNDROME (ANEURYSM OF INTERNAL CAROTID ARTERY SYNDROME)

General

Most commonly caused by congenital aneurysm involving the intradural portion of the carotid artery.

Ocular

Periorbital pain; ptosis; oculomotor paralysis with ptosis, diplopia and internal ophthalmoplegia; cranial nerves IV and VI may be involved; homonymous hemianopia (occasionally); loss of pupillary reflexes for light and accommodation; papilledema; optic atrophy.

Clinical

Meningism; mental disturbances; unilateral frontal or orbital headache; migraine attacks.

Laboratory

Computed tomography (CT), MRI, angiography, magnetic resonance angiography (MRA).

Treatment

Endovascular balloon occlusion.

Bibliography

1. Dailey EJ, Holloway JA, Murto RE, et al. Evaluation of ocular signs and symptoms in cerebral aneurysms. Arch Ophthalmol. 1964;71:463-74.
2. Geeraets WJ. Ocular Syndromes, 3rd edition. Philadelphia: Lea & Febiger; 1976.
3. Misra M, Mohanty AB, Rath S. Giant aneurysm of internal carotid artery presenting features of retrobulbar neuritis. Indian J Ophthalmol. 1991; 39:28-9.

561. FORSIUS-ERIKSSON SYNDROME (ALAND DISEASE)

General

Associated with the natives of the Aland Islands; sex-linked inheritance; consanguinity versus mutant gene; affects males only; it has been considered a variety of incomplete congenital stationary night blindness.

Ocular

Microphthalmos; irregular latent nystagmus; myopia; astigmatism; dyschromatopsia; tapeto-retinal degeneration; primary foveal hypoplasia or dysplasia; nystagmus.

Clinical

Prematurity; impaired hearing; mental retardation; epilepsy.

Laboratory

Diagnosis is made by clinical findings.

Treatment

Genetic counseling.

Bibliography

1. Forsius H, Eriksson AW. Ein Neues Augensyndrom mit X-chromosomaler Transmission. Eine Sippe mit Fundusalbinismus, Foveahypoplasie, Nystagmus, Myopic, Astigmatismus und Dyschromatopsie. Klin Monatsbl Augenheilkd. 1964;144:447.
2. McKusick VA. Mendelian Inheritance in Man: A Catalog of Human Genes and Genetic Disorders, 12th edition. Baltimore: The Johns Hopkins University Press; 1998.

562. FOSTER KENNEDY SYNDROME (BASAL-FRONTAL SYNDROME; GOWERS-PATON-KENNEDY SYNDROME)

General

Caused by tumor in base of frontal lobe or sphenoidal meningioma.

Ocular

Central scotoma may be present on side of optic atrophy; enlarged blind spot and peripheral contraction of field (opposite eye); homolateral descending optic atrophy due to compression of the ipsilateral optic nerve at the optic foramen; contralateral papilledema due to increased intracranial pressure; ipsilateral proptosis.

Clinical

Anosmia; headache; dizziness; vomiting; memory loss; psychic changes; also may be caused by an olfactory groove tumor (usually a meningioma) or pituitary adenoma.

Laboratory

Computed tomography (CT) scan and MRI allow definitive diagnosis.

Treatment

Microsurgical resection usually can be curative, radiotherapy may be necessary with partial resection.

Bibliography

1. Banerjee T, Meagher JN. Foster Kennedy syndrome, aqueductal stenosis and empty sella. Am Surg. 1974;40:552-4.
2. Kennedy F. Retrobulbar neuritis as an exact diagnostic sign of certain tumors and abscesses in the frontal lobes. Am J Med Sci. 1911;142:355-68.
3. Ruben S, Elston J, Hayward R. Pituitary adenoma presenting as the Foster-Kennedy syndrome. Br J Ophthalmol. 1992;76:117-9.
4. Yildizhan A. A case of Foster Kennedy syndrome without frontal lobe or anterior cranial fossa involvement. Neurosurg Rev. 1992;15:139-42.

563. FOURTH NERVE PALSY (TROCHLEAR NERVE PALSY)

General

Paralysis of the IV cranial nerve which can be congenital or acquired. Etiology is obscure for congenital disease. Head trauma, diabetes, atherosclerosis, tumor, aneurysm, multiple sclerosis and hypertension are causes for acquired disease.

Clinical

History of head trauma, diabetes, tumor, aneurysm, multiple sclerosis, hypertension, atherosclerosis.

Ocular

Vertical diplopia, head tilt, superior oblique muscle depression which causes abduction of the globe and intorts, V-pattern esotropia, torticollis.

Laboratory

Diagnosis is made by clinical findings.

Treatment

Prisms may be useful for small deviations. Botulinum toxin may also be useful. For deviation greater than 15 prism diopters, strabismus surgery may be required.

Additional Resource

1. Sheik ZA (2012). Trochlear Nerve Palsy. [online] Available from http://www.emedicine. medscape.com/article/1200187-overview [Accessed April, 2012].

564. FOVEAL HYPOPLASIA AND PRESENILE CATARACT SYNDROME (O'DONNELL-PAPPAS SYNDROME)

General

Autosomal dominant.

Ocular

Foveal hypoplasia; nystagmus; presenile cataract; peripheral corneal pannus.

Clinical

None

Laboratory

Diagnosis is made by clinical findings.

Treatment

Cataract: Change in glasses can sometimes improve a patient's visual function temporarily; however, the most common treatment is cataract surgery.

Bibliography

1. O'Donnell FE, Pappas HR: Autosomal dominant foveal hypoplasia and presenile cataracts: a new syndrome. Arch Ophthalmol 1982;100:279-281.

565. FOVILLE SYNDROME (FOVILLE PEDUNCULAR SYNDROME)

General

Pontine area tumor, hemorrhage, tuberculoma, multiple sclerosis or unilateral obstruction of paramedian branches may cause clinical manifestations.

Ocular

Paralysis of cranial nerve VI; paralysis of conjugate movement to the side of the lesion; abduction or horizontal gaze deficit.

Clinical

Peripheral facial palsy; contralateral hemiplegia; headache; ipsilateral: facial weakness, loss of taste, facial analgesia, Homer syndrome and deafness.

Laboratory

Computed tomography and MRI.

Treatment

Consult neurologist.

Bibliography

1. Bedi HK, Devpura JC, Bomb BS. Clinical tuberculoma of pons presenting as Foville's syndrome. J Indian Med Assoc. 1973;61:184-5.
2. Foville ALF. Note sur une Paralysie Peu Connue des Certains Muscles de l'Oeil, et Sa Liaison avec Quelques Points de l'Anatomie et la Physiologic de la Protuberance Annulaire. Bull Soc Anat (Paris). 1858;33:393.
3. Geeraets WJ. Ocular Syndromes, 3rd edition. Philadelphia: Lea & Febiger; 1976.
4. Newman NJ. Third, fourth, and sixth nerve lesions and the cavernous sinus. In: Albert DM, Jakobiec FA (Eds). Principles and Practice of Ophthalmology. Philadelphia: WB Saunders; 1994. p. 2458.

566. FRAGILE X SYNDROME

General

X-linked recessive; primarily affects males.

Ocular

Strabismus; nystagmus; high myopia; adult-onset glaucoma; blepharospasm; congenital optic atrophy; hyperopia; astigmatism; cataract; ptosis; corneal dystrophy.

Clinical

Mental retardation; dysmorphism; epilepsy; macroorchidism.

Laboratory

Diagnosis is made by clinical findings.

Treatment

Glaucoma: Its medication should be the first plan of action. If medication is unsuccessful, a filtering surgical procedure with or without antimetabolites may be beneficial.

Cataract: Change in glasses can sometimes improve a patient's visual function temporarily; however, the most common treatment is cataract surgery.

Ptosis: If visual acuity is affected most cases require surgical correction, and there are several procedures that may be used including levator resection, repair or advancement and Fasanella-Servat.

Corneal dystrophy: Mild cases can be observed and soft contact lenses are helpful, penetrating keratoplasty may be necessary, graft recurrences treated by superficial keratectomy, phototherapeutic keratectomy or repeat penetrating keratoplasty.

Bibliography

1. Harley RD (Ed). Pediatric Ophthalmology, 4th edition. Philadelphia: WB Saunders; 1998.
2. McKusick VA. Mendelian Inheritance in Man: A Catalog of Human Genes and Genetic Disorders, 12th edition. Baltimore: The Johns Hopkins University Press; 1998.

567. FRANCESCHETTI DISEASE (FUNDUS FLAVIMACULATUS)

General

Affects both sexes; onset between the ages of 10 and 25 years; autosomal recessive; genetic linkage analysis has assigned the disease locus to chromosome 1p21–p13.

Ocular

Irregular yellowish deposit in and around the macula lutea forming a garland; impaired central vision with intact peripheral retinal function; bilateral retinal dystrophy; progressive subretinal fibrosis; chorioretinal punched-out spots in the posterior pole and midperiphery of the retina.

Clinical

None

Laboratory

Diagnosis is made by clinical findings.

Treatment

Ocular/None.

Bibliography

1. Magalini SI, Scrascia E. Dictionary of Medical Syndromes, 2nd edition. Philadelphia: JB Lippincott; 1981.
2. Parodi MB. Progressive subretinal fibrosis in fundus flavimaculatus. Acta Ophthalmol. 1994; 72:260-4.

568. FRANCESCHETTI SYNDROME [BERRY SYNDROME; BERRY-FRANCESCHETTI-K1EIN SYNDROME; BILATERAL FACIAL AGENESIS; EYELID-MALAR-MANDIBLE SYNDROME; FRANCESCHETTI-K1EIN SYNDROME; FRANCESCHETTI SYNDROME (II); FRANCESCHETTI-ZWAHLEN SYNDROME; FRANCESCHETTI-ZWAHLEN-K1EIN SYNDROME; MANDIBULOFACIAL DYSOSTOSIS; MANDIBULOFACIAL SYNDROME; TREACHER COLLINS SYNDROME; OCULOVERTEBRAL SYNDROME; TREACHER COLLINS-FRANCESCHETTI SYNDROME; WEYERS-THIER SYNDROME ZWAHLEN SYNDROME]

General

Irregular dominant inheritance; Weyers-Thier syndrome has similar features, except it is a unilateral variant; prevalent in Caucasians.

Ocular

Microphthalmia; oblique position of eyes with lateral downward slope of palpebral fissures; temporal lower lid coloboma; lack of cilia on middle third of lower lid; iris coloboma; underdeveloped orbicularis oculi muscle; cataract; optic disk hypoplasia.

Clinical

Fish-like face with sunken cheek bones, receding chin, and large, wide mouth; absent or malformed external ears with auricular appendages; high palate and possible harelip; hypoplastic zygomatic arch with absence of normal malar eminences; prolonged hairline on the cheek; deafness; micrognathia; glossoptosis; cleft palate.

Laboratory

Full craniofacial CT scan (axial and coronal slices from the top of the skull through the cervical spine), brain MRI.

Treatment

Operative repair is based upon the anatomic deformity and timing of correction is done according to physiologic need and development.

Additional Resource

1. Tolarova MM (2012). Mandibulofacial Dysostosis (Treacher Collins Syndrome). [online] Available from http://www.emedicine.com/ped/TOPIC1364.HTM [Accessed April, 2012].

569. FRANCESCHETTI SYNDROME (I)

General

Inborn disease occurring at birth; etiology unknown.

Ocular

Deep punctate dystrophy of cornea with ichthyosis dystrophia (punctiformis profunda corneae with congenital ichthyosis).

Clinical

Dry, scaly skin; follicular hyperkeratotic lesions; atopic dermatitis; pruritus.

Laboratory

Diagnosis is made by clinical findings.

Treatment

None/Ocular.

Bibliography

1. Jablonski S. Eponymic Syndromes and Diseases. Philadelphia: WB Saunders; 1969.
2. Stewart WD, Danto JL, Maddin S. Dermatology, 4th edition. St. Louis: CV Mosby; 1978.

570. FRANCESCHETTI-THIER SYNDROME

General

Autosomal recessive inheritance.

Ocular

Corneal dystrophy.

Clinical

Multiple lipomas; mental retardation.

Laboratory

Diagnosis is made by clinical findings.

Treatment

Treatment is primarily surgical; treatment of amblyopia and optical therapy can be helpful.

Bibliography

1. Franceschetti A, Thier CJ. Hornhautdystrophien bei Genodermatosen unter besonderen Beruck-sichtigung der Palmoplantarkeratosen. Graefes Arch Clin Exp Ophthalmol. 1961;162:610-70.
2. Magalini SI, Scrascia E. Dictionary of Medical Syndromes, 2nd edition. Philadelphia: JB Lippincott; 1981. p. 294.

571. FRANCOIS (1) DYSTROPHY (CENTRAL CLOUDY DYSTROPHY CLOUDY CENTRAL CORNEAL DYSTROPHY; FRANCOIS-NEETENS SYNDROME)

General

Autosomal dominant; etiology unknown; not progressive; isolated keratocytes contain elevated amounts of glycosaminoglycans and lipids.

Ocular

Bilateral dystrophy of central third of cornea; snowflake patches covering the pupil; lesions show no definite structure or limits; more dense near Descemet's membrane and becoming less toward the anterior surface toward the periphery; associated with central cloudy dystrophy; keratoconus; limbal dermoid; pseudoxanthoma elasticum; lenticular opacities; reduced corneal sensation.

Laboratory

Diagnosis is made by clinical findings.

Treatment

Treatment is primarily surgical; treatment of amblyopia and optical therapy can be helpful.

Additional Resource

1. Scheinfeld NS (2011). Congenital Clouding of the Cornea. [online] Available from http://www.emedicine.com/oph/TOPIC771.HTM [Accessed April, 2012].

572. FRANCOIS (2) DYSTROPHY (FRANCOIS-EVENS SYNDROME; SPECKLED CORNEAL DYSTROPHY)

General

Etiology unknown; congenital; nonprogressive; autosomal dominant, but sporadic cases have been reported.

Ocular

Corneal dystrophy is characterized by minute punctate opacities found in all layers of the cornea; varies in size, form and degree of opacity but is identical in both eyes; anterior limiting membrane is always intact.

Laboratory

Diagnosis is made by clinical findings.

Treatment

Treatment is primarily surgical; treatment of amblyopia and optical therapy can be helpful.

Bibliography

1. Bron AJ. The corneal dystrophies. Curr Opin Ophthalmol. 1990;1:333-46.
2. Francois J. Heredity in Ophthalmology. St. Louis: CV Mosby; 1961.
3. Magalini SI, Scrascia E. Dictionary of Medical Syndromes, 2nd edition. Philadelphia: JB Lippincott; 1981.

573. FRANCOIS SYNDROME (2)
(DYSTROPHIA DERMACHONDROCORNEALIS FAMILIARIS)

General

Autosomal recessive.

Ocular

Central superficial corneal dystrophy with subepithelial opacities.

Clinical

Distal osteochondral dystrophy of the extremities; cutaneous xanthomas.

Laboratory

Diagnosis is made by clinical findings.

Treatment

Treatment is primarily surgical; treatment of amblyopia and optical therapy can be helpful.

Bibliography

1. Caputo R, Sambvani N, Monti M, et al. Dermochondrocorneal dystrophy (Francois' syndrome). Report of a case. Arch Dermatol. 1988;124:424-8.
2. Francois J. Dystrophic Dermo-Chondro-Corneenne Familiale. Ann Ocul (Paris). 1949;182:409-42.
3. Jablonski S. Eponymic Syndromes and Diseases. Philadelphia: WB Saunders; 1969.
4. McKusick VA. Mendelian Inheritance in Man: A Catalog of Human Genes and Genetic Disorders, 12th edition. Baltimore: The Johns Hopkins University Press; 1998.

574. FRANKL-HOCHWART SYNDROME
(PINEAL-NEUROLOGIC-OPHTHALMIC SYNDROME)

General

Pineal tumor, usually in early adulthood; poor prognosis.

Ocular

Limitation of upward gaze; concentric field constriction; papilledema; lack of pupillary reaction; nystagmus.

Clinical

Bilateral deafness; ataxia; weakness; headache; vomiting; polydipsia; polyphagia; convulsions; facial paralysis; tremor; Romberg sign; hypertonia; tendon hyperreflexia; Babinski sign.

Laboratory

Measurements of serum and CSF tumor markers, MRI with gadolinium, angiography.

Treatment

Stereotactic biopsy has been described as the procedure of choice for obtaining a tissue diagnosis, radiotherapy and chemotherapy.

Additional Resource

1. Bruce JN (2011). Pineal Tumors. [online] Available from http://www.emedicine.com/med/TOPIC2911.HTM [Accessed April, 2012].

---

575. FRASER SYNDROME (CRYPTOPHTHALMIA SYNDROME; CRYPTOPHTHALMOS SYNDACTYLY SYNDROME)

General

Autosomal recessive.

Ocular

Microphthalmia; epibulbar dermoid; cryptophthalmos; enophthalmia; eyebrows partially or completely missing; skin from forehead completely covers one or both eyes, but the globes can be palpated beneath the skin; in unilateral cases, the fellow eye may present lid coloboma; buphthalmos; conjunctival sac partially or totally obliterated; absence of trabeculae, Schlemm canal and ciliary muscles; cornea is differentiated from the sclera; lens anomalies from complete absence to hypoplasia, dislocation and calcification.

Clinical

Syndactyly (finger, toes) (about 40%); coloboma of alae nasi and nostrils; urogenital abnormalities, including pseudohermaphroditism and renal hypoplasia; abnormal, bizarre hairline; narrow external auditory meatus and malformation of ossicles; cleft lip and palate may occur; atresia or hypoplasia of larynx in some cases; hoarse voice; dysplastic pinna; meatal stenosis; glottic web and subglottic stenosis.

Laboratory

Antenatal ultrasonography; radiography of the abdomen; contrast enema; rectal biopsy.

Treatment

Management of the congenital defects.

Additional Resource

1. Rosen NG (2010). Atresia, Stenosis, and Other Obstruction of the Colon. [online] Available from http://www.emedicine.com/ped/TOPIC2928.HTM [Accessed April, 2012].

---

576. FREEMAN-SHELDON SYNDROME (CRANIOCARPOTARSAL DYSPLASIA; WHISTLING FACE SYNDROME)

General

Rare; autosomal dominant and recessive inheritance as well as sporadic cases (genetic heterogeneity).

Ocular

Eyes deeply sunken (enophthalmos); hypertelorism; blepharophimosis; ptosis; antimongoloid slanting of lid fissures; esotropia.

Clinical

Small nose with narrow nostrils and long philtrum; alae nasi often bent, simulating colobomas; nasolabial folds present only near the nose; microstomia; high-arched palate and small mandible; flexion contractures of fingers; excessive bulging of central part of cheeks when whistling.

Laboratory

No specific laboratory studies, imaging or diagnostic procedures are valuable.

Treatment

Various reconstructive procedures may be necessary.

Bibliography

1. Freeman EA, Sheldon JH. Cranio-carpo-tarsal dystrophy. Arch Dis Child. 1938;13:277-83.
2. McKusick VA. Mendelian Inheritance in Man: A Catalog of Human Genes and Genetic Disorders, 12th edition. Baltimore: The Johns Hopkins University Press; 1998.
3. O'Keefe M, Crawford JS, Young JD, et al. Ocular abnormalities in the Freeman-Sheldon syndrome. Am J Ophthalmol. 1986;102:346-8.
4. Wang TR, Lin SJ. Further evidence for genetic heterogeneity of whistling face or Freeman-Sheldon syndrome in a Chinese family. Am J Med Genet. 1987;28:471-5.
5. Weinstein S, Gorlin RJ. Cranio-carpo-tarsal dysplasia or the whistling face syndrome. I. Clinical considerations. Am J Dis Child. 1969;117: 427-33.

577. FRENKEL SYNDROME (ANTERIOR SEGMENT TRAUMATIC SYNDROME; OCULAR CONTUSION SYNDROME)

General

Minor blunt trauma to the anterior segment of the globe.

Ocular

Sluggish pupil reaction; traumatic mydriasis; iris dialysis; heavy pigment deposits on the vitreous surface; subluxation of the lens; transient posterior cortical lens opacities; permanent anterior or posterior capsular opacities; coronary opacities; late anterior cortical rosette; late total traumatic cataract; Vossius ring following hyphema; peripheral pigment disturbance resembling atypical retinitis pigmentosa; macular edema; retinal detachment.

Clinical

None

Laboratory

Diagnosis is made by clinical findings.

Treatment

Cataract surgery, retinal detachment surgery may be necessary.

Bibliography

1. Frenkel H. Sur la Valeur Medico-Legale du Syndrome Traumatique du Segment Anterieur. Arch Ophthalmol. 1931;48:5.
2. Magalini SI, Scrascia E. Dictionary of Medical Syndromes, 2nd edition. Philadelphia: JB Lippincott; 1981.

578. FRIEDREICH ATAXIA (SPINOCEREBELLAR ATAXIA)

General

Etiology unknown, either autosomal recessive or dominant; progressive; incapacitating by age 20 years; death from secondary diseases or cardiac failure; prevalent in males.

Ocular

Nystagmus; optic atrophy; there is a form of Friedreich ataxia (FA) associated with congenital glaucoma.

Clinical

Kyphoscoliosis; tremor; dysmetria; asynergia; slow ataxic speech; paresthesias; Babinski sign; headache; retarded growth; mental retardation; polyuria; polydipsia; deformity of feet (onset in the first year of life); clumsy gait and difficult to turn arms, head and trunk; deafness.

Laboratory

Magnetic resonance imaging (MRI) is the study of choice in the evaluation of the atrophic changes.

Treatment

Results of treating ataxia in FA have generally been disappointing. No therapeutic measures are known to alter the natural history of the neurological disease.

Additional Resource

1. Chawla J (2010). Friedreich Ataxia. [online] Available from http://www.emedicine.com/neuro/TOPIC139.HTM [Accessed April, 2012].

---

579. FRÖHLICH SYNDROME (DYSTROPHIA ADIPOSOGENITALIS)

General

Caused by chromophobe adenoma of pituitary, Rathke pouch tumors; craniopharyngiomas; suprasellar tumors; encephalitis; trauma; more frequent in Jewish families; manifestations occur in childhood, often during puberty.

Ocular

Bitemporal hemianopsia; impaired scotopic vision; papilledema; optic nerve atrophy (with increased intracranial pressure).

Clinical

Adiposity; genital hypoplasia; in females, menstruation fails to appear or may cease in postpubertal period; in males, voice remains high-pitched, undescended testes, absent facial hair and feminine pubic line; possible retarded growth; polyuria; polydipsia.

Laboratory

Magnetic resonance imaging (MRI), CT, nuclear medicine.

Treatment

Three options are available for the management of pituitary adenomas: (1) surgery, (2) medical therapy and (3) radiation therapy.

Additional Resource

1. Khan AN (2011). Pituitary Adenoma Imaging. [online] Available from http://www.emedicine.com/radio/TOPIC557.HTM [Accessed April, 2012].

---

580. FRONTOMETAPHYSEAL DYSPLASIA (FMD)

General

Sex-linked; rare; bony dysplasia.

Ocular

Strabismus; supraorbital deformity; hyperopia; hypertelorism; prominent supraorbital ridges.

Clinical

Agenesis of frontal sinuses; underdevelopment of mandible; metaphysis of tubular bones; deafness; hirsutism; teeth abnormalities; bony overgrowth at base of nose resulting in nasal obstruction and mouth breathing; facial nerve paralysis; normal intelligence.

Laboratory

Diagnosis is made by clinical findings.

Treatment

Strabismus: Equalized vision with correct refractive error; surgery may be helpful in patient with diplopia.

Hypertelorism: Minor degrees of deformity (referred to as telecanthus) can be corrected by removing a small amount of bone in the midline. A limited frontal craniotomy is performed in the midline osteotomy.

Bibliography

1. McKusick VA. Mendelian Inheritance in Man: A Catalog of Human Genes and Genetic Disorders, 12th edition. Baltimore: The Johns Hopkins University Press; 1998.
2. McKusick-Nathans Institute for Genetic Medicine, Johns Hopkins University and National Center for Biotechnology Information, National Library of Medicine. (2007). Online Mendelian Inheritance in Man (OMIM). [online] Available from http://www.ncbi.nlm.nih.gov/omim [Accessed April, 2012].
3. Reardon W, Hall CM, Dillon MJ, et al. Sibs with mental retardation, supraorbital sclerosis, and metaphyseal dysplasia: frontometaphyseal dysplasia, craniometaphyseal dysplasia, or a new syndrome? J Med Genet. 1991;28:622-6.

581. FRONTONASAL DYSPLASIA SYNDROME (MEDIAN CLEFT FACE SYNDROME)

General

Congenital disorder without genetic background; condition may present a variety of facial malformations, depending on the stage of embryonic development at which interference occurs.

Ocular

Hypertelorism; anophthalmia or microphthalmia; significant refractive errors; strabismus; nystagmus; eyelid ptosis; optic nerve hypoplasia; optic nerve colobomas; cataract; corneal dermoid; inflammatory retinopathy.

Clinical

Broad nasal root may be associated with median nasal groove and cleft of nose and/or upper lip; cleft of ala nasi (unilateral or bilateral); V-shaped hair prolongation into forehead.

Laboratory

Computed tomography (CT), MRI and physical examination.

Treatment

Reconstruction surgery may be warranted.

Bibliography

1. Kinsey JA, Streeten BW: Ocular abnormalities in the median cleft face syndrome. Am J Ophthalmol. 1977;83:261-6.
2. Roarty JD, Pron GE, Siegel-Bartelt J, et al. Ocular manifestations of frontonasal dysplasia. Plast Reconstr Surg. 1994;93:25-30.
3. Sedano HO, Cohen MM, Jirasek J, et al. Frontonasal dysplasia. J Pediatr. 1970;76:906-13.
4. Weaver DF, Bellinger DH. Bifid nose associated with midline cleft of the upper lip. Arch Otolaryngol. 1946;44:480-2.

582. FUCHS DELLEN (FACETS, FUCHS DIMPLES)

General

Lid unable to totally wipe across the cornea causing a depression at the corneal limbus.

Clinical

None

Ocular

Paralimbal corneal ulcerations that occur at base of abnormal conjunctiva or corneal elevation.

Laboratory

Diagnosis is made by clinical findings.

Treatment

Pressure dressing to control abnormal conjunctival elevation. Topical corticosteroids, ocular lubricants and antibiotic drops.

Bibliography

1. Roy FH, Fraunfelder FW, Fraunfelder FT. Roy and Fraunfelder's Current Ocular Therapy, 6th edition. Philadelphia: WB Saunders; 2008.

583. FUCHS (1) SYNDROME (HETEROCHROMIC CYCLITIS SYNDROME)

General

Etiology unknown; mild infective cyclitis is the most likely cause; etiology remains unclear, although it is likely to be autoimmune; positive epidemiologic association with ocular toxoplasmosis has been investigated.

Ocular

Secondary glaucoma; unilateral hypochromic heterochromia; painless cyclitis with absence of synechiae and little or no ciliary injection; secondary cataract; vitreous opacities; small white discrete keratic precipitates with fine filaments between the precipitates; corneal epithelium may be slightly edematous; peripheral choroiditis occasionally; keratoconus.

Clinical

Occasional dysraphia of the cervical cord.

Laboratory

Diagnosis is made by clinical findings.

Treatment

Generally no treatment is necessary. Occasionally discomfort and ciliary injection is treated with topical steroids. With cataract surgery there is a higher rate of vitreous debri and hemorrhage. Glaucoma surgery may be indicated and rubeotic glaucoma may require enucleation.

Additional Resource

1. Arif M (2011). Fuchs Heterochromic Uveitis. [online] Available from http://www.emedicine.com/oph/TOPIC432.HTM [Accessed April, 2012].

584. FUCHS-LYELL SYNDROME (DEBRÉ-LAMY-LYELL SYNDROME; TOXIC EPIDERMAL NECROLYSIS)

General

Allergic reaction with severe manifestations; similar to Fuchs-Salzmann-Terrien syndrome (see Fuchs-Salzmann-Terrien Syndrome); may result as a reaction to *Staphylococcus aureus* toxin in children or associated with certain medications, including penicillin, sulfa, nonsteroidal anti-inflammatory agents and allopurinol.

Ocular

Obstruction of nasolacrimal duct; cicatricial changes in conjunctiva and cornea; conjunctivitis; symblepharon; corneal ulceration and possible perforation.

Clinical

Inflammation of mucous membrane with ulcerations; general epidermolysis; cicatricial changes, especially of orifices.

Laboratory

Hematology studies, chemistry to assess fluid and electrolyte losses, liver enzyme tests, coagulation studies.

Treatment

Management requires prompt detection and withdrawal of all potential causative agents, evaluation and largely supportive care.

Additional Resource

1. Cohen V (2011). Toxic Epidermal Necrolysis. [online] Available from http://www.emedicine.com/med/TOPIC2291.HTM [Accessed April, 2012].

585. FUCHS-SALZMANN-TERRIEN SYNDROME

General

Features similar to those of Fuchs-Lyell syndrome; both are based on drug allergies (antibiotics, sulfonamides, arsenic preparations) (see Fuchs-Lyell Syndrome).

Ocular

Features of Salzmann nodular dystrophy; superficial punctate keratitis; marginal degeneration of the cornea; intraocular hemorrhages; choroidal hemorrhages.

Clinical

Allergic cutaneous lesions with erythema and degrees of exfoliative dermatitis.

Laboratory

Hematology studies, chemistry to assess fluid and electrolyte losses, liver enzyme tests, coagulation studies.

Treatment

Management requires prompt detection and withdrawal of all potential causative agents, evaluation and largely supportive care.

Bibliography

1. Duke-Elder S (Ed). System of Ophthalmology. St. Louis: CV Mosby; 1965.
2. Fuchs E. Uber knotchenformige Hornhauttrubung. Graefes Arch Clin Exp Ophthalmol. 1902;53:423.

586. FUCHS' CORNEAL DYSTROPHY (COMBINED DYSTROPHY OF FUCHS, ENDOTHELIAL DYSTROPHY OF THE CORNEA, EPITHELIAL DYSTROPHY OF FUCHS, FUCHS' EPITHELIAL-ENDOTHELIAL DYSTROPHY; FUCHS' ENDOTHELIAL DYSTROPHY OF THE CORNEA)

General

Bilateral, slowly progressive, primary corneal disease which results in vision loss due to corneal edema. Autosomal dominant and usually not clinically evident until the fourth or fifth decade of life.

Clinical

None

Ocular

Central corneal guttae; gray, thickened appearance of Descemet's membrane; stromal edema; subepithelial edema; decreased visual acuity.

Laboratory

Diagnosis is made by clinical findings. The characteristics include endothelium producing an abnormal, banded, posterior layer of Descemet's membrane with charactertistic central guttae excrescences which are a hallmark of this disease.

Treatment

Early intervention includes sodium chloride 5% solution or ointment and the use of a hair dryer on low heat setting for tear film evaporation and corneal deturgescence. Surgical intervention includes corneal transplantation, endothelial keratoplasty (EK), deep lamellar endothelial keratoplasty (DLEK) and Descemet's stripping endothelial keratoplasty (DSEK).

Additional Resource

1. Singh D (2012). Fuchs Endothelial Dystrophy. [online] Available from http://www.emedicine.com/oph/TOPIC91.HTM [Accessed April, 2012].

587. FUNGAL ENOPHTHALMITIS

General

Rare, intraocular fungal infection.

Clinical

None

Ocular

Conjunctival injection, pain, mildly decreased vision, fibrinous membranes in anterior chamber, white fluffy retinal infiltrates.

Laboratory

Fungal tests on anterior chamber aspirates and vitreous cavity aspirates.

Treatment

Topical, subconjunctival, intravitreal antifungal agents. Pars plana vitrectomy.

Additional Resource

1. Wu L (2010). Endophthalmitis, Fungal. [online] Available from http://www.emedicine.com/oph/TOPIC706.HTM [Accessed April, 2012].

588. FUNGAL KERATITIS

General

It can occur following trauma or in immuno-suppressed individuals.

Clinical

None

Ocular

Central or pericentral corneal ulcer, photophobia, pain.

Laboratory

Corneal smear—Giemsa, KOH or Gomori's methenamine silver stain, Cuture—Sabouraud's dextrose agar, brain-heart infusion broth.

Treatment

Yeast—amphotericin hourly while awake for 48 hours then every 2 hours. Fungal—natamycin 5% every hour for 48 hours then every 2 hours. Excisional keratoplasty may be necessary.

Bibliography

1. Shi W, Wang T, Xie L, et al. Risk factors, clinical features, and outcomes of recurrent fungal keratitis after corneal transplantation. Ophthalmology. 2010;117:890-6.

Additional Resource

1. Singh D (2011). Fungal Keratitis. [online] Available from http://www.emedicine.com/oph/TOPIC99.HTM [Accessed April, 2012].

589. FUSOBACTERIUM

General

Gram-negative; normal inhabitant of mouth and respiratory, intestinal and urogenital tracts; usually secondary to an underlying disease, surgical procedure, or therapy that impairs the defense of the host; nonspore forming, nonmotile Gram-negative anaerobic bacilli.

Ocular

Conjunctivitis; dacryocystitis; orbital abscess; orbital cellulitis; corneal ulcer; tenonitis; lid edema; panophthalmitis; gangrene of conjunctiva; cavernous sinus thrombosis; cranial nerve palsy.

Clinical

Brain abscess; pneumonia; liver abscess; endocarditis; sepsis; tissue necrosis.

Laboratory

Gram stain of a smear of the specimen provides important preliminary information regarding types of organisms present.

Treatment

Patient's recovery from anaerobic infection depends on prompt and proper treatment according to the following principles: (1) neutralizing toxins produced by anaerobes, (2) preventing local bacterial proliferation by changing the environment and (3) limiting the spread of bacteria.

Additional Resource

1. Brook I (2011). Peptostreptococcus Infection. [online] Available from http://www.emedicine.com/med/TOPIC1777.HTM [Accessed April, 2012].

590. G SYNDROME (HYPERTELORISM ESOPHAGEAL ABNORMALITY AND HYPOSPADIAS; HYPOSPADIAS-DYSPHAGIA SYNDROME)

General

Neuromuscular defect; autosomal dominant; prevalent in males; males more severely affected (see BBB Syndrome).

Ocular

Retinitis pigmentosa; hypertelorism; narrow palpebral fissures; epicanthal folds; telecanthus.

Clinical

Defect of esophagus; hoarseness; hypospadias; cryptorchidism; imperforate anus; defect of lingual frenulum; deafness; mild mental retardation; dysphagia; anosmia; swallowing difficulties; nasal bridge broad and flat; stridor; aspiration; prominent forehead; cleft lip and palate; laryngotracheal esophageal clefts.

Laboratory

Diagnosis is made by clinical findings.

Treatment

Retinitis pigmentosa: Vitamin A 15,000 IU/day is thought to slow the decline of retinal function, dark sunglasses for outdoor use, surgery for cataract, genetic counseling.

Additional Resource

1. Telander DG (2012). Retinitis Pigmentosa. [online] Available from http://www.emedicine.com/oph/TOPIC704.HTM [Accessed April, 2012].

591. GAISBOCK SYNDROME (EMOTIONAL POLYCYTHEMIA; STRESS ERYTHROCYTOSIS)

General

Prevalent in men, heavy smokers; associated with emotional tension and stress.

Ocular

Afferent pupillary defect; conjunctivitis; central retinal vein occlusion; cystoid macular edema; peripapillary retinal hemorrhage; glaucoma.

Clinical

Obesity; hypertension; stress; vascular disease; plethora.

Laboratory

Bone marrow studies are not necessary to establish the diagnosis, but the finding of hypercellularity and hyperplasia of the erythroid, granulocytic, and megakaryocytic cell lines or myelofibrosis supports the diagnosis of a myeloproliferative process.

Treatment

Phlebotomy or bloodletting has been the mainstay of therapy for this disease process for a long time.

Additional Resource

1. Kooragayala LM (2011). Central Retinal Vein Occlusion. [online] Available from http://www.emedicine.medscape.com/article/1223746-overview [Accessed April, 2012].

592. GALACTOSYLCERAMIDE LIPIDOSIS [GLOBOID CELL LEUKODYSTROPHY; INFANTILE GLOBOID CELL LEUKODYSTROPHY; KRABBE (1) SYNDROME; KRABBE DISEASE]

General

Defect in metabolism of galactocerebroside; genetically determined demyelinating disease that is fatal in early childhood; both sexes affected; onset usually in the first year of life; ambiguous onset; autosomal recessive; onset age 4–6 months, although some late-onset cases have been reported; diagnosis is made after identification of "globoid cells" in brain tissue.

Ocular

Photophobia; cortical blindness; optic atrophy; nystagmus.

Clinical

Hypersensitivity to external stimuli; rigidity; vomiting; seizures; episodic fever; mental retardation; death.

Laboratory

Diagnosis is dependent upon demonstration of specific enzymatic deficiency in peripheral blood leukocytes or cultured fibroblasts.

Treatment

Treatment primarily is directed at symptomatic relief.

Additional Resource

1. Tegay DH (2010). Krabbe Disease. [online] Available from http://www.emedicine.com/ped/TOPIC2892. HTM [Accessed April, 2012].

593. GANGLIOSIDOSIS GM1 TYPE 2 (JUVENILE GANGLIOSIDOSIS)

General

Absence of B and C isoenzymes of beta-galactosidase results in neural and visceral deposition of gangliosides and visceral deposition of mucopolysaccharides; autosomal recessive; defective hexosaminidase A; defect localized to chromosome 15 (15q22–15q25.1).

Ocular

Optic atrophy; pigmentary retinopathy; strabismus; macular cherry-red spot; late optic atrophy.

Clinical

Cerebral degeneration; skeletal changes; visceromegaly; psychomotor deterioration; death between the ages of 3 and 4 years; abnormal acousticomotor reaction; hypotonia; variable hepatosplenomegaly; abnormal hexosaminidases A and B; defect localized to chromosome 5 (5q13).

Laboratory

Diagnosis is dependent upon demonstration of specific enzymatic deficiency in peripheral blood leukocytes or cultured fibroblasts.

Treatment

Treatment primarily is directed at symptomatic relief.

Additional Resource

1. Ierardi-Curto L (2010). Lipid Storage Disorders. [online] Available from http://www.emedicine. com/ped/TOPIC1310.HTM [Accessed April, 2012].

594. GANGLIOSIDOSIS GM1 TYPE 1 [GENERALIZED GANGLIOSIDOSIS (INFANTILE); NORMAN-LANDING SYNDROME; PSEUDO-HURLER LIPOIDOSIS]

General

Absence of A, B and C isoenzymes of beta-galactosidase visceral tissue and mucopolysaccharides in visceral tissues; both sexes affected; autosomal recessive; onset from birth; death from 6 months to 2 years of age; defect has been localized to chromosome 3 (3p12–3p13).

Ocular

Macular cherry-red spots; optic disk pallor; nystagmus; esotropia; corneal clouding; retinal artery tortuosity and narrowing; retinitis pigmentosa; macular cherry-red spot found in 50% of patients with this disorder.

Clinical

Cerebral degeneration combined with visceromegaly and skeletal dysplasia; mental and motor retardation; seizures; deafness; spastic quadriplegia; feeding difficulties; recurrent bronchopneumonia; broad nose; frontal bossing; prominent maxilla; hepatosplenomegaly.

Laboratory

Diagnosis is dependent upon demonstration of specific enzymatic deficiency in peripheral blood leukocytes or cultured fibroblasts.

Treatment

Treatment primarily is directed at symptomatic relief.

Additional Resource

1. Ierardi-Curto L (2010). Lipid Storage Disorders. [online] Available from http://www.emedicine.com/ped/TOPIC1310.HTM [Accessed April, 2012].

595. GANSER SYNDROME (NONSENSE SYNDROME; PRISON PSYCHOSIS SYNDROME; PSEUDODEMENTIA)

General

Found in prisoners and patients with schizophrenia; disparity between the person's complaints and mental alertness.

Ocular

Patient pretends that he or she cannot see or read; no objective findings on examination of visual function.

Clinical

Patient pretends not to know how to do simple things previously familiar to him or her (not to know his or her age, how to spell or read, etc.); mild degree of mental deficiency; amnesia; analgesia; confusion; lethargy; apathetic indifference; headache.

Laboratory

Computed tomography scan or MRI to rule out possible cerebral pathology, electroencephalogram can be performed to rule out seizure disorder.

Treatment

Psychotherapy and monitoring by a psychiatrist is recommended.

Additional Resource

1. Schneider D (2011). Ganser Syndrome. [online] Available from http://www.emedicine.com/med/TOPIC840.HTM [Accessed April, 2012].

596. GANSSLEN SYNDROME (FAMILIAL HEMOLYTIC ICTERUS; HEMATOLOGIC-METABOLIC BONE DISORDER)

General

Autosomal dominant inheritance; occurs mainly in Caucasians.

Ocular

Hypertelorism; microphthalmos; epicanthus; narrowing of palpebral fissure; lid hemorrhages; myopia; dyschromatopsia; hypochromic heterochromia; scleral icterus; conjunctival hemorrhages; retinal pallor and edema in advanced stages; dilated retinal arteries and veins; round retinal hemorrhages in deeper retinal layers; retinal exudates and macular star.

Clinical

Splenomegaly; hemolytic crises; dental deformities; brachydactyly; polydactyly; congenital hip luxation; oxycephaly; deformities of the outer ear and otosclerosis.

Laboratory

Indirect Coombs test and direct antibody test results are positive in the mother and affected newborn, serial maternal antibody titers are monitored until a critical titer of 1:32, which indicates that a high risk of fetal hydrops.

Treatment

Early exchange transfusion with type-O Rh-negative fresh RBCs with intensive phototherapy is usually required.

Bibliography

1. Ganser SJ. Uber Einen Eigenartigen Hysterischen Dammerzustand. Arch Psychiatr Nervenkr. 1898; 30:633-40.
2. Magalini SI, Scrascia E. Dictionary of Medical Syndromes, 2nd edition. Philadelphia: JB Lippincott; 1981.

597. GAPO SYNDROME (ALOPECIA, GROWTH RETARDATION OPTIC ATROPHY SYNDROME, PSEUDOANODONTIA)

General

Autosomal recessive.

Ocular

Progressive optic atrophy; glaucoma; keratoconus.

Clinical

Growth retardation; alopecia; pseudoanodontia; frontal bossing; high forehead; midfacial hypoplasia; wide-open anterior fontanelle; retarded bone age; premature aged appearance; hypogonadism; hepatomegaly; muscular body build.

Laboratory

Erythrocyte sedimentation rate (ESR).

Treatment

The initial dose is 40–60 mg/d of prednisone, depending on the size of the patient and the severity of the disease.

Bibliography

1. Gagliardi AR, González CH, Pratesi R. GAPO syndrome: report of three affected brothers. Am J Med Genet. 1984;19:217-23.
2. McKusick VA. Mendelian Inheritance in Man: A Catalog of Human Genes and Genetic Disorders, 12th edition. Baltimore: The Johns Hopkins University Press; 1998.

598. GARCIN SYNDROME (HALF-BASE SYNDROME; SCHMINCKE TUMOR-UNILATERAL CRANIAL PARALYSIS)

General

Causes include tumors of nasopharynx, rapidly progressing growth of a sarcoma of base of skull, meningitis and cranial polyneuritis; cranial nerves VIII (vestibulocochlear), IX (glossopharyngeal), X (vagus), XI (accessory) and XII (hypoglossal) are most frequently involved.

Ocular

Ptosis (unilateral); unilateral external ophthalmoplegia; papilledema.

Clinical

Difficulties in swallowing; impairment of speech; hearing defect; respiratory difficulties; sensory disturbances; hoarseness.

Laboratory

Magnetic resonance imaging (MRI) with gadolinium and fat suppression is the radiologic modality of choice, transnasal biopsy of nasopharyngeal mass.

Treatment

Radiation therapy is the primary mode of management of nasopharyngeal carcinoma.

Bibliography

1. Bruce JN, Fetell MR. Tumors of the skull and cranial nerves. In: Rowland LP (Ed). Merritt's Textbook of Neurology, 9th edition. Baltimore: Williams & Wilkins; 1995. pp. 320-9.

599. GARDNER SYNDROME

General

Autosomal dominant; both sexes affected; average age of onset is 20 years.

Ocular

Exophthalmos; congenital hypertrophy of retinal pigment epithelium (RPE); multiple lesions of the eye; bilateral occurrence; orbital osteoma; highly pleomorphic pigmentation; unilateral or bilateral retinal lesions; pilomatrixoma-like epidermal cysts; presence of pigmented fundus lesions appears to cluster within families.

Clinical

Intestinal polyps; dermoid tumors; neurofibrous osteomatosis; colon cancer; supernumerary teeth.

Laboratory

Diagnosis is made by clinical findings.

Treatment

Etiology of exophthalmos or proptosis is established, the appropriate specialists should partake in the patient's care.

Additional Resource

1. Mercandetti M (2010). Exophthalmos. [online] Available from http://www.emedicine.com/oph/TOPIC616.HTM [Accessed April, 2012].

600. GASTROCUTANEOUS SYNDROME

General

Combination of symptoms including peptic ulcer, hiatal hernia, multiple lentigines, cafe-au-lait spots, hypertelorism, myopia, acute or chronic; occurs in people with stress who smoke and use ulcerogenic drugs.

Ocular

Hypertelorism; myopia; nystagmus.

Clinical

Upper abdominal pain regularly occurs about 1–2 hours after eating; pain at night, when gastric secretion is at its peak; nausea; vomiting; excessive salivation.

Laboratory

Diagnosis is made by clinical findings.

Treatment

Hypertelorism: Minor degrees of deformity (referred to as telecanthus) can be corrected by removing a small amount of bone in the midline. A limited frontal craniotomy is performed in the midline osteotomy.

Bibliography

1. Kasper DL, Braunwald E, Fauci AS, Hauser SL, Longo DL, Jameson JL (Eds). Harrison's Principles of Internal Medicine, 16th edition. New York: McGraw-Hill; 2005.

2. McKusick VA. Mendelian Inheritance in Man: A Catalog of Human Genes and Genetic Disorders, 12th edition. Baltimore: The Johns Hopkins University Press; 1998.

3. McKusick-Nathans Institute for Genetic Medicine, Johns Hopkins University and National Center for Biotechnology Information, National Library of Medicine. (2007). Online Mendelian Inheritance in Man (OMIM). [online] Available from http://www.ncbi.nlm.nih.gov/omim [Accessed April, 2012].

601. GAUCHER SYNDROME (CEREBROSIDE LIPIDOSIS; GLUCOCEREBROSIDE STORAGE DISEASE; GLUCOSYLCERAMIDE LIPIDOSIS)

General

Storage of glucocerebroside in the reticuloendothelial system; autosomal recessive; occurs frequently in Jewish families; onset at any age; onset usually sudden in the infantile form; disease belongs to group of lipid storage disturbances such as ganglioside (Tay-Sachs), sphingomyelin (Niemann-Pick) and ceramide trihexoside (Fabry) (see Tay-Sachs Syndrome; Niemann-Pick Syndrome; Fabry Syndrome); caused by glucosylceramide beta-glucosidase (glucocerebrosidase) deficiency; psychomotor deterioration apparent before age 6 months.

Ocular

Strabismus; brown-yellowish, wedge-shaped pinguecula; corneal clouding; oculomotor paralysis; gaze palsies.

Clinical

Infantile form: generalized hypertonia, opisthotonus, dysphagia, vomiting, laryngeal spasm, dyspnea; chronic form: hepatosplenomegaly, lymphadenopathy, mild-to-moderate anemia, yellowish-brown patchy skin pigmentation.

Laboratory

Infiltration by cells with "onion-peel" cytoplasm, called Gaucher cells, is caused by a lipid storage disorder (i.e. glucosylceramide lipidosis). Gaucher cells clog or infiltrate the bone marrow, spleen and liver.

Treatment

Treat the underlying disease and provide supportive measures for symptomatic patients. Treat anemia with packed red blood cell transfusions.

Additional Resource

1. Besa EC (2011). Myelophthisic Anemia. [online] Available from http://www.emedicine.com/med/TOPIC1562.HTM [Accessed April, 2012].

---

602. GELINEAU SYNDROME (NARCOLEPTIC SYNDROME)

General

Etiology not well understood; causes include subthalamic lesions, multiple sclerosis and tumor of third ventricle; onset in adolescence or early adulthood; male preponderance (6:1); most characteristic sign is sudden attack of sleep that cannot be resisted and may last from only a few minutes to half an hour.

Ocular

Transient blurred vision; inability to read between attacks; bilateral diplopia; spontaneous eyelid closing; flickering vision.

Clinical

Diurnal attacks of short episodes of uncontrollable sleep (usually several times a day); cataplexy with decreased or absent muscle tone and paralysis caused by an upset emotional state; hallucinations.

Laboratory

An overnight polysomnogram followed by a multiple sleep latency test (MSLT).

Treatment

Sleep hygiene is important. Most patients improve if they maintain a regular sleep schedule, usually 7.5–8 hours of sleep per night. Scheduled naps during the day may also help. CNS stimulants.

Additional Resource

1. Bozorg AM (2010). Narcolepsy. [online] Available from http://www.emedicine.com/neuro/TOPIC522.HTM [Accessed April, 2012].

---

603. GENERAL FIBROSIS SYNDROME (CONGENITAL ENOPHTHALMOS WITH OCULAR MUSCLE FIBROSIS AND PTOSIS; CONGENITAL FIBROSIS SYNDROME; CONGENITAL FIBROSIS OF THE INFERIOR RECTUS WITH PTOSIS; STRABISMUS FIXUS; VERTICAL RETRACTION SYNDROME)

General

Present from birth; familial history; apparent autosomal dominant transmission; sex-linked recessive transmission also reported.

Ocular

Ptosis; enophthalmos; disk hypoplasia; astigmatism; esotropia; exotropia; hypotropia; nystagmus; visual loss; positive forced duction test;

may be associated with Marcus Gunn jaw-winking and synergistic divergence in attempted right gaze.

Clinical

None

Laboratory

Neuroimaging is the most essential laboratory study.

Treatment

Surgically approximating normal orbital bone positions before addressing soft tissue volume loss.

Additional Resource

1. Charles NS Soparkar (2010). Enophthalmos. [online] Available from http://www.emedicine. com/oph/TOPIC617.HTM [Accessed April, 2012].

---

604. GERLIER DISEASE (KUBISAGARI; LE TOURNIQUET; PARALYTIC VERTIGO)

General

Cranial nerve dysfunction suggests a basal lesion such as epidemic paralyzed vertigo; infective agent suspected, small Gram-negative coccus from spinal fluid; contact with cows or horses in warm summer months in contaminated stables; pathology unknown; possible brainstem lesion.

Ocular

During attack: hyperemia of fundus oculi, fundus normal and eyesight normal; between attacks: ptosis, dimness of vision, vertigo and diplopia.

Clinical

Attack of palsies precipitated by severe exertion, bright light, warmth, hunger or looking at a moving object (optokinetic irritation); attacks last approximately 10 minutes and may follow each other at very short intervals; mild form not incapacitating; severe form incapacitating; pains in back of neck; nodding of head during attack; hyperreflexia at intervals; attack of temporary palsy muscles, levator palpebrae superior, muscles of back of neck, extension limbs, face, pharynx and larynx.

Laboratory

Diagnosis is made by clinical findings.

Treatment

Ptosis: If visual acuity is affected most cases require surgical correction, and there are several procedures that may be used including levator resection, repair or advancement and Fasanella-Servat.

Bibliography

1. Gerlier E. Une Epidemie de Vertige Paralysant. Rev Med Suisse Romande. 1887;7:5-29.
2. Magalini SI, Scrascia E. Dictionary of Medical Syndromes, 2nd edition. Philadelphia: JB Lippincott; 1981.

---

605. GERMAN SYNDROME (FETAL TRIMETHADIONE; TRIDIONE)

General

Both sexes affected; prenatal onset; occurs when trimethadione or paramethadione is taken during pregnancy.

Ocular

Eyebrows up-slanted, epicanthal folds.

Clinical

Mild brachycephaly; short upturned nose; prominent forehead; cleft lip and palate; micrognathia; ear abnormalities; tetralogy of Fallot; genital abnormalities; hypospadias; hypertrophic clitoris; abnormalities of skin, gastrointestinal, renal and skeletal systems.

Laboratory

Diagnosis is made by clinical findings.

Treatment

None

Bibliography

1. German J, Kowal A, Ehlers KH. Trimethadione and human teratogenesis. Teratology. 1970;3: 349-62.

---

606. GERSTMANN SYNDROME (DOMINANT HEMISPHERE SYNDROME; LEFT ANGULAR GYRUS SYNDROME)

General

Most frequently caused by tumors of dominant hemisphere in which the angular gyrus is involved; may follow an ischemic posterior cerebellar artery (PCA) lesion affecting the inferior parietal lobule and resulting in jargon aphasia, dyscalculia, agraphia right-left confusion, constructional dyspraxia and alexia.

Ocular

Homonymous hemianopsia; visual agnosia for colors.

Clinical

Agraphia (inability to write); finger agnosia; anosognosia; aciculae (difficulties in or inability to perform serial number projects); confusion (mainly between left and right).

Laboratory

Computed tomography (CT) and MRI.

Treatment

Consult neurologist.

Additional Resource

1. Haddad G (2011). Meningioma. [online] Available from http://www.emedicine.medscape.com/article/1156552-overview [Accessed April, 2012].

---

607. GHOST CELL GLAUCOMA

General

Usually follows vitreous hemorrhage when the presence of blood debris in the anterior chamber clogs the trabecular meshwork resulting in elevated intraocular pressure.

Clinical

Vitreous hemorrhage sometimes associated with diabetes.

Ocular

Elevated intraocular pressure, vitreous hemorrhage, corneal edema, decreased visual acuity, posterior vitreous detachment.

Laboratory

Cytologic examination of the aqueous humor, B-scan ultrasonography.

Treatment

Usually involves surgical intervention with lavage of the anterior chamber or vitrectomy.

Bibliography

1. Campbell DG, Essigmann EM. Hemolytic ghost cell glaucoma. Arch Ophthalmol. 1979;97:2141-6.
2. Montenegro MH, Simmons RJ. Ghost cell glaucoma. Int Ophthalmol Clin. 1995;35:111-5.
3. Rojas L, Ortiz G, Gutierrez M, et al. Ghost cell glaucoma related to snake poisoning. Arch Ophthalmol. 2001;119:1212-3.

608. GIANT FORNIX SYNDROME

General

Enlarged upper fornix with buildup of mucopurulent debri and persistent discharge.

Ocular

Bacterial conjunctivitis; blepharospasm; enlarged fornix; secondary ptosis.

Clinical

Recurrent chronic conjunctivitis.

Laboratory

Diagnosis is made by clinical findings.

Treatment

The mainstay of medical treatment of bacterial conjunctivitis is topical antibiotic therapy.

Additional Resource

1. Yeung KK (2011). Bacterial Conjunctivitis. [online] Available from http://www.emedicine.com/oph/TOPIC88.HTM [Accessed April, 2012].

609. GIANT PAPILLARY CONJUNCTIVITIS SYNDROME

General

Commonly associated with contact lenses (hard and soft), foreign bodies and ocular prosthesis; immunologic in origin.

Ocular

Ocular irritation; itching of the eye; decreased visual acuity; increased mucous production; papillary changes of the upper tarsal conjunctiva; contact lens coatings; may appear after a lens change from one style to another or by replacement of the previous design; aging of a lens, particularly of a soft contact lens, may be associated; usually bilateral, although it can be markedly asymmetrical.

Clinical

None

Laboratory

Diagnosis is made by clinical findings.

Treatment

Stop wearing contact lens for 4 weeks, replace contact lens every 6–12 months, topical lubricants and nonsteroidal anti-inflammatory drops.

Additional Resource

1. Weissman BA (2011). Giant Papillary Conjunctivitis. [online] Available from http://www.emedicine.com/oph/TOPIC87.HTM [Accessed April, 2012].

---

610. GIARDIASIS

General

Multiflagellate protozoan; parasite of human duodenum; encystation occurs in transit through colon.

Ocular

Uveitis; retinal hemorrhages; central serous retinopathy; palpebral edema.

Clinical

Nausea; flatulence; epigastric pain; abdominal cramps; diarrhea; weight loss; malabsorption.

Laboratory

The traditional basis of diagnosis is identification of *Giardia lamblia* trophozoites or cysts in the stool of infected patients via a stool ova and parasite examination.

Treatment

Metronidazole is the most commonly prescribed antibiotic for this condition.

Additional Resource

1. Mukherjee S (2011). Giardiasis. [online] Available from http://www.emedicine.com/med/TOPIC868.HTM [Accessed April, 2012].

---

611. GILLUM-ANDERSON SYNDROME

General

Genetic defect responsible for weakness in the orbital connective tissue; proposed connective tissue defect of sclera, zonules and levator aponeurosis.

Ocular

Dislocated lenses; high myopia; bilateral ptosis typical for levator disinsertions; ectopia lentis.

Laboratory

Diagnosis is made by clinical findings.

Treatment

Treatment of a lens dislodged into the anterior chamber is initially pharmacological with mydriasis/cycloplegia (to permit posterior migration of the lens behind the iris) in conjunction with ocular massage through a closed lid to promote this posterior migration. Surgical treatment will then be needed to prevent further complications.

Additional Resource

1. Eifrig CW (2011). Ectopia Lentis. [online] Available from http://www.emedicine.com/oph/TOPIC55.HTM [Accessed April, 2012].

612. GITELMAN SYNDROME

General

Autosomal recessive, renal tubulopathy characterized by hypokalemia, hypomagnesemia, metabolic alkalosis, hypocalciuria and hypernatremia.

Ocular

Sclerochoroidal calcification.

Clinical

Patients may have arthralgias, seizures, episodes of tetany, muscular weakness or paresthesia; also may be asymptomatic.

Laboratory

Blood and urine chemistries, renal ultrasonography.

Treatment

The cornerstones of medical therapy are the administration of indomethacin and potassium supplementation.

Additional Resource

1. Devarajan P (2011). Pediatric Bartter Syndrome. [online] Available from http://www.emedicine.com/ped/TOPIC210.HTM [Accessed April, 2012].

613. GALACTOSEMIA (GALACTOKINASE DEFICIENCY; GALACTOSE-1-PHOSPHATE URIDYL TRANSFERASE DEFICIENCY; GALACTOSE-6-PHOSPHATE EPIMERASE DEFICIENCY)

General

Autosomal recessive disorder resulting from an error of galactose metabolism caused by a deficiency of any one of three enzymes: (1) transferase, (2) galactokinase or (3) epimerase.

Clinical

Escherichia coli sepsis, hypoglycemia, hyperbilirubinemia, jaundice, hypoparathyroidism.

Ocular

"Oil droplet" cataracts, vitreous hemorrhage.

Laboratory

Newborn blood screening of GALT enzyme activity and quantify total red blood cell galactose-1-phosphate concentration and galactose.

Treatment

Immediate dietary restriction of all lactose-containing foods and medications.

Bibliography

1. Roy FH, Fraunfelder FW, Fraunfelder FT. Roy and Fraunfelder's Current Ocular Therapy, 6th edition. Philadelphia: WB Saunders; 2008.

614. GLANDER SYNDROME

General

Serious infection caused by *Malleomyces mallei*; no naturally acquired infections in the United States since 1938; transmission from equine animals to man; caused by traumatic inoculations or inhalations; either acute, gangrenous or chronic ulcerative; fatal usually in 7–10 days.

Ocular

Conjunctivitis; dacryocystitis; ulcerating granulomatous orbital lesions; photophobia; lacrimation.

Clinical

Systemic erythematous pustules; inhalation infection; fever; rigors; generalized myalgia lymphangitis; fatigue, headache; pleuritic chest pain; diarrhea; lymphadenopathy; splenomegaly; mild leukocytosis; multiple subcutaneous and intramuscular abscesses (often arms and legs); visceral involvement, including pulmonary, pleural, skeletal, hepatic, splenic, meningeal and intracranial.

Laboratory

WBC may be minimally elevated. Elevated liver enzyme levels in glanders may signify hepatic abscess formation.

Treatment

Initiate rapid administration of supportive care and intravenous antibiotic therapy for severe disease.

Additional Resource

1. Rega PP (2011). CBRNE - Glanders and Melioidosis. [online] Available from http://www.emedicine.com/emerg/TOPIC884.HTM [Accessed April, 2012].

---

615. GLAUCOMA ASSOCIATED WITH ANTERIOR UVEITIS

General

Glaucoma related to anterior uveitis.

Clinical

None

Ocular

Increased IOP associated with iritis, cells and flare in the anterior chamber, keratitic precipitates.

Laboratory

Serology, skin test, chest X-ray, conjunctival biopsy.

Treatment

Identify and treat the underlying cause of ocular inflammation. Anti-inflammatory medications (topical, periocular and systemic) and immunosuppressive agents are useful. Glaucoma should be treated with topical antiglaucoma agents.

Additional Resource

1. Herndon L (2010). Uveitic Glaucoma. [online] Available from http://www.emedicine.com/oph/TOPIC145.HTM [Accessed April, 2012].

---

616. GLAUCOMA ASSOCIATED WITH ELEVATED VENOUS PRESSURE

General

Systemic disorders that raise the venous pressure to the eye and may cause glaucoma.

Clinical

Elevated episcleral venous pressure as venous obstruction, carotid cavernous fistula and Sturge Weber syndrome.

Ocular

Prominent veins under the conjunctiva help diagnose this condition.

Laboratory

Diagnosis is made by clinical findings.

Treatment

Topical antiglaucoma agents. Filtering procedure if topical treatment is not affective.

Additional Resource

1. Dahl AA (2010). Glaucoma, Intraocular Tumors. [online] Available from http://www.emedicine.com/oph/TOPIC143.HTM [Accessed April, 2012].

617. GLAUCOMA ASSOCIATED WITH INTRAOCULAR TUMORS (ANGLE-CLOSURE GLAUCOMA, MELANOMALYTIC GLAUCOMA, NEOVASCULAR GLAUCOMA TUMOR RELATED GLAUCOMA)

General

Unilateral, closed-angle glaucoma secondary to intraocular tumor.

Clinical

Systemic hamartomatoses, lymphoid tumors, leukemias.

Ocular

Glaucoma in one eye primarily caused by tumor of eye. Primary tumors of uvea, retina, and pigmented and nonpigmented epithelium.

Laboratory

Ultrasonography, fluorescein angiography or iridocyanine green angiography, MRI and CT scan of orbit, liver function tests (LFTs), liver imaging test, general oncologist evaluation.

Treatment

Benign tumor—treat glaucoma medically, malignant tumor—treat tumor first, antiglaucoma drops and systemic carbonic anhydrase inhibitors are instituted as necessary. Iris and ciliary body tumors—observation initially. Uveal metastases and choroidal melanoma treatment consists of serial observation, photocoagulation, transpupillary thermotherapy, radiotherapy, local resection, enucleation and even orbital exenteration. Retinoblastoma may require an enucleation. Irradiation and chemotherapy should be used at the discretion of the oncologist.

Bibliography

1. Roy FH, Fraunfelder FW, Fraunfelder FT. Roy and Fraunfelder's Current Ocular Therapy, 6th edition. Philadelphia: WB Saunders; 2008.

618. GLAUCOMA, CONGENITAL

General

Autosomal recessive; occurs more frequently in males; can occur isolated or associated with other systemic or ocular malformations (dysgenesis of iris, angle and peripheral cornea).

Ocular

Buphthalmos; corneal haze; glaucoma; epiphora.

Clinical

None

Laboratory

Tonometry, corneal measurements, gonioscopy and ophthalmoscopy should be performed in the operating room and carefully documented. Intraocular pressures recorded under general anesthesia are usually lower than those obtained in the office because of the effects of the anesthetic agents.

Treatment

Primary congenital glaucoma almost always is managed surgically, both goniotomy and trabeculectomy may be useful. When multiple goniotomies and/or trabeculectomies fail, the surgeon usually resorts to a filtering procedure.

Bibliography

1. Ben-Zion I, Tomkins O, Moore DB, et al. Surgical results in the management of advanced primary congenital glaucoma in a rural pediatric population. Ophthalmology. 2011;118:231-5.
2. Bowman RJ, Dickerson M, Mwende J, et al. Outcomes of goniotomy for primary congenital glaucoma in East Africa. Ophthalmology. 2011; 118:236-40.

Additional Resource

1. Cibis GW (2011). Primary Congenital Glaucoma. [online] Available from http://www.emedicine.com/oph/TOPIC138.HTM [Accessed April, 2012].

---

619. GLAUCOMA FOLLOWING PENETRATING KERATOPLASTY

General

Second most common cause for graft failure; etiology varies greatly and includes postoperative inflammation, viscoelastic substances in the chamber, hyphema, operative technique, pre-existing glaucoma, misdirected aqueous, epithelial downgrowth and others.

Clinical

None

Ocular

Elevated intraocular pressure; progressive visual field changes; graft edema; graft failure.

Laboratory

Accurate measurement of the intraocular pressure with a Mackay-Marg electronic applanation tonometer, the pneumatic applanation tonometer, the Tononpen or the dyanamic contour tonometer.

Treatment

Treatment is controversial because of the high risk of graft failure. Medical management with topical drops and systemic pills is the treatment of choice; surgical therapy may be necessary and include trabeculoplasty, trabeculectomy, drainage device and cyclodestructive procedures.

Additional Resource

1. Shetty R (2012). Glaucoma and Penetrating Keratoplasty. [online] Available from http://www.emedicine.medscape.com/article/1208228-overview [Accessed April, 2012].

620. GLAUCOMA, GONIODYSGENESIS (DYSGENIC GLAUCOMA; STEROID GLAUCOMA)

General

Autosomal dominant; use of topical dexamethasone under the two-allele system; three genotypes; (1) high, (2) intermediate and (3) low; more prominent in blacks; mechanism may be related to morphologic changes in the trabecular meshwork.

Ocular

Glaucoma; cataracts.

Clinical

None

Laboratory

Diagnosis is made by clinical findings.

Treatment

Discontinuation of corticosteroids if possible. If it is not possible to discontinue the corticosteroids then traditional drops for IOP control should be started.

Additional Resource

1. Rhee DJ (2012). Drug-Induced Glaucoma. [online] Available from http://www.emedicine.com/oph/TOPIC124.HTM [Accessed April, 2012].

621. GLAUCOMA, HEREDITARY JUVENILE

General

Autosomal dominant, present at birth; there has been linkage with chromosome 1q21–q23; age at diagnosis is 5–30 years; positive family history; male-to-female ratio of 2:1.

Ocular

Dysgenesis of the iris and iridocorneal angle; glaucoma; hypoplasia of iris; dark-colored irides; myopia; smooth iris; prominent iris processes; grayish-pale color of trabecular meshwork.

Clinical

None

Laboratory

Tonometry, corneal measurements, gonioscopy and ophthalmoscopy should be performed in the operating room and carefully documented. Intraocular pressures recorded under general anesthesia are usually lower than those obtained in the office because of the effects of the anesthetic agents.

Treatment

Congenital glaucoma: Primary congenital glaucoma almost always is managed surgically, both goniotomy and trabeculectomy may be useful. When multiple goniotomies and/or trabeculectomies fail, the surgeon usually resorts to a filtering procedure.

Additional Resource

1. Walton DS (2011). Juvenile Glaucoma. [online] Available from http://www.emedicine.com/oph/TOPIC333.HTM [Accessed April, 2012].

622. GLAUCOMA WITH ELEVATED EPISCLERAL VENOUS PRESSURES

General

Autosomal dominant. Systemic disorders that raise the venous pressure to the eye and may cause glaucoma.

Clinical

Elevated episcleral venous pressure as venous obstruction, carotid cavernous fistula and Sturge Weber Syndrome.

Ocular

Open-angle glaucoma; elevated episcleral venous pressure; dilated episcleral veins.

Treatment

Topical medications are the first therapy. Oral medication such as carbonic anhydrase inhibitors can be used if topical medications fail. Surgical options include laser-trabeculoplasty or incisional-filtering or shunt procedures.

Bibliography

1. Minas TF, Podos SM. Familial glaucoma associated with elevated episcleral venous pressure. Arch Ophthalmol. 1968;80:202-8.

623. CHRONIC ANGLE-CLOSURE GLAUCOMA

General

Portion of the anterior chamber angle closed with peripheral anterior synechiae; five types: (1) CACG, (2) combined mechanism, (3) mixed mechanism, (4) plateau iris and (5) miotic therapy induced.

Clinical

Asymptomatic due to the slow onset of the disease.

Ocular

Elevated intraocular pressure; peripheral anterior synechiae; deposits of pigment in the angle; plateau iris.

Laboratory

Measurement of intraocular pressure; gonioscopy; optic nerve head and retinal nerve fiber layer assessments; visual field testing and slit lamp examination.

Treatment

Iridotomy is the treatment of choice. Argon laser peripheral iridoplasty and goniosynechialysis may be necessary.

Additional Resource

1. Tham CC (2010). Glaucoma, Angle Closure, Chronic. [online] Available from http://www.emedicine.medscape.com/article/1205154-overview [Accessed April, 2012].

624. GLAUCOMA, HYPHEMA

General

Collection of red blood cells in the anteior chamber.

Clinical

Most common following trauma; bleeding disorders; sickle cell disease.

Ocular

Blood in the anterior chamber, corneal blood-staining; pupillary block; rubeosis iridis; intraocular tumors, older style intraocular lens (2L and 4L Binkhorst styles).

Laboratory

Slit lamp examination; measurement of intraocular pressure; history of trauma, CT scan and ultrasonography to exclude orbital fracture and other associated eye injuries.

Treatment

Limiting activities that cause rapid movement of the globe; sleeping with head elevated; topical and oral ocular hypotensive medications; cycloplegia and topical steroids; avoiding medications such as aspirin that thin the blood.

Additional Resource

1. Irak-Dersu I (2010). Glaucoma, Hyphema. [online] Available from http://www.emedicine. medscape.com/article/1206635-overview [Accessed April, 2012].

---

625. GLOBE RETRACTION

General

Displacement of the globe deeper into the globe than normal position. The etiology may be from a variety of causes which include Duane retraction syndrome, blowout fractures and metastatc orbital tumors.

Clinical

Facial trauma, breast, prostate and lung carcinoma.

Ocular

Duane retraction syndrome, lack of full range of eye movements, diplopia, globe displacement, narrowing of palpebral fissure, ptosis, decreased visual acuity, optic nerve compression, traumatic optic neuropathy, abnormal head position.

Laboratory

Diagnosis is made by clinical findings, CT scan and B-scan of orbit.

Treatment

Treatment depends on the etiology.

Additional Resource

1. Yen MT (2011). Globe Retraction. [online] Available from http://www.emedicine.medscape.com/article/1200002-overview [Accessed April, 2012].

---

626. GLUCAGONOMA SYNDROME

General

Alpha-cell islet tumor of pancreas with retrobulbar neuritis first sign and necrolytic migratory erythema early signs.

Ocular

Central scotoma; retrobulbar neuritis.

Clinical

Necrolytic migratory erythema; diabetes; hypoaminoacidemia and hyperglucagonemia secondary to alpha-cell islet tumor of pancreas; anemia; glossitis; weight loss; angular stomatitis; onycholysis; diarrhea; monochromic monocytic anemia; recurrent venous thrombosis (associated with alpha-cell tumor).

Laboratory

Determining the level of glucagonemia by means of radioimmunoassay (RIA) test is mandatory. A positive test result for glucagonoma exceeds 1,000 pg/mL (reference range is 50–200 pg/mL).

Treatment

Surgical resection, which is the only curative therapy.

Additional Resource

1. Santacroce L (2011). Glucagonoma. [online] Available from http://www.emedicine.com/med/TOPIC896.HTM [Accessed April, 2012].

627. GLUTATHIONE SYNTHETASE DEFICIENCY

General

Rare, autosomal-recessive inborn error of glutathione metabolism.

Clinical

Metabolic acidosis, hemolytic anemia, progressive neurologic symptoms, seizures, spasticity, cerebellar symptoms.

Ocular

Retinitis pigmentosa, rod-cone dystrophy, decreased visual acuity, crytalline opacities in the lens, visual field defects.

Laboratory

Diagnosis of glutathione synthetase (GS) deficiency is confirmed by the presence of a large peak of 5-oxoproline in the urine. Diagnosis can be confirmed through enzyme analysis of GS (which is found to be deficient) in cultured skin fibroblasts. Blood gases may be needed to diagnose acidiosis and CBC may help to diagnose anemia.

Treatment

Supplements of vitamin A, C and E may be useful to correct acidosis. Sodium citrate and citric acid may also be useful.

Additional Resource

1. Adams DJ (2012). Glutathione Synthetase Deficiency. [online] Available from http://www.emedicine.medscape.com/article/944368-diagnosis [Accessed April, 2012].

628. GOLDBERG DISEASE

General

Unclassified syndrome with features of mucopolysaccharidoses, sphingolipidoses and mucolipidoses; deficiency of neuraminidase; located in chromosome 20q 13.1.

Ocular

Macular cherry-red spot; corneal clouding; cerebromacular degeneration.

Clinical

Dwarfism; gargoyle facies; mental retardation; seizures; hearing disorder.

Laboratory

Diagnosis is made by clinical findings.

Treatment

For patients with bilateral and visually disabling corneal opacity, penetrating keratoplasty (PK) is recommended.

Additional Resources

1. Scheinfeld NS (2011). Congenital Clouding of the Cornea. [online] Available from http://www.emedicine.com/oph/TOPIC771.HTM [Accessed April, 2012].

2. Banikazemi M (2012). Genetics of Mucopolysaccharidosis Type I. [online] Available from http://www.emedicine.com/ped/TOPIC2052.HTM [Accessed April, 2012].

629. GOLDENHAR SYNDROME (GOLDENHAR-GORLIN SYNDROME; OCULOAURICULOVERTEBRAL DYSPLASIA)

General

Most cases have been sporadic, but cases of autosomal dominant and recessive inheritance have been reported; male preponderance (60%); present at birth.

Ocular

Anophthalmia; colobomata of choroid, iris and eyelid; antimongolian slant of lid fissure; epibulbar dermoid or lipodermoids of conjunctiva, cornea and orbit; tilted optic disk; nerve hypoplasia; microphthalmia; macular heterotopia; tortuous retinal vessels.

Clinical

Frontal bulging of the skull; receding chin; malar hypoplasia; micrognathia and macrostomia; auricular appendices (single or multiple); multiple vertebral anomalies; preauricular fistulas; mental retardation.

Laboratory

Diagnosis is made by clinical findings.

Treatment

Dermoid: Surgery for function or cosmesis.

Additional Resource

1. Tewfik TL (2011). Manifestations of Craniofacial Syndromes. [online] Available from http://www.emedicine.com/ent/TOPIC319.HTM [Accessed April, 2012].

630. GOLDSCHEIDER SYNDROME (DOMINANT EPIDERMOLYSIS BULLOSA DYSTROPHICA ALBOPAPULOIDEA; EPIDERMOLYSIS BULLOSA; WEBER-COCKAYNE SYNDROME)

General

Rare; Weber-Cockayne syndrome, inherited as an autosomal dominant trait, is actually a milder form without scar formation, whereas Goldscheider syndrome, inherited either autosomal dominant or recessive, shows dystrophic changes with scarring; consanguinity frequent.

Ocular

Blepharitis; shrinkage of conjunctiva; pseudomembrane formation with symblepharon; conjunctivitis; bullous keratitis and subepithelial blisters lead to erosions with subsequent ulcerations and corneal opacities or even perforation; sclera may be similarly involved; lagophthalmos, cicatricial lacrimal stenosis; retinal detachment; cataract; pannus.

Clinical

Vesicular and bullous skin lesions and similar lesions of mucous membranes occur spontaneously or after mild trauma; keloid scars and contraction after healing are common in the dystrophic forms, whereas in the mild form the lesions heal without scarring but may leave some skin pigmentation; growth and mental retardation may be present in the group with recessive inheritance; stenosis of the larynx due to scarring may occur.

Laboratory

Obtain a skin biopsy following a thorough history and physical examination.

Treatment

Wound healing and prevention of infection is the preferred strategy. Esophageal lesions can be managed with phenytoin and oral steroid elixirs to reduce the symptoms of dysphagia. In addition, if oral candidiasis is present, an anticandidal medication is helpful. Patients can experience recurrent blepharitis in one or both eyes along with bullous lesions of the conjunctiva, corneal ulcerations, corneal scarring, obliteration of tear ducts, eyelid lesions and cicatricial conjunctivitis. Corneal erosions are treated with antibiotic ointment and use of cycloplegic agents to reduce ciliary spasm and provide comfort. Avoid using tape to patch the eye because of frequent blistering of the skin under the adhesive. Chronic blepharitis can result in cicatricial ectropion and exposure keratitis. Moisture chambers and ocular lubricants are used commonly for management. This disorder also has been treated with full-thickness skin grafting to the upper eyelid.

Additional Resource

1. Marinkovich MP (2010). Epidermolysis Bullosa. [online] Available from http://www.emedicine.com/derm/TOPIC124.HTM [Accessed April, 2012].

631. GOLTZ SYNDROME (FOCAL DERMAL HYPOPLASIA SYNDROME)

General

X-linked dominant inheritance; lethal in males; skin manifestations present at birth.

Ocular

Microphthalmia; strabismus; coloboma of iris and/or choroid; epiphora; blue sclera; nystagmus; anophthalmos; keratoconus.

Clinical

Skin atrophy and linear pigmentation; telangiectasias of trunk and extremities; superficial, localized fatty skin deposits; multiple papillomas of mucous membranes and periorificial skin (oral, genital, anal); anomalies of extremities with syndactyly, oligodactyly, adactyly; hypohidrosis; paper-thin nails may be present; spina bifida; hypoplasia of right clavicle; umbilical or inguinal hernia.

Laboratory

Radiography may reveal osteopathia striata.

Treatment

Flashlamp-pumped pulsed dye laser may ameliorate the pruritic symptoms that sometimes are noted in affected skin and improve the clinical appearance of the telangiectatic and erythematous skin lesions. Papillomas frequently require repeated surgical intervention.

Additional Resource

1. Goltz RW (2010). Focal Dermal Hypoplasia Syndrome. [online] Available from http://www.emedicine.com/derm/TOPIC155.HTM [Accessed April, 2012].

632. GONORRHEA

General

Caused by *Neisseria gonorrhoeae*, which is transmitted sexually.

Ocular

Conjunctivitis; eyelid edema; keratitis; uveitis.

Clinical

Pelvic inflammatory disease; arthritis; dermatitis; carditis; meningitis.

Laboratory

Gram stain smear demonstrates Gram-negative diplococci with polymorphonuclear leukocytes in conjunctival exudates.

Treatment

Therapy consists of systemic antibiotics; topical antibiotics are relatively ineffective in the treatment of eye disease. It is important to treat all sexual partners simultaneously to prevent reinfection.

Additional Resource

1. Bashour M (2010). Gonococcus. [online] Available from http://www.emedicine.com/oph/TOPIC497.HTM [Accessed April, 2012].

633. GOOD ACUITY PLUS PHOTOSENSITIVITY (GAPP), TRACK RELATED IRIDIOCYCLITIS AND SCLERITIS (TRISC), TRANSIENT LIGHT SENSITIVITY (TLS)

General

Use of intralase to perform LASIK.

Ocular

Photophobia; glare; uveitis; iridocyclitis; scleritis.

Clinical

Associated with refractive surgery and the use of Intralase technology; starts 6–8 weeks postoperatively and resolves by 4–5 months.

Laboratory

Diagnosis is made by clinical findings.

Treatment

Medical management generally consists of topical or systemic corticosteroids and often cycloplegics.

Additional Resource

1. Janigian RH (2011). Uveitis Evaluation and Treatment. [online] Available from http://www.emedicine.medscape.com/article/1209123-overview [Accessed April, 2012].

634. GOODPASTURE SYNDROME

General

Chronic, relapsing pulmonary hemosiderosis, often in association with fatal glomerulonephritis; rare; occurs in young males.

Ocular

Episcleritis; juxtapapillary subretinal neovascular membranes; superficial retinal hemorrhages; bilateral peripheral retinoschisis; hemorrhagic and/or exudative retinopathy; nonrhegmatogenous retinal detachment (rare).

Clinical

Cough with recurrent hemoptysis; dyspnea; pulmonary infiltrates; hypochromic iron deficiency anemia; glomerulonephritis; progressive renal failure; diffuse hemorrhagic inflammation of lung.

Laboratory

Assessments of antinuclear antibody (ANA), C3, and C4 levels and of the Westergren sedimentation rate are recommended. Chest radiography is the most useful imaging test available to document the presence of pulmonary hemorrhage.

Treatment

Plasma exchange for antibody removal, corticosteroids therapy, sodium restriction and fluid restriction.

Additional Resource

1. Valentini RP (2012). Pediatric Anti-GBM Disease (Goodpasture Syndrome). [online] Available from http://www.emedicine.com/ped/TOPIC888.HTM [Accessed April, 2012].

635. GOPALAN SYNDROME (BURNING FEET SYNDROME; NUTRITIONAL MELALGIA SYNDROME)

General

Female preponderance; onset between the ages of 20 and 40 years; pantothenic acid deficiency; lack of nicotinic acid and low-protein diet are contributory factors; found in malnourished populations, detainees in prison camps and chronic alcoholics.

Ocular

Decreased vision; central or paracentral scotomata.

Clinical

Hyperalgesia; hyperesthesia; severe burning of palms and soles (more pronounced at night); excessive sweating; circulatory insufficiency; tachycardia; muscle atrophy.

Laboratory

History is the key to diagnosing a nutritional deficiency.

Treatment

Nutritional supplements, discontinue alcohol.

Additional Resource

1. Sewell RA (2010). Nutritional Neuropathy. [online] Available from http://www.emedicine.com/neuro/TOPIC278.HTM [Accessed April, 2012].

636. GORLIN-CHAUDHRY-MOSS SYNDROME

General

Etiology unknown.

Ocular

Microphthalmia; hypertelorism; depressed supraorbital ridges; inability to open or close lids fully because of incomplete lid development; antimongoloid, oblique palpebral fissures; sparse eyelash development; lid defect (notching); horizontal nystagmus at extreme lateral gaze; limited upper gaze; astigmatism; marked hyperopia; corneal scars (possibly due to exposure keratitis); keratoconus.

Clinical

Craniofacial dysostosis; saddled appearance of upper face; high-arched, narrow palate; dental anomalies (size, number, position); hypertrichosis; hypoplasia of labia majora; patent ductus arteriosus; normal mental development; fatigue; frontal headache.

Laboratory

Diagnosis is made by clinical findings.

Treatment

Patients with bilateral and visually disabling corneal opacity, penetrating keratoplasty (PK) is recommended.

Additional Resource

1. Scheinfeld NS (2011). Congenital Clouding of the Cornea. [online] Available from http://www.emedicine.com/oph/TOPIC771.HTM [Accessed April, 2012].

637. GOUT (HYPERURICEMIA)

General

Genetic disease of purine metabolism and renal excretion of uric acid.

Ocular

Conjunctivitis; episcleritis; posterior scleritis; ocular motor disturbances; iritis; band keratopathy; interpalpebral paralimbal nodules.

Clinical

Acute inflammatory arthritis; accumulation of sodium urate deposits; uric acid nephrolithiasis; renal failure; tophi in any body tissue; marked swelling of feet and ankles.

Laboratory

Serum uric acid is used in diagnosing this condition and in monitoring the treatment process.

Treatment

Treatment is directed at reducing both hyperuricemia and ocular inflammation. Treatment involves hydration, colchicine for prevention and acute treatment, nonsteroidal and steroidal anti-inflammatory drugs, uricosuric agents (e.g. probenecid) and antihyperuricemic drugs.

Additional Resource

1. Rothschild BM (2012). Gout and Pseudogout. [online] Available from http://www.emedicine.com/oph/TOPIC506.HTM [Accessed April, 2012].

638. GRADENIGO SYNDROME (LANNOIS-GRADENIGO SYNDROME; TEMPORAL SYNDROME)

General

Caused by extradural abscess of the petrous portion of the temporal bone; good prognosis.

Ocular

Ipsilateral paralysis (cranial nerve VI); transient involvement of cranial nerves III and IV occasionally present; severe pain in area of ophthalmic branch (cranial nerve V); photophobia; lacrimation; reduced corneal sensitivity; optic nerve involvement occasionally present.

Clinical

Inner ear infection with deafness; mastoiditis; facial paresis possible; temperature may be elevated; meningeal signs possible; can occur rarely as a complication of otitis media.

Laboratory

Computed tomography (CT) and MRI.

Treatment

Consult otolaryngologist.

Bibliography

1. de Graaf J, Cats H, de Jager AE. Gradenigo's syndrome: a rare complication of otitis media. Clin Neurol Neurosurg. 1988;90:237-9.
2. Gradenigro G. A special syndrome of endocranial otitic complications. Ann Otol Rhinol Laryngol. 1904;13:637.
3. Joffe WS. Clinical nerve disease. Int Ophthalmol Clin. 1967;7:823-38.

639. GRAFT VERSUS HOST DISEASE

General

Major complication of bone marrow transplantation; donor T lymphocytes attack recipient's cells; targets are skin, liver, intestine, oral mucosa, conjunctiva, lacrimal gland, vaginal mucosa and esophageal mucosa.

Ocular

Keratoconjunctivitis; photophobia; hemorrhagic conjunctivitis; proptosis; intraretinal hemorrhages; nerve palsy; herpes simplex/herpes zoster manifestations; uveitis; corneal epithelial denudement; conjunctival scarring; dry eye syndrome; corneal melt; dacryoadenitis; keratoconjunctivitis sicca; cataract; retinitis.

Clinical

Leukemia; aplastic anemia; exanthematous dermatitis; hepatitis; enteritis; scleroderma-like involvement of skin; chronic liver dysfunction; recurrent bacterial infections.

Laboratory

Diagnosis is made by clinical findings.

Treatment

Keratoconjunctivitis: Ocular lubricants, nonsteroidal anti-inflammatory and steroid drops, oral nonsteroidal anti-inflammatory or steroids. Supratarsal steroids. Surgical excision, cryotherapy and beta-irradiation of papillae.

Proptosis: Reversing the problem, which is causing the exophthalmos, is the treatment of choice and will minimize the ocular complications. Ocular lubricants are beneficial for control of the corneal exposure.

Additional Resource

1. Chang-Godinich A (2011). Atopic Keratoconjunctivitis. [online] Available from http://www.emedicine.com/oph/TOPIC102.HTM [Accessed April, 2012].

640. GRANULAR CORNEAL DYSTROPHY

General

Autosomal dominant inheritance affecting the corneal stroma.

Clinical

None

Ocular

Corneal dystrophy has four types: (1) granular corneal dystrophy (GCD) I—classic, Groenouw; (2) GCD II—Avellino dystrophy, combined lattice/granular; (3) GCD III—superficial, Reis-Bücklers corneal dystrophy, affecting the Bowman's layer and (4) GCD IV—French variant similar to GCD III.

Laboratory

Diagnosis is made by clinical findings.

Treatment

Mild cases—observation and recurrent erosion therapy, soft contact lenses are helpful, penetrating keratoplasty may be necessary, graft recurrences treated by superficial keratectomy, phototherapeutic keratectomy or repeat penetrating keratoplasty.

Additional Resource

1. Afshari N (2010). Granular Dystrophy. [online] Available from http://www.emedicine.com/oph/TOPIC92.HTM [Accessed April, 2012].

641. GRANULOMA ANNULARE

General

Benign; self-limited dermatosis; etiology unknown but reported to follow insect bites, sun exposure, trauma, viral infection and psoralen ultraviolet radiation therapy; hereditary predisposition; seen in children and young adults.

Ocular

Granuloma of lid; predilection for lateral upper lid and outer canthus; lesions are clinically similar to the subcutaneous nodules of rheumatoid arthritis.

Clinical

Skin lesions localized, generalized, subcutaneous, perforating or arcuate dermal erythema; papules often arranged in a complete or half circle.

Laboratory

Diagnosis is made by clinical findings. Biopsy is recommended for a subcutaneous lesion and for an atypical presentation with respect to history or location of lesion.

Treatment

Localized lesions have been treated with potent topical corticosteroids. Cryotherapy using liquid nitrogen or nitrous oxide may be useful. Isotretinoin or phototherapy with oral psoralen and UV-A (PUVA) as first-line options for generalized granuloma annulare (GA).

Additional Resource

1. Ghadially R (2012). Granuloma Annulare. [online] Available from http://www.emedicine.com/derm/TOPIC169.HTM [Accessed April, 2012].

642. GRANULOMA FACIALE

General

Uncommon disease; etiology unknown; characterized by single or multiple cutaneous nodules usually occurring on the face; asymptomatic; most common in males; seen in whites, rarely in blacks and Japanese.

Ocular

Unusual eyelid nodules.

Clinical

Cutaneous nodules most often on face but may appear anywhere; lesions are soft, elevated, well-circumscribed nodules, from a few millimeters to several centimeters in size; extrafacial lesions are extremely rare but have been reported.

Laboratory

Skin biopsy of a representative lesion.

Treatment

A variety of surgical procedures may be used in the management of granuloma faciale (GF). Scarring may occur with many of these, so the pulsed dye laser is preferred.

Additional Resource

1. Wiederkehr M (2011). Granuloma Faciale. [online] Available from http://www.emedicine.com/derm/TOPIC170.HTM [Accessed April, 2012].

643. GRANULOMA VENEREUM

General

Donovania granulomatis; infective venereal disease; prevalent in black women; *Chlamydia trachomatis* is an intracellular bacterium lacking respiratory enzymes that has an affinity for mucosal epithelium; serotypes A through C have been epidemiologically associated with trachoma; serotypes E through K have been associated with genital infection and keratoconjunctivitis in sexually active adults and neonates; other serotypes have been associated with lymphogranuloma venereum and Reiter syndrome.

Ocular

Lid and orbit granulomas.

Clinical

Painless primary lesions; painful secondarily infected ulcers.

Laboratory

Culturing the organism with best results obtained using aspirates from an involved inguinal lymph node and from bacterial typing of the culture after growth.

Treatment

Recommended treatment is with doxycycline (100 mg PO bid) or erythromycin (500 mg qid). Continue treatment for 3 weeks, combined with aspiration of the lymph nodes if needed.

Additional Resource

1. Plaza JA (2012). Dermatologic Manifestations of Lymphogranuloma Venereum. [online] Available from http://www.emedicine.com/derm/TOPIC617.HTM [Accessed April, 2012].

644. GRAY IRIS SYNDROME

General

Excessive trauma of iris at time of lens implantation with loss of posterior iris pigment; originally had blue irides.

Ocular

Pigmentary glaucoma; gray iris; massive pigment deposits in chamber angle; nonfixated intraocular lens.

Clinical

None

Laboratory

Diagnosis is made by clinical findings.

Treatment

If glaucoma occurs topical glaucoma drops can be used, laser trabeculoplasty, laser iridectomy, filtering surgery may be necessary.

Additional Resource

1. Ritch R (2010). Glaucoma, Pigmentary. [online] Available from http://www.emedicine.com/oph/TOPIC136.HTM [Accessed April, 2012].

645. GRAYSON-WILBRANDT SYNDROME (CORNEAL DYSTROPHY OF REIS-BUECKLERS; REIS-BUECKLERS SYNDROME)

General

Onset at the end of the first decade; infrequent episodes of eye redness and pain; autosomal dominant trait; electron microscopy reveals peculiar curly material in the subepithelial fibrous tissue that parallels the distribution of attachment proteins.

Ocular

Corneal changes variable from a mottled scarring to gray macular opacities of the anterior limiting membrane of the cornea; strabismus.

Clinical

None

Laboratory

Diagnosis is made by clinical findings.

Treatment

Penetrating keratoplasty (PK) is recommended if decrease in acuity occurs.

Additional Resource

1. Scheinfeld NS (2011). Congenital Clouding of the Cornea. [online] Available from http://www.emedicine.com/oph/TOPIC771.HTM [Accessed April, 2012].

646. GREIG SYNDROME (HYPERTELORISM; HYPERTELORISM OCULARIS; OCULAR HYPERTELORISM SYNDROME; PRIMARY EMBRYONIC HYPERTELORISM)

General

Condition is rare; sporadic or hereditary; autosomal dominant or sex linked; if not associated with mental deficiency, then adequate mental and physical development is found.

Ocular

Hypertelorism (wide spacing of orbits); enophthalmos; epicanthus; deformities of eyelids and brows; defects of the palpebral fissure; bilateral sixth nerve paralysis; esotropia; astigmatism;

optic atrophy by tension on the optic nerve; strabismus.

Clinical

Skull may show mild malformations, including bitemporal eminences and decreased antero-posterior diameter; harelip; high-arched palate; cleft palate; broad and flat nasal root; mental impairment.

Laboratory

Diagnosis is made by clinical findings.

Treatment

Minor degrees of deformity (referred to as telecanthus) can be corrected by removing a small amount of bone in the midline. A limited frontal craniotomy is performed in the midline osteotomy.

Additional Resource

1. Jackson IT (2012). Congenital Syndromes. [online] Available from http://www.emedicine.com/plastic/TOPIC183.HTM [Accessed April, 2012].

647. GRÖNBLAD-STRANDBERG SYNDROME (DARIER-GRÖNBLAD-STRANDBERG SYNDROME; ELASTORRHEXIS; PSEUDOXANTHOMA ELASTICUM; SYSTEMIC ELASTODYSTROPHY)

General

Autosomal recessive; female-to-male ratio of 2:1; inheritance is usually autosomal recessive, but it also has reported as autosomal dominant.

Ocular

"Angioid streaks" of the retina; macular hemorrhages and transudates not infrequent; choroidal sclerosis; retinal detachment; keratoconus; cataract; paralysis of extraocular muscles (secondary to vascular lesions of central nervous system); subluxation of lens; exophthalmos; optic atrophy; vitreous hemorrhages; Salmon spot multiple atrophic peripheral retinal pigment epithelium (RPE) lesions; reticular pigment dystrophy of the macula; optic disk drusen; multiple small crystalline bodies associated with atrophic RPE changes.

Clinical

Pseudoxanthoma elasticum with thickening, softening and relaxation of the skin; skin changes are symmetrical in skin folds near large joints (axilla, elbow, inguinal region, lower abdomen, neck); flattening of the pulse curve and peripheral vascular disturbances; gastrointestinal hemorrhages.

Laboratory

Characteristic skin and retinal findings. Fluorescein angiography to detect angioid streaks and choroidal neovascular membranes.

Treatment

Dietary calcium and phosphorus restriction to minimum daily requirement levels has shown arrest in progression of the disease.

Additional Resource

1. Dahl AA (2010). Ophthalmologic Manifestations of Pseudoxanthoma Elasticum. [online] Available from http://www.emedicine.com/oph/TOPIC475.HTM [Accessed April, 2012].

648. GROUPED PIGMENTATION OF THE MACULA

General

Autosomal recessive.

Ocular

Grouped pigmentation limited to foveal area; metamorphopsia; pigmented spots around a clear hole in the foveal area.

Clinical

None

Laboratory

Diagnosis is made by clinical findings.

Treatment

None/Ocular.

Bibliography

1. Forsius H, Eriksson A, Nuutila A, et al. A genetic study of three retinal disorders: dystrophia retinae dysacusis syndrome, X-chromosomal retinoschisis and grouped pigments of the retina. Birth Defects Orig Artic Ser. 1971;7:83-98.
2. McKusick VA. Mendelian Inheritance in Man: A Catalog of Human Genes and Genetic Disorders, 12th edition. Baltimore: The Johns Hopkins University press; 1998.

649. GRUNER-BERTOLOTTI SYNDROME

General

Various causes, including pineal tumor, supranuclear lesions, thrombosis of anterior choroidal artery, aneurysm or tumor; combination of Parinaud and von Monakow syndromes (see Parinaud Syndrome; von Monakow Syndrome).

Ocular

Hemianopia; lid retraction; ptosis; extraocular muscle paralysis; papilledema.

Clinical

Vertigo; hemiplegia; sensory disturbances; brain tumors.

Laboratory

Diagnosis is made by clinical findings.

Treatment

Ptosis: If visual acuity is affected most cases require surgical correction, and there are several procedures that may be used including levator resection, repair or advancement and Fasanella-Servat.

Lid retraction: Identify systemic abnormalities such as thyroid. Treatment must be given for 6 months for stabilizing before performing eyelid surgery. Local-ocular lubrication (drops or ointment). Botulism type A may also be useful.

Papilledema: Underlying cause should be determined and treated. Systemic acetazolamide is the medical therapy of choice.

Bibliography

1. Magalini SI, Scrascia E. Dictionary of Medical Syndromes, 2nd edition. Philadelphia: JB Lippincott; 1981.
2. Parinaud H. Paralysie des mouvements associés des yeux. Arch Neurol. 1883;5:145-72.

650. GUILLAIN-BARRÉ SYNDROME (ACUTE FEBRILE POLYNEURITIS; ACUTE IDIOPATHIC POLYNEURITIS; ACUTE INFECTIOUS NEURITIS; ACUTE POLYRADICULITIS; INFLAMMATORY POLYRADICULONEUROPATHY; LANDRY-GUILLAIN-BARRÉ-STROHL SYNDROME; LANDRY PARALYSIS; POSTINFECTIOUS POLYNEURITIS)

General

Etiology unknown; occurs from age 16 to 50 years; Fisher syndrome is a variant (see Fisher Syndrome).

Ocular

Facial nerve paralysis with paralytic ectropion of the lower eyelid; mild-to-complete external ophthalmoplegia; optic neuritis; papilledema; ptosis; anisocoria; nystagmus; dyschromatopsia; scotoma; bilateral tonic pupils.

Clinical

Polyneuritis involving facial peripheral motor nerves and spinal cord; facial diplegia; bladder incontinence; variable degrees of paralysis, usually beginning in lower extremities; tendon reflexes absent; involvement of respiratory muscles possible; paresthesia (symmetrical).

Laboratory

Cytomegalovirus, Epstein-Barr virus and human immunodeficiency virus (HIV) have been most closely associated with this condition.

Treatment

Plasma exchange has shown to be beneficial. Corneal exposure is treated with topical therapy or lateral tarsorrhaphies if warranted.

Additional Resource

1. Andary MT (2011). Guillain-Barre Syndrome. [online] Available from http://www.emedicine.com/pmr/TOPIC48.HTM [Accessed April, 2012].

651. GYRATE ATROPHY (ORNITHINE KETOACID AMINOTRANSFERASE DEFICIENCY)

General

Deficiency of the enzyme ornithine aminotransferase; autosomal recessive; chronic, progressive dystrophy; responsible human gene has been localized to chromosome 10.

Ocular

Chorioretinal atrophy; crystalline deposits associated with brown pigment in fundus; myopia; cataract; keratoconus; night blindness; constricted visual fields; axial hypermetropia; cobblestone-like peripheral lesions; blunting of ciliary processes; iris atrophy.

Clinical

Absence of enzyme ornithine ketoacid transaminase; elevated levels of amino acid ornithine in body fluids; seizures; abnormal electroencephalography; eosinophilic subsarcolemmal deposits are seen on muscle biopsy; massive cystinuria and lysinuria; diabetes.

Laboratory

Visual field test, electroretinography (ERG) and electro-oculography (EOG).

Treatment

Cataract: Change in glasses can sometimes improve a patient's visual function temporarily; however, the most common treatment is cataract surgery.

Keratoconus: Spectacle correction, hard contacts and avoid eye rubbing may be useful. If hydrops occurs discontinue contact lens, use NaCl drops and ointment, patching and short course of steroids. As the disease advances penetrating keratoplasty, deep anterior lamellar keratoplasty, intacs with laser grooves or collagen stabilization of cornea.

Additional Resource

1. Weissman BA (2011). Keratoconus. [online] Available from http://www.emedicine.com/oph/TOPIC104.HTM [Accessed April, 2012].

---

652. HAEMOPHILUS AEGYPTIUS (KOCH-WEEKS BACILLUS)

General

Caused by Gram-negative Koch-Weeks bacillus in warm-climate regions; characterized by a 24–48 hour incubation period; now classified as *Haemophilus influenzae* biotype III; *H. influenzae* is divided into biotypes based on biochemical reactions (indole production, urease activity, ornithine decarboxylase activity) and into serotypes based on their capsular polysaccharides; common cause of purulent conjunctivitis and preseptal cellulitis in children.

Ocular

Conjunctivitis; corneal opacity; corneal ulcer; phlyctenular keratoconjunctivitis; keratitis; cellulitis of lid; pseudoptosis; uveitis; petechial subconjunctival hemorrhages.

Clinical

Coryza; systemic symptoms are rare.

Laboratory

Poorly staining Gram-negative bacilli or coccobacilli. Culture on chocolate agar.

Treatment

Antibiotics are the mainstay of treatment. Invasive and serious infections are best treated with an intravenous third-generation cephalosporin until antibiotic sensitivities are available.

Additional Resource

1. Devarajan VR (2012). Haemophilus Influenzae Infections. [online] Available from http://www.emedicine.com/med/TOPIC936.HTM [Accessed April, 2012].

---

653. HAEMOPHILUS INFLUENZAE

General

Gram-negative rod.

Ocular

Conjunctivitis; cellulitis; tenonitis; uveitis; vitreous opacity; pannus; corneal opacity.

Clinical

Pharyngitis; epiglottitis; laryngotracheitis; pneumonia; bronchitis; otitis media; meningitis; cellulitis; septic arthritis; sinusitis.

Laboratory

Gram-negative coccobacillus with 8 biotypes and 6 serotypes. Gram stain and culture.

Treatment

Antibiotics are the mainstay of treatment. Invasive and serious infections are best treated with an intravenous third-generation cephalosporin until antibiotic sensitivities are available.

Additional Resource

1. Devarajan VR (2012). Haemophilus Influenzae Infections. [online] Available from http://www.emedicine.com/med/TOPIC936.HTM [Accessed April, 2012].

---

654. HAJDU-CHENEY SYNDROME

General

Rare; autosomal dominant; disorder of bone metabolism.

Ocular

Bilateral visual loss; choroidal folds; optic nerve head swelling; optic neuropathy; optic nerve meningocele.

Clinical

Facial dysmorphism; progressive platybasia; syringomyelia; curvature of the spine; aplasis of facial sinuses.

Laboratory

Diagnosis is made by clinical findings.

Treatment

The initial dose is 40–60 mg/d of prednisone, depending on the size of the patient and the severity of the disease followed by tapering off the medication can be useful for the treatment of optic neuropathy.

Bibliography

1. Di Rocco F, Oi S. Spontaneous regression of syringomyelia in Hajdu-Cheney syndrome with severe platybasia. Case report. J Neurosurg. 2005;103:194-7.
2. Golnik KC, Kersten RC. Optic nerve head swelling in the Hadju-Cheney syndrome. J Neuroophthalmol. 1998;18:60-5.

---

655. HALLERMANN-STREIFF SYNDROME [AUDRY I SYNDROME; DOHNA SYNDROME; DYSCEPHALIC-MANDIBULO-OCULO-FACIAL SYNDROME; DYSCEPHALY-TEETH ABNORMALITY-DWARFISM; DYSCEPHALIA OCULOMANDIBULARIS-HYPOTRICHOSIS; FRANCOIS SYNDROME (1); FRANCOIS DYSCEPHALIC SYNDROME; FRANCOIS-HALLERMANN-STREIFF SYNDROME; FREMERY-DOHNA SYNDROME; HALLERMANN-STREIFF-FRANCOIS SYNDROME; MANDIBULO-OCULAR DYSCEPHALIA HYPOTRICHOSIS; MANDIBULO-OCULO-FACIAL DYSCEPHALY SYNDROME; OCULO-MANDIBULO-FACIAL DYSCEPHALY; OCULO-MANDIBULO-DYSCEPHALY; ULLRICH-FREMERY-DOHNA SYNDROME]

General

Rare; familial occurrence and consanguinity; males and females equally affected.

Ocular

Microphthalmos (bilateral); proptosis; nystagmus; strabismus; cataracts; bilateral optic atrophy; coloboma of optic disk, choroid and iris; keratoglobus; microcornea; antimongoloid slant; iris atrophy; uveitis; blue sclera; persistent pupillary membrane; secondary glaucoma.

Clinical

Malformations of skull (brachycephaly), facial skeleton and jaws; erupted teeth at birth; diminished hair growth; hyperextensibility of joints; short stature; skin atrophy; mental deficiency; predisposition to upper airway compromise; obstructive sleep apnea.

Laboratory

Diagnosis is made by clinical findings.

Treatment

Cataract: Change in glasses can sometimes improve a patient's visual function temporarily; however, the most common treatment is cataract surgery.

Strabismus: Equalized vision with correct refractive error; surgery may be helpful in patient with diplopia.

Uveitis: Topical steroids and cycloplegic medication should be the initial treatment of choice. Oral steroids if not responsive to topical steroids, immunosuppressants if bilateral disease that does not respond to oral steroids, periocular steroids for unilateral or posterior uveitis. Vitrectomy can be used for severe vitreous opacification. Cryotherapy and laser photocoagulation may be used for localized pars plana exudates.

Glaucoma: Its medication should be the first plan of action. If medication is unsuccessful, a filtering surgical procedure with or without antimetabolites may be beneficial.

Bibliography

1. Francois J, Victoria-Troncoso V. Francois' dyscephalic syndrome and skin manifestations. Ophthalmologica. 1981;183:63-7.
2. Roy FH, Fraunfelder FW, Fraunfelder FT. Roy and Fraunfelder's Current Ocular Therapy, 6th edition. Philadelphia: WB Saunders; 2008.
3. Hallermann W. Vogelgesicht und Cataracta Congenita. Klin Monatsbl Augenheilkd. 1948;113:315.
4. Ronen S, Rozenmann Y, Isaacson M, et al. The early management of baby with Hallermann-Streiff-Francois syndrome. J Pediatr Ophthalmol Strabismus. 1979;16:119-21.
5. Spaepen A, Schrander-Stumpel C, Fryns JP, et al. Hallermann-Streiff syndrome: clinical and psychological findings in children. Nosologic overlap with oculodentodigital dysplasia? Am J Med Genet. 1991;41:517-20.
6. Streiff EB. Dysmorphic Mandibulo-faciale (Tete d'Oiseau) et Alterations Oculaires. Ophthalmologica. 1950;120:79-83.

656. HALLERVORDEN-SPATZ SYNDROME (PIGMENTARY DEGENERATION OF GLOBUS PALLIDUS; PROGRESSIVE PALLIDAL DEGENERATION SYNDROME)

General

Etiology unknown; autosomal dominant; onset between the ages of 7 and 9 years; globus pallidus and pars reticularis of the substantia nigra are involved with demyelinization and degenerative processes; perhaps a form of iron storage disease.

Ocular

Nystagmus; retinitis pigmentosa; optic nerve atrophy; degeneration of photoreceptors; retinal gliosis; narrowing and obliteration of blood vessels with perivascular cuffing; degeneration of retinal pigment epithelial cells.

Clinical

Slowly progressing spasticity and rigidity of the extremities; emotional disturbances (pseudobulbar type); dementia; clubfoot; dysphagia; athetosis; dysphonia; choreoathetosis; rigidity; seizures; pyramidal signs; generalized dystonia.

Laboratory

Radionuclide scan reveals increased uptake of iron by the basal ganglia, Bone marrow histiocytes and peripheral lymphocytes may demonstrate the presence of abnormal cytosomes.

Treatment

Treatment remains directed toward symptomatic findings. Systemic chelating agents such as des-ferrioxamine have been used in an attempt to remove excess iron from the brain, but these have not proved beneficial.

Additional Resource

1. Hanna PA (2012). Hallervorden-Spatz Disease. [online] Available from http://www.emedicine.com/neuro/TOPIC151.HTM [Accessed April, 2012].

657. HALLGREN SYNDROME (RETINITIS PIGMENTOSA-DEAFNESS-ATAXIA SYNDROME; USHER SYNDROME TYPE I)

General

Autosomal recessive inheritance.

Ocular

Horizontal nystagmus (10%); cataract; retinitis pigmentosa; retinal atrophy; narrow retinal vessels; optic atrophy; keratoconus.

Clinical

Congenital deafness (complete or at least severe auditory impairment); mental deficiency (25%); vestibulocerebellar ataxia (90%); schizophrenia-like symptoms (25%).

Laboratory

Diagnosis is made by clinical findings.

Treatment

Low-vision evaluation. Vitamin A 15,000 IU/day is thought to slow the decline of retinal function, dark sunglasses for outdoor use, surgery for cataract, genetic counseling.

Additional Resource

1. Telander DG (2012). Retinitis Pigmentosa. [online] Available from http://www.emedicine.com/oph/TOPIC704.HTM [Accessed April, 2012].

658. HAMMAN-RICH SYNDROME (ALVEOLAR CAPILLARY BLOCK SYNDROME; DIFFUSE PULMONARY FIBROSIS SYNDROME; RHEUMATOID LUNG SYNDROME)

General

Etiology unknown; insidious onset with progressive exertional dyspnea; association with rheumatoid arthritis or scleroderma; autosomal recessive; occurs between the ages of 40 and 50 years.

Ocular

Xerophthalmia; keratomalacia; retinal venous congestion and engorgement; ischemic retinopathy; cystic macular changes.

Clinical

Cyanosis; dyspnea; cough; weight loss; clubbing of fingers; high sodium and chloride concentrations in sweat; heart failure.

Laboratory

Most patients have abnormal chest radiography findings. Bilateral diffuse reticular or reticulo-nodular infiltrates are observed.

Treatment

Oxygen therapy should be prescribed for patients with documented hypoxemia. Pulmonary specialist should be involved.

Additional Resource

1. Godfrey A (2012). Idiopathic Pulmonary Fibrosis. [online] Available from http://www.emedicine.com/med/TOPIC1960.HTM [Accessed April, 2012].

659. HANEY-FALLS SYNDROME (CONGENITAL KERATOCONUS POSTICUS CIRCUMSCRIPTUS SYNDROME)

General

Etiology unknown; autosomal dominant or recessive.

Ocular

Hypertelorism (mild); lateral canthi are displaced upward; myopic astigmatism; sharply localized posterior curvature of the cornea; corneal nebulae.

Clinical

Mental retardation; retarded growth; broad nose; brachydactyly; pterygium colli; barrel chest.

Laboratory

Corneal topography.

Treatment

Rigid contact lenses (CLs) are the mainstay of treatment, intrastromal corneal rings (Intacs) may be of benefit and in extreme cases corneal transplant may be necessary.

Additional Resource

1. Weissman BA (2011). Keratoconus. [online] Available from http://www.emedicine.com/oph/TOPIC104.HTM [Accessed April, 2012].

660. HANHART SYNDROME (RECESSIVE KERATOSIS PALMOPLANTARIS; RICHNER SYNDROME; PSEUDODENDRITIC KERATITIS; PSEUDOHERPETIC KERATITIS; RICHNER-HANHART SYNDROME; TYROSINEMIA II; TYROSINOSIS)

General

Autosomal recessive; consanguinity.

Ocular

Excess tearing; photophobia; dendritic lesions of the cornea with corneal sensitivity not affected; keratitis; papillary hypertrophy of conjunctiva; corneal haze; neovascularization of cornea; cataract; nystagmus.

Clinical

Dyskeratosis palmoplantaris; diffuse keratosis; dystrophy of nails; hypotrichosis; mental retardation (usually pronounced); sensorineural hearing loss.

Laboratory

Serum—plasma tyrosine 16–62 mg/dL; urine—tyrosinuria and tyrosyluria; liver biopsy—decreased cTAT activity.

Treatment

Topical keratolytics, topical retinoids, potent topical steroids with or without keratolytics in dermatoses with an inflammatory component.

Additional Resource

1. Lee RA (2011). Keratosis Palmaris et Plantaris. [online] Available from http://www.emedicine.com/derm/TOPIC589.HTM [Accessed April, 2012].

---

661. HANSEN DISEASE (LEPROSY)

General

Communicable disease caused by *Mycobacterium leprae*.

Ocular

Keratitis; leukoma; pannus; corneal ulcer; uveitis; iris atrophy; dacryocystitis; anisocoria; multiple pupils; decreased or absent pupillary reaction to light; paralysis of seventh nerve; episcleritis; blepharospasm; lagophthalmos; madarosis; secondary glaucoma; decreased intraocular pressure; subconjunctival fibrosis; punctate epithelial keratopathy; posterior subcapsular cataract; corneal hypesthesia; prominent corneal nerves; iridocyclitis; foveal avascular keratitis; scleritis; interstitial keratitis; iris pearls; dry eye.

Clinical

Disease affects primarily the skin, mucous membrane and peripheral nerves.

Laboratory

Skin biopsy specimens contain vacuolated macrophages, few lymphocytes and numerous acid-fast bacilli often in clumps or globi.

Treatment

The WHO recommends multiple drug therapy (MDT) for all forms of leprosy. MDT 14 consists of rifampin, ofloxacin and minocycline.

Additional Resource

1. Kim EC (2011). Ocular Manifestations of Leprosy. [online] Available from http://www.emedicine.com/oph/TOPIC743.HTM [Accessed April, 2012].

---

662. HAPPY PUPPET SYNDROME (PUPPET CHILDREN)

General

Etiology unknown; very rare form of infantile epilepsy.

Ocular

Optic atrophy; deficiency of choroidal pigment; lightly colored irides; Brushfield spots; retinal pigment epithelium abnormalities; heterotropia; blindness.

Clinical

Mental retardation; seizures; puppet-like ataxia; paroxysms of laughter; absent speech; microcephaly; horizontal occipital depression; brachycephaly; prognathism, abnormal electroencephalographic findings.

Laboratory

Electroencephalography.

Treatment

Antiepileptic drugs, such as valproic acid, benzodiazepines, ethosuximide, levetiracetam and lamotrigine are preferred.

Additional Resource

1. Kaddurah AK (2011). Benign Childhood Epilepsy. [online] Available from http://www.emedicine.com/neuro/TOPIC641.HTM [Accessed April, 2012].

663. HARBOYAN SYNDROME (CONGENITAL CORNEAL DYSTROPHY AND SENSORINEURAL HEARING LOSS; CONGENITAL HEREDITARY ENDOTHELIAL; CORNEAL DYSTROPHY, MAUMENEE SYNDROME)

General

Autosomal recessive; both sexes affected; corneal edema present at birth; slow and progressive; both dominant and recessive forms of this disorder have been described.

Ocular

Bluish-white opacities of cornea with normal sensitivity and no vascularization; nystagmus; keratoconus.

Clinical

Sensorineural hearing loss with childhood onset.

Laboratory

Diagnosis is made by clinical findings.

Treatment

Corneal dystrophy: Mild cases can be observed and soft contact lenses are helpful, penetrating keratoplasty may be necessary, graft recurrences treated by superficial keratectomy, phototherapeutic keratectomy or repeat penetrating keratoplasty.

Keratoconus: Spectacle correction, hard contacts and avoid eye rubbing may be useful. If hydrops occurs discontinue contact lens, use NaCl drops and ointment, patching and short course of steroids. As the disease advances penetrating keratoplasty, deep anterior lamellar keratoplasty, intacs with laser grooves or collagen stabilization of cornea.

Additional Resource

1. Scheinfeld NS (2011). Congenital Clouding of the Cornea. [online] Available from http://www.emedicine.com/oph/TOPIC771.HTM [Accessed April, 2012].

664. HARLEQUIN SYNDROME (BULLOUS ICHTHYOSIFORM ERYTHRODERMA; COLLODION BABY; CONGENITAL ICHTHYOSIS; EPIDERMOLYTIC HYPERKERATOSIS; ICHTHYOSIS; ICHTHYOSIS VULGARIS; LAMELLAR ICHTHYOSIS; NONBULLOUS ICHTHYOSIFORM ERYTHRODERMA; XERODERMA; X-LINKED ICHTHYOSIS)

General

Autosomal inherited disorder; affects both sexes; normal at birth; onset within first 7 days.

Ocular

Keratopathy; corneal scarring; keratitis; conjunctivitis; lagophthalmos; photophobia; ectropion; lid erythema; lacrimation.

Clinical

At birth, the skin surface is moist, red and tender; within several days, thick verrucous scales form.

Laboratory

Diagnosis is made by clinical findings.

Treatment

Treatment is primarily surgical. Patients with bilateral and visually disabling corneal opacity, penetrating keratoplasty (PK) is recommended.

Bibliography

1. Chua CN, Ainsworth J. Ocular management of harlequin syndrome. Arch Ophthalmol. 2001;119: 454-5.
2. Roy FH, Fraunfelder FW, Fraunfelder FT. Roy and Fraunfelder's Current Ocular Therapy, 6th edition. Philadelphia: WB Saunders; 2008.
3. Frost P. Disorders of cornification. In: Moschella SL, Pillsbury DM, Hurley HJ. (Eds). Dermatology. Philadelphia: WB Saunders; 1975. pp. 1056-84.
4. Magalini SI, Scrascia E. Dictionary of Medical Syndromes, 2nd edition. Philadelphia: JB Lippincott; 1981.
5. Orth DH, Fretzin DF, Abramson V. Collodion baby with transient bilateral lid ectropion. Review of ocular manifestations of ichthyosis. Arch Ophthalmol. 1974;91:206-7.

665. HARTNUP SYNDROME (H DISEASE; NIACIN DEFICIENCY; PELLAGRA-CEREBELLAR ATAXIA-RENAL AMINOACIDURIA SYNDROME)

General

Recessive; inborn error in amino acid metabolism with abnormal metabolism of tryptophan; both sexes affected; presents from infancy.

Ocular

Ectropion; symblepharon; nystagmus; scleral ulcers; corneal leukoma; photophobia; diplopia during attacks.

Clinical

Dermatitis (similar to pellagra) with skin eruptions; progressive mental retardation; cerebellar ataxia.

Laboratory

Therapeutic response to niacin in a patient with the typical symptoms and signs of establishes the diagnosis.

Treatment

Oral therapy with nicotinamide or niacin usually is effective in reversing the clinical manifestations.

Additional Resource

1. Hegyi V (2010). Dermatologic Manifestations of Pellagra. [online] Available from http://www.emedicine.com/derm/TOPIC621.HTM [Accessed April, 2012].

666. HAYS-WELLS SYNDROME (AEC SYNDROME; ANKYLOBLEPHARON-ECTODERMAL DEFECTS-CLEFT LIP/PALATE SYNDROME)

General

Autosomal dominant disease, as initially described, but may exist as an autosomal recessive disorder.

Ocular

Ankyloblepharon; filiforme adnatum (fused eyelids).

Clinical

Coarse, wiry and sparse hair; dystrophic nails; slight hypohidrosis; scalp infections; hypodontia; maxillary hypoplasia; cleft lip and palate.

Laboratory

Sweat pore counts, skin biopsy, orthopantography at an early age if hypodontia or dental abnormalities are present.

Treatment

Care of affected patients depends on which ectodermal structures are involved.

Additional Resource

1. Shah KN (2012). Ectodermal Dysplasia. [online] Available from http://www.emedicine.com/derm/ TOPIC114.HTM [Accessed April, 2012].

---

667. HEAD-RIDDOCH SYNDROME

General

Occurs in quadriplegics; caused by distention of a viscus below the level of spinal cord lesion; seen most frequently in people with high cervical cord lesion; may follow catheter obstruction, fecal impaction, bladder calculi, urinary infection or decubiti.

Ocular

Dilated pupils; blurred vision.

Clinical

Sweating; flushing; pilomotor activity; nasal stuffiness; headaches; generalized seizures; bradycardia; hypertension.

Laboratory

Diagnosis is made by clinical findings.

Treatment

Treat underlying problem.

Additional Resource

1. Ing E (2010). Neuro-Ophthalmic Examination. [online] Available from http://www.emedicine. medscape.com/article/1820707-overview [Accessed April, 2012].

---

668. HEADACHE NEUROLOGIC DEFECTS AND CEREBROSPINAL FLUID LYMPHOCYTOSIS SYNDROME

General

Age range from 7 years to 52 years; no gender bias.

Ocular

Papillema; homonymous hemianopia; photopsias; VI nerve palsy.

Clinical

Headache; hemisensory defects; muscle weakness; aphasia; elevated intracranial pressure.

Laboratory

Lumbar puncture reveals elevated opening pressure without leukocytosis or abnormalities in glucose or protein concentration.

Treatment

Carbonic anhydrase inhibitors decrease the production of CSF.

Bibliography

1. Morrison DG, Phuah HK, Reddy AT, et al. Ophthalmologic involvement in the syndrome of headache, neurologic deficits, and cerebrospinal fluid lymphocytosis. Ophthalmology. 2003;110: 115-8.

---

669. HEADACHE, CHILDREN

General

Generally migraine type in nature; headache occurrence increases with age; before puberty males are affected slightly more than females, after puberty females are affected more.

Clinical

Headache; nausea; vomiting; dizziness; hypotension; bradycardia; diarrhea; sensitivity to sound and smell.

Ocular

Ocular migraine; scotoma; photophobia; hallucinations.

Laboratory

Neuroimaging may rarely be necessary.

Treatment

Acetaminophen and antihistimines may be beneficial. Prophylactic treatment may be necessary if the frequency and severity of the headache worsens.

Additional Resource

1. Lenaerts ME (2010). Ophthalmologic Manifestations of Pediatric Headache. [online] Available from http://www.emedicine.medscape.com/article/1214702-overview [Accessed April, 2012].

---

670. HEERFORDT SYNDROME (UVEOPAROTITIS; UVEOPAROTID FEVER UVEOPAROTITIC PARALYSIS)

General

Occurs in young adults, more frequently in females than in males; usual cause is sarcoidosis.

Ocular

Band keratopathy; keratoconjunctivitis sicca; uveitis; optic atrophy; papilledema; episcleritis; snowball opacity of vitreous; retinal vasculitis; proptosis; cataract; paralysis of seventh nerve; sarcoid nodules of eyelid, iris, ciliary body, choroid and sclera; dacryoadenitis.

Clinical

Parotid gland swelling; facial paralysis; lymphadenopathy; splenomegaly; cutaneous nodules; facial nerve palsy.

Laboratory

Biopsy of liver, skin, lymph nodes or conjunctiva shows noncaseating epithelioid cell follicles; X-ray lung changes; low tuberculin sensitivity; elevated angiotension-converting enzyme level.

Treatment

Systemic corticosteroids are the treatment of choice.

Additional Resource

1. Dahl AA (2011). Ophthalmologic Manifestations of Sarcoidosis. [online] Available from http://www.emedicine.com/oph/TOPIC451.HTM [Accessed April, 2012].

671. HEMANGIOMA

General

Can occur throughout the body, but particularly in the head; primary intraosseous orbital hemangiomas are rare; capillary hemangioma of the orbit and eyelids generally is unilateral.

Ocular

Hemangiomas of lids or orbit; ptosis; strabismus; amblyopia; proptosis; optic atrophy; hypermetropia; cavernous hemangiomas are the most common benign orbital tumors of adults.

Clinical

Ipsilateral hemangiomas of the brain and meninges.

Laboratory

Neuroimaging can be of great assistance in making the diagnosis.

Treatment

Most of these lesions regress on their own, there is no need to intervention. If spontaneous regression does not occur corticosteroids, in various formulations, may be considered. Topical application of timolol has been useful in some cases.

Bibliography

1. Karmel M. Topical Timolol for Capillary Hemangioma. EyeNet. June, 2010.

Additional Resource

1. Seiff S (2011). Capillary Hemangioma. [online] Available from http://www.emedicine.com/oph/ TOPIC691.HTM [Accessed April, 2012].

672. HEMANGIOMA, CAPILLARY

General

Benign orbital tumors of infancy; rapid growth; thought to be of placental origin due to a unique microvascular phenotype shared by juvenile hemangiomas and human placenta.

Clinical

Kasabach-Merritt syndrome; congestive heart failure; nasopharyngeal obstruction; thrombocytopenia; hemolytic anemia.

Ocular

Red, thickened spot in the periorbital area, lid or brow; amblyopia; anisometropia.

Laboratory

Neuroimaging studies are useful to establish the diagnosis; CT, MRI and ultrasound may be beneficial.

Treatment

Corticosteroids topically, systemically and injected are the first line of treatment. Interferon may also be used in resistant cases. Laser and incisional surgical techniques have had variable success.

Additional Resource

1. Seiff S (2011). Capillary Hemangioma. [online] Available from http://www.emedicine.medscape. com/article/1218805-overview [Accessed April, 2012].

673. HEMANGIOMA, CAVERNOUS

General

Most common intraorbital tumors found in adults; benign, vascular lesions; slow growing; usually unilateral; first symptoms include bulging of the globe and eyelid fullness; usually found in the intraconal space between the optic nerve and extraocular muscles.

Clinical

Neurosurgical or otolarynologic issues may be present of the hemangioma extends to the facial sturcture outside of the orbit.

Ocular

Decreased visual acuity and visual field; diplopia; proptosis; extraocular and pupillary dysfunction; lagophthalmos; exposure keratopathy; keratitis; corneal perforation.

Laboratory

Computed tomography (CT), MRI scan and ultrasound studies are commonly used to make the diagnosis.

Treatment

Most require no intervention; some cases do require surgical treatment.

Additional Resource

1. Cohen AJ (2011). Cavernous Hemangioma. [online] Available from http://www.emedicine medscape.com/article/1218120-overview [Acessed April, 2012].

674. HEMERALOPIA

General

Autosomal dominant.

Ocular

Complete loss of the outer quadrant of visual field bilaterally; visual fields become progressively more constricted until blindness occurs; corneal ulcers; photoreceptor dysfunction.

Clinical

None

Laboratory

Visual field examination.

Treatment

Low vision aids and counseling.

Bibliography

1. Gehrs K, Tiedeman J. Hemeralopia in an older adult. Surv Ophthalmol. 1992;37:185-9.
2. McKusick VA. Mendelian Inheritance in Man: A Catalog of Human Genes and Genetic Disorders, 12th edition. Baltimore: The Johns Hopkins University Press; 1998.

675. HEMIFACIAL HYPERPLASIA WITH STRABISMUS (BENCZE SYNDROME)

General

Autosomal dominant; abnormal growth of facial skeleton, soft tissue and viscera; left side prominent.

Ocular

Strabismus; amblyopia.

Clinical

Facial asymmetry; submucous cleft palate.

Laboratory

X-ray, CT and MRI.

Treatment

Silastic implants remain one of the most common materials used for malar and submalar augmentation.

Bibliography

1. Bencze J, Schnitzler A, Walawska J. Dominant inheritance of hemifacial hyperplasia associated with strabismus. Oral Surg Oral Med Oral Pathol. 1973;35:489-500.
2. McKusick VA. Mendelian Inheritance in Man: A Catalog of Human Genes and Genetic Disorders, 12th edition. Baltimore: The Johns Hopkins University Press; 1998.
3. McKusick-Nathans Institute for Genetic Medicine, Johns Hopkins University and National Center for Biotechnology Information, National Library of Medicine. (2007). Online Mendelian Inheritance in Man (OMIM). [online] Available from http://www.ncbi.nlm.nih.gov/omim [Accessed April, 2012].

676. HEMIFACIAL MICROSOMIA SYNDROME (FRANCOIS-HAUSTRATE SYNDROME; OTOMANDIBULAR DYSOSTOSIS; UNILATERAL FACIAL AGENESIS)

General

No inheritance pattern; left side of face seems to be more frequently involved; facial asymmetry usually most obvious finding; both sexes affected; alteration of intrauterine environment is possible cause.

Ocular

Microphthalmos; congenital cystic ophthalmia; enophthalmos; strabismus; cataract; colobomata of iris, choroid and retina.

Clinical

Microtia; macrostomia; failure of development of mandibular ramus and condyle; external auditory meatus may be absent; single or numerous ear tags; hypoplasia of facial muscles unilaterally; pulmonary agenesis (ipsilateral side); associated with Goldenhar syndrome.

Laboratory

X-ray, CT and MRI.

Treatment

Silastic implants remain one of the most common materials used for malar and submalar augmentation.

Bibliography

1. Francois J, Haustrate L. Anomalies Colobomateuses du Globe Oculaire et Syndrome du Premier arc. Ann Ocul. 1954;187:340-68.
2. Geeraets WJ. Ocular Syndromes, 3rd edition. Philadelphia: Lea & Febiger; 1976.
3. Kobrynski L, Chitayat D, Zahed L, et al. Trisomy 22 and facioauriculovertebral (Goldenhar) sequence. Am J Med Genet. 1993;46:68-71.
4. Magalini SI, Scrascia E. Dictionary of Medical Syndromes, 2nd edition. Philadelphia: JB Lippincott; 1981.

677. HEMIMACROSOMIA SYNDROME (HEMIGIGANTISM; HEMIFACIAL OR UNILATERAL HYPERTROPHY; STEINER SYNDROME)

General

Occasionally hereditary, although true etiology is obscure; right side affected more frequently than left side; slight male preponderance.

Ocular

Dilated pupil on the affected side; eccentric pupillary location; hypochromic heterochromia.

Clinical

Unilateral facial enlargement may be associated with enlargement of half of entire body to varied extent and degree; thickened skin over involved area with increased activity of sebaceous and sweat glands; telangiectasias and multiple nevi; polydactyly; syndactyly; macrodactyly; scoliosis.

Laboratory

Diagnosis is made by clinical findings.

Treatment

Ocular/None.

Bibliography

1. Curtius F. Kongenitaler Partieller Riesenwuchs mit Endokrinen Storungen. Dtsch Arch Klin Med. 1925;147:310.
2. Geeraets WJ. Ocular Syndromes, 3rd edition. Philadelphia: Lea & Febiger; 1976.
3. Stafne EC, Lovestedt SA. Congenital hemihypertrophy of the face (facial gigantism). Oral Surg Oral Med Oral Pathol. 1962;15:184-9.

678. HEMOCHROMATOSIS

General

Iron metabolism disorder; genetically determined, but mode of inheritance unknown; male preponderance (10:1); inheritance is autosomal recessive.

Ocular

Eyelid hyperpigmentation; diabetic retinopathy.

Clinical

Hemosiderin pigment deposition in many tissues; diabetes mellitus; cutaneous hyperpigmentation; cirrhosis of the liver; hypermelanotic pigmentation of skin; heart failure.

Laboratory

Detect iron metabolism defect.

Treatment

Diabetic retinopathy: Glucose control with diet, exercise and medication, daily dose of aspirin (650 mg), laser photocoagulation, intravitreal injections of triamcinolone, Avastin and Lucentis can be used. The use of Avastin and Lucentis is off label. Vitrectomy and cryotherapy may also be necessary.

Additional Resource

1. Duchini A (2011). Hemochromatosis. [online] Available from http://www.emedicine.com/med/TOPIC975.HTM [Accessed April, 2012].

679. HEMOLYTIC ANEMIA OF NEWBORNS (ERYTHROBLASTOSIS FETALIS; ICTERUS GRAVIS NEONATORUM)

General

Rh-positive/negative infant carried by an Rh-positive/negative mother; isoimmunization of the mother by her fetus of different blood group.

Ocular

Retinal hemorrhages; ophthalmoplegia; optic atrophy; yellow conjunctiva and lids.

Clinical

Jaundice; edema; liver and spleen palpable; cutaneous purpura; bleeding from mucosa.

Laboratory

Rh testing.

Treatment

Normalize antibody levels in patients with primary defective antibody synthesis. They prevent and treat certain bacterial and viral infections and reduce the immune-mediated hemolysis and phagocytosis.

Additional Resource

1. Wagle S (2011). Hemolytic Disease of Newborn. [online] Available from http://www.emedicine.com/ped/TOPIC959.HTM [Accessed April, 2012].

680. HENNEBERT SYNDROME (LUETIC-OTITIC-NYSTAGMUS SYNDROME)

General

Caused by congenital syphilis; manifestations in childhood; when a fistula in the labyrinth exists, compression of the external auditory meatus will produce nystagmus of a wide amplitude (diagnostic of fistula).

Ocular

Spontaneous nystagmus when the column of air in the auditory canal is compressed; interstitial keratitis; disseminated syphilitic chorioretinitis may be present.

Clinical

Vertigo; fistula in the labyrinth; deafness; other clinical manifestations of congenital syphilis may be present, such as "saddle" nose and Hutchinson teeth.

Laboratory

Serologic testing is commonly used to confirm a diagnosis of syphilis.

Treatment

Penicillin remains the treatment of choice.

Additional Resource

1. Waseem M (2011). Pediatric Syphilis. [online] Available from http://www.emedicine.com/ped/TOPIC2193.HTM [Accessed April, 2012].

681. HENOCH-SCHÖNLEIN PURPURA (ANAPHYLACTOID PURPURA; PURPURA)

General

Occurs chiefly in children, although it can affect persons of any age; frequently follows an upper respiratory tract infection within 3 weeks.

Ocular

Retinal hemorrhages; iritis; optic neuritis.

Clinical

Purpuric skin rash; concentrated on lower extremities; joint pain; abdominal pain; hematuria; central nervous system involvement.

Laboratory

Diagnosis is made by clinical findings.

Treatment

Consult hematologist.

Bibliography

1. Harley RD (Ed). Pediatric Ophthalmology, 4th edition. Philadelphia: WB Saunders; 1998.
2. Lorentz WB, Weaver RG. Eye involvement in anaphylactoid purpura. Am J Dis Child. 1980;134:524-5.
3. Ryder HG, Marcus O. Henoch-Schonlein purpura: a case report. S Afr Med J. 1976;50:2005-6.

682. HEPATIC FAILURE

General

Liver failure from infections or from toxic or inflammatory causes.

Ocular

Visual field defects; scleral icterus; night blindness; abnormal color vision; eyelid retraction; lid lag; Kayser-Fleischer ring; yellow discoloration of the conjunctiva.

Clinical

Bilirubin accumulation; reduced vitamin A levels.

Laboratory

Diagnosis is made by clinical findings.

Treatment

Consult internist.

Additional Resource

1. Nazer H (2011). Pediatric Fulminant Hepatic Failure. [online] Available from http://www.emedicine.com/ped/TOPIC808.HTM [Accessed April, 2012].

683. HEREDITARY ECTODERMAL DYSPLASIA SYNDROME (ANHIDROTIC ECTODERMAL DYSPLASIA; CHRIST-SIEMENS-TOURAINE SYNDROME; HYPOHIDROTIC ECTODERMAL DYSPLASIA; ICHTHYOSIS FOLLICULARIS; KERATOSIS FOLLICULARIS SPINULOSA SYNDROME; SIEMENS SYNDROME; WEECH SYNDROME)

General

Autosomal recessive inheritance; strong male preponderance (about 95%); linked to X chromosome.

Ocular

Complete loss of eyebrows (madarosis); follicular keratosis; blepharitis; entropion or ectropion;

reduced tear formation or epiphora; myopia; keratoconjunctivitis; corneal erosions and ulcers (recurrent); corneal dystrophy; cataract; increased periorbital pigmentation; mongoloid lid slant; photophobia; absence of iris; luxation of lens; papillary abnormalities.

Clinical

Mental retardation; dry skin and anhidrosis (reduced number of sweat glands); hypotrichosis; follicular hyperkeratosis (neck, palms, soles); hypohidrosis.

Laboratory

Diagnosis is made by clinical findings.

Treatment

Corneal dystrophy: Mild cases can be observed and soft contact lenses are helpful, penetrating keratoplasty may be necessary, graft recurrences treated by superficial keratectomy, phototherapeutic keratectomy or repeat penetrating keratoplasty.

Cataract: Change in glasses can sometimes improve a patient's visual function temporarily; however, the most common treatment is cataract surgery.

Additional Resource

1. Shah KN (2012). Ectodermal Dysplasia. [online] Available from http://www.emedicine.com/derm/TOPIC114.HTM [Accessed April, 2012].

684. HEREDITARY MICROCORNEA, GLAUCOMA, AND ABSENT FRONTAL SINUSES

General

Autosomal dominant.

Ocular

Microcornea; glaucoma; epicanthal folds; optic cupping.

Clinical

Thickened palmar skin; torus palatinus; frontal sinus hypoplasia.

Laboratory

Diagnosis is made by clinical findings.

Treatment

Glaucoma: Its medication should be the first plan of action. If medication is unsuccessful, a filtering surgical procedure with or without antimetabolites may be beneficial.

Bibliography

1. Holmes LB, Walton DS. Hereditary microcornea, glaucoma, and absent frontal sinuses: a family study. J Pediatr. 1969;74:968-72.
2. McKusick VA. Mendelian Inheritance in Man: A Catalog of Human Genes and Genetic Disorders, 12th edition. Baltimore: The Johns Hopkins University Press; 1998.

685. HERMANSKY-PUDLAK SYNDROME (OCULOCUTANEOUS ALBINISM AND HEMORRHAGIC DIATHESIS)

General

Autosomal recessive; mostly affects children or young adults; tyrosinase-positive oculocutaneous albinism; abnormal platelets; increased ceroid-like material in the reticuloendothelial system.

Ocular

Translucent irides; minimally pigmented ocular fundi; nystagmus; foveal hypoplasia; large refractive errors; strabismus; fundus hypopigmentation.

Clinical

Gingival bleeding; epistaxis; easy bruisability; pale skin; interstitial lung disease; defect in platelet function; "imperfect" oculocutaneous albinism; restrictive lung disease; ulcerative colitis.

Laboratory

Hair bulb incubation test classifies patients into tyrosinase negative or tyrosinase positive.

Treatment

Ophthalmologists should try to avoid retrobulbar blocks in patients with the syndrome. Whenever possible, patients may benefit from general endotracheal anesthesia. Phacoemulsification may help prevent intraoperative and postoperative bleeding in patients with the syndrome. Prolonged bleeding has been reported following strabismus surgery in patients with the syndrome.

Additional Resource

1. Izquierdo NJ (2010). Hermansky-Pudlak Syndrome. [online] Available from http://www.emedicine.com/oph/TOPIC713.HTM [Accessed April, 2012].

---

686. HERMIT SYNDROME

General

Seen in alcoholic men in their 60s and 70s living in relative social isolation; secondary to history of sun exposure or chronic irritation; high prevalence in the tropics or developing countries; masquerades as conjunctivitis or orbital cellulitis; develops from carcinoma in situ (see Bowen Disease).

Ocular

Squamous cell carcinoma of conjunctiva; proptosis; erythema of eyelids; edema of eyelids; conjunctival hyperemia; vitreous hemorrhage; ciliary body hemorrhage; choroidal hemorrhage; paresis of extraocular muscles; ocular pain; orbital cellulitis.

Clinical

Vitamin A deficiency; nutritional disorders; recurrent infections; actinic keratoses.

Laboratory

Diagnosis is made by clinical findings.

Treatment

Squamous cell carcinoma of conjunctiva: Excisional biopsy is the treatment of choice. Careful monitoring is necessary to look for orbital invasion. Oncologist should be consulted if metastatic disease is suspected.

Bibliography

1. Gamel JW, Eiferman RA, Guibor P. Mucoepidermoid carcinoma of the conjunctiva. Arch Ophthalmol. 1984;102:730-1.
2. Li WW, Pettit TH, Zakka KA. Intraocular invasion by papillary squamous cell carcinoma of the conjunctiva. Am J Ophthalmol. 1980;90:697-701.
3. Rootman J, Roth AM, Crawford JB, et al. Extensive squamous cell carcinoma of the conjunctiva presenting as orbital cellulitis: the hermit syndrome. Can J Ophthalmol. 1987;22:40-4.

687. HERPES SIMPLEX

General

Large, complex deoxyribonucleic acid (DNA) virus.

Ocular

Conjunctivitis; keratitis; iridocyclitis; corneal ulcer; uveitis; hyphema; hypopyon; iris atrophy; cataract; scleritis; dacryoadenitis; blepharitis; acute retinal necrosis.

Clinical

Recurrent skin vesicles on lids, perioral area, nose and genitalia; meningitis; encephalitis.

Laboratory

Viral cultures.

Treatment

Antiviral therapy, topical or oral, is an effective treatment of epithelial herpes infection.

Additional Resource

1. Wang JC (2010). Ophthalmologic Manifestations of Herpes Simplex Keratitis. [online] Available from http://www.emedicine.com/oph/TOPIC100. HTM [Accessed April, 2012].

688. HERPES SIMPLEX MASQUERADE SYNDROME

General

Acanthamoeba keratitis occurs in those who wear soft contact lenses daily; confused with herpes simplex; *Acanthamoeba culbertsoni, Acanthamoeba castellanii* and *Acanthamoeba polyphaga* are causative agents; agents found in distilled water, hot tubs and swimming pools (see Acanthamoeba).

Ocular

Keratitis; corneal ulcer; corneal cysts; stromal infiltrates and necrosis; scleritis; uveitis; epiphora; pseudodendrites.

Clinical

None

Laboratory

Corneal smears and cultures.

Treatment

Antibiotics are used to treat the ulcer, lubrication, oral tetracycline, proper wear of contact lens.

Bibliography

1. Berger ST, Hoft RH, Mondino BJ, et al. Successful medical management of Acanthamoeba keratitis. Am J Ophthalmol. 1990;110:395-403.
2. John KJ, O'Day DM, Head WS, et al. Herpes simplex masquerade syndrome: acanthamoeba keratitis. Curr Eye Res. 1987;6:207-12.
3. Moore MB, McCulley JP, Luckenbach M, et al. Acanthamoeba keratitis associated with soft contact lenses. Am J Ophthalmol. 1985;100:396-403.
4. Samples JR, Binder PS, Luibel FJ, et al. Acanthamoeba keratitis possibly acquired from a hot tub. Arch Ophthalmol. 1984;102:707-10.
5. Wilhelmus KR. Parasitic keratitis and conjunctivitis. In: Smolin G, Thoft RA (Eds). The Cornea, 3rd edition. Boston: Little, Brown and Company; 1994. pp. 262-6.

689. HERPES ZOSTER

General

Caused by varicella-zoster virus; about 75% of cases occur in persons over age 45 years; condition is more frequent with advancing age and in patients who are immunocompromised by drugs or disease; in particular, an increasing number of patients with herpes zoster ophthalmicus are immunosuppressed.

Ocular

Conjunctivitis; keratitis; recurrent corneal ulcer; neuralgia; zoster rash of eyelids; uveitis; iris atrophy; scleritis; cataract; optic neuritis; paralysis of third nerve; proptosis; paralysis of lids; orbital apex syndrome; retinitis; neurotrophic keratitis; acute retinal necrosis; progressive outer retinal necrosis; ocular motor nerve pareses; tonic pupil; encephalitis; vasculitis.

Clinical

Local lesions involving the posterior or root ganglia; nerve damage; tissue scarring.

Laboratory

Diagnosed mostly on the basis of the characteristic pain and appearance of the dermatomal rashes.

Treatment

Antiviral agents, systemic corticosteroids, antidepressants and adequate pain control. Immunocompetent adults aged 60 years or older, benefit from receipt of the herpes zoster vaccine and have a lower incidence of herpes zoster.

Bibliography

1. Tseng HF, Smith N, Harpaz R, et al. Herpes zoster vaccine in older adults and the risk of subsequent herpes zoster disease. JAMA. 2011;305:160-6.

Additional Resource

1. Diaz MM (2011). Herpes Zoster Ophthalmicus. [online] Available from http://www.emedicine.com/oph/TOPIC257.HTM [Accessed April, 2012].

690. HERRICK SYNDROME (DRESBACH SYNDROME; DREPANOCYTIC ANEMIA; SICKLE CELL DISEASE)

General

Usually occurs in members of the black race; poor prognosis.

Ocular

Secondary glaucoma; telangiectasis of conjunctival vessels; scleral icterus; vitreous hemorrhages; cataract; retinal hemorrhages, exudates and neovascularization; retinitis proliferans; microaneurysms; thrombosis of retinal venules; retinal vascular sheathing; central vein occlusion; angioid streaks; retinopathy with "black sunburst sign" in patients with SS hemoglobin; "sea fan sign" in patients with SC hemoglobin; comma signs of conjunctiva; fan-shaped neovascularization of iris; sector ischemic atrophy of iris; optic atrophy; white cotton mass of vitreous; retinal holes; color vision defects; central retinal artery obstruction; branch retinal artery obstruction; white without pressure; venous tortuosity; sickling maculopathy.

Clinical

Severe anemia with hemolytic crises; bone and joint aches; hemarthrosis; jaundice; hepatosplenomegaly.

Laboratory

Blood—sickling of red blood cells, newborn screening for hemoglobin disorders.

Treatment

Transfusion is required in an aplastic crisis. Erythrocytapheresis is an automated red cell exchange and bone marrow transplantation may be useful. Pain is the hallmark of sickle cell disease. While frequency and severity vary greatly, most patients have interval symptoms. Once pain has begun, no therapy reverses the process. Analgesics may provide a reasonable degree of comfort. While certain dosing guidelines are available, the amount of drug given should be titrated to the degree of pain experienced. Vitrectomy may be necessary.

Additional Resource

1. Maakaron JE (2012). Sickle Cell Anemia. [online] Available from http://www.emedicine.com/ped/TOPIC2096.HTM [Accessed April, 2012].

691. HETEROCHROMIA IRIDIS

General

Autosomal dominant; can be associated with Horner, Waardenburg and Marfan syndromes; may occur as an isolated phenomenon.

Ocular

Different pigmentation in the two irides or in the sectors of one iris (heterochromia iridium).

Clinical

None

Laboratory

Diagnosis is made by clinical findings.

Treatment

None

Bibliography

1. Gladstone RM. Development and significance of heterochromia of the iris. Arch Neurol. 1969;21:184-91.
2. McKusick VA. Mendelian Inheritance in Man: A Catalog of Human Genes and Genetic Disorders, 12th edition. Baltimore: The Johns Hopkins University Press; 1998.

692. HIE SYNDROME (HYPERIMMUNOGLOBULINEMIA E SYNDROME)

General

Mononuclear cells inhibit normal neutrophil and monocyte chemotaxis; caused by *Staphylococcus aureus* and *Candida trachomatis*; autosomal dominant phenotype; onset age 1–8 weeks; marked elevation of immunoglobulin E.

Ocular

Atopic keratitis; keratoconjunctivitis; photophobia; corneal ulcer; chorioretinal scars; lid edema.

Clinical

Pruritic dermatitis; dry skin; skin abscesses; pneumonia; upper respiratory infections; reduced resistance; coarse facial features.

Laboratory

Computed tomography (CT) of the lungs, An IgE level greater than two standard deviations higher than normal limits.

Treatment

The first-line antistaphylococcal antibiotics are dicloxacillin or trimethoprim-sulfamethoxazole.

Additional Resource

1. Jyonouchi H (2011). Hyperimmunoglobulinemia E (Job) Syndrome. [online] Available from http://www.emedicine.com/ped/TOPIC1074.HTM [Accessed April, 2012].

---

693. HILDING SYNDROME (DESTRUCTIVE IRIDOCYCLITIS AND MULTIPLE JOINT DISLOCATIONS)

General

Atrophy of body cartilages and joint dislocations without destruction of bone or joint surfaces.

Ocular

Severe ocular hypotony; severe plastic iridocyclitis; iris atrophy; corneal endothelial precipitates; mature cataracts; retrolental inflammatory membrane.

Clinical

Multiple joint dislocations; hyperlaxity of joint capsules; generalized cartilage destruction with nose and ear deformities.

Laboratory

Diagnosis is made by clinical findings.

Treatment

Cataract: Change in glasses can sometimes improve a patient's visual function temporarily; however, the most common treatment is cataract surgery.

Uveitis: Topical steroids and cycloplegic medication should be the initial treatment of choice. Oral steroids if not responsive to topical steroids, immunosuppressants if bilateral disease that does not respond to oral steroids, periocular steroids for unilateral or posterior uveitis. Vitrectomy can be used for severe vitreous opacification. Cryotherapy and laser photocoagulation may be used for localized pars plana exudates.

Bibliography

1. Geeraets WJ. Ocular Syndromes, 3rd edition. Philadelphia: Lea & Febiger; 1976.
2. Hilding AC. Syndrome of cartilage pathology, destructive iridocyclitis, multiple joint dislocations: comparison with concurrent eye and joint diseases described in literature. AMA Arch Ophthalmol. 1952;48:420-7.

---

694. HIRSCHSPRUNG DISEASE

General

Occurs in 1 out of every 5,000 live births. Cause is unknown but involves the incomplete development of the intestinal nerve cells. More common in males and in children with Down syndrome.

Clinical

Constipation, loss of appetitie, gradual onset of vomiting, delayed growth, bloating of the abdomen.

Ocular

Partial or sector heterochromia.

Laboratory

Abdominal X-ray, barium enema, anorectal manometry and biopsy of the rectum or large intestine.

Treatment

Surgical removal of the affected colon or for intestinal obstruction is usually required. Colostomy either parital or permanent is usually necessary.

Additional Resource

1. Lee SL (2012). Hirschsprung Disease. [online] Available from http:/www.emedicine.medscape. com/article/178493-overview [Accessed April, 2012].

---

695. HISTIDINEMIA (HYPERHISTIDINEMIA; HISTIDASE DEFICIENCY)

General

Autosomal recessive; abnormality of amino acid metabolism due to lack of enzyme histidine ammonia lyase; the histidine gene has been assigned to 12q22–q23 in situ hybridization techniques.

Ocular

Nystagmus; hypopigmentation of the macula.

Clinical

Speech defects; mental retardation; head nodding movements; dysarthria; defective hand grip.

Laboratory

Blood analysis for ammonia levels, amino acids and organic acids; neuroimaging study.

Treatment

Cobalamin (Cbl) supplementation, restriction of protein to 1.5 g/kg/day, and carnitine supplementation are suggested.

Bibliography

1. Dhir SP, Shisku MW, Krewi A. Ocular involvement in histidinaemia. Ophthalmic Paediatr Genet. 1987;8:175-6.
2. McKusick VA. Mendelian Inheritance in Man: A Catalog of Human Genes and Genetic Disorders, 12th edition. Baltimore: The Johns Hopkins University Press; 1998.
3. Taylor RG, García-Heras J, Sadler SJ, et al. Localization of histidase to human chromosome region 12q22–q24.1 and mouse chromosome region 10C2-D1. Cytogenet Cell Genet. 1991;56: 178-81.

---

696. HISTIOCYTOSIS X (ACUTE HISTIOCYTOSIS X; EOSINOPHILIC GRANULOMA; HAND-SCHULLER-CHRISTIAN SYNDROME; LETTERER-SIWE SYNDROME; LIPOID GRANULOMA; RETICULOENDOTHELIOSIS SYNDROME; SCHULLER-CHRISTIAN-HAND SYNDROME; XANTHOMATOUS GRANULOMA SYNDROME)

General

The term histiocytosis X has been proposed to include Letterer-Siwe disease, Hand-Schuller-Christian disease and eosinophilic granuloma of bone; there are sufficient grounds to treat Hand-Schuller-Christian and Letterer-Siwe together as different phases of the same disease process; eosinophilic granuloma most likely represents a reaction pattern, sharing some histologic features with the first two but nonetheless carrying a more benign prognosis; Letterer-Siwe disease is referred to as acute differentiated histiocytosis; Hand-Schuller-Christian disease is referred to as

Laboratory

Magnetic resonance imaging (MRI) shows mal-development of dorsomedial pontine structures including VI cranial nerve nuclei and medial longitudinal fasciculus (MLF).

Treatment

No eye treatment.

Additional Resources

1. Mehlman CT (2012). Idiopathic Scoliosis. [online] Available from http://www.emedicine.com/orthoped/TOPIC504.HTM [Accessed April, 2012].
2. Ehrenhaus MP (2012). Abducens Nerve Palsy. [online] Available from http://www.emedicine.com/oph/TOPIC158.HTM [Accessed April, 2012].

704. HORNER SYNDROME (BERNARD-HORNER SYNDROME; CERVICAL SYMPATHETIC PARALYSIS SYNDROME; CLAUDE-BERNARD-HORNER SYNDROME; HORNER OCULOPUPILLARY SYNDROME)

General

Paralysis of cervical sympathetic; hypothalamic lesion with first neuron involved or lesion in the pons or cervical portion of cord; syndrome present in Babinski-Nageotte, Cestan-Chenais, Dejerine-Klumpke, Pancoast, Raeder and Wallenberg syndromes (see Babinski-Nageotte Syndrome; Cestan-Chenais Syndrome; Dejerine-Klumpke Syndrome; Pancoast Syndrome; Raeder Syndrome; Wallenberg Syndrome).

Ocular

Enophthalmos; ptosis or narrowing of palpebral fissure; ocular hypotony; miosis (degree of miosis depends on site of lesion; most pronounced when roots of cranial nerves VII and VIII and first thoracic nerve are involved); hypochromic heterochromia (children more than adults); pupil does not dilate with cocaine.

Clinical

Anhidrosis on ipsilateral side of face and neck; transitory rise in facial temperature; hemifacial atrophy; may result from a variety of conditions, including cluster headache, parasellar neoplasms or aneurysms, internal carotid dissection or occlusion, and Tolosa-Hunt syndrome.

Laboratory

Pharmacologic testing is very helpful in the diagnosis of Horner syndrome. Cocaine or apraclonidine instilled in an eye with intact sympathetic innervation causes the pupil to dilate. A sympathetically denervated pupil dilates poorly to cocaine, regardless of the level of the sympathetic interruption because of the absence of endogenous norepinephrine in the synapse.

Treatment

Surgical and medical care is dependent upon the particular etiology. Potential surgical care includes neurosurgical care for aneurysm-related Horner syndrome and vascular surgical care for etiologies such as carotid artery dissection/aneurysm.

Additional Resource

1. Bardorf CM (2012). Horner Syndrome. [online] Available from http://www.emedicine.com/oph/TOPIC336.HTM [Accessed April, 2012].

705. HUNT SYNDROME (GENICULATE NEURALGIA; HERPES ZOSTER AURICULARIS; RAMSAY-HUNT SYNDROME)

General

Herpes of the geniculate ganglion; course is prolonged; characterized by severe pain that frequently precedes skin and mucosal lesions and may persist for sometime after lesions have disappeared; immunocompromised individuals.

Ocular

Diminished lacrimation; absence of motor corneal reflex on affected side, whereas consensual reflex of noninvolved eye remains normal.

Clinical

Herpes zoster lesions of external ear and oral mucosa; severe pain in area of external auditory meatus and pinna; diminished hearing; tinnitus; vertigo, facial palsy; diminution or total loss of superficial and deep facial reflexes; zoster lesions may involve the scalp, face and neck; hoarseness; absence of auricular lesions has been reported; progressive dementia; extensive frontal white matter change; myoclonus; ataxia; facial paralysis; tinnitus; hearing loss; hyperacusis; vertigo; dysgeusia; seizures; cerebellar ataxia; schizophrenia-like symptoms.

Laboratory

Diagnosed mostly on the basis of the characteristic pain and appearance of the dermatomal rashes.

Treatment

Antiviral agents, systemic corticosteroids, antidepressants and adequate pain control.

Bibliography

1. Adour KK. Otological complications of herpes zoster. Ann Neurol. 1994;35:S62-4.
2. Blackley B, Friedmann I, Wright I. Herpes zoster auris associated with facial nerve palsy and auditory nerve symptoms: a case report with histopathological findings. Acta Otolaryngol. 1967;63:533-50.
3. Collins JF. Handbook of Clinical Ophthalmology. New York: Masson; 1982.
4. Hori T, Mizukami K, Suzuki T, et al. Ramsay Hunt syndrome with mental disorder. Jpn J Psychiatry Neurol. 1991;45:873-7.
5. Hunt JR. On herpetic inflammations of the geniculate ganglion: a new syndrome and its complications. J Nerv Ment Dis. 1907;34:73-96.
6. Kobayashi K, Morikawa K, Fukutani Y, et al. Ramsay Hunt syndrome: progressive mental deterioration in association with unusual cerebral white matter change. Clin Neuropathol. 1994;13:88-96.
7. Shapiro BE, Slattery M, Pessin MS. Absence of auricular lesions in Ramsay Hunt syndrome. Neurology. 1994;44:773-4.

706. HUNTER SYNDROME (MPS II SYNDROME; MUCOPOLYSACCHARIDOSIS II; SYSTEMIC MUCOPOLYSACCHARIDOSIS TYPE II)

General

Sex-linked recessive inheritance; clinically less severe than Hurler syndrome (MPS I) with a longer life span (into adulthood); similar to MPS I (Hurler syndrome), with chondroitin sulfate B and heparitin sulfate excreted in excess in the urine (see Sanfilippo-Good Syndrome; Morquio-Brailsford Syndrome; Scheie Syndrome; Maroteaux-Lamy Syndrome); X-linked recessive inheritance; decreased iduronate sulfatase.

Ocular

Visual fields may be constricted; splitting or absence of Bowman's membrane in the periphery;

stromal haze may be present; pigmentary degeneration of the retina; night blindness; narrowed retinal vessels and central choroidal sclerosis; bushy eyebrows; coarse eyelashes; ptosis; optic atrophy; papilledema; proptosis; angle-closure glaucoma; corneal clouding; scleral thickening; uveal effusion.

Clinical

Dwarfism; stiff joints; hepatosplenomegaly; gargoyle-like facies.

Laboratory

Urine—dermatan and heparin sulfate; serum—assay of IDS activity; assay for activity of sulfoiduronate sulfatase in fibroblasts.

Treatment

The relevant enzyme [IDS in the case of mucopolysaccharidosis type II (MPS II)] can be given in the form of enzyme replacement therapy (ERT) or by bone marrow transplantation (BMT). Surgical intervention for chronic hydrocephalus, nerve entrapment (carpal tunnel syndrome), abdominal wall hernias, tracheostomy and joint contractures.

Additional Resource

1. Braverman NE (2011). Genetics of Mucopolysaccharidosis Type II. [online] Available from http://www.emedicine.com/ped/TOPIC1029.HTM [Accessed April, 2012].

---

707. HURLER-SCHEIE SYNDROME (MPS I H/S)

General

Clinical disorder with severity midway between the Hurler and Scheie syndromes; genetic compound of the two alleles H and S; autosomal recessive.

Ocular

Corneal clouding; chronically elevated optic disk; diminished or extinguished electroretinogram; pigmentary retinopathy; glaucoma; optic atrophy; retinal pigmentary degeneration.

Clinical

Shares some clinical features of both MPS IH (Hurler) and MPS IS (Scheie); Severe bone involvement; minor intellectual impairment (see Hurler Syndrome; Scheie Syndrome); cardiac failure; cardiomyopathy; conduction defects; valvular heart disease.

Laboratory

Blood smears—abnormal cytoplasmic inclusions in lymphocytes; urine—increased excretion dermatan sulfate and heparin sulfate.

Treatment

Enzyme replacement therapy with laronidase.

Bibliography

1. Frangiegh GT, Traboulsi EI, Kenyon KR. Mucopolysaccharidoses. In: Gold DH, Weingest TA (Eds). The Eye in Systemic Disease. Philadelphia: JB Lippincott; 1990. pp. 372-6.
2. Roy FH, Fraunfelder FW, Fraunfelder FT. Roy and Fraunfelder's Current Ocular Therapy, 6th edition. Philadelphia: WB Saunders; 2008.
3. Karpati G, Carpenter S, Eisen AA, et al. Multiple peripheral nerve entrapments. An unusual phenotypical variant of the Hunter syndrome (mucopolysaccharidosis II) in a family. Arch Neurol. 1974;31:418-22.
4. Kenyon KR, Quigley HA, Hussels IE, et al. The systemic mucopolysaccharidoses. Ultrastructural and histochemical studies of conjunctiva and skin. Am J Ophthalmol. 1972;73:811-33.
5. Klintworth GK, Hawkins HK, Smith CF. Acridine orange particles in cultured fibroblasts. A comparative study of macular corneal dystrophy, systemic mucopolysaccharidoses types I-H and II, and normal controls. Arch Pathol Lab Med. 1979;103:297-9.

708. HURLER SYNDROME (DYSOSTOSIS MULTIPLEX; GARGOYLISM; MPS IH SYNDROME; MUCOPOLYSACCHARIDOSIS IH; PFAUNDLER-HURLER SYNDROME; SYSTEMIC MUCOPOLYSACCHARIDOSIS TYPE IH)

General

Autosomal recessive inheritance; in addition to corneal opacities and enlargement of the head at birth, other symptoms become apparent at the end of the first year; death occurs usually before age 20 years; gross excess of chondroitin sulfate B and heparitin sulfate in the urine (see Hunter Syndrome; Sanfilippo-Good Syndrome; Morquio-Brailsford Syndrome; Scheie Syndrome; Maroteaux-Lamy Syndrome). Jensen suggested that the pathogenesis of the various mucopolysaccharidoses is the same but that the variations in the defective enzymes cause the different types; most common mucopolysaccharidosis, decreased alpha-iduronidase.

Ocular

Proptosis; hypertelorism; thick, enlarged lids; esotropia; diffuse haziness of the cornea at birth progressive to milky opacity; retinal pigmentary changes may exist; macular edema and absence of foveal reflex; optic atrophy; megalocornea; bushy eyebrows; coarse eyelashes; mucopolysaccharide deposits of iris, lens and sclera; enlarged optic foramen; retinal detachment; anisocoria; buphthalmos; nystagmus; secondary open-angle glaucoma; progressive retinopathy with vascular narrowing; hyperpigmentation of the fundus; bone spicule; papilledema.

Clinical

Dorsolumbar kyphosis; head deformities with depressed nose bridge; short cervical spine; short limbs; macroglossia; enlarged liver and spleen; short stature; facial dysmorphism; progressive psychomotor retardation.

Laboratory

Blood smears—abnormal cytoplasmic inclusions in lymphocytes; urine—increased excretion of dermatan sulfate and heparin sulfate.

Treatment

Macular edema: Uses of corticosteroids, carbonic anhydrase inhibitors and NSAIDs are the mainstay of treatment. If traditional therapy is not effective, intraocular injections of Avastin may be helpful. In cases that have vitreous strand tugging against the macula, pars plana vitrectomy may be necessary.

Retinal detachment: Scleral buckle, pneumatic retinopexy and vitrectomy may be used to close all the breaks.

Glaucoma: Its medication should be the first plan of action. If medication is unsuccessful, a filtering surgical procedure with or without antimetabolites may be beneficial.

Papilledema: Underlying cause should be determined and treated. Systemic acetazolamide is the medical therapy of choice.

Additional Resource

1. Banikazemi M (2012). Genetics of Mucopolysaccharidosis Type I. [online] Available from http://www.emedicine.com/ped/TOPIC1031.HTM [Accessed April, 2012].

709. HUTCHINSON-GILFORD SYNDROME (PROGERIA)

General

Inheritance unknown; belongs to group of ectodermal dysplasias (see Werner Syndrome-Progeria of Adults); elevated hyaluronic acid of unknown etiology, likely sporadic dominant mutation.

Ocular

Microphthalmia; hypotrichosis; microcornea; cataract.

Clinical

Appearance of "old age" in children; short stature to dwarfism; dyscephaly; atrophy of skin and subcutaneous adipose tissue; aplasia of maxilla; oligodontia; arteriosclerosis (premature); progeria.

Laboratory

Radiography findings usually manifest within the first or second year of life and most commonly involve the skull, thorax, long bones and phalanges.

Treatment

No effective therapy is available. Careful monitoring and referral to the proper specialists is important.

Additional Resource

1. Shah KN (2011). Hutchinson-Gilford Progeria. [online] Available from http://www.emedicine.com/derm/TOPIC731.HTM [Accessed April, 2012].

710. HUTCHINSON SYNDROME (ADRENAL CORTEX NEUROBLASTOMA WITH ORBITAL METASTASIS; PEPPER SYNDROME)

General

Metastatic infraorbital neuroblastoma after hematogenous dissemination of primary tumor; occurs in infants and children up to age 6 years; poor prognosis; in children neuroblastoma commonly involves the orbit; 15% of patients with neuroblastoma had proptosis and ecchymosis.

Ocular

Exophthalmos; lid hematoma; extraocular muscle palsy; subconjunctival hemorrhages; choroidal metastatic tumor; papilledema; optic atrophy.

Clinical

Severe anemia; increased sedimentation rate; urinary excretion of 3-methoxy-4-hydroxy mandelic acid.

Laboratory

Computed tomography (CT) and MRI are diagnostic.

Treatment

Chemotherapy and bone marrow or stem cell transplantation are used for therapy.

Bibliography

1. Volpe NJ, Albert DM. Metastases to the uvea. In: AlbertDM, Jakobiec FA (Eds). Principles and Practice of Ophthalmology. Philadelphia: WB Saunders; 1994. p. 3260.

711. HYDATID CYST (ECHINOCOCCOSIS)

General

Caused by *Echinococcus granulosus* acquired by contact with a dog host.

Ocular

Conjunctivitis; keratitis; exophthalmos; phthisis bulbi; optic atrophy; optic neuritis; papilledema; abscesses of orbit and cornea; retinal detachment; retinal hemorrhages; cataract; hypopyon; secondary glaucoma; hydatid cysts of the conjunctiva, eyelid, orbit and lacrimal system; acute visual loss; vitreous mass.

Clinical

Pruritus; urticaria; pulmonary cysts; brain cysts; anaphylactic shock; death.

Laboratory

Plain orbital radiographs may show enlarged orbital diameters and increased soft-tissue density. Ultrasonography demonstrates a cystic lesion without internal reflectivity computed tomography discloses a well-defined cystic mass.

Treatment

Echinococcosis is rare and can be severe. Refer patients to reference centers to confirm their diagnosis and to obtain advice on therapeutic strategy.

Additional Resource

1. Vuitton DA (2011). Echinococcosis. [online] Available from http://www.emedicine.com/med/TOPIC326.HTM [Accessed April, 2012].

712. HYDRANENCEPHALY

General

Rare; development disorder in which cerebral hemispheres are replaced by a cystic space filled with cerebrospinal fluid, covered by intact meninges; short life expectancy of weeks to months, but adulthood is possible; positive association with cocaine.

Ocular

Pupillary abnormalities; strabismus; nystagmus; ptosis; optic nerve hypoplasia; chorioretinitis; retinal vessel attenuation; incomplete anterior chamber cleavage; microphthalmia; blepharospasm.

Clinical

Irritability; convulsions; muscular rigidity; decerebrate posturing; increasing head circumference; quadriplegia; psychomotor retardation.

Laboratory

Computed tomography (CT) and MRI the key to distinguishing hydrocephalus from hydranencephaly is the presence of a thin rim of residual cerebral cortical tissue in hydrocephalus that is not present in hydranencephaly. Most cases of hydranencephaly can be detected with prenatal ultrasonography.

Treatment

If the patient's head circumference is increasing because of concomitant hydrocephalus, shunting may be needed for clinical management.

Additional Resource

1. Wagner AL (2011). Imaging in Hydranencephaly. [online] Available from http://www.emedicine.com/radio/TOPIC351.HTM [Accessed April, 2012].

713. HYDROA VACCINIFORME

General

Sensitivity to sunlight.

Ocular

Conjunctivitis; corneal vesiculae; keratitis; cicatricial ectropion.

Clinical

Vesicular skin eruptions in areas exposed to sunlight.

Laboratory

Repetitive, broad-spectrum, UV-A phototesting.

Treatment

Consult a dermatologist for evaluation and management of hydroa vacciniforme (HV).

Additional Resource

1. Sebastian QL (2011). Hydroa Vacciniforme. [online] Available from http://www.emedicine.com/derm/TOPIC181.HTM [Accessed April, 2012].

714. HYDROPHOBIA (LYSSA; RABIES)

General

Acute viral zoonosis of the central nervous system.

Ocular

Lid retraction; widening of palpebral fissure; retinal hemorrhages; mydriasis; paralysis of third, fourth, fifth or seventh nerve; bilateral optic neuritis; branch retinal artery occlusion; vaccine-induced autoimmune demyelinative optic neuritis.

Clinical

Fever; headache; nausea; numbness; tingling; acute sensitiveness to sound and light; laryngeal and pharyngeal spasms; increased muscle tonus; convulsions; delirium; coma; death.

Laboratory

Saliva can be tested by virus isolation or reverse transcription followed by polymerase chain reaction. Suspected infections, animal should be quarantined for 10 days.

Treatment

Before the onset of symptoms, both passive and active immunizations are effective for preventing progression to full-blown rabies. In exposures to high-risk species, initiate treatment immediately pending laboratory examination of the animal, if it is caught.

Additional Resource

1. Gompf SG (2011). Rabies. [online] Available from http://www.emedicine.com/med/TOPIC1374.HTM [Accessed April, 2012].

715. HYPERAMMONEMIA I (CARBAMYL PHOSPHATE SYNTHETASE DEFICIENCY; HYPERAMMONEMIA II; HYPERAMMONEMIA-HYPERORNITHINEMIA-HOMOCITRULLINURIA SYNDROME; ORNITHINE TRANSCARBAMYLASE DEFICIENCY)

General

Hyperammonemias I and II are due to errors at or near the "start" of the urea cycle; in hyperammonemia I, a decrease in the activity of the enzyme carbamyl phosphate synthetase, responsible for the first step of the cycle, results in the accumulation of excess ammonia; in hyperammonemia II, the defect is in ornithine transcarbamylase; type II occurs only in infants.

Ocular

Ptosis and visual loss; retinal depigmentation and chorioretinal thinning.

Clinical

Vomiting; screaming; confusion; lethargy; ataxia; mental retardation; atrophy of cerebral cortex; decreased vibration sense; bucco-faciolingual dyspraxia; learning difficulties; widespread manifestations in the central and peripheral nervous systems.

Laboratory

Plasma ornithine is increased at the time of presentation, which differentiates hyperornithinemia-hyperammonemia-homocitrullinemia (HHH) syndrome from other urea cycle disorders.

Treatment

Ornithine supplementation, arginine supplementation, sodium benzoate and sodium phenylacetate may reduce ammonia levels, crisis might be managed with short-term protein restriction and intravenous fluids that contain large amounts of glucose.

Additional Resource

1. Frye RE (2012). Genetics of Hyperammonemia-Hyperornithinemia-Homocitrullinemia Syndrome. [online] Available from http://www.emedicine.com/ped/TOPIC1058.HTM [Accessed April, 2012].

716. HYPERKALEMIC FAMILIAL PERIODIC PARALYSIS (ADYNAMIA EPISODICA HEREDITARIA)

General

Recurrent paralysis of skeletal muscles; occurs by age 10 years; usually occurs during the day when patient is sitting in a chair without exercise; attacks last 30 minutes to 2 hours.

Ocular

Transient attacks of staring with lid elevation in younger children; sclera above cornea is visible in adults when they look down; lid lag is present during attacks but repeated up-and-down movements of eyes help.

Clinical

Muscle weakness; difficulty swallowing and coughing; tremor; episodes of quadriparesis lasting 2–3 weeks; salt craving; intense thirst; stomach pain.

Treatment

Ocular lubricants are beneficial for control of the corneal exposure.

Additional Resource

1. Sripathi N (2010). Periodic Paralyses. [online] Available from http://www.emedicine.com/neuro/TOPIC308.HTM [Accessed April, 2012].

717. HYPERLIPOPROTEINEMIA

General

Metabolic disorder characterized by abnormally elevated concentrations of specific lipoprotein particles in the plasma.

Ocular

Arcus; lipid keratopathy; xanthelasma; lipemia retinalis; lipemia of limbal vessels; xanthomata of choroid, conjunctiva, eyelids, iris and retina; central retinal vein occlusion; Schnyder crystalline corneal dystrophy (association).

Clinical

Deposition of lipids at various sites throughout the body, such as skin, tendons and vascular system.

Laboratory

A standard serum lipid profile consists of total cholesterol, triglycerides and HDL cholesterol.

Measure plasma lipid and lipoprotein levels while the patient is on a regular diet after an overnight fast of 12–16 hours.

Treatment

Drugs are used to lower cholesterol and triglyceride levels.

Additional Resource

1. Roy H (2011). Hyperlipoproteinemia. [online] Available from http://www.emedicine.com/oph/TOPIC505.HTM [Accessed April, 2012].

718. HYPEROPIA, HIGH

General

Defect in eyesight in which the focal point falls behind the retina, resulting in farsightedness; autosomal recessive; eye shorter than normal.

Ocular

Farsightedness

Clinical

None

Laboratory

Diagnosis is made by clinical findings.

Treatment

Glasses, contact lens, conductive keratoplasty, LASIK and phakic IOL.

Additional Resource

1. Roque MR (2011). Conductive Keratoplasty Hyperopia and Presbyopia. [online] Available from http://www.emedicine.com/oph/TOPIC736.HTM [Accessed April, 2012].

719. HYPEROPIA LASIK

General

Farsightedness corrected with a surgical procedure LASIK which is done, cutting a corneal flap and using an excimer laser to steepen the cornea to correct the hyperopia.

Clinical

None

Ocular

Inability to see well distance or near without correction. Possible complications include displaced flap, corneal perforation, interface debris and diffuse lamellar keratitis.

Laboratory

Corneal topography; corneal pachymetry; keratometry; cycloplegic refraction; slit lamp examination.

Treatment

Glasses or contact lens can be used to correct hyperopia. If patient is unhappy with glasses or contact lens, LASIK can be considered.

Additional Resource

1. Gulani AC (2011). LASIK Hyperopia Treatment & Management. [online] Available from http://www.emedicine.medscape.com/article/1221098-treatment [Accessed April, 2012].

---

720. HYPEROPIA, PHAKIC IOL

General

Farsightedness corrected with a surgical procedure, phakic IOL. It is used more frequently in individuals with higher degree of hyperopia.

Clinical

None

Ocular

Inability to see well distance or near without correction.

Laboratory

Corneal topography; corneal pachymetry; keratometry; cycloplegic refraction; slit lamp examination; IOL power calculation.

Treatment

Glasses or contact lens can be used to correct hyperopia. If patient is unhappy with glasses or contact lens, phakic IOL can be considered.

Additional Resource

1. Singh D (2011). Phakic IOL Hyperopia. [online] Available from http://www.emedicine.medscape.com/article/1221201-overview [Accessed April, 2012].

---

721. HYPERPARATHYROIDISM

General

Increased secretion of parathyroid hormone.

Ocular

Glasslike crystals of conjunctiva; band keratopathy; optic atrophy; papilledema; vascular engorgement of retina; ptosis; scleral thinning; ectopic calcifications in the choroid and sclera; unilateral visual loss; ischemic optic neuropathy.

Clinical

Hypercalcemia; hypophosphatemia; brown tumor.

Laboratory

Diagnosis is made based on hypercalcemia and elevated parathyroid hormone levels. Other abnormal laboratory findings may include elevated BUN and creatinine levels, hyperchloremic acidosis, reduced serum bicarbonate levels due to renal bicarbonate casting, hypophosphatemia, elevated alkaline phosphatase levels and hypercalciuria.

Treatment

Surgical removal of the pathologic gland or glands. Medical management of hyperparathyroidism is generally reserved for patients with poor medical conditions.

Additional Resource

1. LaBagnara J (2011). Hyperparathyroidism in Otolaryngology and Facial Plastic Surgery. [online] Available from http://www.emedicine.com/ent/TOPIC299.HTM [Accessed April, 2012].

722. HYPERPIGMENTATION OF EYELIDS

General

Autosomal dominant; causes may include drugs, sun or too little adrenaline.

Ocular

Unusual darkening of eyelids.

Clinical

None

Laboratory

Diagnosis is made by clinical findings. If malignancy is suspected biopsy should be performed.

Treatment

Benign pigmented lesions of the eyelids do not require any medical therapy. Benign lesion that affects vision should be excised with primary reconstruction. Surgical therapy may be performed for cosmetic reasons or suspicion of malignancy in benign pigmented lesions.

Additional Resource

1. Bashour M (2011). Pigmented Lesions of the Eyelid. [online] Available from http://www.emedicine.com/oph/TOPIC715.HTM [Accessed April, 2012].

723. HYPERTENSION

General

Elevated blood pressure.

Ocular

Retinal arterial narrowing; arteriosclerosis; hemorrhages; retinal edema; cotton-wool spots; fatty exudates; optic disk edema; exudative retinal detachment; optic neuropathy; swollen optic nerve; central retinal vein occlusion; branch retinal vein occlusion; choroidal ischemia.

Clinical

Systemic hypertension; patchy loss of muscle tone in vessel walls; vascular decompensation.

Laboratory

Diagnosis is made from clinical findings, CBC, serum electrolytes, serum creatinine, serum glucose, uric acid, and urinalysis, Lipid profile [total cholesterol, low-density lipoprotein (LDL), high-density lipoprotein (HDL), and triglycerides].

Treatment

Lifestyle modifications—weight loss, stop smoking, exercise, reduce stress, limit alcohol intake, reduce sodium intake, maintain adequate calicium and potassium intake. Refer to internist for drug therapy.

Additional Resource

1. Riaz K (2012). Hypertension. [online] Available from http://www.emedicine.com/med/TOPIC1106.HTM [Accessed April, 2012].

724. HYPERTRICHOSIS (HIRSUTISM)

General

Excessive hair growth due to endocrinologic or physiologic states.

Ocular

Keratitis; excessive cilia; ectropic cilia; monilethrix; pili torti; polytrichosis; reduplication of ciliary follicles; trichomegaly; association between congenital hypertrichosis lanuginosa and congenital glaucoma.

Clinical

Excessive hair growth on any part of the body except palms and soles; eczema; psoriasis; lupus erythematosus; association with acquired immunodeficiency syndrome.

Laboratory

Diagnosis is made by clinical findings.

Treatment

The use of eflornithine (Vaniqa cream), 13.9% or hair removal by means of repeated shaving, depilatory methods (e.g. chemical, electric methods) or bleaching can improve the patient's appearance.

Additional Resource

1. Taylor SK (2012). Congenital Hypertrichosis Lanuginosa. [online] Available from http://www.emedicine.com/derm/TOPIC811.HTM [Accessed April, 2012].

725. HYPERTRICHOSIS CUBITI (HAIRY ELBOW SYNDROME)

General

Autosomal dominant; occurs in childhood and regresses spontaneously in puberty; long vellus hair on extensor surface of the distal third of the upper arms and proximal third of the forearms.

Ocular

Facial dysmorphias.

Clinical

Mental retardation; short stature.

Laboratory

Diagnosis is made by clinical findings.

Treatment

The use of eflornithine (Vaniqa cream), 13.9% or hair removal by means of repeated shaving, depilatory methods (e.g. chemical, electric methods) or bleaching can improve the patient's appearance.

Additional Resource

1. Taylor SK (2012). Congenital Hypertrichosis Lanuginosa. [online] Available from http://www.emedicine.com/derm/TOPIC811.HTM [Accessed April, 2012].

726. HYPERTROPHIC NEUROPATHY

General

Autosomal recessive.

Ocular

Cataract

Clinical

Elevated spinal fluid protein; severe distal sensory and motor loss.

Laboratory

Diagnosis is made by clinical findings.

Treatment

Cataract surgery is the treatment of choice and should be performed when patients are younger than 17 weeks to ensure minimal or no visual deprivation.

Bibliography

1. Gold GN, Hogenhuis LA. Hypertrophic interstitial neuropathy and cataracts. Neurology. 1968;18: 526-33.
2. McKusick VA. Mendelian Inheritance in Man: A Catalog of Human Genes and Genetic Disorders, 12th edition. Baltimore: The Johns Hopkins University Press; 1998.

727. HYPERVITAMINOSIS A

General

Excessive vitamin A ingestion.

Ocular

Papilledema; congenital cataract; congenital anophthalmos; night blindness; diplopia; exophthalmos; "hourglass" cornea and iris with reduplicated lens.

Clinical

Elevation of cerebrospinal fluid pressure; migratory polyarthritis; hepatosplenomegaly; skin changes.

Laboratory

Diagnosis is usually based on a high index of suspicion in children who are malnourished or in patients with predisposing factors for its development.

Treatment

Oral administration of vitamin A 200,000 IU at presentation, the following day, and a third dose one week later is recommended. Infants should receive half doses.

Additional Resource

1. Schwartz RA (2012). Dermatologic Manifestations of Vitamin A Deficiency. [online] Available from http://www.emedicine.com/derm/TOPIC794. HTM [Accessed April, 2012].

728. HYPERVITAMINOSIS D

General

Excessive vitamin D ingestion.

Ocular

Band keratopathy; epicanthal folds; osteosclerosis of orbital bones; nystagmus; papilledema; iritis; cataract; sluggish pupillary reaction.

Clinical

Hypercalcemia; calcium deposition in body tissues.

Laboratory

Serum calcium, X-ray, CT and MRI may be helpful.

Treatment

Initial treatment involves hydration to improve urinary calcium output. Isotonic sodium chloride solution is used, because increasing sodium excretion increases calcium excretion. Addition of a loop diuretic inhibits tubular reabsorption of calcium, with furosemide having been used up to every 2 hours.

Bibliography

1. Kasper DL, Braunwald E, Fauci AS, Hauser SL, Longo DL, Jameson JL (Eds). Harrison's Principles of Internal Medicine, 16th edition. New York: McGraw-Hill; 2005.

2. Collins JF. Handbook of Clinical Ophthalmology. New York: Masson; 1982.

3. Duke-Elder S (Ed). System of Ophthalmology. St. Louis: CV Mosby; 1976. p. 75.

4. Jacobus CH, Holick MF, Shao Q, et al. Hypervitaminosis D associated with drinking milk. N Engl J Med. 1992;326:1173-7.

729. HYPHEMA (TRAUMATIC HYPHEMA)

General

Trauma although bleeding may occur spontaneously in conditions, such as rubeosis iridis, leukemia, hemophilia, anticoagulation therapy, retinoblastoma or juvenile xanthogranuloma of iris.

Clinical

None

Ocular

Tear and bleeding from the iris, ciliary body, or elevated intraocular pressure may occur.

Laboratory

Diagnosis is made by clinical findings.

Treatment

Cycloplegia decreased the inflammation and discomfort associated with traumatic iritis. Topical beta-adreneric antagonists are the therapy of choice for elevated intraocular pressures.

Additional Resource

1. Sheppard JD (2011). Hyphema. [online] Available from http://www.emedicine.com/oph/TOPIC765. HTM [Accessed April, 2012].

730. HYPOCALCEMIA

General

Serum calcium level depressed; secondary hypocalcemia can result following foscarnet treatment for cytomegalovirus retinitis in patients with acquired immunodeficiency syndrome.

Ocular

Conjunctivitis; blepharitis; blepharospasm; madarosis; ptosis; cataract; papilledema; strabismus.

Clinical

Chronic renal failure; hypoparathyroidism; hypoproteinemia; hypomagnesemia; malabsorption; acute pancreatitis; osteoblastic metastases; rickets; osteomalacia; medullary carcinoma of the thyroid; neuromuscular abnormalities.

Laboratory

Serum calcium and magnesium levels, serum electrolyte and glucose levels, phosphorus levels and parathyroid hormone (PTH) levels.

Treatment

Intravenous treatment is usually indicated in patients having seizures, those who are critically ill, and those who are planning to have surgery. Oral calcium therapy is used in asymptomatic patients and as follow-up to intravenous calcium therapy.

Additional Resource

1. Ferry RJ (2011). Pediatric Hypocalcemia. [online] Available from http://www.emedicine.com/ped/TOPIC1111.HTM [Accessed April, 2012].

731. HYPOGONADISM-CATARACT SYNDROME

General

Autosomal recessive.

Ocular

Cataracts

Clinical

Elevated follicle-stimulating hormone levels; myotonic dystrophy; infertility.

Laboratory

Diagnosis is made by clinical findings.

Treatment

Cataract surgery is the therapy of choice if there is visual limitation.

Bibliography

1. Lubinsky MS. Cataracts and testicular failure in three brothers. Am J Med Genet. 1983;16:149-52.
2. McKusick VA. Mendelian Inheritance in Man: A Catalog of Human Genes and Genetic Disorders, 12th edition. Baltimore: The Johns Hopkins University Press; 1998.

732. HYPOLIPIDEMIA SYNDROME (HOOFT SYNDROME)

General

Autosomal recessive inheritance; disorder of tryptophan metabolism; normal glycolysis disturbed, which in turn interferes with normal fat synthesis; low levels of serum phospholipids, present from birth.

Ocular

Tapetoretinal degeneration of the posterior pole with irregular, small areas of grayish-yellow discoloration scattered over posterior aspect of the retina; increased shiny reflection from the macular region, with "wet" and shiny appearance.

Clinical

Mental retardation; disturbance in normal growth; anomalies of hair, nails and teeth; erythematous squamous skin rash (mainly face, arms and legs).

Laboratory

Lipids can be routinely measured individually as TC, TGs or HDL-C.

Treatment

Rare and will need to be followed by an internist.

Bibliography

1. Collins JF. Handbook of Clinical Ophthalmology. New York: Masson; 1982.
2. Francois J. Ocular manifestations in certain congenital errors of metabolism. Symposium on Surgical and Medical Management of Congenital Anomalies of the Eye. St. Louis: CV Mosby; 1968. p. 171.
3. Hooft C, De Laey P, Herpol J, et al. Familial hypolipidaemia and retarded development without steatorrhea: another inborn error of metabolism? Helv Paediatr Acta. 1962;17:1-23.

733. HYPOMELANOSIS OF ITO SYNDROME (INCONTINENTIA PIGMENTI ACHROMIANS; SYSTEMATIZED ACHROMIC NEVUS)

General

Probable autosomal dominant transmission; cutaneous abnormality consisting of bizarre, patterned, macular hypopigmentation over variable portions of the body with multiple associated defects in other body systems; abnormal chromosome constitutions.

Ocular

Iridal heterochromia; myopia; esotropia; microphthalmia; hypertelorism; nystagmus; strabismus; corneal opacity; choroidal atrophy; exotropia; small optic nerve; hypopigmentation of the fundus; corneal asymmetry; pannus; atrophic irides with irregular pupillary margins; cataract; retinal detachment.

Clinical

Cutaneous manifestations consisting of macular hypopigmented whorls, streaks and patches in a bilateral or unilateral distribution affecting almost any portion of the body surface; 50% have associated noncutaneous abnormalities, including central nervous system dysfunction (seizure, delayed development) and musculoskeletal anomalies.

Laboratory

Diagnosis is made by clinical findings.

Treatment

No treatment is necessary for the cutaneous findings except makeup for cosmetic purposes. Other symptoms should be treated by specific specialists.

Additional Resource

1. Ratz JL (2012). Hypomelanosis of Ito. [online] Available from http://www.emedicine.com/derm/TOPIC186.HTM [Accessed April, 2012].

734. HYPOPARATHYROIDISM

General

Deficient secretion of parathyroid hormone.

Ocular

Keratitis; blepharospasm; ptosis; cataract; madarosis; optic neuritis; papilledema; conjunctivitis; myopia; ocular colobomata.

Clinical

Decreased blood calcium; increased serum phosphate; tetany; muscle cramps; stridor; carpopedal spasms; convulsions; lethargy; personality changes; mental retardation; intracranial calcification; choreoathetosis; hemiballismus; renal agenesis.

Laboratory

Diagnosis made rests on the functional capacity of the adrenal cortex to synthesize cortisol. This is accomplished primarily by use of the rapid ACTH stimulation test (Cortrosyn, cosyntropin or Synacthen).

Treatment

Endocrinologist should be consulted for the acute care and chronic care.

Additional Resource

1. Gonzalez-Campoy JM (2012). Hypoparathyroidism. [online] Available from http://www.emedicine.com/med/TOPIC1131.HTM [Accessed April, 2012].

---

735. HYPOPHOSPHATASIA (PHOSPHOETHANOLAMINURIA)

General

Inborn error of metabolism that entails increased urinary excretion of phosphoethanolamine and associated with low alkaline phosphatase and hypercalcemia; prevalent in females; may result from absence or abnormal circulating factor regulating expression of alkaline phosphatase.

Ocular

Papilledema; optic atrophy; exophthalmos; blue sclera; conjunctival calcification; lid retraction; cataract; corneal subepithelial calcifications.

Clinical

Defect in true bone formation associated with widespread skeletal abnormalities; low serum alkaline phosphatase activity; hypercalcemia; nausea; vomiting; bowing of legs; convulsions; premature loss of teeth.

Laboratory

Assess the alkaline phosphatase levels. The levels are low in all types of hypophosphatasia. Fasting laboratory evaluations should include levels of calcium, phosphorus, magnesium, alkaline phosphatase, creatinine, parathyroid hormone (PTH), 25(OH) vitamin D and 1,25(OH)2 vitamin D. Levels of PLP, PPi, and PEA in serum and urine determine the diagnosis.

Treatment

No medical therapy is available. Supportive care is necessary to decrease the morbidity associated with hypophosphatasia. Regularly examine infants and children to check for evidence of increased intracranial pressure. Observe fractures closely. Adult pseudofractures may require orthopedic care to heal properly. A dentist should closely monitor all individuals with hypophosphatasia.

Additional Resource

1. Plotkin H (2010). Hypophosphatasia. [online] Available from http://www.emedicine.com/ped/TOPIC1126.HTM [Accessed April, 2012].

736. HYPOPROTEINEMIA SYNDROME (KWASHIORKOR SYNDROME; MALNUTRITION SYNDROME; PLURIDEFICIENCY SYNDROME)

General

Manifested in children aged 4–5 years; widespread in underdeveloped countries; lack of adequate intake of protein; good prognosis with adequate diet therapy, otherwise fatal outcome; pseudomotor cerebri.

Ocular

Dullness of cornea and conjunctiva; thick, sticky and foamy conjunctival excretion; corneal infiltrations and cloudiness; corneal ulcers (minimally inflammatory); keratomalacia possible in prolonged cases without therapy, eventually leading to panophthalmitis.

Clinical

Muscle atrophy; generalized edema; anorexia; vomiting; diarrhea; hepatosplenomegaly; dermatitis with desquamation; pigmentation and dyspigmentation; irritability; apathy; changes in hair color; hair becomes straight; hepatomegaly; failure to grow; weak cry.

Laboratory

Hematological studies and laboratory studies evaluating protein status.

Treatment

Identification of the underlying etiology and dietary intervention.

Additional Resource

1. Shashidhar HR (2011). Malnutrition. [online] Available from http://www.emedicine.com/ped/TOPIC1360.HTM [Accessed April, 2012].

737. HYPOTHALAMIQUE CARREFOUR SYNDROME (CARREFOUR HYPOTHALAMIQUE SYNDROME)

General

Onset is sudden with hemiplegia; etiology unknown.

Ocular

Visual loss.

Clinical

Hypertension; hemianesthesia; apraxia; astereognosia; asynergias.

Laboratory

Electromyography, neurolysis, MRI.

Treatment

Neuromuscular electrical stimulation, physical therapy.

Bibliography

1. Geeraets WJ. Ocular Syndromes, 3rd edition. Philadelphia: Lea & Febiger; 1976.
2. Ramirez F, Arana Iniguez R. Sindrome de la Encrucijada Hipotalamica (The "Carrefour Hypothalamique" Syndrome). Ann Fac Med (Montevideo). 1952;37:109.

738. HYPOTHERMAL INJURY (CRYOINJURY; FROSTBITE)

General

Loss of body heat to the point of local cold injury or freezing of tissue.

Ocular

Localized cryoinjury that can cause choroidal atrophy, retinal hemorrhages, hyperpigmentation of retina, uveitis, corneal edema, neovascularization of cornea, ectropion, lid edema, madarosis, pseudoepitheliomatous hyperplasia, iris atrophy and paresis of extraocular muscles.

Clinical

Vesicles and blebs of affected tissue, especially ears, fingers, toes and nose; contractures; dry gangrene of affected tissues.

Laboratory

Diagnosis is made by clinical findings.

Treatment

The management of frostbite may be divided into 3 phases: (1) field management, (2) rewarming and (3) post-rewarming management. Rewarm the affected area in warm water at 40–42ºC (104–108ºF) for 15–30 minutes or until thawing is complete by clinical assessment. Debridement of white or clear blisters and topical treatment is necessary in the post-rewarming management.

Additional Resource

1. Bjerke HS (2012). Frostbite. [online] Available from http://www.emedicine.com/med/TOPIC2815. HTM [Accessed April, 2012].

739. HYPOTRICHOSIS WITH JUVENILE MACULAR DYSTROPHY SYNDROME (HJMD)

General

Rare; autosomal recessive.

Ocular

Macular dystrophy; hypotrichosis; vitreous hemorrhage in newborns.

Clinical

Early hair loss.

Laboratory

Diagnosis is made by clinical findings.

Treatment

Ocular lubrication, corneal erosion therapy including patching, bandage contact lens and topical ointments. Excessive corneal erosions or a mild visual decrease can be treated with excimer laser phototherapeutic keratectomy (PTK).

Bibliography

1. Dana MR, Werner MS, Viana MA, et al. Spontaneous and traumatic vitreous hemorrhage. Ophthalmology. 1993;100:1377-83.
2. Leibu R, Jermans A, Hatim G, et al. Hypotrichosis with juvenile macular dystrophy. Ophthalmology. 2006;113:841-7.

740. HYPOVITAMINOSIS A (XEROPHTHALMIA)

General

Deficient serum levels of vitamin A; principal cause of infantile blindness in the world; due to insufficient intake of vitamin A or interference with its absorption from the intestinal tract; transport or storage in the liver; obstruction of biliary tract or pancreatic ducts.

Ocular

Bitot spot; xerosis; keratomalacia; keratitis; corneal perforation and ulcer; corneal opacity; hyperkeratosis; retinal degeneration; scotoma.

Clinical

Inadequate dietary intake or interference with absorptive storage or transport capacities, as occurs in liver disease, sprue, regional enteritis and chronic gastroenteritis; respiratory infection; diarrhea; reduced childhood mortality.

Laboratory

Serum vitamin A levels.

Treatment

Oral administration of vitamin A 200,000 IU at presentation, the following day, and a third dose one week later is recommended. Infants should receive half doses.

Additional Resource

1. Schwartz RA (2012). Dermatologic Manifestations of Vitamin A Deficiency. [online] Available from http://www.emedicine.com/derm/TOPIC794.HTM [Accessed April, 2012].

741. HYSTERIA (MALINGERING; OPHTHALMIC FLAKE SYNDROME)

General

Willful or unwillful exaggeration or simulation of symptoms of an illness without physiologic cause; frequently secondary to a state of anxiety; may be seen more in children; physical or sexual abuse may be a predisposing factor.

Ocular

Anxiety-induced angiospastic or central serous retinopathy; self-induced conjunctivitis; traumatic epithelial erosions; herpetic keratitis; angioneurotic edema; contact dermatitis; ptosis; recurrent herpetic vesicles; anisocoria; peculiar pupillary reflexes; accommodative spasm; amaurosis fugax; anxiety-induced optic neuritis; disturbance of conjugate movement; dyschromatopsia; facial tic; hypersecretion glaucoma; increased or decreased tear secretion; night blindness; nystagmus; photophobia; strabismus; visual loss; psychogenic amaurosis with headaches.

Clinical

Aphonia; deafness; paralysis of limb; hemiplegia; dissociative state; anxiety; insomnia; tachycardia; shortness of breath; fatigue; vertigo, chest pains.

Laboratory

Eye examination to rule out pathology. Visual evoked responses, electroretinopathy and electro-oculography all should be normal.

Treatment

Psychiatric intervention is required in severe cases.

Bibliography

1. Barris MC, Kaufman DI, Barberio D. Visual impairment in hysteria. Doc Ophthalmol. 1992;82:369-82.
2. Catalono RA, Simon JW, Krohel GB, et al. Functional visual loss in children. Ophthalmology. 1986;93:385-90.
3. Roy FH, Fraunfelder FW, Fraunfelder FT. Roy and Fraunfelder's Current Ocular Therapy, 6th edition. Philadelphia: WB Saunders; 2008.
4. Kramer KK, La Piana FG, Appleton B. Ocular malingering and hysteria: diagnosis and management. Surv Ophthalmol. 1979;24:89-96.
5. Miller BW. A review of practical tests for ocular malingering and hysteria. Surv Ophthalmol. 1973;17:241-6.
6. Ziegler DK, Schlemmer RB. Familial psychogenic blindness and headache: a case study. J Clin Psychiatry. 1994;55:114-7.

---

742. IMPETIGO

General

Superficial primary pyoderma caused by streptococci and *Staphylococcus aureus*.

Ocular

Pustular, crusting lesions of eyelids and eyebrows; conjunctivitis; corneal ulcer; cicatricial ankyloblepharon.

Clinical

Thin-roofed vesicles that develop a thin amber crust occur on face and exposed areas of the extremities; extremely common skin infections caused by *S. aureus* in patients infected with human immunodeficiency virus (HIV).

Laboratory

Diagnosis is made by clinical findings.

Treatment

Antibiotics are the mainstay of therapy and the chosen agent must provide coverage against both *S. aureus* and *S. pyogenes*. Topical antibiotics are used in patients with small or few lesions.

Additional Resource

1. Lewis LS (2011). Impetigo. [online] Available from http://www.emedicine.com/derm/TOPIC195.HTM [Accessed April, 2012].

---

743. INCIPIENT PRECHIASMAL OPTIC NERVE COMPRESSION SYNDROME

General

Caused by an expansive prechiasmal tumor or other lesion slowly compressing the optic nerve; frequently unilateral.

Ocular

Gradually progressive dimming of vision with near-normal acuity; reduced color perception (dyschromatopsia); subtle monocular field defects (progressive); positive Marcus Gunn pupillary sign (afferent pupillary light defect); optic nerve atrophy, depending on duration of compression before removal of the lesion; central or hemicentral scotoma.

Clinical

None

Laboratory

Computed tomography (CT) scans and MRIs are useful for determining the cause of optic nerve compression.

Treatment

Radiation therapy often is appropriate for malignant lesions, surgical excision or decompression as a treatment option when orbital tumors compress the optic nerve.

Additional Resource

1. Kim JW (2011). Compressive Optic Neuropathy. [online] Available from http://www.emedicine.com/oph/TOPIC167.HTM [Accessed April, 2012].

---

744. INFANTILE NEUROAXONAL DYSTROPHY [SEITELBERGER DISEASE (2); SPASTIC AMAUROTIC AXONAL IDIOCY]

General

Axonal disease; occurs chiefly in female infants, less frequently in older children; etiology possibly vitamin E deficiency; autosomal recessive; selective axonal degeneration in the retina.

Ocular

Nystagmus; blindness; degeneration of optic pathways and long tracts.

Clinical

Muscular hypotonia; decreased pain sense; arrest of development in late infancy; areflexia; atonic bladder; dementia; spasticity; ataxia; spread of axonal lesions in the posterior gray horns of spinal cord, restiform bodies and tegmentum of the lower brainstem; atrophy of the cerebral cortex; degeneration of the caudate nucleus and putamen with accumulation of lipids in these nuclei and in the globus pallidus may be associated; accumulation of iron-containing pigment in the globus pallidus and putamen occurs.

Laboratory

Bone marrow histiocytes and peripheral lymphocytes may demonstrate the presence of abnormal cytosomes including fingerprint, granular and multilaminated bodies. MRI may also be useful.

Treatment

Dystonia is the most prominent and disabling symptom and responds to a modest extent to dopaminergic agents such as levodopa and bromocriptine. A multidisciplinary team approach involving physical, occupational and speech therapists may be needed in selected patients with a protracted course to improve functional skills and communication.

Additional Resource

1. Hanna PA (2012). Hallervorden-Spatz Disease. [online] Available from http://www.emedicine.com/neuro/TOPIC151.HTM [Accessed April, 2012].

745. INFANTILE TYPE OF NEURONAL CEROID LIPOFUSCINOSIS (CEROID LIPOFUSCINOSIS; HAGBERG-SANTAVUORI SYNDROME; HALTIA-SANTAVUORI SYNDROME; SANTAVUORI-HALTIA SYNDROME)

General

Age of onset varies between 8 and 18 months; autosomal recessive; widespread loss of photoreceptor function; cerebral deterioration; death occurs at age 5–9 years (see Ceroid Lipofuscinosis).

Ocular

Visual failure simultaneously with or before neurologic signs; blindness; brownish macula and other signs of macular degeneration with narrow retinal vessels; atrophic optic disk; hypopigmented dystrophic peripheral retina without pigments; nystagmus; exotropia; formed and unformed visual hallucinations.

Clinical

Psychomotor deterioration; generalized muscular hypotonia; ataxia; myoclonic jerks; "knitting" hyperkinesia; microcephaly; convulsions (rare).

Laboratory

Lipid profile with possible protein electrophoresis.

Treatment

Maximize the vision with refraction and low-vision evaluation.

Bibliography

1. Berson EL. Retinitis pigmentosa and allied diseases. In: Albert DM, Jakobiec FA (Eds). Principles and Practice of Ophthalmology. Philadelphia: WB Saunders; 1999. p. 548.
2. Lanska DJ, Lanska MJ. Visual release hallucinations in juvenile neuronal ceroid-lipofuscinosis. Pediatr Neurol. 1993;9:316-7.

746. INFECTIOUS MONONUCLEOSIS (ACUTE; ACUTE EPSTEIN-BARR VIRUS, EPSTEIN-BARR VIRUS, GLANDULAR FEVER; MONONUCLEOSIS)

General

Asymptomatic in childhood; manifested in late adolescence of early adulthood; associated with Burkitt lymphoma and nasopharyngeal carcinoma.

Ocular

Conjunctivitis; ptosis; hippus; dacryocystitis; episcleritis; hemianopsia; nystagmus; retinal and subconjunctival hemorrhages; optic neuritis; orbital edema; scotoma; paralysis of extraocular muscles; uveitis; peripheral choroiditis; keratitis; papilledema; scleritis; retrobulbar neuritis, Sjögren syndrome; retinitis; choroiditis.

Clinical

Fever; widespread lymphadenopathy; pharyngitis; hepatic involvement; presence of atypical lymphocytes and heterophile antibodies in the blood; fatigue.

Treatment

A self-limited illness that does not usually require specific therapy. If splenic rupture is an acute abdominal emergency that usually requires surgical intervention.

Additional Resource

1. Cunha BA (2011). Infectious Mononucleosis. [online] Available from http://www.emedicine.com/med/TOPIC1499.HTM [Accessed April, 2012].

747. INFERIOR RECTUS MUSCLE PALSY

General

Rare, usually associated with abnormalities of one or more additional extraocular muscles.

Clinical

Myasthenia gravis, blowout fracture.

Ocular

Chronic progressive external ophthalmoplegia, orbital neoplasm, rectus muscle myositis.

Laboratory

Diagnosis is made by clinical findings.

Treatment

Prisms, monocular occlusion and surgical management of inferior rectus muscle.

Bibliography

1. Roy FH, Fraunfelder FW, Fraunfelder FT. Roy and Fraunfelder's Current Ocular Therapy, 6th edition. Philadelphia: WB Saunders; 2008.

748. INFLAMMATORY OPTIC NEUROPATHIES

Condition	Clinical	Laboratory	Treatment
Autoimmune optic neuritis	Bilateral severe progressive visual loss, positive ANA (antinuclear antibody)	MRI of orbits and brain, CSF examination, ANA	Corticosteroids Azathioprine Chlorambucil
Behçet's disease	Bilateral simultaneous visual loss, uveitis, retinal vasculitis, genital ulceration, acneiform nodules	MRI of orbits and brain, CSF examination, ANA, biopsy of ulcerated lesion	Costicosteroids Ciclosporin
Chronic relapsing inflammatory optic neuropathy (CRION)	Bilateral simultaneous visual loss, no evidence of sarcoid or vasculitis	MRI of orbits and brain, CSF examination, serum and CSF ACE, ANA, chest X-ray, gallium scan	Corticosteroids Azathioprine Methotrexate
Neuromyelitis optica (NMO) or Devic's disease	Bilateral simultaneous visual loss, transverse myelitis, monophasic or relapsing course	MRI of orbits and brain, and spinal cord, CSF examination, serum NMO-IgG	Corticosteroids Plasma exchange Azathioprine Rituximab
Neuroretinitis	Swollen optic disk with macular star, spontaneous recovery, although relapsing	Bartonella, Borrelia, Syphilis and Toxoplasma serology	Corticosteroids Azathioprine Antibiotics
Optic perineuritis	Arcuate or paracentral scotoma often with spared central vision, circumferential optic nerve sheath	MRI of orbits and brain, CSF examination	Corticosteroids Azathioprine
Postinfectious postimmunization acute disseminated encephalomyelitis	Bilateral optic neurology, often in childhood, good prognosis	MRI of orbits and brain, CSF examination	Corticosteroids

| Sarcoidosis | Bilateral simultaneous visual loss, isolated optic neuropathy, common in African, Afro-Caribbean or African-American populations | MRI of orbits and brain, CSF examination, serum and CSF ACE, chest X-ray, Gallium scan, biopsy of involved organ | Corticosteroids Methotrexate Infliximab |
| Systemic lupus erythematosus | Bilateral simultaneous visual loss in patient with known SLE or systemic features of the disease | MRI of orbits and brain, CSF examination, ANA | Corticosteroids Cyclophosphamide |

Bibliography

1. Roy FH, Fraunfelder FW, Fraunfelder FT. Roy and Fraunfelder's Current Ocular Therapy, 6th edition. Philadelphia: WB Saunders; 2008.

749. INFLUENZA

General

Acute respiratory infection of specific viral etiology which includes H1N1.

Ocular

Conjunctivitis; subconjunctival hemorrhages; keratitis; tenonitis; ptosis; cellulitis of orbit and lid; dacryocystitis; retinal hemorrhage; cataract; episcleritis; hypopyon; optic neuritis; uveitis; panophthalmitis; vitreal hemorrhage; paralysis of third or fourth nerve; uveitis following vaccination for influenza.

Clinical

Headache; fever; malaise; muscular aching; substernal soreness; nasal stuffiness; nausea.

Laboratory

The criterion standard for diagnosing influenza A and B is a viral culture of nasopharyngeal samples, throat samples, or both.

Treatment

Prevention is the most effective therapy. Two new drugs have been marketed recently for treatment of influenza A and B. These are the neuraminidase inhibitors oseltamivir and zanamivir.

Additional Resource

1. Derlet RW (2012). Influenza. [online] Available from http://www.emedicine.com/med/TOPIC1170.HTM [Accessed April, 2012].

750. INTERNAL ORBITAL FRACTURES (BLOWOUT FRACTURE)

General

Trauma that involves the walls of the orbit leaving the bony rim intact.

Clinical

Tripod fracture of the zygoma.

Ocular

Proptosis, enophthalmos, diplopia.

Laboratory

Computed tomography.

Treatment

The transconjunctival approach with lateral canthotomy and cantholysis is preferred to expose the orbital floor, nasal approach to further expose the medial wall.

Additional Resource

1. Cohen AJ (2012). Orbital Floor Fractures (Blowout). [online] Available from http://www.emedicine.com/plastic/TOPIC485.HTM [Accessed April, 2012].

751. INTERSTITIAL KERATITIS

General

Nonsuppurative inflammation characterized by cellular in filtrates, usually caused by syphilis but can be secondary to bacterial, viral, parasitic and autoimmune causes.

Clinical

Syphilis; tuberculosis; leprosy; Lyme disease; acathamoeba; leishmania; Epstein-Barr; mumps; Cogan syndrome.

Ocular

Decreased vision; photophobia; tearing; blepharospasm; dense, white stromal necrosis of the cornea.

Laboratory

Clinical findings; serologic testing to determine the cause.

Treatment

Treat the underlying disorder. Ocular—topical of corticosteroids; if permanent corneal opacity occurs, corneal transplant may be necessary.

Additional Resource

1. Majmudar PA (2011). Interstitial Keratitis Overview of Interstitial Keratitis. [online] Available from http://emedicine.medscape.com/article/1194376-overview [Accessed April, 2012].

752. INTRAOCULAR EPITHELIAL CYSTS

General

Anterior chamber epithelial cysts develop when implanted epithelial cells proliferate centripetally.

Clinical

None

Ocular

Perforated corenal ulcer, glaucoma and uveitis.

Laboratory

Diagnosis is made from clinical findings.

Treatment

Surgical intervention is required if complications obstruct the visual axis.

Bibliography

1. Roy FH, Fraunfelder FW, Fraunfelder FT. Roy and Fraunfelder's Current Ocular Therapy, 6th edition. Philadelphia: WB Saunders; 2008.

753. INTRAOCULAR FOREIGN BODY — NONMAGNETIC CHEMICALLY INERT

General

Intraocular foreign bodies that are nonmagnetic and chemically inert.

Clinical

None

Ocular

Endopthalmitis and ocular laceration.

Laboratory

Computed tomography to localize foreign body and B-scan ultrasonography.

Treatment

Topical antibiotics are recommended. Topical steroid may be useful with traumatic uveitis. Repair of ocular laceration. Vitrectomy may be needed.

Additional Resource

1. Kuhn F (2011). Intraocular Foreign Body. [online] Available from http://www.emedicine.com/oph/ TOPIC648.HTM [Accessed April, 2012].

754. INTRAOCULAR FOREIGN BODY: STEEL OR IRON

General

Intraocular foreign body of either steel or iron. Foreign bodies are the major cause of ocular trauma legal blindness.

Clinical

None

Ocular

Subconjunctival hemorrhage or edema, iris defect, lens disruption, retinal hemorrhage, inflammation or edema, endophthalmitis.

Laboratory

Computed tomography (CT) to define and localize the foreign body and B-scan ultrasonography.

MRI is contraindicated because it may shift the position of the foreign body.

Treatment

Antibiotics via IV are recommended to prevent endophthalmitis, intravitreal antibiotics, repair of laceration and other ocular injury. Vitrectomy may be needed.

Additional Resource

1. Kuhn F (2011). Intraocular Foreign Body. [online] Available from http://www.emedicine.com/oph/ TOPIC648.HTM [Accessed April, 2012].

755. INVERTED Y SYNDROME

General

Etiology unknown.

Ocular

Partial A syndrome with additional deviation occurring only in downgaze; occurs primarily with exodeviation.

Clinical

None

Laboratory

Diagnosis is made by clinical findings.

Treatment

The medial rectus muscles are moved toward the direction of vertical gaze where the convergence is greater (upward); this loosens the muscle in upgaze and tightens the muscle in downgaze, which results in a relative weakening of adduction in upgaze and strengthening in downgaze.

Additional Resource

1. Plotnik JL (2011). A-Pattern Esotropia and Exotropia. [online] Available from http://www.emedicine.com/oph/TOPIC560.HTM [Accessed April, 2012].

756. IRIDAL ADHESION SYNDROME (IRIDOCORNEAL ENDOTHELIAL SYNDROME, IRIS ADHESION SYNDROME)

General

Surgically related phenomenon following intra-ocular surgery in which iris pigment epithelium proliferates and adheres to cut edge of anterior capsule, drawing iris posteriorly to posterior and anterior capsules.

Ocular

Posterior synechiae; irregular pupil.

Clinical

None

Laboratory

Diagnosis is made by clinical findings.

Treatment

Aqueous suppressants can be tried but usually surgery is required.

Bibliography

1. Dickerson D. Surgery-related iridal adhesion syndrome. Ophthalmol Times. 1984;9:6.
2. Teekhasaenee C, Ritch R. Iridocorneal endothelial syndrome in Thai patients. Arch Ophthalmol. 2000;118:187-92.

757. IRIDOGONODYSGENESIS (IRIS HYPOPLASIA WITH GLAUCOMA)

General

Autosomal dominant; similar to Rieger syndrome or hereditary juvenile glaucoma.

Ocular

Stroma of iris hypoplastic; light irides; congenital glaucoma; optic atrophy; microphthalmia; opacities in Descemet's membrane.

Clinical

None

Laboratory

Diagnosis is made by clinical findings.

Treatment

Glaucoma medications may temporally control IOP but usually surgery is required. Goniotomy or traditionally filtering procedures may be necessary.

Additional Resource

1. Walton DS (2011). Juvenile Glaucoma. [online] Available from http://www.emedicine.com/oph/TOPIC333.HTM [Accessed April, 2012].

---

758. IRIS BOMBE

General

Peripheral iris bowed forward while the central iris remains deep. Most commonly seen as primary pupillary block.

Clinical

Pain, nausea.

Ocular

Bowing forward of the peripheral iris, corneal edema, ciliary, pain, elevated IOP.

Laboratory

Diagnosis is made by clinical findings.

Treatment

Systemic IV Mannitol, IV or oral acetazolamide, topical antiglaucoma agents, YAG laser peripheral iridotomy.

Bibliography

1. Roy FH, Fraunfelder FW, Fraunfelder FT. Roy and Fraunfelder's Current Ocular Therapy, 6th edition. Philadelphia: WB Saunders; 2008.

---

759. IRIS CYSTS

General

Intraepithelial cyst originating between the epithelial layers and stromal cysts that are congenital or caused by surgery or trauma.

Clinical

None

Ocular

Keratopathy, iridocyclitis, glaucoma, iris cysts.

Laboratory

Diagnosis is made by clinical findings.

Treatment

Chemical cauterization, laser photocoagulation, diathermy, cryocoagulation and block excision with corneoscleral transplant.

Bibliography

1. Roy FH, Fraunfelder FW, Fraunfelder FT. Roy and Fraunfelder's Current Ocular Therapy, 6th edition. Philadelphia: WB Saunders; 2008.

760. IRIS LACERATIONS AND IRIS HOLES, AND IRIDODIALYSIS

General

Partial or full thickness iris defects that are most often caused by trauma. Iridodialysis is a separation of the thin, weak iris root from its attachment to the ciliary body and sclera spur.

Clinical

None

Ocular

Transillumination defects, corneal edema, traumatic cataract, hyphema, retinal tears, vitreous hemorrhage, retinal detachment, choroidal rupture and traumatic optic neuropathy.

Laboratory

Diagnosis is made by clinical findings.

Treatment

Cycloplegics and steroid drops for traumatic iritis.

Bibliography

1. Roy FH, Fraunfelder FW, Fraunfelder FT. Roy and Fraunfelder's Current Ocular Therapy, 6th edition. Philadelphia: WB Saunders; 2008.

761. IRIS MELANOMA

General

Malignant neoplasm.

Clinical

None

Ocular

Iris melanoma, ectropion uveae, sector cataract, sentinel vessels, heterochromia, hyphema, chronic uveitis, glaucoma.

Laboratory

Diagnosis is made by clinical findings.

Treatment

Resection with iridectomy/iridocyclectomy or radiotherapy and enucleation.

Additional Resource

1. Waheed NK (2012). Iris Melanoma. [online] Available from http://www.emedicine.com/oph/TOPIC405.HTM [Accessed April, 2012].

762. IRIS NEOVASCULARIZATION WITH PSEUDOEXFOLIATION SYNDROME

General

Anoxia secondary to iris vessel obstruction; electron microscopic studies reveal endothelial thickening with decreased lumen size and fenestration of vessel walls.

Ocular

Material found on posterior and anterior iris surface, anterior lens surface, ciliary processes, zonules and anterior hyaloid membranes; neovascularization of iris stroma; increased permeability of iris vessels.

Clinical

None

Laboratory

Diagnosis is made by clinical findings.

Treatment

Patients with pseudoexfoliation syndrome should have annual eye examinations for early detection of glaucoma.

Additional Resource

1. Pons ME (2011). Pseudoexfoliation Glaucoma. [online] Available from http://www.emedicine. com/oph/TOPIC140.HTM [Accessed April, 2012].

763. IRIS NEVUS SYNDROME (CHANDLER SYNDROME; COGAN-REESE SYNDROME; ICE SYNDROME; IRIDOCORNEAL ENDOTHELIAL SYNDROME)

General

Usually unilateral but may be bilateral; usually in young adult women; nonfamilial; cause unknown; Chandler, Cogan-Reese and iridocorneal endothelial syndromes have been considered three separate syndromes but are now recognized as a single spectrum of diseases.

Ocular

Unilateral glaucoma in eyes with peripheral anterior synechiae; multiple iris nodules; ectopic Descemet's membrane; corneal edema; stromal iris atrophy; iris pigment epithelial atrophy; ectropion uveae; ectopic pupil; keratoconus; herpes simplex virus DNA has been detected in patients with iridocorneal endothelial syndrome from corneal specimens.

Clinical

Glasslike membrane covering the anterior iris surface; corneal endothelial degeneration and accompanying ectopic endothelial membranes are responsible for occlusion of the filtration meshwork and subsequent pressure increase.

Laboratory

Diagnosis is made by clinical findings.

Treatment

This disease does not usually respond to medications and trabeculectomy operations. Glaucoma drainage devices create an alternate aqueous pathway by channeling aqueous from the anterior chamber through a tube to an equatorial plate inserted under the conjunctiva that promotes bleb formation.

Bibliography

1. Alvarado JA, Underwood JL, Green WR, et al. Detection of herpes simplex viral DNA in the iridocorneal endothelial syndrome. Arch Ophthalmol. 1994;112:1601-9.
2. Buckley RJ. Pathogenesis of the ICE syndrome. Br J Ophthalmol. 1994;78:595-6.
3. Chandler PA. Atrophy of the stroma of the iris; endothelial dystrophy, corneal edema, and glaucoma. Am J Ophthalmol. 1956;41:607-15.
4. Cogan DG, Reese AB. A syndrome of iris nodules, ectopic Descemet's membrane, and unilateral glaucoma. Doc Ophthalmol. 1969;26:424-33.
5. Radius RL, Herschler J. Histopathology in the iris-nevus (Cogan-Reese) syndrome. Am J Ophthalmol. 1980;89:780-6.
6. Rodrigues MM, Stulting RD, Waring GO. Clinical, electron microscopic, and immunohistochemical study of the corneal endothelium and Descemet's membrane in the iridocorneal endothelial syndrome. Am J Ophthalmol. 1986;101:16-27.

764. IRIS PIGMENT LAYER CLEAVAGE

General

Autosomal dominant; cleavage of pigment of iris and ciliary body.

Ocular

Cataracts; reduced sagittal and spherical lens diameters; glaucoma; retinal detachment; microphakia; spherophakia.

Clinical

None

Laboratory

Diagnosis is made by clinical findings.

Treatment

Cataract: Change in glasses can sometimes improve a patient's visual function temporarily; however, the most common treatment is cataract surgery.

Glaucoma: Its medication should be the first plan of action. If medication is unsuccessful, a filtering surgical procedure with or without antimetabolites may be beneficial.

Retinal detachment: Scleral buckle, pneumatic retinopexy and vitrectomy may be used to close all the breaks.

Bibliography

1. Kafer O. Dominant Vererbte Spaltung des Pigmentblattes van Iris und Ciliarkoeper mit Consekutiver Microphakie, Ectopia Lentis and Cataract. Graefes Arch Klin Exp Ophthalmol. 1977;202:133-41.
2. McKusick VA. Mendelian Inheritance in Man: A Catalog of Human Genes and Genetic Disorders, 12th edition. Baltimore: The Johns Hopkins University Press; 1998.
3. McKusick-Nathans Institute for Genetic Medicine, Johns Hopkins University and National Center for Biotechnology Information, National Library of Medicine. (2007). Online Mendelian Inheritance in Man (OMIM). [online] Available from http://www.ncbi.nlm.nih.gov/omim [Accessed April, 2012].

765. IRIS PROLAPSE

General

Uncommon intraoperative or postoperative complication of intraocular surgery or a penetrating injury.

Clinical

None

Ocular

Floppy iris, papillary block, retrorbital or expulsive hemorrhage, poor wound healing.

Laboratory

Diagnosis is made by clinical findings.

Treatment

Reduce wound leak, decrease the wound size by placing sutures, excision of prolapsed iris.

Additional Resource

1. Giri G (2011). Iris Prolapse. [online] Available from http://www.emedicine.com/oph/TOPIC584.HTM [Accessed April, 2012].

766. IRIS RETRACTION SYNDROME (POSTERIOR SYNECHIAE AND IRIS RETRACTION SYNDROME)

General

Rhegmatogenous retinal detachment, hypotony and retrodisplacement of the iris with seclusion of the pupil, often associated with ciliochoroidal detachment, inflammation and posterior vitreous retraction; caused by lowering of pressure behind iris partially due to posterior removal of fluid from subretinal space.

Ocular

Retinal detachment; hypotony; iris retraction; angle-closure glaucoma; iris bombs; cataract; vitreous retraction; seclusion of the pupil; following intraocular surgery.

Clinical

None

Laboratory

Diagnosis is made by clinical findings.

Treatment

The surgical goals are to identify and close all the breaks with minimum iatrogenic damage. Scleral buckles, scleral implant, vitrectomy and pneumatic retinopexy may be useful.

Additional Resource

1. Wu L (2011). Rhegmatogenous Retinal Detachment. [online] Available from http://www.emedicine.com/oph/TOPIC410.HTM [Accessed April, 2012].

767. IRON DEFICIENCY ANEMIA (MICROCYTIC HYPOCHROMIC ANEMIA)

General

Conjunctival pallor; small retinal hemorrhages; diplopia; visual field defects; fixed and dilated pupil; swelling or pallor of optic disk; retrobulbar neuritis; optic atrophy; it represents a state of inadequate body stores of iron; diagnosis of iron deficiency anemia is the *sine qua non* of chronic iron loss; most usual source is the gastrointestinal tract.

Clinical

Lethargy; increased susceptibility to infections; lymphadenopathy; hepatomegaly; splenomegaly.

Laboratory

Serum iron, total iron-binding capacity (TIBC) and serum ferritin.

Treatment

In most patients, the iron deficiency should be treated with oral iron therapy, and the underlying etiology should be corrected so the deficiency does not recur.

Additional Resource

1. Harper JL (2012). Iron Deficiency Anemia. [online] Available from http://www.emedicine.com/med/TOPIC1188.HTM [Accessed April, 2012].

768. IRVINE SYNDROME (HRUBY-IRVINE-GASS SYNDROME IRVINE-GASS SYNDROME)

General

Failing vision after uneventful cataract extraction; caused by spontaneous rupture of vitreous face with vitreous adhesions to the wound followed by macular edema; no gender or race preference; more common in older adults; positive association with other systemic vascular disease; may follow neodymium:yttrium-aluminum-garnet (Nd:YAG) laser posterior capsulotomy.

Ocular

Failing improvement or decrease in visual acuity after cataract surgery, due to macular changes; permanent impairment if the condition is not restored before secondary degenerative changes occur; vitreous opacities; rupture of the hyaloid face (spontaneous); vitreous adhesions to the wound; cystoid macular edema (CME); papilledema; optic atrophy.

Clinical

None

Laboratory

Fluorescein angiography and optical coherence tomography.

Treatment

Treatment is aimed at the underlying etiology; however, several of the common treatments may help different causes of CME. Corticosteroids are the primary treatment and can be administered topically or orally; they can also be injected intra-vitreally or injected into the sub-Tenon's space, and topical NSAIDs may be useful. Surgical therapy includes pars plana vitrectomy.

Additional Resource

1. Telander DG (2010). Macular Edema, Pseudophakic (Irvine-Gass). [online] Available from http://www.emedicine.com/oph/TOPIC400.HTM [Accessed April, 2012].

769. ISCHEMIC OPTIC NEUROPATHIES

General

Rare, result of shock usually from injury or surgery in combination with compartment syndrome.

Clinical

Headaches, low-grade fever, weight loss, arthralgias, jaw claudication.

Ocular

Sudden visual loss, optic disk edema, amaurosis fugax, diplopia.

Laboratory

Erythrocyte sedimentation rate, C-reactive protein, CBC and temporal artery biopsy.

Treatment

Systemic corticosteroids.

Additional Resource

1. Younge BR (2012). Anterior Ischemic Optic Neuropathy. [online] Available from http://www.emedicine.com/oph/TOPIC161.HTM [Accessed April, 2012].

770. ISCHEMIC ORBITAL COMPARTMENT SYNDROME

General

Associated with spine surgery in the prone position.

Ocular

Proptosis; elevated intraocular pressure; decreased vision; periocular pain; ischemic optic atrophy.

Clinical

Facial swelling; spinal stenosis or other diagnosis that would require long surgical procedures on the prone position.

Laboratory

Computed tomography (CT) scan or MRI of the orbit may help to identify the etiology of compression.

Treatment

Osmotic agents, carbonic anhydrase inhibitors and high-dose steroid therapy are standard of care.

Additional Resource

1. Peak DA (2011). Acute Orbital Compartment Syndrome. [online] Available from http://www.emedicine.com/emerg/TOPIC881.HTM [Accessed April, 2012].

771. ISOTRETINOIN TERATOGEN SYNDROME

General

Maternal ingestion of isotretinoin (accutane) during early pregnancy.

Ocular

Small palpebral fissures; deep orbits; systemic treatment with isotretinoin has been associated with blepharitis and conjunctivitis.

Clinical

Prominent forehead; low-set, small and undifferentiated ears; depressed nasal bridge; small chin.

Laboratory

Diagnosis is made by clinical findings.

Treatment

No treatment for palpebral fissures and orbits.

Additional Resource

1. Draper JC (2011). Teratology and Drug Use During Pregnancy. [online] Available from http://www.emedicine.com/med/TOPIC3242.HTM [Accessed April, 2012].

772. IVIC SYNDROME (HEARING IMPAIRMENT, INTERNAL OPHTHALMOPLEGIA, RADIAL RAY DEFECTS, THROMBOCYTOPENIA)

General

Autosomal dominant; Institute Venezolano de Investigacionas Cientificas (IVIC); observed in 1800s from Canary Islands in Venezuela; has been observed in descendants of a family that migrated to Venezuela from the Canary Islands.

Ocular

Strabismus; internal ophthalmoplegia.

Clinical

Malformed upper limb; short distal phalanx; hearing loss; thrombocytopenia; leukocytosis; imperforate anus; radial ray defect.

Laboratory

Diagnosis is made by clinical findings.

Treatment

Traditional surgery for esotropia or exotropia.

Bibliography

1. Arias S, Penchaszadeh VB, Pinto-Cisternas J, et al. The IVIC syndrome: a new autosomal dominant complex pleiotropic syndrome with radial ray hypoplasia, hearing impairment, external ophthalmoplegia, and thrombocytopenia. Am J Med Genet. 1980;6:25-59.
2. Czeizel A, Göblyös P, Kodaj I. IVIC syndrome: report of a third family. Am J Med Genet. 1989; 33:282-3.
3. McKusick-Nathans Institute for Genetic Medicine, Johns Hopkins University and National Center for Biotechnology Information, National Library of Medicine. (2007). Online Mendelian Inheritance in Man (OMIM). [online] Available from http://www.ncbi.nlm.nih.gov/omim [Accessed April, 2012].

773. JABS SYNDROME (GRANULOMATOUS UVEITIS, AND CRANIAL NEUROPATHIES, SYNOVITIS)

General

Autosomal dominant.

Ocular

Granulomatous uveitis; iritis; VI nerve palsy.

Clinical

Granulomatous synovitis; corticosteroid responsive hearing loss; boggy polysynovitis; boutonneuse deformities; granulomatous arthritis; skin involvement; fever; hypertension; large-vessel vasculitis.

Laboratory

Diagnosis is made by clinical findings.

Treatment

Cycloplegics, corticosteroids, aqueous suppressant if the IOP is elevated.

Additional Resource

1. Al-Fawaz A (2010). Uveitis, Anterior, Granulomatous. [online] Available from http://www.emedicine.com/oph/TOPIC586.HTM [Accessed April, 2012].

774. JACOBS SYNDROME (SUPER FEMALE SYNDROME; TRIPLE X SYNDROME; XXX SYNDROME)

General

Caused by sex chromosomal anomaly with 44 autosomal and 3X sex chromosomes; due to nondisjunction; often associated with autosomal trisomies; majority of cases are asymptomatic.

Ocular

Hypertelorism; epicanthus; mongoloid slanted lid fissure; strabismus.

Clinical

Microcephaly; oligophrenia, occasionally with secondary amenorrhea; abnormal dentition; high-arched palate; hypogenitalism; occasionally mental retardation; early menopause.

Laboratory

Diagnosis is made by clinical findings.

Treatment

Strabismus can be treated with appropriate surgical procedure.

Bibliography

1. Jacobs PA, Baikie AG, Brown WM, et al. Evidence for the existence of the human "super female". Lancet. 1959;2:423-5.
2. Kohn G, Winter JS, Mellman WJ. Trisomy X in three children. J Pediatr. 1968;72:248-52.

775. JACOBSEN-BRODWALL SYNDROME

General

Syndrome consists of inborn defect in erythropoiesis; dysplastic kidneys; eye lesions; malformation of the teeth; impaired hearing; etiology unknown; features of Alport, Fanconi and Lowe syndromes do not conform with the findings in this syndrome.

Ocular

Loss of vision progressing to blindness; secondary glaucoma; vitreous opacities; cataract; macular changes; retinal hemorrhages and exudates.

Clinical

Anemia; atypical development of teeth, with caries and resorption of permanent teeth; kidney dysplasia; hearing defect.

Laboratory

Diagnosis is made by clinical findings.

Treatment

Monitor and treat for glaucoma. If glaucoma develops, intraocular pressure-lowering agents must be used. Often, these patients require surgical intervention with goniotomy, trabeculectomy or a drainage filtration device. Congenital cataracts should be removed, ideally in the first 6 weeks of life, to optimize the visual potential.

Additional Resource

1. Phillpotts BA (2011). Vitreous Hemorrhage. [online] Available from http://www.emedicine. com/oph/TOPIC421.HTM [Accessed April, 2012].

776. JACOD SYNDROME (NEGRI-JACOD SYNDROME; PETROSPHENOIDAL SPACE SYNDROME)

General

Lesion involving cranial nerves II (optic) to VI (abducens); most frequently a malignant nasopharyngeal tumor originating in lateropharyngeal area.

Ocular

Ophthalmoplegia; unilateral blindness; trigeminal neuralgia (ophthalmic branch); descending optic atrophy if cranial nerve II is involved; amaurosis fugax.

Clinical

Trigeminal neuralgia (at the beginning the first and second divisions of nerve V are involved; later the third division is affected as well); unilateral or bilateral enlargement of cervical lymph nodes (30%); deafness; palatal muscle paralysis.

Laboratory

Magnetic resonance imaging (MRI) with gadolinium and fat suppression is the radiologic modality of choice. Transnasal biopsy of nasopharyngeal mass may also be necessary.

Treatment

External beam radiation therapy is the primary mode of management. Chemotherapeutic approaches have been devised to improve the response rates.

Additional Resource

1. Lin HS (2012). Malignant Nasopharyngeal Tumors. [online] Available from http://www.emedicine. com/ent/TOPIC269.HTM [Accessed April, 2012].

777. JADASSOHN-LEWANDOWSKY SYNDROME (PACHYONYCHIA CONGENITA)

General

Autosomal dominant inheritance; three variants: (1) Type I has symmetric keratoses of hands and feet and follicular keratosis of body; (2) Type II same as Type I, plus leukokeratosis and (3) Type III same as Type I with corneal changes; gene for this disorder has been found to be closely linked to the keratin gene cluster on 17q12–q21; disorder usually develops in early infancy.

Ocular

Dyskeratosis of the cornea; bilateral cataract.

Clinical

Keratosis and hyperhidrosis of palms and soles, whereas the remaining skin is usually rather dry; bullous lesions may occur with secondary infections, mainly during warm seasons; leukokeratosis of oral mucosa (mainly tongue); follicular keratosis; congenital pachyonychia (nails not only may be thickened but also may be frequently inflamed and lost with aggravation at sites of regrowth); hoarse voice; epidermoid cysts; oral leukokeratosis.

Laboratory

Electron microscopy can be performed by using plantar or palmar skin samples. Electron microscopy shows thickened and clumped intermediate filaments, as well as enlarged keratohyaline granules.

Treatment

The thickened nail plate can be softened by using 20% salicylic acid ointment or 20–40% urea and 10% salicylic acid in an emulsifying ointment with occlusive dressings. The affected nails can be removed under local or general anesthesia; however, unless the nail matrix is partially removed, nails regrow.

Additional Resource

1. George SJ (2010). Pachyonychia Congenita. [online] Available from http://www.emedicine. com/derm/TOPIC812.HTM [Accessed April, 2012].

778. JANSEN DISEASE (METAPHYSEAL DYSOSTOSIS)

General

Affects both sexes; etiology unknown; autosomal dominant.

Ocular

Exophthalmos

Clinical

Mental retardation; muscular atrophy; flat nose; large mouth; dwarfism; deafness; metaphyses of all bones affected with marked widening.

Laboratory

Conventional radiographic examination remains the most useful means of studying the dysplastic skeleton. CT scan and MRI of the skull and brain can reveal concurrent brain anomalies.

Treatment

Medical care should be directed at preventing neurologic and orthopedic complications due to spinal cord compression, joint instability and long bone deformity.

Bibliography

1. Jansen M. Ubex Atypische Condrodystrophie (Achondroplasic) und Uber Eine Noch Nicht Beschriebene Angeborene Washstumsstoring des Knochensystems Metaphysare Dysostosis. Orthop Chir. 1934;61:253-86.
2. Magalini SI, Scrascia E. Dictionary of Medical Syndromes, 2nd edition. Philadelphia: JB Lippincott; 1981. p. 434.
3. McKusick VA. Mendelian Inheritance in Man: A Catalog of Human Genes and Genetic Disorders, 12th edition. Baltimore: The Johns Hopkins University Press; 1998.
4. McKusick-Nathans Institute for Genetic Medicine, Johns Hopkins University and National Center for Biotechnology Information, National Library of Medicine. (2007). Online Mendelian Inheritance in Man (OMIM). [online] Available from http://www.ncbi.nlm.nih.gov/omim/ [Accessed April, 2012].

779. JAPANESE RIVER FEVER (MITE-BORNE TYPHUS; RURAL TYPHUS; SCRUB TYPHUS; TROPICAL TYPHUS; TSUTSUGAMUSHI DISEASE; TYPHUS)

General

Acute febrile illness by *Orientia tsutsugamushi* (formerly *Rickettsia tsutsugamushi*); transmitted by the larval form of a mite.

Ocular

Keratitis; uveitis; paracentral scotoma; vitreous opacity; nystagmus; retinal hemorrhages; exudates; edema.

Clinical

Chills; fever; malaise; headache; lymphadenopathy; generalized aching.

Laboratory

The confirmatory tests are the indirect immunoperoxidase test and the immunofluorescent assay. An infection is confirmed by a 4-fold increase in antibody titers between acute and convalescent serum specimens.

Treatment

Treatment must be initiated early in the course of the disease, based on presumptive diagnosis, to reduce morbidity and mortality. Doxycycline and chloramphenicol are both effective.

Additional Resource

1. Cennimo DJ (2012). Pediatric Scrub Typhus. [online] Available from http://www.emedicine.com/ped/TOPIC2710.HTM [Accessed April, 2012].

---

780. JENSEN DISEASE (JUXTAPAPILLARY RETINOPATHY)

General

Etiology unknown.

Ocular

Circumscribed inflammatory changes of the choroid; visual field defect.

Clinical

None

Laboratory

Diagnosis is made by clinical findings.

Treatment

None/Ocular.

Bibliography

1. Harley RD (Ed). Pediatric Ophthalmology, 4th edition. Philadelphia: WB Saunders; 1998.
2. Magalini SI, Scrascia E. Dictionary of Medical Syndromes, 2nd edition. Philadelphia: JB Lippincott; 1981.

---

781. JEUNE DISEASE (ASPHYXIATING THORACIC DYSTROPHY; THORACIC-PELVIC-PHALANGEAL DYSTROPHY)

General

Autosomal recessive; similar to Ellis-van Creveld syndrome; positive associations of this disorder with cystinuria has been reported in two sisters.

Ocular

Retinal dysfunction; granular pigmentation of the choroid; nystagmus; small white patches in peripheral fundus; retinal degeneration; coloboma of iris; eyes symmetrically involved; retinal aplasia; photophobia; strabismus; pigmentary retinopathy.

Clinical

Long, narrow thorax; short anteriorly clubbed ribs forming a continuous tube with the abdominal cavity; dwarfing skeletal dysplasia; progressive renal failure; liver abnormalities; severe respiratory insufficiency; long, narrow trunk; dystrophic rib cage with respiratory distress; short limbs; polydactyly.

Laboratory

Newborn and infant radiography show small and bell-shaped thorax with reduced transverse and anteroposterior diameter. Urinalysis may show hematuria and proteinuria.

Treatment

Chest reconstruction and enlargement of the thoracic cage by sternotomy and fixation with bone grafts or a methylmethacrylate prosthesis plate provides patients with the time needed for thoracic cage growth may be necessary.

Additional Resource

1. Chen H (2011). Genetics of Asphyxiating Thoracic Dystrophy (Jeune Syndrome). [online] Available from http://www.emedicine.com/ped/TOPIC1224.HTM [Accessed April, 2012].

782. JOHNSON SYNDROME (ADHERENCE SYNDROME; ADHERENT LATERAL RECTUS SYNDROME)

General

Congenital delayed development; most frequent in children below age 3 years; spontaneous disappearance possible; two principal types of disturbances: (1) adhesions between sheaths of external rectus and inferior oblique with resulting limits in abduction and (2) adhesions between sheaths of superior rectus and superior oblique with resulting limits in elevation.

Ocular

Forced muscle duction test may prove presence or absence of adherence versus paralysis.

Clinical

None

Laboratory

Diagnosis is made by clinical findings.

Treatment

Strabismus: Equalized vision with correct refractive error; surgery may be helpful in patient with diplopia.

Additional Resource

1. Ehrenhaus MP (2012). Abducens Nerve Palsy. [online] Available from http://www.emedicine.com/oph/TOPIC158.HTM [Accessed April, 2012].

783. JONES SYNDROME (CHERUBISM; MANDIBULAR CYSTIC DYSPLASIA)

General

Etiology unknown; both sexes affected; present at birth.

Ocular

White line beneath the iris on sclera; hypertelorism; optic atrophy.

Clinical

Rounded cheeks; jaw fullness; submandibular region swelling; narrow, V-shaped palate.

Laboratory

Diagnosis is made by clinical findings.

Treatment

Optic atrophy: Intravenous steroids may be used with optic neuritis or ischemic neuropathy. Stem cell treatment may be the future treatment of choice.

Additional Resource

1. Goldman KE (2011). Mandibular Cysts and Odontogenic Tumors. [online] Available from http://www.emedicine.com/ent/TOPIC681.HTM [Accessed April, 2012].

---

784. JOUBERT SYNDROME (FAMILIAL CEREBELLAR VERMIS AGENESIS)

General

Autosomal recessive; both sexes affected; onset in early infancy.

Ocular

Choroidal coloboma; nystagmus; ocular fibrosis; telecanthus.

Clinical

Episodic hyperpnea; apnea; ataxia; psychomotor retardation; rhythmic protrusion of tongue; mental retardation; micrognathia; complex cardiac malformation; cutaneous dimples over wrists and elbows.

Laboratory

Urine culture, renal ultrasonography, dimercaptosuccinic acid (DMSA) renal scanning.

Treatment

Lifetime follow-up is required whether or not involution has occurred or a nephrectomy.

Additional Resource

1. Swiatecka-Urban A (2011). Multicystic Renal Dysplasia. [online] Available from http://www. emedicine.com/ped/TOPIC1493.HTM [Accessed April, 2012].

---

785. JUGULAR FORAMEN SYNDROME (VERNET SYNDROME)

General

Injuries, aneurysms and tumors (more commonly due to metastatic lesion than primary neoplasms) affecting the foramen jugulare are the primary causes for the syndrome to develop; if sympathetic fibers surrounding the carotid artery are involved, this will produce Horner triad; note similarity of clinical findings of Villaret syndrome or "retroparotid space syndrome", which may include epiphora and lagophthalmos and in which cranial nerves IX to XII and the cervical sympathetics are involved.

Ocular

Enophthalmos; ptosis; miosis.

Clinical

Paralysis of the IX, X and XI cranial nerves with resulting impairment of related function, i.e. dysphagia, loss of taste on the posterior third of the tongue and nasal regurgitation; anhidrosis; paralysis of the sternocleidomastoid muscle and part of the trapezium (upper portion); hoarseness; tachycardia; dysarthria; weight loss.

Laboratory

Computed tomography (CT), MRI, carotid arteriography.

Treatment

Anticoagulation or thrombolytic therapy is useful. Severe neurological deterioration may require open thrombectomy and local thrombolytic therapy.

Additional Resource

1. McElveen WA (2011). Cerebral Venous Thrombosis. [online] Available from http://www.emedicine.com/neuro/TOPIC642.HTM [Accessed April, 2012].

786. JUNIUS-KUHNT SYNDROME [KUHNT-JUNIUS DISEASE; MACULAR SENILE DISCIFORM DEGENERATION (I); MACULA LUTEA JUVENILE DEGENERATION (2)]

General

Onset in advanced age or in juvenile period; etiology unknown; possible autosomal dominant or recessive inheritance.

Ocular

Impairment of central vision; central scotoma; atrophic macular degeneration surrounded by retinal hemorrhages, resulting in mountlike lesion; exudative and atrophic reaction with deposit in and about macula.

Clinical

None

Laboratory

Diagnosis is made by clinical findings.

Treatment

Macular degeneration: No treatment available for non-neovascular age-related macular degeneration (AMD). Preventative therapy includes no smoking, control of hypertension, cholesterol, and blood sugar, exercise and vitamins. Neovascular AMD treatment consists of laser, Avastin and Lucentis.

Bibliography

1. Deutman AF. Hereditary dystrophies of the central retina and choroid. In: Winkelman JE, Crone RA (Eds). Perspectives in Ophthalmology, Amsterdam: Excerpta Medica; 1970.
2. Deutman AF. Macular dystrophies. In: Ryan SJ (Ed). Retina, 2nd edition. St. Louis: Mosby; 1994.
3. Kimura SJ, Caygill WM (Eds). Retinal Diseases. Philadelphia: Lea & Febiger; 1966.
4. Magalini SI, Scrascia E. Dictionary of Medical Syndromes, 2nd edition. Philadelphia: JB Lippincott; 1981. p. 440.

787. JUVENILE CORNEAL EPITHELIAL DYSTROPHY (MEESMAN'S CORNEAL DYSTROPHY)

General

Autosomal dominant inheritance, rare, infrequently causes discomfort and minimal visual loss.

Clinical

None

Ocular

Epithelial corneal cysts, irregular astigmatism and superficial haze.

Laboratory

Slit lamp examination is diagnostic.

Treatment

Usually no treatment. Bandage soft contact lens can be used to reduce discomfort.

Bibliography

1. Roy FH, Fraunfelder FW, Fraunfelder FT. Roy and Fraunfelder's Current Ocular Therapy, 6th edition. Philadelphia: WB Saunders; 2008.

788. JUVENILE DIABETES-DWARFISM-OBESITY SYNDROME (DWARFISM-HEPATOMEGALY-OBESITY-JUVENILE DIABETES SYNDROME; MAURIAC SYNDROME)

General

Etiology is obscure, although nutritional deficiencies, metabolic disorders and deficiency in insulin have been considered; develops slowly, with slow growth and difficulties in management of diabetic condition.

Ocular

Cataract; diabetic retinopathy with retinal hemorrhages, exudates, microaneurysms, neovascularization, vaso and glial proliferation (grades I to IV diabetic retinopathy; hypertensive retinopathy); occasional optic neuritis.

Clinical

Hepatomegaly; diminished growth; osteoporosis; hypertension; arteriosclerosis; obesity (with moon face); juvenile diabetes; abdominal colic.

Laboratory

Random plasma glucose level of greater than 200 mg/dL is adequate to establish the diagnosis of diabetes.

Treatment

Insulin therapy, self-monitor blood glucose levels, diabetic diet and education.

Additional Resource

1. Khardori R (2012). Type 1 Diabetes Mellitus. [online] Available from http://www.emedicine.com/emerg/TOPIC133.HTM [Accessed April, 2012].

789. JUVENILE GLAUCOMA

General

Group of glaucomas occurring in later childhood or early adulthood.

Clinical

None

Ocular

Chronic open-angle glaucoma. If mild cases of infantile glaucoma may have mild corenal enlargement and breaks in Descemet's membrane.

Laboratory

Testing for Juvenile rheumatic arthritis, sarcoidosis, ankylosing spondylitis, herpes zoster, syphilis and turberculosis.

Treatment

Trial topical medical therapy. If IOPs are uncontrolled, iridectomy, goniotomy, trabeculectomy, filtration surgery or cyclodestructive may be necessary.

Additional Resource

1. Walton DS (2011). Juvenile Glaucoma. [online] Available from http://www.emedicine.com/oph/TOPIC333.HTM [Accessed April, 2012].

---

790. JUVENILE RHEUMATOID ARTHRITIS (JRA; STILL DISEASE)

General

Onset before age 16 years; greater occurrence of systemic manifestations, monoarticular and oligoarticular joint involvement, and iridocyclitis.

Ocular

Hypopyon; band keratopathy; uveitis; cataract; papillitis; glaucoma; macular edema; ocular pain; vitreous cells; synechiae; scleritis; presumed to have an autoimmune etiology; antiocular antibodies, including iris protein antibodies, have been found in the sera of patients.

Clinical

Salmon pink macular rash; arthritis; hepatosplenomegaly; leukocytosis; chronic pain; joint swelling; low-grade fever; anemia; rheumatoid nodules.

Laboratory

Antinuclear antibody, rheumatoid factor, human leukocyte antigen B27 (HLA-B27), X-ray imaging of joints.

Treatment

Uveitis is initially treated with topical corticosteroids. Systemic immunomodulatory agents may be useful for patients with limited or no response to topical or systemic corticosteroids.

Additional Resource

1. Roque MR (2010). Uveitis, Juvenile Idiopathic Arthritis. [online] Available from http://www.emedicine.com/oph/TOPIC675.HTM [Accessed April, 2012].

---

791. JUVENILE XANTHOGRANULOMA (JXG; NEVOXANTHOENDOTHELIOMA)

General

Childhood disease; unknown etiology.

Ocular

Uveal tract tumor presenting as spontaneous hyphema; secondary glaucoma; uveitis; corneal, lid and epibulbar tumors; proptosis; retinal and choroidal lesions (rare).

Clinical

Multiple benign tumors, primarily of the skin; usually appear in the first 3 years of life; lesions appear as yellow-to-brown papules or nodules.

Laboratory

Diagnostic techniques include biomicroscopy, high frequency ultrasound and cytologic examination of anterior chamber parencentesis material.

Treatment

Topical, subconjunctival, intralesional and systemic corticosteroids are useful. Low-dose radiation may be the treatment of choice for diffuse uveal lesions. Glaucoma medications should be used in the setting of hyphema and increased intraocular pressure.

Additional Resource

1. Curtis T (2010). Juvenile Xanthogranuloma. [online] Available from http://www.emedicine.com/oph/TOPIC588.HTM [Accessed April, 2012].

---

792. KABUKI MAKE-UP SYNDROME (NIIKAWA-KUROKI SYNDROME)

General

Etiology unknown; originally termed Kabuki make-up syndrome because dysmorphic facies resembled the stylized make-up worn by Kabuki actors; also seen in ethnic groups other than Japanese.

Ocular

Ectropion of lower eyelid; long palpebral fissures; sparse lateral half of eyebrows; highly arched eyebrows.

Clinical

Prominent ears; cleft or highly arched palates; brachydactyly; dermatoglyphics; padlike swelling of fingertips; short stature; mental retardation; susceptibility to infection; characteristic facies; developmental delay; mental and growth retardation with specific craniofacial malformations including a depressed nasal tip; musculoskeletal abnormalities, evolving phenotype over time suggesting an underlying defect of the connective tissue.

Laboratory

Diagnosis is made by clinical findings.

Treatment

Lubrication and moisture shields are helpful if significant corneal exposure exists from the ectropion. If symptoms warrant a surgical procedure may be necessary for the ectropion. Lateral tarsal strip—horizontal lid laxity is a component of most ectropion cases.

Bibliography

1. Kaiser-Kupfer MI, Mulvihill JJ, Klein KL, et al. The Niikawa-Kuroki (Kabuki make-up) syndrome in an American black. Am J Ophthalmol. 1986;102: 667-8.
2. Kuroki Y, Suzuki Y, Chyo H, et al. A new malformation syndrome of long palpebral fissures, large ears, depressed nasal tip, and skeletal anomalies associated with postnatal dwarfism and mental retardation. J Pediatr. 1981;99:570-3.
3. Niikawa N, Matsuura N, Fukushima Y, et al. Kabuki make-up syndrome: a syndrome of mental retardation, unusual facies, large and protruding ears, and postnatal growth deficiency. J Pediatr. 1981;99:565-9.
4. Shiekh TM, Qazi QH, Beller E. Niikawa-Kuroki syndrome. Pediatr Res. 1986;20:340A.

793. KAHLER DISEASE (MULTIPLE MYELOMA; MYELOMATOSIS)

General

Disseminated malignancy of plasma cells located predominantly in the bone marrow.

Ocular

Tumor of orbit common, with proptosis or displacement of globe; conjunctival sledging and segmentation; crystalline deposits of cornea and conjunctiva; cotton-wool spots; retrobulbar neuritis; occlusion of central retinal artery and vein; palsy of sixth nerve; vitreous hemorrhage; dilated veins and hemorrhages; retinal microaneurysms; choroidal detachment; amaurosis fugax; myeloma infiltrates in orbit, iris, choroid, retina, sclera and optic nerve; corneal opacities; ciliary body cysts; iritis; glaucoma; subluxation of lens; papilledema; corneal edema; cavernous sinus syndrome; bilateral superficial punctate keratitis; central retinal vein occlusion; crystalline keratopathy in a vortex distribution; spontaneous endocapsular hematoma.

Clinical

Bone pain; fractures; dehydration; hypercalcemia; hyperuricemia; proteinuria; inclination to infection; hyperviscosity.

Laboratory

Comprehensive metabolic panel to assess a patient's total protein, albumin and globulin, BUN, creatinine, and uric acid, MRI scan, bone marrow aspirate and biopsy.

Treatment

Bone marrow transplantation and radiation may be beneficial. Patients often benefit from the expertise of an orthopedic surgeon versed in oncologic management because prophylactic fixation of impending pathologic fractures is occasionally warranted.

Additional Resource

1. Seiter K (2012). Multiple Myeloma. [online] Available from http://www.emedicine.com/med/TOPIC1521.HTM [Accessed April, 2012].

794. KALLMANN SYNDROME (HYPOGONADOTROPIC HYPOGONADISM-ANOSMIA SYNDROME)

General

Disorder of hypothalamic function involving the control of releasing factors, with hypogonadism and anosmia as the clinical signs; agenesis of olfactory bulbs; midline cranial anomalies (cleft lip, cleft palate, imperfect fusion); autosomal recessive phenotype.

Ocular

Color blindness (variable occurrence).

Clinical

Failure of sexual maturation; decrease in primary and secondary sex characteristics; loss of smell; hypertension; mental retardation; schizophrenia.

Laboratory

Patients with idiopathic hypogonadotropic hypogonadism secondary to *DAX1* gene mutations typically present with early-onset adrenocortical insufficiency and may have hyponatremia and hyperkalemia before specific treatment is begun. MRI may also be helpful.

Treatment

Gonadal steroid replacement therapy. Medical therapies are used to treat associated conditions, including osteoporosis, adrenocortical insuffi-

ciency, congenital heart disease and neurologic disorders.

Additional Resource

1. Tritos NA (2011). Kallmann Syndrome and Idiopathic Hypogonadotropic Hypogonadism. [online] Available from http://www.emedicine. com/med/TOPIC1216.HTM [Accessed April, 2012].

795. KAPOSI DISEASE (KAPOSI HEMORRHAGIC SARCOMA; KAPOSI SARCOMA; KAPOSI VARICELLIFORM ERUPTION; MULTIPLE IDIOPATHIC HEMORRHAGIC SARCOMA)

General

Vascular tumor of unknown cause; seen most often in males, Jews, and those from eastern Europe, the southern Mediterranean and Africa; human immunodeficiency virus-related Kaposi syndrome is the most common type of cancer seen in acquired immunodeficiency syndrome patients.

Ocular

Ocular adnexa, varicelliform eruption, including lids, conjunctivae, lacrimal glands and orbit, may be involved; hemorrhage; extensive injection and thickening of conjunctival tissues; conjunctival involvement more evident in bulbar conjunctiva.

Clinical

Vascular sarcomas usually occur on the legs, although widespread cutaneous and visceral tumors may develop; secondary malignancies are very common; lymphedema.

Laboratory

Diagnosis is histopathologic.

Treatment

Cutaneous or conjunctival biopsy of the lesion may be necessary for a definitive diagnosis.

Additional Resource

1. Freudenthal J (2010). Ophthalmologic Manifestations of Kaposi Sarcoma. [online] Available from http://www.emedicine.com/oph/TOPIC481.HTM [Accessed April, 2012].

796. KARSCH-NEUGEBAUER SYNDROME (NYSTAGMUS-SPLIT HAND SYNDROME)

General

Autosomal dominant.

Ocular

Horizontal nystagmus; strabismus; cataract; fundus changes.

Clinical

Split hand and split foot deformities; monodactylous hands.

Laboratory

Diagnosis is made by clinical findings.

Treatment

Baclofen has been effective in treating the periodic alternating nystagmus. Retrobulbar or intramuscular injection of botulinum toxin (BOTOX®) has been demonstrated to abolish nystagmus temporarily. Strabismus surgery is used in patients with certain forms of nystagmus with varying degrees of success.

Bibliography

1. Karsch J. Erbliche Augenmissbildung in Verbendung mit Spalthand Und-Fuss. Z Augenhulk. 1936;89:274-9.

2. McKusick VA. Mendelian Inheritance in Man: A Catalog of Human Genes and Genetic Disorders, 12th edition. Baltimore: The Johns Hopkins University Press; 1998.

3. McKusick-Nathans Institute for Genetic Medicine, Johns Hopkins University and National Center for Biotechnology Information, National Library of Medicine. (2007). Online Mendelian Inheritance in Man (OMIM). [online] Available from http://www.ncbi.nlm.nih.gov/omim/ [Accessed April, 2012].

4. Neugebauer H. Splathand Und-Fuss mit Familiaerer Besonderheit. Z Orthop. 1962;95:500-6.

797. KARTAGENER SYNDROME (BRONCHIECTASIS-DEXTROCARDIA-SINUSITIS; KARTAGENER TRIAD; SINUSITIS-BRONCHIECTASIS-SITUS INVERSUS SYNDROME)

General

Autosomal recessive; onset in early infancy; occasionally dominant; finding of various structural defects in patients with this condition suggests that there are several genetic determinants.

Ocular

Myopia; glaucoma; conjunctival melanosis; iris coloboma; tortuous and dilated retinal vessels; retinal pigmentary degeneration; pseudopapillitis.

Clinical

Immotile cilia; situs inversus; bronchiectasis; sinusitis; various cardiovascular and renal abnormalities; dyspnea; productive cough; recurrent respiratory infections; palpitation; otitis media; nasal speech; conductive hearing loss; nasal polyps; situs inversus viscerum with hepatic dullness on left side.

Laboratory

High-resolution CT scan of the chest is the most sensitive modality for documenting early and subtle abnormalities within airways and pulmonary parenchyma when compared to routine chest radiographs.

Treatment

Antibiotics, intravenous or oral and continuous or intermittent, are used to treat upper and lower airway infections. Obstructive lung disease, if present, should be treated with inhaled bronchodilators and aggressive pulmonary toilet. Tympanostomy tubes are required to reduce conductive hearing loss and recurrent infections.

Additional Resource

1. Bent JP (2011). Kartagener Syndrome. [online] Available from http://www.emedicine.com/med/TOPIC1220.HTM [Accessed April, 2012].

798. KASABACH-MERRITT SYNDROME (CAPILLARY ANGIOMA-THROMBOCYTOPENIA; HEMANGIOMA-THROMBOCYTOPENIA; THROMBOCYTOPENIA PURPURA-HEMANGIOMA)

General

Angioma causing sequestration of platelets and platelet deficiency.

Ocular

Capillary hemangiomas of the orbit; retinal detachments.

Clinical

Extraorbital hemangiomas found on trunk, extremities and palate or in subglottic space; thrombocytopenia; found in infants; purpura and bleeding.

Laboratory

B-scan ultrasound, CT and MRI.

Treatment

Corticosteroids (topical, injectable and systemic) are the treatment of choice. Interferon alpha-2a has emerged as a new modality. Laser surgery and incisional surgical techniques may be necessary.

Additional Resource

1. Seiff S (2011). Capillary Hemangioma. [online] Available from http://www.emedicine.com/oph/TOPIC691.HTM [Accessed April, 2012].

799. KAUFMAN OCULOCEREBROFACIAL SYNDROME

General

Autosomal recessive; significant positive and negative features.

Ocular

Hypertelorism; epicanthal folds; ptosis; mongoloid obliquity; microcornea; pale optic disk; laterally broad eyebrows sparse.

Clinical

Flat philtrum; congenital hypotonia; micrognathia; respiratory distress; high narrow palate; lordosis; constipation; flat feet.

Laboratory

Diagnosis is made by clinical findings.

Treatment

Ptosis: If visual acuity is affected most cases require surgical correction, and there are several procedures that may be used including levator resection, repair or advancement and Fasanella-Servat.

Bibliography

1. Kaufman RL, Rimoin DL, Prensky AL, et al. An oculocerebrofacial syndrome. Birth Defects Orig Artic Ser. 1971;7:135-8.
2. McKusick VA. Mendelian Inheritance in Man: A Catalog of Human Genes and Genetic Disorders, 12th edition. Baltimore: The Johns Hopkins University Press; 1998.

800. KBG SYNDROME

General

Rare condition characterized by typical facial dysmorphism, macrodontia, costovertebral anomalies and developmental delay. Etiology unknown.

Clinical

Short stature, hearing loss, palatal defects, congenital heart defects, wide eyebrows, mild synophrys, prominent and high nasal bridge, anteverted ears, macrodontia of upper central incisors, skeletal anomalies, delayed psychomotor development, low birth weight.

Ocular

Telecantus, strabismus, hypertelorism.

Laboratory

Diagnosis is made by clinical findings.

Treatment

Genetic counseling and referral to appropriate specialists for treatment of the varying characteristics.

Bibliography

1. Dowling PA, Fleming P, Gorlin RJ, et al. The KBG syndrome, characteristics dental findings: a case report. Int J Paediatr Dent. 2001;11:131-4.
2. Smithson SF, Thompson EM, McKinnon AG, et al. The KBG syndrome. Clin Dysmorphol. 2000;9:87-91.

801. KEARNS-SAYRE SYNDROME (KEARNS DISEASE; KEARNS-SHY SYNDROME; OPHTHALMOPLEGIA PLUS SYNDROME)

General

Etiology unknown; sporadic (nonhereditary); onset before age 20 years; external ophthalmoplegia; complete heart block.

Ocular

Pigmentary degeneration of retina; progressive external ophthalmoplegia; corneal decompensation; optic neuritis.

Clinical

Abnormal mitochondria with paracrystalline inclusion in muscle cell; heart block; limb weakness; hyperglycemic acidotic coma; death; cerebellar dysfunction.

Laboratory

Best means of achieving definitive diagnosis is via analysis of a muscle biopsy specimen, with quantification of the level of deletion using Southern blot analysis.

Treatment

No disease-modifying therapy exists for Kearns-Sayre syndrome but symptoms can be treated traditionally.

Additional Resource

1. Basu AP (2010). Kearns-Sayre Syndrome. [online] Available from http://www.emedicine.com/ped/TOPIC2763.HTM [Accessed April, 2012].

802. KENNY SYNDROME

General

Congenital syndrome.

Ocular

Nanophthalmos with hyperopia; papilledema; vascular tortuosity; macular crowding; bilateral optic atrophy.

Clinical

Dwarfism; thickened long bone cortex; transient hypocalcemia.

Laboratory

The diagnosis is supported by hypocalcemia, hyperphosphatemia and low parathyroid hormone levels in the absence of renal failure or intestinal malabsorption.

Treatment

The main goal of treatment is to restore serum calcium levels to alleviate symptoms of acute hypocalcemia. Care to prevent long-term complications from hypocalcemia or hypercalcemia should be coordinated with an endocrinologist.

Additional Resource

1. Gliwa A (2012). Hypoparathyroidism in Emergency Medicine. [online] Available from http://www.emedicine.com/emerg/TOPIC276.HTM [Accessed April, 2012].

803. KERATITIS FUGAX HEREDITARIA

General

Autosomal dominant; onset from 4 to 12 years of age; characterized by acute attacks of keratitis.

Ocular

Keratitis; corneal opacities.

Clinical

None

Laboratory

Diagnosis is made by clinical findings.

Treatment

Initiate broad-spectrum antibiotics with the following: tobramycin every hour alternating with fortified cefazolin (50 mg/mL) 1 drop every hour. If the corneal ulcer is small, peripheral and no impending perforation is present, intensive monotherapy with fluoroquinolones is an alternative treatment.

Additional Resource

1. Mills TJ (2011). Corneal Ulceration and Ulcerative Keratitis in Emergency Medicine. [online] Available from http://www.emedicine.com/emerg/TOPIC115.HTM [Accessed April, 2012].

804. KERATOACANTHOMA

General

Benign epithelial tumor that arises on hair follicles in exposed skin of caucasians.

Clinical

Keratoacanthoma can occur in other parts of the body.

Ocular

Conjunctival nodules may result in foreign body sensation and tearing.

Laboratory

Biopsy of lesion can be diagnostic.

Treatment

Excisional biopsy, curettage, cryotherapy, radiation.

Bibliography

1. Roy FH, Fraunfelder FW, Fraunfelder FT. Roy and Fraunfelder's Current Ocular Therapy, 6th edition. Philadelphia: WB Saunders; 2008.

805. KERATOCONJUNCTIVITIS SICCA AND SJÖGREN SYNDROME

General

Autoimmune disease, seen more frequently in females.

Clinical

Xerostomia (dry mouth), dry nasal and genital mucosa.

Ocular

Severe dry eyes, corneal ulceration, corneal perforation, corneal scarring and vascularization.

Laboratory

Biopsy of lip and lacrimal gland positive, antinuclear antibody rheumatoid factor (RF), anti-Ro (Sjögren's specific A) and anti-La (Sjögren specific B). Elevated IgG level—positive predication for positive biopsy.

Treatment

Severe cases—immunosuppressive agents as cyclosporine A and corticosteroids. Frequent application of tear substitutes, steroids, punctal plugs, bandage contacts and partial tarsorrhaphy.

Additional Resource

1. Foster CS (2012). Dry Eye Syndrome. [online] Available from http://www.emedicine.com/oph/TOPIC597.HTM [Accessed April, 2012].

806. KERATOCONUS

General

Noninflammatory corneal disorder, usually bilateral.

Clinical

None

Ocular

Thinning corneal stroma in central or inferior corneal, astigmatism.

Laboratory

Corneal topography.

Treatment

Spectacle correction, hard contacts and avoid eye rubbing may be useful. If hydrops occurs discontinue contact lens, use NaCl drops and ointment, patching and short course of steroids. As the disease advances penetrating keratoplasty, deep anterior lamellar keratoplasty, intacs with laser grooves or collagen stabilization of cornea.

Bibliography

1. Kymionis GD, Kounis GA, Portaliou DM, et al. Intraoperative pachymetric measurements during corneal collagen cross-linking with riboflavin and ultraviolet A irradiation. Ophthalmology. 2009; 116:2336-9.

Additional Resource

1. Weissman BA (2011). Keratoconus. [online] Available from http://www.emedicine.com/oph/ TOPIC104.HTM [Accessed April, 2012].

807. KERATOCONUS POSTICUS CIRCUMSCRIPTUS (KPC; KPC ASSOCIATED WITH MALFORMATIONS)

General

Autosomal recessive; rare; abnormality in corneal curvature centrally localized on its posterior surface in association with opacification of the overlying stroma; may be an anterior chamber cleavage defect with failure of normal separation of the lens and iris from the cornea.

Ocular

Corneal opacities; retinal coloboma; ptosis; hyperopia; iridocorneal adhesions; hypertelorism.

Clinical

Cleft lip; cleft palate; neck webbing; short stature; mental retardation; inguinal hernia; undescended testes; tight heel cords; vertebral anomalies; delayed bone age; double ureters; cone-shaped epiphyses; stubby limbs and digits; limitation of extension and supination of the elbows; brachydactyly; fifth finger clinodactyly; frequent urinary tract infections; prominent nose; mild maxillary hypoplasia; low posterior hairline; short, broad feet with bilateral pes cavus; bilateral ureteric reflux.

Laboratory

Corneal topography.

Treatment

Rigid contact lenses (CLs) are the mainstay of treatment, intrastromal corneal rings (Intacs) have shown some success and corneal graft is sometimes necessary.

Bibliography

1. McKusick VA. Mendelian Inheritance in Man: A Catalog of Human Genes and Genetic Disorders, 12th edition. Baltimore: The Johns Hopkins University Press; 1998.
2. McKusick-Nathans Institute for Genetic Medicine, Johns Hopkins University and National Center for Biotechnology Information, National Library of Medicine. (2007). Online Mendelian Inheritance in Man (OMIM). [online] Available from http:// www.ncbi.nlm.nih.gov/omim/ [Accessed April, 2012].
3. Young ID, Macrae WG, Hughes HE, et al. Keratoconus posticus circumscriptus, cleft lip and palate, genitourinary abnormalities, short stature, and mental retardation in sibs. J Med Genet. 1982;19:332-6.

808. KERATODERMIA PALMARIS ET PLANTARIS (KERATOSIS PALMOPLANTARIS; PALMOPLANTAR KERATODERMIA)

General

Autosomal recessive; hereditary disorder; diffuse or focal thickening of the palms and soles.

Ocular

Hyperkeratosis of lid and cornea; ectropion; leukoma; corneal ulceration; pronounced photophobia; hereditary optic atrophy; epiphora; conjunctivitis.

Clinical

Localized or disseminated hyperkeratotic changes of the palms and soles with a tendency toward fissure and secondary infection.

Laboratory

Diagnosis is made by clinical findings.

Treatment

Ectropion: Topical ocular lubricants. Congenital-full thickness skin graft with canthal tendon tightening. Involutional-tighten lid by resecting full thickness wedge-medial spindle procedure for punctal eversion. Paralytic may require a fascia lata sling procedure if does not resolve in 3–6 months.

Corneal ulcer: Corneal cultures may be taken and treatment initiated. Treatment includes a broad spectrum of antibiotics and cycloplegic drops.

Additional Resource

1. Lee RA (2011). Keratosis Palmaris et Plantaris. [online] Available from http://www.emedicine.com/derm/TOPIC589.HTM [Accessed April, 2012].

809. KERATOPATHY, NEUROTROPHIC

General

Degenerative disease characterized by poor corneal sensitivity and healing. It can be a result of herpes zoster, trauma to the trigeminal nerve, ocular surgery or systemic disease such as diabetes.

Ocular

Decreased corneal sensitivity, poor corenal healing, decreased tearing, ulceration, corneal melting and decreased vision.

Clinical

Herpes zoster, surgical or traumatic injury to the trigeminal nerve, diabetes mellitus acoustic neuroma.

Laboratory

Corneal esthesiometry to measure corneal sensitivity is crucial for diagnosis. MRI of brain and orbits may be necessary to diagnose neurologic deficit. Diagnosis is made by clinical findings.

Treatment

Preservative-free topical lubrication, discontinue ocular medications with preservatives, discontinue systemic drugs such as antihistamines and antipsychotics if possible. In some cases surgical intervention may be necessary which includes lateral tarsorrhaphy, conjunctival flap, and lamellar or penetrating keratoplasty.

Additional Resource

1. Graham RH (2012). Neurotrophic Keratopathy. [online] Available from http://emedicine.medscape.com/article/1194889-overview [Accessed April, 2012].

810. KILOH-NEVIN SYNDROME (MUSCULAR DYSTROPHY OF EXTERNAL OCULAR MUSCLES; OCULAR MYOPATHY)

General

Etiology unknown; autosomal dominant.

Ocular

Ptosis; orbicularis muscle weakness; ocular myopathy; diplopia progressing to bilateral myopathic ophthalmoplegia; may be associated with pigmentary retinopathy and heart block (see Kearns-Sayre syndrome).

Clinical

Progressive muscular dystrophy in which facial muscles may be involved; occasionally, hereditary ataxia; pain; myokymia.

Laboratory

Diagnosis is made by clinical findings.

Treatment

Topical keratolytics, systemic and topical retinoids, potent topical steroids.

Bibliography

1. Kiloh LG, Nevin S. Progressive dystrophy of the external ocular muscles. Brain. 1951;74:115-43.
2. Duszowa J, Koraszewska-Matuszewska B, Niebrój TK. The Kiloh-Nevin syndrome. Klin Oczna. 1974;44:805-7.

811. KIMMELSTIEL-WILSON SYNDROME (DIABETIC GLOMERULOSCLEROSIS; DIABETES MELLITUS-HYPERTENSION-NEPHROSIS SYNDROME; DIABETES-NEPHROSIS SYNDROME; INTERCAPILLARY GLOMERULOSCLEROSIS; RENAL GLOMERULOHYALINOSIS-DIABETIC SYNDROME)

General

Occurs in patients with diabetes mellitus of several years' duration.

Ocular

Retinal lesions, including hemorrhages, exudates, and neovascularization.

Clinical

Hypertension; proteinuria; edema; glomerulonephrosis; arteriosclerosis; capillary or intercapillary glomerulosclerosis; eosinophilic nodules; hyaline degeneration of the renal arterioles.

Laboratory

Serum—hyperglycemia; urine—glycosuria.

Treatment

Pharmacologic therapy allowing glycemic control, diet modification and weight loss is the main therapy for diabetes.

Additional Resource

1. Khardori R (2012). Type 2 Diabetes Mellitus. [online] Available from http://www.emedicine.com/med/TOPIC547.HTM [Accessed April, 2012].

812. KINSBOURNE SYNDROME (DANCING EYES SYNDROME; OPSOCLONUS-MYOCLONUS SYNDROME)

General

Etiology unknown; occurs in infancy and early childhood; myoclonic encephalopathy; has been reported as the only manifestation of a postinfectious syndrome without evidence of encephalitis.

Ocular

Twitching of lids and eyebrows on occasion, more pronounced with activity than at rest; irregular vertical movements, jerky in appearance and sometimes with some lateral nystagmic components.

Clinical

Sporadic, jerky movements of head, trunk and limbs, usually more pronounced when the child is active; lack of coordination; ataxia; irritability; mental retardation; chronic neurologic deficits.

Laboratory

Diagnosis is made by clinical findings.

Treatment

Nystagmus: See-saw nystagmus—visual field to consider neoplastic or vascular etiologies. Upbeat nystagmus—may indicate multiple sclerosis, cerebellar degeneration, tumors or infarcts. Treatment is directed toward identification and resolution of underlying cause. Downbeat nystagmus—affects the cerebellum or craniocervical junction including Arnold-Chiari malformation, multiple sclerosis, trauma, tumor, infarction and many toxic metabolic entities. MRI may indicate a surgically correctable lesion. Periodic alternating nystagmus is continuous horizontal nystagmus from stroke, tumor, multiple sclerosis, trauma, infection and drug intoxication. Can occur from cataract, vitreous hemorrhage or optic atrophy.

Bibliography

1. Bhatia K, Thompson PD, Marsden CD. "Isolated" postinfectious myoclonus. J Neurol Neurosurg Psychiatry. 1992;55:1089-91.
2. Geeraets WJ. Ocular Syndromes, 3rd edition. Philadelphia: Lea & Febiger; 1976.
3. Kinsbourne M. Myoclonic encephalopathy of infants. J Neurol Neurosurg Psychiatry. 1962;25: 271-6.
4. Koh PS, Raffensperger JG, Berry S, et al. Long-term outcome in children with opsoclonus-myoclonus and ataxia and coincident neuroblastoma. J Pediatr. 1994;125:712-6.

813. KIRK SYNDROME

General

Etiology unknown; raised hereditary masses over central cornea; rare, only one family known to be affected.

Ocular

Photophobia; excessive lacrimation; amyloid corneal deposits.

Clinical

None

Laboratory

Diagnosis is made by clinical findings.

Treatment

Phototherapeutic keratectomy (PTK) with the excimer laser may be useful in removing opacities. If the visual acuity drops and the opacities are deep, a lamellar or full-thickness corneal transplant can be performed.

Bibliography

1. Kirk HQ, Rabb M, Hattenhauer J, et al. Primary familial amyloidosis of the cornea. Trans Am Acad Ophthalmol Otolaryngol. 1973;77:411-7.

814. KJELLIN SYNDROME

General

Autosomal recessive disorder; progressive.

Ocular

Yellow retinal flecks that lie at the pigment epithelial level; poor visual perceptual skills; central retinal degeneration.

Clinical

Spastic paraparesis; dementia; progressive lower extremity weakness; dysarthric speech; muscle atrophy.

Laboratory

Diagnosis is made by clinical findings.

Treatment

None/Ocular.

Bibliography

1. Puech B, Lacour A, Stevanin G, et al. Kjellin syndrome: long-term neuro-ophthalmologic follow-up and novel mutations in the *SPG11* gene. Ophthalmology. 2011;118:564-73.

Additional Resource

1. Chawla J (2010). Neurological Manifestations of Vascular Dementia. [online] Available from http://www.emedicine.com/neuro/TOPIC227.HTM [Accessed April, 2012].

815. KLEIN SYNDROME

General

Autosomal dominant; belongs to the group of iridodermatoauditive dysplasias.

Ocular

Hypertelorism; blepharophimosis; hypertrichosis; blue irides; heterochromia.

Clinical

Bilateral labyrinthine deafness; mandibular retrognathism; skull deformities and arched palate; partial albinism of skin and hair; syndactylism (cutaneous).

Laboratory

Diagnosis is made by clinical findings.

Treatment

None/Ocular.

Additional Resource

1. Jackson IT (2012). Congenital Syndromes. [online] Available from http://www.emedicine.com/plastic/TOPIC183.HTM [Accessed April, 2012].

816. KLINEFELTER SYNDROME (GYNECOMASTIA-ASPERMATOGENESIS SYNDROME; XXY SYNDROME; XXXY SYNDROME; XXYY SYNDROME; REIFENSTEIN-ALBRIGHT SYNDROME)

General

Occurrence in 1% of retarded males; phenotypically males with positive female sex chromatin; karyotype shows 47 chromosomes, 44 autosomes and 3 sex chromosomes with the complement XXY.

Ocular

Anophthalmos; coloboma; corneal opacities.

Clinical

Testicular hypoplasia; sterility; gynecomastia; eunuchoid physique; mental retardation; association with progressive systemic sclerosis and systemic lupus erythematosus.

Laboratory

It may be diagnosed prenatally based on cytogenetic analysis of a fetus. If not diagnosed prenatally, the 47,XXY karyotype may manifest as various subtle age-related clinical signs that may prompt chromosomal evaluation.

Treatment

Treatment should address three major facets of the disease: (1) hypogonadism, (2) gynecomastia and (3) psychosocial problems.

Additional Resource

1. Chen H (2011). Klinefelter Syndrome. [online] Available from http://www.emedicine.com/ped/TOPIC1252.HTM [Accessed April, 2012].

817. KLIPPEL-FEIL SYNDROME (CONGENITAL BREVICOLLIS; SYNOSTOSIS OF CERVICAL VERTEBRA)

General

Autosomal recessive inheritance; females more commonly affected; progressive paraplegia may develop late in life.

Ocular

Esotropia; hypertropia combined with torticollis; occasional horizontal nystagmus.

Clinical

Platybasia; congenital upward displacement of scapula (Sprengel deformity); brevicollis; immobility of neck (painless); low posterior hairline; peculiar facies; cleft palate; short stature; congenital brevicollis; vertebral abnormalities; autosomal dominant mode of inheritance has been reported.

Laboratory

Plain radiography is the basis for the diagnosis. CT and MRI may also be helpful.

Treatment

Medical therapy depends on the congenital anomalies present in the syndrome. Consulta-tions with cardiogist, urologist, audiologist and nephrologist may be necessary.

Additional Resource

1. Sullivan JA (2012). Klippel-Feil Syndrome. [online] Available from http://www.emedicine.com/or-thoped/TOPIC408.HTM [Accessed April, 2012].

---

818. KLIPPEL-TRENAUNAY-WEBER SYNDROME (ANGIO-OSTEO-HYPERTROPHY SYNDROME; PARKES-WEBER SYNDROME)

General

Most frequently inherited as irregular dominant; however, reported to be recessive with parent consanguinity; association of Klippel-Trenaunay-Weber syndrome and Sturge-Weber syndrome has been reported.

Ocular

Enophthalmos; unilateral hydrophthalmos; con-junctival telangiectasia; atypical iris coloboma; cataract; irregular and dilated retinal vessels; choroidal angiomas; exudative outer retinal vas-cular masses.

Clinical

Vascular nevi; varicose vessels; capillary angio-mas; lymphangioma; arteriovenous aneurysm; hypertrophy of soft tissues and bones (local); phlebitis; thrombosis; syndactyly; polydactyly; early eruption of teeth; hemifacial hypertrophy.

Laboratory

Ultrasound, MRI, angiography and X-ray.

Treatment

Compression stockings or pneumatic pumps are usually successful. Surgical intervention (resection or ligation of abnormal blood vessels) is sometimes necessary.

Additional Resource

1. Buehler B (2009). Genetics of Klippel-Trenaunay-Weber Syndrome. [online] Available from http://www.emedicine.com/ped/TOPIC1253.HTM [Accessed April, 2012].

---

819. KLOEPFER SYNDROME

General

Rare autosomal recessive disease; manifestations at age 2 months; death between the ages of 21 and 30 years.

Ocular

Progressive loss of vision to complete blindness associated with progressive dementia.

Clinical

Severe blistering in sunlight; no increase in weight and height after erythema subsides at age 5–6 years; mental age does not progress beyond the level of imbeciles; progressive degenerative dementia occurs during or immediately after adolescence.

Laboratory

Diagnosis is made by clinical findings.

Treatment

None/Ocular.

Additional Resource

1. Horner KL (2012). Leiomyoma. [online] Available from http://www.emedicine.com/derm/TOPIC217.HTM [Accessed April, 2012].

---

820. KLÜVER-BUCY SYNDROME (TEMPORAL LOBECTOMY BEHAVIOR SYNDROME)

General

Occurs after temporal lobectomy, carried out therapeutically for temporal lobe epilepsy.

Ocular

"Psychic blindness" or visual agnosia.

Clinical

Changes in emotional behavior (possible rage reactions); hypersexuality; bulimia (changes in dietary habits); loss of recognition of people; strong oral tendencies (i.e. licking, biting, chewing); deficiency of memory; psychic blindness; aberrant sexual behavior; hypermetamorphosis; aphasia; visual agnosia; memory deficit; speech disturbance; syndrome in adults is commonly associated with neurodegenerative conditions, following radiation therapy, or after temporal lobectomy; syndrome in children has been recognized almost exclusively in association with acute bitemporal injury or dysfunction.

Laboratory

Diagnosis is made by clinical findings.

Treatment

Treatment is symptomatic and supportive, and may include drug therapy.

Bibliography

1. Hooshmand H, Sepdham T, Vries JK. Kluver-Bucy syndrome. Successful treatment with carbamazepine. JAMA. 1974;229:1782.
2. Kluver H, Bucy PC. Psychic blindness and other symptoms following bilateral temporal lobectomy in rhesus monkeys. Am J Physiol. 1937;119:352-3.
3. Lanska DJ, Lanska MJ. Kluver-Bucy syndrome in juvenile neuronal ceroid lipofuscinosis. J Child Neurol. 1994;9:67-9.

821. KNIEST DYSPLASIA (METATROPIC DWARFISM TYPE II)

General

Autosomal dominant disease; Swiss cheese pattern on cartilage biopsy specimen; due to either alteration metabolism of proteoglycans or abnormality in collagen synthesis; both sexes affected; collagen type II collagenopathy; produced by a single amino acid substitution in the type II collagen triple helix.

Ocular

Retinal detachment; severe myopia; cataracts; dislocated lenses; blepharoptosis; vitreoretinal degeneration; vitreous traction; congenital glaucoma; hypertelorism; mild synophrys; epicanthal folds; perivascular lattice degeneration, white without pressure.

Clinical

Severe short stature; typical facies with flat nasal bridge; cleft palate; hearing loss; joint contractures; lordosis; kyphosis.

Laboratory

Computed tomography (CT), MRI, X-ray and ultrasound.

Treatment

Retinal detachment, cataract and congenital glaucoma surgery.

Additional Resource

1. Khan AN (2011). Achondroplasia Imaging. [online] Available from http://www.emedicine.com/radio/TOPIC809.HTM [Accessed April, 2012].

822. KNOBLOCH SYNDROME

General

Autosomal recessive; retinal detachment with occipital encephalocele.

Ocular

High myopia; retinal detachment; vitreoretinal degeneration; persistent papillary membrane; posterior vitreous detachment; retinochoroidal staphylomas.

Clinical

Occipital encephalocele; normal intelligence; congenital midline scalp defect; unusual plantar creases.

Laboratory

Computed tomography (CT), MRI, ultrasound and angiography.

Treatment

Prenatal diagnosis should be discussed with the parents, because in most pregnancies, termination is chosen. If the diagnosis is made later in pregnancy, cesarean delivery may be considered when neonatal surgery is planned.

Additional Resource

1. Khan AN (2011). Encephalocele Imaging. [online] Available from http://www.emedicine.com/radio/TOPIC246.HTM [Accessed April, 2012].

823. KOBY SYNDROME (FLORIFORM CATARACT)

General

Autosomal dominant; both sexes affected.

Ocular

Multiple opacities of different shapes (annular, floriform and polychromatic); found especially around embryonic nucleus.

Clinical

None

Laboratory

Diagnosis is made by clinical findings.

Treatment

Cataract surgery should be considered if visual acuity is decreased.

Additional Resource

1. Bashour M (2011). Congenital Cataract. [online] Available from http://www.emedicine.com/oph/TOPIC45.HTM [Accessed April, 2012].

824. KOERBER-SALUS-ELSCHNIG SYNDROME (NYSTAGMUS RETRACTORIUS SYNDROME; SYLVIAN AQUEDUCT SYNDROME)

General

Caused by tumor or inflammation in region of aqueduct of Sylvius, third and fourth ventricle, or corpora quadrigemina.

Ocular

Lid retraction may be associated with midbrain lesions above the posterior commissure; paresis of vertical gaze; tonic spasm of convergence on attempted upward gaze; clonic convergence movements or convergence nystagmus; vertical nystagmus on gaze up or down; nystagmus retractorius with spasmodic retraction of the eyes when an attempt is made to move them in any direction; occasional extraocular muscle paresis.

Clinical

Headaches; dizziness; hypertension; possible hemiparesis; ataxia; hemitremor; Babinski's sign.

Laboratory

Computed tomography (CT) and MRI.

Treatment

Lid retraction: Identify systemic abnormalities such as thyroid. Treatment must be given for 6 months for stabilizing before performing eyelid surgery. Local-ocular lubrication (drops or ointment). Botulism type A may also be useful.

Bibliography

1. Elschnig A. Nystagmus Retractorius, ein Cerebrales Herdsymptom. Med Klin. 1913;9:8-11.
2. Geeraets WJ. Ocular Syndromes, 3rd edition. Philadelphia: Lea & Febiger; 1976.

825. KOMOTO SYNDROME (CONGENITAL EYELID TETRAD; CET)

General

Autosomal dominant; all races affected; most patients are of normal intelligence.

Ocular

Ptosis; epicanthus inversus; blepharophimosis; telecanthus.

Clinical

None

Laboratory

Diagnosis is made by clinical findings.

Treatment

Ptosis: If visual acuity is affected most cases require surgical correction, and there are several procedures that may be used including levator resection, repair or advancement and Fasanella-Servat.

Bibliography

1. Bergin DJ, La Piana FG. Natural history of the congenital eyelid tetrad (Komoto's syndrome). Ann Ophthalmol. 1981;13:1145-8.
2. Komoto J. Veber die Operation be; Hereditaren Phimosis Congenita mit Ptosis. Nippon Ganka Gakkai. 1920;24, and Klin Monatsbl Augenheilkd. 1921;66:952.

826. KRABBE (2) SYNDROME (GALACTOCEREBROSIDASE DEFICIENCY; STURGE-WEBER-KRABBE SYNDROME)

General

Etiology unknown; some evidence of irregularly dominant transmission; variant of Sturge-Weber syndrome; both sexes affected; present from birth; appears that the GALC locus lies somewhere in the region 14q21–q31.

Ocular

Buphthalmos; conjunctival angiomas; choroidal angiomatosis; retinal aneurysm.

Clinical

Cerebral angiomas (possible calcium deposition); flat angioma of the skin in the distribution area of the trigeminal nerve (V) (nevus flammeus); mental deterioration due to progressive atrophy of the brain; contralateral hemiplegia; facial hemiatrophy.

Laboratory

GALC activity measurement can help confirm a diagnosis, CT, EEG, EMG.

Treatment

Hematopoietic stem cell transplantation should be considered in individuals with late-onset or slowly progressive disease.

Additional Resource

1. Tegay DH (2010). Krabbe Disease. [online] Available from http://www.emedicine.com/ped/TOPIC2892.HTM [Accessed April, 2012].

827. KRAUSE SYNDROME (CONGENITAL ENCEPHALO-OPHTHALMIC DYSPLASIA; ENCEPHALO-OPHTHALMIC SYNDROME)

General

No hereditary factors involved; no predilection for either sex; more frequent in premature infants; death frequently from intercurrent infections.

Ocular

Microphthalmos; enophthalmos; ptosis; strabismus; secondary glaucoma; iris atrophy; anterior and posterior synechiae; scleral atrophy; persistent remnants of hyaloids artery; intraocular hemorrhages and exudates; cyclitic membranes; cataracts; retinal hypoplasia and hyperplasia; choroidal and retinal malformation; retinal glial membranes; retinal detachment; choroidal atrophy; optic nerve malformation; optic atrophy.

Clinical

Congenital cerebral dysplasia; hydrocephalus or microcephaly; mental retardation; heterotopia.

Laboratory

Diagnosis is made by clinical findings.

Treatment

Ptosis: If visual acuity is affected most cases require surgical correction, and there are several procedures that may be used including levator resection, repair or advancement and Fasanella-Servat.

Strabismus: Equalized vision with correct refractive error; surgery may be helpful in patient with diplopia.

Glaucoma: Its medication should be the first plan of action. If medication is unsuccessful, a filtering surgical procedure with or without antimetabolites may be beneficial.

Cataract: Change in glasses can sometimes improve a patient's visual function temporarily; however, the most common treatment is cataract surgery.

Vitreous hemorrhage: If possible the source of the bleeding needs to be isolated and treated with laser. Vitrectomy may be necessary.

Retinal detachment: Scleral buckle, pneumatic retinopexy and vitrectomy may be used to close all the breaks.

Bibliography

1. Krause AC. Congenital encephalo-ophthalmic dysplasia. Arch Ophthalmol. 1946;36:387.
2. Miller M, Robbins J, Fishman R, et al. A chromosomal anomaly with multiple ocular defects. Am J Ophthalmol. 1963;55:901.

828. KUFS DISEASE (ADULT CHRONIC GM2 GANGLIOSIDOSIS; GANGLIOSIDOSIS GM2 ADULT TYPE; HALLERVORDEN-KUFS SYNDROME)

General

Autosomal recessive; hexosaminase A decrease; onset in the third and fourth decades of life; slow death within 19 or 20 years of onset; very rare type of adult neuronal ceroid lipofuscinosis; autosomal recessive and dominant inheritance have been reported.

Ocular

Retinal storage; ocular lesions usually are absent; rare macular discoloration; no pigmentary degeneration of the retina.

Clinical

Dementia and behavioral changes; progressive gait and postural deterioration; mild ataxia; dysarthria; ascending muscular atrophy; pes cavus; cerebral degeneration; apathy; progressive myoclonus epilepsy; aphasia; facial dyskinesias; lipid infiltration of the brain cells is the principal pathologic feature (see Ceroid Lipofuscinosis).

Laboratory

Electromyographic abnormalities may be noted, and creatine phosphokinase isoenzyme levels may be elevated. Muscle biopsy may be useful.

Treatment

None/Ocular.

Additional Resource

1. Tegay DH (2012). GM2 Gangliosidoses. [online] Available from http://www.emedicine.com/ped/TOPIC3016.HTM [Accessed April, 2012].

829. KUGELBERG-WELANDER SYNDROME (JUVENILE MUSCULAR ATROPHY)

General

Autosomal recessive; juvenile spinal muscular atrophy; affects both sexes; onset in late childhood or adolescence.

Ocular

Ptosis; ophthalmoplegia; exotropia; orbicularis oculi paresis.

Clinical

Slowly progressive proximal muscle atrophy; lower extremities usually are affected first, with the upper limbs being affected late; frequently, fasciculation; proximal muscle weakness, especially of the lower extremities; elevated serum creatine kinase levels.

Laboratory

Routine genetic testing only detects patients with the homozygous deletion. Ultrasound of the muscles had been used to assess for neurogenic atrophy.

Treatment

No cure is known treatment is focused on symptomatic control and preventative rehabilitation.

Additional Resource

1. Oleszek JL (2011). Kugelberg-Welander Spinal Muscular Atrophy. [online] Available from http://www.emedicine.com/pmr/TOPIC62.HTM [Accessed April, 2012].

830. KURU SYNDROME (LAUGHING DEATH)

General

Restricted to Fore tribe of Eastern New Guinea; prevalent in children and adult women; etiology unknown, possibly related to the tribe's practice of cannibalism; uncertain whether significant genetic factors also are involved.

Ocular

Strabismus; nystagmus.

Clinical

Ataxia; trembling leg muscles; incoordination; exaggeration of voluntary movements; jerks; slurred speech; fecal incontinence; aphonia; dysphagia.

Laboratory

Diagnosis is made by clinical findings.

Treatment

Nystagmus: See-saw nystagmus—visual field to consider neoplastic or vascular etiologies. Up-beat nystagmus—may indicate multiple sclerosis, cerebellar degeneration, tumors or infarcts. Treatment is directed toward identification and resolution of underlying cause. Downbeat nystagmus—affects the cerebellum or craniocervical junction including Arnold-Chiari malformation, multiple sclerosis, trauma, tumor, infarction and many toxic metabolic entities. MRI may indicate a surgically correctable lesion. Periodic alternating nystagmus is continuous horizontal nystagmus from stroke, tumor, multiple sclerosis, trauma, infection and drug intoxication. Can occur from cataract, vitreous hemorrhage or optic atrophy.

Additional Resource

1. Khan ZZ (2010). Kuru. [online] Available from http://www.emedicine.com/med/TOPIC1248. HTM [Accessed April, 2012].

831. LANZIERI SYNDROME

General

Developmental anomaly that belongs to group of craniofacial malformations; present from birth.

Ocular

Microphthalmia; anophthalmos; iris coloboma; cataracts; retinal and choroidal coloboma; optic nerve coloboma.

Clinical

Dwarfism; dyscephalia; dental anomalies; hypertrichosis; skin atrophy; absence of fibula, some tarsal and metatarsal bones.

Laboratory

Diagnosis is made by clinical findings.

Treatment

Cataract: Change in glasses can sometimes improve a patient's visual function temporarily; however, the most common treatment is cataract surgery.

Bibliography

1. Geeraets WJ. Ocular Syndromes, 3rd edition. Philadelphia: Lea & Febiger; 1976.
2. Lanzieri M. On a rare association of craniofacial malformative syndrome and congenital absence of the fibula. Ann Ottalmol Clin Ocul. 1961;87: 667-78.
3. Magalini SI, Scrascia E. Dictionary of Medical Syndromes, 2nd edition. Philadelphia: JB Lippincott; 1981.

832. LARON SYNDROME

General

Autosomal recessive; insulin-like growth factor I (IGF-I) hormone resistance.

Ocular

Microphthalmia; reduced retinal vascularization; optic nerve hypoplasia; pseudopapilledema.

Clinical

Short stature; abnormally small extremities; subnormal head circumference, increased body fat and delayed sexual development.

Laboratory

Diagnosis is made by clinical findings.

Treatment

None/Ocular.

Additional Resource

1. http://www.emedicine.medscape.com/article/922902-overview

833. LARSEN SYNDROME

General

Etiology unknown; autosomal recessive; possibly dominant in some cases.

Ocular

Hypertelorism; bilateral chronic keratitis; corneal neovascularization; lower lid entropion.

Clinical

Frontal bossing; depressed nasal bridge; flat face; flat and broad thumbs; skeletal dysplasia with multiple joint dislocations; unusual faces; long, cylindrical fingers; spatulate thumbs; dental abnormalities; cardiac defects; hydrocephalus; laryngotracheomalacia; dislocation of the cervical spine; tracheomalacias; heart disease; severe respiratory infection; clubfeet; multiple joint deformities; hydrocephalus; tracheal stenosis.

Laboratory

Diagnosis is made by clinical findings.

Treatment

Keratitis: Local treatment is used for prevention and reduction of corneal damage. Systemic therapy is used for controlling the underlying disease. Tissue adhesives may be necessary for impending perforation. Keratectomy, conjunctival resection, amniotic membrane transplantation and keratoplasty may necessary.

Entropion: Topical antibiotics and lubricants, temporary sutures to evert the eyelid, lateral cantholysis with subconjunctival incision just inferior to the tarsus. Inferior retractors are isolated and reattached to anteroinferior portion of tarsus with multiple interrupted sutures.

Bibliography

1. Laville JM, Lakermance P, Limouzy F. Larsen's syndrome: review of the literature and analysis of thirty-eight cases. J Pediatr Orthop. 1994;14:63-73.
2. Magalini SI, Scrascia E. Dictionary of Medical Syndromes, 2nd edition. Philadelphia: JB Lippincott; 1981.

Additional Resource

1. http://www.emedicine.medscape.com/article/1467286-overview

834. LASEK

General

Laser assisted subepithelial keratectomy is a procedure specifically used to correct astigmatism, hyperopia and myopia. LASEK is done with surface ablation.

Clinical

None

Ocular

Refractive error; severe dry eyes.

Laboratory

Diagnosis is made by clinical observation.

Treatment

After epithelium is removed, with a mixture of alcohol and water, and a flap is formed, the laser is used to obliterate the specified amount of tissue. The flap is then rolled back over the area of ablation.

Additional Resource

1. Roque MR (2012). PRK Astigmatism. [online] Available from http://www.emedicine.medscape.com/article/1220845-overview [Accessed April, 2012].

835. LASIK MYOPIA

General

LASIK is a surgical technique that involves the creation of a hinged lamellar corneal flap, after which an excimer laser is used to make a refractive cut on the underlying stromal bed.

Clinical

None

Ocular

Unstable refractive error, active collagen vascular disease, conjunctivitis, severe dry eye, keratoconus.

Laboratory

None

Treatment

The combined suction ring and microkeratome is placed on the eye and centered over the limbus with slight nasal displacement. Intraocular pressure with the suction ring applied is between 60 and 90 mm Hg. High pressure is necessary to hold suction ring in place. A corneal flap is made, and a spatula is placed between the flap and the stromal bed. The laser is focused and centered, and the planned refractive ablation takes place.

Additional Resource

1. Taravella M (2012). LASIK Myopia Treatment & Management. [online] Available from http://www.emedicine.medscape.com/article/1221604-treatment [Accessed April, 2012].

836. LATERAL SINUS THROMBOSIS (SIGMOID SINUS THROMBOSIS)

General

Predominant in children; acute onset secondary to chronic otitic infections; high mortality rate without treatment; any microorganism may be responsible for infection and secondary thrombosis; associated with oral contraceptive usage.

Ocular

Pain behind the eye; muscle palsies; papilledema (50%).

Clinical

Fever; headaches; nausea; vomiting; swelling over mastoid region; intracranial hypertension; seizures; hemiplegia.

Laboratory

The diagnosis of lateral sinus thrombosis is usually suspected on clinical grounds, but radiology is essential to confirm it. CT scanning and MRI are the current imaging tools of choice in making the diagnosis.

Treatment

Combination of antibiotics and surgery is usually necessary. Surgery includes mastoid exploration, exposure of sinus, incision and drainage, and removal of as much clot as possible.

Additional Resource

1. Viswanatha B (2012). Otogenic Lateral Sinus Thrombosis. [online] Available from http://www.emedicine.com/ent/TOPIC1048625.HTM [Accessed April, 2012].

837. LATTICE CORNEAL DYSTROPHY (AVELLINO DYSTROPHY, BIBER-HAAB-DIMMER DYSTROPHY, FAMILIAL MYLOID POLYNEUROPATHY TYPE IV, LATTICE DYSTROPHY TYPE I, LATTICE DYSTROPHY TYPE II, LATTICE DYSTROPHY TYPE III, LCD-I, LCD-II, LCD-III, MERETOJA'S SYNDROME)

General

LCD I—autosomal dominant; LCD II—autosomal dominant onset third decade (Scandinavia) and LCD III—autosomal dominant onset third decade (Japan).

Clinical

None

Ocular

Corneal dystrophy, thin lines in corneal stroma.

Laboratory

Diagnosis is made by clinical findings.

Treatment

Topical—lubricants, soft contacts, pressure patching. Surgical—phototherapeutic keratectomy (PTK) may be useful in superficial lesions. Penetrating keratoplasty may be necessary.

Bibliography

1. Roy FH, Fraunfelder FW, Fraunfelder FT. Roy and Fraunfelder's Current Ocular Therapy, 6th edition. Philadelphia: WB Saunders; 2008.

838. LATTICE DEGENERATION AND RETINAL DETACHMENT

General

Autosomal dominant; progressive; lattice degeneration precedes retinal detachment by about 20 years; familial occurrence of lattice degeneration in nonmyopes has been reported.

Ocular

Myopia; retinoschisis; peripheral retinal degeneration; lattice degeneration.

Clinical

None

Laboratory

Diagnosis is made by clinical findings.

Treatment

Laser photocoagulation, cryotherapy, scleral buckling procedure and/or pars plana vitrectomy and gas administration.

Additional Resource

1. Sarraf D (2010). Lattice Degeneration. [online] Available from http://www.emedicine.com/oph/TOPIC397.HTM [Accessed April, 2012].

839. LAURENCE-MOON-BARDET-BIEDL SYNDROME (BARDET-BIEDL SYNDROME; RETINITIS PIGMENTOSA-POLYDACTYLY-ADIPOSOGENITAL SYNDROME)

General

Recessive, dominant autosomal, and recessive sex-linked gene; male preponderance; onset in childhood; cases of Laurence-Moon belong to the group of heredoataxias.

Ocular

Ptosis; epicanthus; nystagmus; strabismus; night blindness; myopia; hypermetropia; iris coloboma; retinitis pigmentosa "bone corpuscles"; macular degeneration; attenuation of retinal vessels; choroidal atrophy; optic nerve atrophy; cataract; microphthalmia; keratoconus.

Clinical

Obesity (Fröhlich type); hypogenitalism; reduced intelligence and mental retardation; turricephaly; shortness of stature; atresia ani; genu valgum; congenital heart disease; polydactyly; body hair scant or absent; pseudogynecomastia.

Laboratory

Chromosomal analysis is recommended to confirm chromosomal sex and to evaluate for associated genetic syndromes.

Treatment

Consultation by pediatric endocrinologist and pediatric urologist is usually necessary. Vitamin A 15,000 IU/day is thought to slow the decline of retinal function, dark sunglasses for outdoor use, surgery for cataract, genetic counseling.

Additional Resource

1. Telander DG (2012). Retinitis Pigmentosa. [online] Available from http://www.emedicine.com/oph/TOPIC704.HTM [Accessed April, 2012].

840. LEAD POISONING

General

Now rare and mostly of industrial origin; cumulative poisoning; excreted slowly; absorption slow by any route; prolonged exposure required for development of symptoms; acute poisoning virtually nonexistent.

Ocular

Sclerosis and obliteration of choroidal vessels; retinal arterial spasms; retrobulbar neuritis; papilledema; optic atrophy; cortical blindness; divergence palsy; papillary paralysis; bilateral abducens paralysis; accommodative palsy; mechanism of ocular pathology with this condition is not well defined, although there is evidence pointing to the level of cyclic adenosine monophosphate.

Clinical

Loss of appetite; weight loss; colic; constipation; insomnia; headache; dizziness; irritability; moderate hypertension; albuminuria; anemia; blue line edge of gum; encephalopathy; peripheral neuropathy leading to paralysis; convulsions; mania; coma.

Laboratory

Whole blood lead level, radiograph of the abdomen.

Treatment

Eliminating the source of lead exposure is the treatment of choice. Chelation is used only when lead level does not drop fast enough or far enough or when the lead level is in the potentially encephalopathogenic level.

Additional Resource

1. Marcus S (2011). Emergent Management of Lead Toxicity. [online] Available from http://www.emedicine.com/emerg/TOPIC293.HTM [Accessed April, 2012].

841. LEBER HEREDITARY OPTIC NEUROPATHY (LEBER SYNDROME; OPTIC ATROPHY AMAUROSIS; PITUITARY SYNDROME)

General

Male preponderance; in acute phase of neuropathy there are three characteristic fundus changes: (1) circumpapillary microangiopathy, (2) pseudoedema around the disk and (3) absence of staining on fluorescein angiography; possibly a toxic metabolic disorder, an abnormality of cyanide metabolism, or an effect of smoking; maternally inherited disease affecting young males presenting with unilateral or bilateral visual loss; second eye becomes involved within weeks to months later; positive association with an inherited mutation in mitochondrial DNA.

Ocular

Sudden severe loss of vision, which usually reaches its maximum after 1 or 2 months; complete blindness rare; central vision remains seriously impaired; occasional considerable visual improvement; sheathing of retinal vessels; circumpapillary telangiectatic microangiopathy; initial low-grade optic neuritis, then bilateral optic atrophy (partial or complete); possible swelling of the disk with hemorrhages and exudates, but usually transitory; nystagmus; macular colobomas; optic disk edema; cataracts; keratoconus; hyperemia of the disk; swelling of peripapillary nerve fiber layer.

Clinical

Headaches and vertigo; Uhthoff sign.

Laboratory

Diagnosis is made by clinical findings.

Treatment

Optic atrophy: Intravenous steroids may be used with optic neuritis or ischemic neuropathy. Stem cell treatment may be the future treatment of choice.

Cataract: Change in glasses can sometimes improve a patient's visual function temporarily; however, the most common treatment is cataract surgery.

Keratoconus: Spectacle correction, hard contacts and avoid eye rubbing may be useful. If hydrops occurs discontinue contact lens, use NaCl drops and ointment, patching and short course of steroids. As the disease advances penetrating keratoplasty, deep anterior lamellar keratoplasty, intacs with laser grooves or collagen stabilization of cornea.

Additional Resource

1. Younge BR (2012). Anterior Ischemic Optic Neuropathy. [online] Available from http://www.emedicine.com/oph/TOPIC161.HTM [Accessed April, 2012].

842. LEBER TAPETORETINAL DYSTROPHY SYNDROME (ALSTROM-OLSEN SYNDROME; AMAUROSIS CONGENITA; DYSGENESIS NEUROEPITHELIALIS RETINAE; PIGMENTARY RETINITIS WITH CONGENITAL AMAUROSIS; RETINAL ABIOTROPHY; RETINAL APLASIA)

General

Autosomal recessive inheritance; consanguinity; occurs from teens to 30 years of age.

Ocular

Nystagmus; keratoconus; narrow retinal arteries; yellowish-brown or gray macular lesions; grayish atrophic retinal lesions; salt and pepper-like retinal pigmentation or typical "bone corpuscle" pigmentary changes; keratoglobus.

Clinical

Mental retardation; microcephaly; mongoloid appearance; oculodigital sign; association with Down syndrome has been reported; hypoplasia of the cerebellar vermis; mild-to-moderate ventriculomegaly.

Laboratory

Diagnosis is made by clinical findings.

Treatment

Keratoconus: Spectacle correction, hard contacts and avoid eye rubbing may be useful. If hydrops occurs discontinue contact lens, use NaCl drops and ointment, patching and short course of steroids. As the disease advances penetrating keratoplasty, deep anterior lamellar keratoplasty, intacs with laser grooves or collagen stabilization of cornea.

Bibliography

1. Elder MJ. Leber congenital amaurosis and its association with keratoconus and keratoglobus. J Pediatr Ophthalmol Strabismus. 1994;31:38-40.
2. Firat T. Clinical and genetic investigations in Leber's tapeto-retinal dystrophy. Ann Ophthalmol. 1970;2:664-73.
3. Hayasaka S, Noda S, Setogawa T, et al. Leber congenital amaurosis in an infant with Down syndrome. Ann Ophthalmol. 1992;24:250-2.
4. Lambert SR, Sherman S, Taylor D, et al. Concordance and recessive inheritance of Leber congenital amaurosis. Am J Med Genet. 1993;4:275-7.
5. Leber T. Uber Retinitis Pigmentosa und Angeborene Amaurose. Arch F Ophthalmol (Berlin). 1869;15:1.

6. Magalini SI, Scrascia E. Dictionary of Medical Syndromes, 2nd edition. Philadelphia: JB Lippincott; 1981.

7. Pau H. Differential Diagnosis of Eye Diseases. New York: Thieme; 1987.

8. Steinberg A, Ronen S, Zlotogorski Z, et al. Central nervous involvement in Leber congenital amaurosis. J Pediatr Ophthalmol Strabismus. 1992;29: 224-7.

843. LECITHIN-CHOLESTEROL ACYLTRANSFERASE DEFICIENCY

General

Lecithin-cholesterol acyltransferase (LCAT) enzyme involved in metabolism of cholesterol deficiency; autosomal recessive; rare.

Ocular

Cloudy cornea; diplopia; photophobia; corneal opacities.

Clinical

Autoimmune hyperlipoproteinemic anemia; renal failure; hypertension.

Laboratory

A definitive diagnosis requires mutational analysis of the *LCAT* gene and a functional analysis of the mutated gene product.

Treatment

Renal replacement by dialysis is necessary in those individuals who develop kidney failure. Kidney transplantation and corneal transplantation may be necessary.

Additional Resource

1. Raghavan VA (2011). Lecithin-Cholesterol Acyltransferase Deficiency. [online] Available from http://www.emedicine.com/med/TOPIC1270. HTM [Accessed April, 2012].

844. LEGG-PERTHES DISEASE (COXA PLANA; LEGG-CALVE-PERTHES DISEASE; LEGG-CALVE-WALDENSTROM SYNDROME; LEGG DISEASE; LEGG-CALVE DISEASE)

General

Etiology not established; occurs in children between the ages of 3 and 12 years; more common in boys; unilateral involvement more common than bilateral; retardation of bone age; occasionally familial; rare in blacks; possible role for protein C and S deficiency, thrombophilia, venous hypertension and hypofibrinolysis in the pathophysiologic mechanism of this disease.

Ocular

Iris processes (pectinate ligaments in the anterior chamber angle).

Clinical

Osteochondrosis of the capitular epiphysis of the femur; limpness associated with muscular spasm.

Laboratory

X-ray, CT, MRI, ultrasound and angiography.

Treatment

Primarily treatment includes analgesia, bracing, or surgery.

Additional Resource

1. Khan AN (2011). Legg-Calve-Perthes Disease Imaging. [online] Available from http://www.emedicine.com/radio/TOPIC387.HTM [Accessed April, 2012].

845. LEIGH SYNDROME (GANGLIOSIDOSIS GM2 TYPE 3; HYPERPYRUVICEMIA WITH HYPER-ALPHA-ALANINEMIA; INFANTILE SUBACUTE NECROTIZING ENCEPHALOMYELOPATHY; SUBACUTE NECROTIZING ENCEPHALOMYELOPATHY)

General

Autosomal recessive; metabolic disease occurring in infancy and childhood with increased levels of serum lactate, serum pyruvates, blood alpha-ketoglutarate, and aminoaciduria; course is remittent with early neuro-ophthalmologic manifestations and psychomotor retardation; the later the onset of clinical manifestations, the longer the survival time; acute form in young infants, subacute form in older infants and chronic course in juveniles; Mutation at nt 8993 of mitochondrial DNA has been reported as a common cause of Leigh syndrome; biochemical analysis revealed cytochrome c oxidase deficiency with this condition.

Ocular

Nystagmoid movements or nystagmus; disconjugate ocular movements due to tegmental involvement of brainstem; degrees of visual impairment, depending on pathologic changes involving optic nerves and tracts; optic nerve atrophy; oculomotor palsy; supranuclear gaze palsy; blindness.

Clinical

Spasticity of extremities; ataxia; muscular weakness; hemiparesis; progressive mental deterioration; hearing defects; dysphagia; dyspnea; mild hypotonia; slow development; intermittent abnormal respiratory rhythm; cranial nerve palsies.

Laboratory

Diagnosis is made by clinical findings.

Treatment

None/Ocular.

Additional Resource

1. Prasad A (2010). Ataxia with Identified Genetic and Biochemical Defects. [online] Available from http://www.emedicine.com/neuro/TOPIC556.HTM [Accessed April, 2012].

846. LEIOMYOMA

General

Rare, benign tumor that arises from smooth muscle; usually well encapsulated.

Ocular

Pigmented tumor of ciliary body; proptosis; distorted pupil; ectropion; iris tumor; glaucoma;

cataract; preferential location: ciliary body, peripheral choroid, supraciliary or suprachoroidal space; has a predilection for younger patients and females.

Clinical

Metastases have not been described.

Laboratory

Diagnosis is made on histologic examination.

Treatment

Excise the leiomyoma from the iris and ciliary body if tumors increase in size.

Additional Resource

1. Roque MR (2010). Leiomyoma, Iris. [online] Available from http://www.emedicine.com/oph/ TOPIC589.HTM [Accessed April, 2012].

---

847. LEISHMANIASIS

General

Caused by protozoa of the genus *Leishmania*.

Ocular

Conjunctivitis; ulcerative keratitis; ulcerating granulomatous lid lesions; lid edema; interstitial keratitis; subacute focal retinitis; retinal hemorrhage; iridocyclitis; unilateral chronic granulomatous blepharitis.

Clinical

Lesions in spleen, liver and large intestine; fever; leukopenia; cutaneous lesions on the face.

Laboratory

Diagnosis of leishmaniasis has been confirmed by isolating, visualizing and culturing the parasite from infected tissue. Over recent years, significant advances in polymerase chain reaction (PCR) techniques have allowed for the highly sensitive and rapid diagnosis of specific *Leishmania* species.

Treatment

Sodium stibogluconate, amphotericin B (AmBisome) and pentamidine, dapsone, ketoconazole and fluconazole are drugs used for treatment. Which drug is best suited is dependent on what part of the world the patient is in.

Additional Resource

1. Stark CG (2011). Leishmaniasis. [online] Available from http://www.emedicine.com/med/TOPIC1275. HTM [Accessed April, 2012].

---

848. LENOBLE-AUBINEAU SYNDROME (NYSTAGMUS-MYOCLONIA SYNDROME)

General

Familial; pathogenesis not known; prevalent in males; manifest during the first year of life; X-linked dominant inheritance has been reported in one family.

Ocular

Congenital nystagmus associated with fasciculations of muscles spontaneously elicited by mechanical stimulation or cold.

Clinical

Tremors of head and limbs; myoclonic movements of extremities and trunk; hypospadias; abnormalities of teeth; facial asymmetry; localized edema.

Laboratory

Diagnosis is made by clinical findings.

Treatment

Baclofen, gabapentin and retrobulbar injection of botulinum toxin may be useful for nystagmus.

Bibliography

1. Lenoble E, Aubineau E. Nystagmus-Myoclonia Syndrome: Une Variete Nouvelle de Myoclonie Congenitale Pouvant Etre Hereditaire et Familiale A Nystagmus Constant. Rev Med (Paris). 1906; 26:471.
2. Magalini SI, Scrascia E. Dictionary of Medical Syndromes, 2nd edition. Philadelphia: JB Lippincott; 1981.
3. McKusick VA. Mendelian Inheritance in Man: A Catalog of Human Genes and Genetic Disorders, 12th edition. Baltimore: The Johns Hopkins University Press; 1998.

849. LENS-INDUCED GLAUCOMA (PHACOLYTIC, LENS PARTICLE, AND PHACOANTIGENIC)

General

Open angle secondary glaucoma can be phacolytic, lens particle, and phacoantigenic. Closed angle secondary lens glaucoma occurs from lens intumescence (phacomorphic glaucoma) or lens dislocation (ectopia lentis).

Clinical

None

Ocular

Open angle or closed angle secondary glaucoma, cataract, retained lens material, uveitis.

Laboratory

Diagnosis is made by clinical findings.

Treatment

Mature or hypermature cataract: Topical steroids, IOP lowering agents, hyperosmotic agents. Removal of cataract will usually restore normal IOP.

Lens particle glaucoma: Topical IOP lowering agents, cycloplegics and steroids. Removal of residual lens material.

Phacoantigenic glaucoma: Topical steroids, IOP lowering agents, and cycloplegics. Pars plana vitrectomy to remove all residual lens material and posterior capsule or removal of capsule manually with forceps after injection of chymotrypsin beneath the iris.

Phacomorphic glaucoma: Topical IOP lowering agents. Argon laser iridoplasty to open angle, laser iridotomy to bypass papillary black, cataract extraction.

Ectopia lentis: Laser iridotomy to bypass papillary block. If lens floats in vitreous treat conservatively.

Additional Resources

1. Sullivan BR (2010). Glaucoma, Lens-Particle. [online] Available from http://www.emedicine.com/oph/TOPIC56.HTM [Accessed April, 2012].
2. Gill H (2010). Glaucoma, Phacomorphic. [online] Available from http://www.emedicine.com/oph/TOPIC58.HTM [Accessed April, 2012].
3. Yi K (2011). Phacolytic Glaucoma. [online] Available from http://www.emedicine.com/oph/TOPIC57.HTM [Accessed April, 2012].

850. LENS-IRIS DIAPHRAGM RETROPULSION SYNDROME

General

Associated with small incision phacoemulsification.

Ocular

Infusion of fluid into the anterior chamber; posterior displacement of the lens-iris diaphragm; posterior iris bowing; pupil dilatation; ocular discomfort.

Clinical

Deep anterior chamber with small incision phacoemulsification.

Laboratory

Diagnosis is made by clinical findings.

Treatment

Consider YAG iridotomy.

Additional Resource

1. Ocampo VVD (2012). Senile Cataract. [online] Available from http://www.emedicine.medscape.com/article/1210914-overview [Accessed April, 2012].

851. LENTICONUS AND LENTIGLOBUS

General

Lenticonus is a circumscribed conical bulge of the anterior or, more commonly, posterior lens capsule and cortex. In lentiglobus, the entire posterior capsule has a globular shape.

Clinical

Alport syndrome; Waardenburg syndrome.

Ocular

Oil droplet appearance; amblyopia; strabismus.

Laboratory

Diagnosis is made by clinical findings.

Treatment

Lens extraction with irrigation-aspiration.

Bibliography

1. Roy FH, Fraunfelder FW, Fraunfelder FT. Roy and Fraunfelder's Current Ocular Therapy, 6th edition. Philadelphia: WB Saunders; 2008.

852. LENZ MICROPHTHALMIA SYNDROME

General

X-linked recessive; female carriers.

Ocular

Microphthalmia; microcornea; ocular coloboma; colobomatous microphthalmia.

Clinical

Skeletal abnormalities of vertebral column, clavicles and limbs; severe renal dysgenesis and hydroureters; dental anomalies; hypospadias and bilateral cryptorchidism; severe speech impairment; shortness of stature; long, cylindrical and thin thorax; sloping shoulders; flat feet.

Laboratory

Diagnosis is made by clinical findings.

Treatment

None/Ocular.

Bibliography

1. Antoniades K, Tzouvelekis G, Doudou A, et al. A sporadic case of Lenz microphthalmia syndrome. Ann Ophthalmol. 1993;25:342-5.
2. Herrmann J, Opitz JM. The Lenz microphthalmia syndrome. Birth Defects. 1969;5:138-48.

---

853. LEPTOMENINGEAL ADHESIVE THICKENING (CHRONIC ADHESIVE ARACHNOIDITIS)

General

Follows a chronic leptomeningeal infection, trauma or subarachnoid hemorrhage; insidious onset.

Ocular

Diplopia

Clinical

Headache; nausea; vomiting; vertigo; epileptic seizures.

Laboratory

Diagnosis is made by clinical findings.

Treatment

None/Ocular.

Additional Resource

1. Zebian RC (2011). Emergent Management of Subarachnoid Hemorrhage. [online] Available from http://www.emedicine.com/emerg/TOPIC559.HTM [Accessed April, 2012].

---

854. LERI SYNDROME (CARPAL TUNNEL SYNDROME; PLEONOSTEOSIS SYNDROME)

General

Autosomal dominant type of congenital osseous dystrophy; early epiphyseal bone formation of extremities; Morton metatarsalgia syndrome may result; onset in early infancy.

Ocular

Microphthalmia; anophthalmia; oculomotor paralysis; corneal clouding; cataract.

Clinical

Dwarfism (disproportionate); articular deformities; cutaneous deformities; carpal tunnel syndrome (median nerve compression); deformities of thumbs and great toes; laryngeal stenosis.

Laboratory

Diagnosis is made by clinical findings.

Treatment

Cataract: Change in glasses can sometimes improve a patient's visual function temporarily; however, the most common treatment is cataract surgery.

Corneal clouding: Check for elevated intraocular pressure. Medical treatment includes the use of hyperosmotic drops, nonsteroidal and steroid eye drops. Corneal transplant may be necessary.

Additional Resource

1. Fuller DA (2010). Orthopedic Surgery for Carpal Tunnel Syndrome. [online] Available from http://www.emedicine.com/orthoped/TOPIC455.HTM [Accessed April, 2012].

855. LERMOYEZ SYNDROME

General

Form of Ménière disease; however, hearing acuity improves during the climax of the vestibular attacks; onset in the third or fourth decade of life.

Ocular

Nystagmus (spontaneous) directed toward opposite side of involved vestibular system or to the side of the increased tonic state.

Clinical

Dizziness; vertigo; tinnitus; improvement of hearing during vestibular attacks; sweating; nausea; tremor; low tone hearing loss.

Laboratory

Computed tomography (CT) and MRI of the brain is used to detect abnormal inner ear anatomy, masses and lesions.

Treatment

Control of vertiginous sensation using the medications such as antiemetics, diuretics, antihistamines and anticholinergics.

Additional Resource

1. Li JC (2011). Meniere Disease (Idiopathic Endolymphatic Hydrops). [online] Available from http://www.emedicine.com/emerg/TOPIC308.HTM [Accessed April, 2012].

856. LEROY SYNDROME

General

Possible mild increase in mucopolysaccharide excretion.

Ocular

Nasal epicanthal folds; corneal opacities.

Clinical

High, narrow forehead; narrow nasal bridge.

Laboratory

Urine spot tests are readily available to screen for mucopolysaccharidoses (MPSs), full skeletal survey.

Treatment

Enzyme replacement therapy (ERT) and bone marrow transplantation can be useful.

Additional Resource

1. Roth KS (2009). I-Cell Disease (Mucolipidosis Type II). [online] Available from http://www.emedicine.com/ped/TOPIC1150.HTM [Accessed April, 2012].

857. LEUKEMIA

General

Acute or chronic blood disorder.

Ocular

Engorgement of conjunctival vessels; papillary hypertrophy; aggregations of tumor cells in conjunctiva, choroid and orbit; secondary glaucoma; retinal venous engorgement and tortuosity with pronounced constrictions; retinal hemorrhages; retinal detachment; cotton-wool spots; macular edema; papilledema; optic atrophy; optic neuritis; paralysis of extraocular muscles; hypopyon; vitreous opacities; retinal sea fans; perilimbal subconjunctival infiltrates; corneal leukemic infiltration (rare); shallow serous retinal detachments; hyphema; iris neovascularization; central retinal vein occlusion; vitreous infiltrates.

Clinical

Frequent involvement of central nervous system (CNS); intracranial hemorrhage; thrombocytopenia; rising white cell count.

Laboratory

Complete blood count and differential, bone marrow aspiration, immunophenotyping, chromosomal analysis.

Treatment

Chemotherapy with or without radiotherapy.

Additional Resource

1. Wu L (2012). Leukemias. [online] Available from http://www.emedicine.com/oph/TOPIC489.HTM [Accessed April, 2012].

858. LEWIS SYNDROME (TUBEROSERPIGINOUS SYPHILID OF LEWIS)

General

Lesions more common on nose and ears but may involve eyelids primarily; clinical manifestations are similar to lupus vulgaris.

Ocular

Lesions most frequently involve the lower eyelids; tear ducts may become involved, with lesions of mouth and nose as a direct extension or via the lymphatic route; granulomatous conjunctival lesions, usually an extension of involvement of buccal and nasal mucosa; iridocyclitis may occur; corneal ulcers as seen in tuberculous granulomatosis.

Clinical

Skin lesions similar to those of the face may be seen on other parts of extremities or trunk.

Laboratory

Diagnosis is made by clinical findings.

Treatment

Corneal ulcer: Corneal cultures may be taken and treatment initiated. Treatment includes a broad spectrum of antibiotics and cycloplegic drops.

Additional Resource

1. Walton RC (2010). Vogt-Koyanagi-Harada Disease. [online] Available from http://www.emedicine.com/oph/TOPIC459.HTM [Accessed April, 2012].

---

859. LICHEN PLANUS

General

Conjunctival disorder associated with dermatologic disorder; disappears spontaneously.

Ocular

Conjunctivitis; cicatrizing conjunctivitis; keratin plaque on bulbar conjunctiva.

Clinical

Grayish-white papules; oral lesions may precede skin lesions.

Laboratory

Diagnosis is made by clinical findings.

Treatment

Topical and systemic corticosteroids, systemic immunomodulators.

Additional Resource

1. Foster CS (2011). Ophthalmologic Manifestations of Cicatricial Pemphigoid. [online] Available from http://www.emedicine.com/oph/TOPIC83.HTM [Accessed April, 2012].

---

860. LID MYOKYMIA

General

Usually unilateral, persist for months, benign, self-limited.

Clinical

Stress, fatigue, excessive caffeine or alcohol intake.

Ocular

Spontaneous fascicular eyelid tremor without muscular atrophy or weakness.

Laboratory

Diagnosis is made by clinical findings.

Treatment

Reassurance and reduction of precipitating factors, botulism toxin type A, oral quinine or baclofen.

Additional Resource

1. Lam BL (2011). Eyelid Myokymia. [online] Available from http://www.emedicine.com/oph/TOPIC607.HTM [Accessed April, 2012].

861. LID RETRACTION

General

Unilateral or bilateral. Cause can be mechanical, neurogenic or myogenic.

Clinical

None

Ocular

Lid retraction, corneal exposure, dry eye syndrome.

Laboratory

Testing to determine cause. If thyroid suspect—total thyroxine, thyroid-stimulating hormone and thyroid-stimulating immunoglobulins.

Treatment

Identify systemic abnormalities such as thyroid. Treatment must be given for 6 months for stabilizing before performing eyelid surgery. Local-ocular lubrication (drops or ointment). Botulism type A may also be useful.

Bibliography

1. Roy FH, Fraunfelder FW, Fraunfelder FT. Roy and Fraunfelder's Current Ocular Therapy, 6th edition. Philadelphia: WB Saunders; 2008.

862. LIDRS SYNDROME (INFUSION DEVIATION SYNDROME)

General

Occurs in highly myopic eyes and postvitrectomy eyes following infusions with the phaco tip or the I & A tip.

Clinical

None

Ocular

Iris sphincter ruptures; iris blocks back against the anterior capsule.

Laboratory

Diagnosis is made by clinical findings.

Treatment

Repressurize the eye by establishing normal chamber depth or depress the anterior capsular rim to equalize the pressure between the anterior and posterior chamber.

Bibliography

1. Osher RH. LIDRS Syndrome. J Cataract Refract Surg. January 2010.

863. LIGNAC-FANCONI SYNDROME (CYSTINOSIS SYNDROME; CYSTINE STORAGE-AMINOACIDURIA-DWARFISM SYNDROME; FANCONI-LIGNAC SYNDROME; NEPHROPATHIC CYSTINOSIS; RENAL RICKETS)

General

Autosomal recessively inherited storage disorder in which nonprotein cystine accumulates within cellular lysosomes; occurs primarily in children; prognosis in children with renal tubular insufficiency and dwarfism poor, with survival past age 10 years rare without renal transplant.

Ocular

Cystine crystals located in conjunctiva, cornea, sclera, iris, ciliary body, lens and perhaps choroid; general clouding of cornea caused by dense deposition of cystine crystals; pupillary block glaucoma; photophobia; band keratopathy; posterior synechiae with thickened stroma of iris; decreased visual function; patchy retinopathy; visual field constriction.

Clinical

Fanconi syndrome with rickets; dwarfism; glomerular dystrophy; renal failure; oral motor dysfunction.

Laboratory

Diagnosis is made based on tests that document the excessive loss of substances in the urine (e.g. amino acids, glucose, phosphate, bicarbonate) in the absence of high plasma concentrations.

Treatment

Replacement of substances lost in the urine. Liver transplantation is sometimes necessary.

Additional Resource

1. Fathallah-Shaykh S (2011). Fanconi Syndrome. [online] Available from http://www.emedicine.com/ped/TOPIC756.HTM [Accessed April, 2012].

864. LIGNEOUS CONJUNCTIVITIS

General

Rare form of recurrent conjunctivitis, usually bilateral in infants or children.

Clinical

None

Ocular

Inflammation is characterized by formation of thick membranes and pseudomembranes to the lid.

Laboratory

Histology, plasminogen activity and plasminogen antigen levels.

Treatment

Surgical excision of conjunctival membrane followed by cautery, cryopexy and grafting with conjunctiva or sclera.

Bibliography

1. Roy FH, Fraunfelder FW, Fraunfelder FT. Roy and Fraunfelder's Current Ocular Therapy, 6th edition. Philadelphia: WB Saunders; 2008.

865. LINEAR IGA DISEASE

General

Bullous dermatosis with pruritic urticarial lesions with overlying vesicles or bullae; skin lesions heal without scarring; homogeneous deposition of immunoglobulin A (IgA) at the dermal-epidermal junction and, rarely, deposition of other immunoglobulin present; heterogeneous disease with regard to its clinical features, target antigens and immunogenetics; association with HLA-B8, DR3, Cw7, and the linked rare tumor necrosis factor-alpha allele; may be induced by amiodarone.

Ocular

Chronic conjunctivitis; subconjunctival fibrosis; symblepharon; chronic progressive conjunctival cicatrization.

Clinical

Recurrent blistering skin disorder consisting of urticarial macules and plaques with vesicular eruptions on trunk and extremities; subepidermal vesiculation.

Laboratory

Diagnosis is made by clinical findings.

Treatment

Conjunctivitis: Symptomatic control may include cold compresses and artificial tears; nonsteroidal and occasionally steroidal drops to relieve itching.

Additional Resource

1. Foster CS (2011). Ophthalmologic Manifestations of Cicatricial Pemphigoid. [online] Available from http://www.emedicine.com/oph/TOPIC83.HTM [Accessed April, 2012].

---

866. LINEAR NEVUS SEBACEOUS OF JADASSOHN (JADASSOHN-TYPE ANETODERMA; NEVUS SEBACEOUS OF JADASSOHNORGANOID NEVUS SYNDROME; SEBACEOUS NEVUS SYNDROME)

General

Skin nevus caused by failure of separation of skin appendages from adjacent epithelium during the third month of gestation.

Ocular

Proptosis; epibulbar lipodermoids; colobomata of eyelids, iris and choroid; antimongoloid fissures; ocular motor palsies; nystagmus; teratomas of orbit and aberrant lacrimal glands; corneal vascularization; vision defects; conjunctival dermolipomas; choristomas of conjunctiva, sclera; corneal vascularization/opacification; colobomas of uvea, retina, optic disk and lids; optic nerve hypoplasia; microphthalmia; anophthalmia; hemangioma of the sclera/conjunctiva.

Clinical

Circumscribed lesions of the face and scalp with excessively large sebaceous glands; papill-omatous epidermal hyperplasia; seizures; skeletal abnormalities, particularly in skull; failure to thrive; convulsion; mental retardation.

Laboratory

Epidermis shows papillomatous hyperplasia. In the dermis, the numbers of mature sebaceous glands are increased. Ectopic apocrine glands are often found in the deep dermis beneath sebaceous glands.

Treatment

Photodynamic therapy with topical aminolevulinic acid. Full-thickness skin excision is usually required, and topical destruction.

Additional Resource

1. Hammadi AA (2010). Nevus Sebaceus. [online] Available from http://www.emedicine.com/derm/TOPIC296.HTM [Accessed April, 2012].

867. LIPODYSTROPHY (KOBBERLING-DUNNIGAN SYNDROME)

General

Disturbance of the fat metabolism; autosomal dominant; affects females predominantly; occurs at puberty.

Ocular

Enophthalmos; lack of eyelid apposition; choroidal atrophy; optic disk pallor; corneal opacity.

Clinical

Progressive symmetrical loss of subcutaneous fat in upper part of body, including face and orbits; fat accumulation of neck, shoulders, buffalo hump and genitalia; hyperthyroidism; lipoatrophic diabetes; hepatosplenomegaly; acanthosis nigricans; hyperlipemia; lean muscular limbs; phlebectasia; insulin resistance; hyperglycemia; type IV lipoproteinemia.

Laboratory

Head MRIs show evidence of fat loss. Skin biopsy findings confirm the diagnosis.

Treatment

Symptomatic therapy should be prescribed as necessary for the treatment of renal complications and associated autoimmune disorders.

Additional Resource

1. Schwartz RA (2011). Progressive Lipodystrophy. [online] Available from http://www.emedicine. com/derm/TOPIC897.HTM [Accessed April, 2012].

868. LIPOSARCOMA

General

Aggressive malignant neoplasms of lipogenic cells; occurs at any age, but rarely before age 30 years and most commonly in the fifth decade; occurs almost exclusively in adults and is found most often in the thigh or retroperitoneum.

Ocular

Paresis of extraocular muscle; proptosis; orbital liposarcoma; eyelid edema.

Clinical

Neoplasms of deeper soft tissues; metastasis to lungs, liver, lymph nodes and periosteum.

Laboratory

Magnetic resonance imaging (MRI) may be diagnostic, ultrasonography helps to separate true orbital cysts from liposarcoma, diagnosis is usually made only after biopsy.

Treatment

Consultation with oncologist as necessary.

Additional Resource

1. Khan AN (2011). Liposarcoma Imaging. [online] Available from http://www.emedicine.com/radio/ TOPIC392.HTM [Accessed April, 2012].

869. LISSENCEPHALY SYNDROME (MILLER-DIEKER SYNDROME)

General

Autosomal recessive; consanguinity; association with deletion of the *LIS1* gene located at chromosome 17p13.

Ocular

Hypertelorism

Clinical

Microcephaly; small mandible; bizarre facies; failure to thrive; retarded motor development; mental retardation; dysphagia; decorticated and decerebrate postures; polydactyly; malformations of brain, heart, kidneys and other organs; spastic paraplegia; agyri-apachygyria; inverted gray-to-white matter ratio; absence of white-gray interdigitations; hypoplastic brainstem; characteristic facial dysmorphism.

Laboratory

Magnetic resonance imaging (MRI), proton magnetic resonance spectroscopic imaging.

Treatment

None/Ocular.

Additional Resource

1. Sheth RD (2011). Neonatal Seizures. [online] Available from http://www.emedicine.medscape.com/article/1177069-overview [Accessed April, 2012].

870. LISTERELLOSIS (LISTERIOSIS)

General

Caused by Gram-positive bacillus Listeria monocytogenes. High mortality among pregnant women, their fetuses and immunocompromised persons with symptoms of abortion, neonatal death, septicemia, meningitis, brain abscesses, endocarditis.

Ocular

Conjunctivitis; keratitis; corneal abscess and ulcer; blepharitis; uveitis; endophthalmitis; cataract; secondary glaucoma.

Clinical

Vomiting; cardiorespiratory distress; diarrhea; hepatosplenomegaly; maculopapular skin lesions.

Laboratory

Histopathology and culture of rash, CT scanning or MRI may be useful in detecting abscesses in the brain or liver.

Treatment

Antibiotics as well as careful monitoring of the patient's temperature, respiratory system, fluid and electrolyte balance, nutrition and cardiovascular support.

Additional Resource

1. Zach T (2011). Listeria Infection. [online] Available from http://www.emedicine.com/ped/TOPIC1319.HTM [Accessed April, 2012].

871. LITTLE SYNDROME (HEREDITARY OSTEO-ONYCHO-DYSPLASIA; HOOD SYNDROME; NAIL-PATELLA SYNDROME)

General

Inherited as autosomal dominant; affects males and females equally.

Ocular

Hypertelorism; ptosis; epicanthus; microcornea; keratoconus; sclerocornea; cataract; microphakia; light pigmentation of iris root with dark pigmented "clover-leaf" spots, referred to as the Lester line, not seen in all cases.

Clinical

Absent or hypoplastic patella; hypoplastic or dislocated head of radius; exostosis of skull bones; bilateral horns of iliac crests; longitudinal ridging of fingernails; glomerulonephritis; renal involvement; bilateral antecubital pterygia; arthrogryposis; disorder has been mapped to the long arm of chromosome 9; sensorineural hearing loss.

Laboratory

Conduct urinalysis, along with a microscopic analysis, to check for proteinuria and hematuria, radiography findings reveal iliac horns, MRI to identify abnormal muscle insertions, renal biopsy.

Treatment

Renal dialysis and transplantation are necessary.

Additional Resource

1. Hoover-Fong J (2012). Genetics of Nail-Patella Syndrome. [online] Available from http://www.emedicine.com/ped/TOPIC1546.HTM [Accessed April, 2012].

872. LOCKED-IN SYNDROME

General

Usually caused by extensive pontine hemorrhage; awake but paralyzed patient; unable to communicate following basilar artery occlusion; trauma.

Ocular

Ocular bobbing; bilateral paresis of horizontal gaze; spared vertical eye movements, and hearing.

Clinical

Paralysis of all four extremities and the lower cranial nerves without interference with consciousness.

Laboratory

Computed tomography (CT) and MRI.

Treatment

Consultation with neurologist or neurosurgeon is recommended.

Additional Resource

1. Liebeskind DS (2011). Intracranial Hemorrhage. [online] Available from http://www.emedicine.com/neuro/TOPIC177.HTM [Accessed April, 2012].

873. LOCKJAW (TETANUS)

General

Acute infectious disease affecting nervous system; causative agent is *Clostridium tetani*; bacteria enters body through a puncture wound, abrasion, cut or burn.

Ocular

Chemosis; keratitis; nystagmus; uveitis; corneal ulcer; cellulitis of orbit; hypopyon; panophthalmitis; pupil paralysis; pseudoptosis; blepharospasm; paralysis of third or seventh nerve; may occur following perforating ocular injuries.

Clinical

Severe muscle spasms; dysphagia; trismus; facial palsy; muscle stiffness; irritability.

Laboratory

Gram-positive spore-forming bacteria, lab studies of little value.

Treatment

Passive immunization with human tetanus immune globulin shortens the course of tetanus and may lessen its severity. Benzodiazepines have emerged as the mainstay of symptomatic therapy for tetanus.

Additional Resource

1. Hinfey PB (2011). Tetanus. [online] Available from http://www.emedicine.com/med/TOPIC2254.HTM [Accessed April, 2012].

874. LOFFLER SYNDROME (EOSINOPHILIC PNEUMONITIS)

General

Etiology unknown, but such considerations as drug hypersensitivity, parasites, mycoses and periarteritis nodosa have been advanced; eosinophilia up to 80%; condition self-limited and benign; may occur after using crack cocaine, after administration of medications such as minocycline or as an idiopathic disorder.

Ocular

Endophthalmitis; retinal infarction with hemorrhages and exudates.

Clinical

Dry cough; shortness of breath; increased body temperature; weight loss; malaise; anorexia; fever; dyspnea; pleural rales; pericardial effusion; prolonged expiration; wheezing.

Laboratory

Parasites and ova can be found in the stool 6–12 weeks after the initial parasitic infection, X-rays usually show peripheral densities, usually of a combined interstitial and alveolar pattern and often a few centimeters in diameter.

Treatment

Consultation with pediatric pulmonologist is usually necessary.

Additional Resource

1. Sharma GD (2012). Loffler Syndrome. [online] Available from http://www.emedicine.com/ped/TOPIC1322.HTM [Accessed April, 2012].

875. LONGFELLOW-GRAETHER SYNDROME

General

Rare; etiology unknown.

Ocular

Grossly dilated retinal veins; intermittent attacks of uniocular blindness.

Clinical

None

Laboratory

Diagnosis is made by clinical findings.

Treatment

Identify cause of intermittent uniocular blindness.

Bibliography

1. Pau H. Differential Diagnosis of Eye Diseases. New York: Thieme; 1987.
2. Roy FH. Ocular Differential Diagnosis, 9th edition. Jaypee Highlights Medical Publisher, New Delhi, India 2012.

876. LOST LENS SYNDROME

General

Occurs when the intraocular lens (IOL) is completely dislocated into the vitreous cavity, caused by luxation of the implant through a zonular disinsertion or an unrecognized opening in the posterior capsule or trauma.

Ocular

Decreased visual acuity; retinal detachment; cystoid macular edema.

Clinical

None

Laboratory

Diagnosis is made by clinical findings.

Treatment

If IOL is mobile options include removal, exchange or repositioning of the IOL. Repositioning of the IOL into the ciliary sulcus or over capsular remnants with less than a total of 6 clock hours of inferior capsular support is not a stable situation, as many of those repositioned IOLs will end up dislocating again. Transscleral suturing or IOL exchange (removal of the dislocated IOL and placement of a flexible open loop ACIOL) is recommended in these cases.

Additional Resource

1. Wu L (2011). Intraocular Lens Dislocation. [online] Available from http://www.emedicine.com/oph/TOPIC392.HTM [Accessed April, 2012].

877. LOUIS-BAR SYNDROME (ATAXIA-TELANGIECTASIA SYNDROME; CEPHALO-OCULOCUTANEOUS TELANGIECTASIS)

General

Autosomal recessive; thymic abnormality leading to an immunologic deficiency has been suggested as the cause; chromosomal translocations are found in 5–10% of peripheral T cells from most patients.

Ocular

Rapid blinking in upward gaze; "pseudo-ophthalmoplegia"; fixational nystagmus (see Roth-Bielschowsky syndrome) halting intermittently, mainly on lateral and upward gaze; on head turning, eyes are involuntarily directed to opposite side with slow return to the primary position; ocular motor apraxic movement; loss of optokinetic responses; poor convergence ability; telangiectasias of anterior segment and sclera; fine, bright, symmetrical red streaks of the temporal and nasal conjunctiva (usually first seen at age 4–6 years); prominent veins in canthal regions of conjunctiva.

Clinical

Progressive cerebellar ataxia; slow and scanning speech; mental retardation; cutaneous telangiectasis and fine spots of pigmentation; recurrent sinopulmonary infections; hypotonia; diminished growth; cutaneous telangiectasis of ears, cheeks, and antecubital space; deficiency of IgA; lymphoreticular malignancy; high cancer risk in children with progressive cerebellar ataxia most commonly lymphoma (B-cell type) or leukemias.

Laboratory

Magnetic resonance imaging (MRI), electrocardiogram (EKG), encephalogram.

Treatment

Monitor and treat respiratory infections.

Additional Resource

1. Dahl AA (2010). Ataxia-Telangiectasia in Ophthalmology. [online] Available from http://www. emedicine.com/oph/TOPIC319.HTM [Accessed April, 2012].

878. LOUPING III SYNDROME

General

Tick-borne disease of sheep; occurs in Britain.

Ocular

Difficulty in blinking; retrobulbar neuritis; transient diplopia.

Clinical

Cerebellar ataxia; mild encephalitis; weak facial muscles.

Laboratory

The diagnosis of human monocytic ehrlichiosis (HME), human granulocytic anaplasmosis (HGA) or human granulocytotropic ehrlichiosis (HGE) rests on a single elevated immunoglobulin G (IgG) immunofluorescent antibody (IFA) Ehrlichia titer or by demonstrating a 4-fold or greater increase between acute and convalescent IFA Ehrlichia titers.

Treatment

The preferred drug is doxycycline and an infectious disease consultation should be considered.

Additional Resource

1. Cunha BA (2011). Ehrlichiosis. [online] Available from http://www.emedicine.com/emerg/TOPIC159.HTM [Accessed April, 2012].

---

879. LOWE SYNDROME (OCULOCEREBRORENAL SYNDROME)

General

Essential enzyme or protein abnormality is unknown; sex-linked recessive trait (male incidence only); onset in early infancy.

Ocular

Nystagmus; congenital glaucoma; miotic pupils; no pupillary reaction; ectropion uveae; malformation of the anterior chamber angle and of the iris; Schlemm canal may be absent with imperfect angle cleavage; blue sclera; cloudy cornea; cataracts; megalocornea; corneal dystrophy; buphthalmos; microphthalmos; microphakia; mydriasis; strabismus; lens punctate cortical opacities.

Clinical

Mental, psychomotor and growth retardation; aminoaciduria; albuminuria; glycosuria; renal tubular acidosis; rickets; osteomalacia; muscular hypotony; hyporeflexia; hyperactivity with bizarre choreoathetoid movements and screaming.

Laboratory

Urine—aminoaciduria, proteinuria, calciuria, phosphaturia; serum—elevated acid phosphate; imaging studies—brain MRI—mild ventriculomegaly (1/3 cases); ocular ultrasound—if dense cataract rule out mass or retinal detachment posterior.

Treatment

Monitor and treat for glaucoma. If glaucoma develops, intraocular pressure-lowering agents must be used. Often, these patients require surgical intervention with goniotomy, trabeculectomy or a drainage filtration device. Congenital cataracts should be removed, ideally in the first 6 weeks of life, to optimize the visual potential.

Additional Resource

1. Alcorn DM (2010). Oculocerebrorenal Syndrome. [online] Available from http://www.emedicine.com/oph/TOPIC516.HTM [Accessed April, 2012].

---

880. LUBARSCH-PICK SYNDROME (AMYLOIDOSIS; IDIOPATHIC AMYLOIDOSIS; PRIMARY AMYLOIDOSIS)

General

Rare condition of unknown etiology; inherited as a dominant trait, with male preponderance; characterized by amyloid accumulation in muscles and in gastrointestinal and genitourinary tracts.

Ocular

Internal and external ophthalmoplegia; diminished lacrimation; amyloid deposits in conjunctival, episcleral and ciliary vessels; vitreous opacities; amyloid deposits in the corneal stroma; retinal hemorrhages and perivascular exudates;

paralysis of extraocular muscles; pseudopodia lentis; strabismus fixus convergence; keratoconus.

Clinical

Peripheral neuropathy (extremities); heart failure; defective hepatic and renal functions with hepatosplenomegaly; waxy skin lesions; muscular weakness (progressive); multiple myeloma; hoarseness; chronic gastrointestinal symptoms.

Laboratory

Biopsy—stain with Congo red demonstrates apple-green birefringence under polarized light. Distinctive fibriller ultrastructure.

Treatment

Deoxydoxorubicin had demonstrated some clinical benefit.

Bibliography

1. Biswas J, Badrinath SS, Rao NA. Primary nonfamilial amyloidosis of the vitreous. A light microscopic and ultrastructural study. Retina. 1992;12:251-3.
2. Goebel HH, Friedman AH. Extraocular muscle involvement in idiopathic primary amyloidosis. Am J Ophthalmol. 1971;71:1121-7.
3. Lubarsch O. Zur Kenntnis Ungewohnlicher Amyloidablagerungen. Virchows Arch Pathol Anat. 1929;271:867-89.
4. Magalini SI, Scrascia E. Dictionary of Medical Syndromes, 2nd edition. Philadelphia: JB Lippincott; 1981.
5. Sharma P, Gupta NK, Arora R, et al. Strabismus fixus convergens secondary to amyloidosis. J Pediatr Ophthalmol Strabismus. 1991;28:236-7.
6. Wong VG, McFarlin DE. A case of primary familial amyloidosis. Arch Ophthalmol. 1967;78:208-13.

881. LYME DISEASE

General

Caused by tick bite; symptoms resolve after treatment.

Ocular

Keratitis may occur up to 5 years after the first episode; diplopia; photophobia; ischemic optic neuropathy; iritis; panophthalmitis; conjunctivitis; exudative retinal detachment; choroiditis; vitreitis; multiple cranial nerve palsies; association with acute, posterior, multifocal, placoid, pigment epitheliopathy; branch retinal artery occlusion.

Clinical

Arthritis; increased intracranial pressure; effusion of knees; swelling of wrists.

Laboratory

Immunofluorescent assay (IFA) and enzyme-linked immunosorbent assay (ELISA).

Treatment

Oral antibiotics for 2–3 weeks: tetracycline 500 mg four times a day, doxycycline 100 mg two times a day, phenoxymethyl penicillin 500 mg four times a day or amoxicillin 500 mg 3–4 times a day.

Additional Resource

1. Zaidman GW (2011). Ophthalmic Aspects of Lyme Disease Overview of Lyme Disease. [online] Available from http://www.emedicine.com/oph/TOPIC262.HTM [Accessed April, 2012].

882. LYMPHADENOSIS BENIGNA ORBITAE

General

Onset from age 18–88 years; localized inflammatory process of undetermined origin; duration usually 2–12 months.

Ocular

Exophthalmos; well-circumscribed painless swelling around the eyes; glaucoma; restricted eye movements.

Clinical

Malignant tumor; insect bites; lymphadenosis benigna cutis.

Laboratory

Biopsy is necessary to establish a diagnosis.

Treatment

When the offending agent is known, its removal results in resolution. Surgical removal, cryosurgery or local irradiation may be necessary. Topical or injected corticosteroids and topical immunomodulators such as tacrolimus have also been useful.

Bibliography

1. Bafverstedt B, Lundmark C, Mossberg H, et al. Lymphadenosis benigna orbitae. Acta Ophthalmol. 1956;34:367-76.

883. LYMPHEDEMA

General

Abnormal accumulation of lymph in the extremities; occurs from multiple causes.

Ocular

Conjunctival chemosis; ectropion; ptosis; strabismus; hyperpigmentation of eyelids; chorioretinal dysplasia; distichiasis; eyelid lymphedema.

Clinical

Abnormal lymphatic drainage; painless swelling; fibrosis of skin and subcutaneous tissues; skin becomes thickened, brown, multiple papillary projections (lymphostatic verrucosis); microcephaly; lymphedema.

Laboratory

Lymphangiography, CT, MRI, Doppler ultrasonography.

Treatment

The goal of conservative therapy is to eliminate protein stagnation and to restore normal lymphatic circulation. Compression garments, intermittent pneumatic pump compression therapy, weight loss, avoiding even minor trauma and avoiding constrictive clothing are all useful.

Additional Resource

1. Revis DR (2011). Lymphedema. [online] Available from http://www.emedicine.com/med/TOPIC2722. HTM [Accessed April, 2012].

884. LYMPHOCYTIC CHORIOMENINGITIS (ASEPTIC MENINGITIS)

General

Virus of which natural host is house mouse; more common in late fall and winter; usually benign.

Ocular

Palpebral edema; optic neuritis; ocular motor palsies; pupillary and accommodative pareses; strabismus; diplopia; conjunctival injection.

Clinical

Fever; meningeal irritation; headaches; confusion; coma; stiffness of neck; Babinski sign; may occur early in the course of human immunodeficiency virus infection; syndrome is considered to be usually viral in origin, with enteroviruses accounting for most cases, but rare bacterial organisms such as *Mycobacterium tuberculosis*, *Leptospira sp*, *Brucella sp*, *Borrelia burgdorferi* and others, may cause aseptic meningitis; drug-induced aseptic meningitis also should be considered.

Laboratory

Cerebrospinal fluid (CSF) evaluation including cell count and differential and glucose and protein levels, focal neurologic signs or any unusual features are present, early CT scan or MRI should be performed.

Treatment

Management is supportive. Administer adequate analgesia. Seizures should be treated with appropriate emergency therapies.

Additional Resource

1. Faust SN (2012). Pediatric Aseptic Meningitis. [online] Available from http://www.emedicine.com/ped/TOPIC3004.HTM [Accessed April, 2012].

885. LYMPHOGRANULOMA VENEREUM (LYMPHOGRANULOMA INGUINALE; NICOLAS-FAVRE DISEASE; TROPICAL BUBO LGV)

General

Venereally transmitted infection caused by *Chlamydia*.

Ocular

Conjunctivitis; chronic lid edema; keratitis; pannus; corneal ulcer; keratoconus; episcleritis; uveitis; tortuosity of retinal vessels; retinal hemorrhages.

Clinical

Enlargement of inguinal lymph nodes; lymphadenitis; lymphogranuloma.

Laboratory

Cerebrospinal fluid (CSF) evaluation including cell count and differential and glucose and protein levels, CT, MRI.

Treatment

Management is supportive. Administer adequate analgesia.

Additional Resource

1. http://www.emedicine.medscape.com/article/220869-overview

886. LYMPHOID HYPERPLASIA (BURKITT LYMPHOMA; LYMPHOID TUMORS; MALIGNANT LYMPHOMA; NEOPLASTIC ANGIOENDOTHELIOMATOSIS PSEUDOLYMPHOMA; PSEUDOTUMOR; REACTIVE LYMPHOID HYPERPLASIA)

General

Occurs in tropical Africa; young children; idiopathic orbital inflammation; systemic disease is rarely associated but occasionally occurs with either vasculitis or lymphomas; etiology of Burkitt lymphoma currently includes three factors: (1) Epstein-Barr virus, (2) malaria and (3) chromosomal translocations activating the *c-myc* oncogene, which induces uncontrolled B-cell proliferation.

Ocular

Proptosis; extraocular motility disturbances; lesions of orbit, lacrimal gland, conjunctiva and uvea; cortical blindness; retinal artery occlusion; retinal vascular and pigment epithelial alterations; vitreitis.

Clinical

Maxillary tumor; Epstein-Barr virus; cranial neuropathy.

Laboratory

Generally diagnosed with a lymph node biopsy.

Treatment

Chemotherapy, monoclonal antibody therapy and bone marrow or stem cell infusions may be chosen as therapy.

Bibliography

1. Brooks HL, Downing J, McClure JA, et al. Orbital Burkitt's lymphoma in a homosexual man with acquired immune deficiency. Arch Ophthalmol. 1984;102:1533-7.
2. Cheung MK, Martin DF, Chan CC, et al. Diagnosis of reactive lymphoid hyperplasia by chorioretinal biopsy. Am J Ophthalmol. 1994;118:457-62.

887. MACROANEURYSM

General

Dilation of the large arterioles of the retina; associated with systemic hypertension and atherosclerotic disease; most commonly seen in the sixth and seventh decades of life.

Clinical

Hypertension; elevated cholesterol; atherosclerosis disease.

Ocular

Retinal edema; sudden painless vision loss; retinal hemorrhage; retinal exudate.

Laboratory

Fluorescein angiography is most helpful in diagnosis.

Treatment

Control hypertension and serum lipids. Many cases resolve without treatment. Laser photocoagulation may be necessary if the disease is persistent or progressive.

Additional Resource

1. Chaum E (2010). Macroaneurysm. [online] Available from http://www.emedicine.medscape.com/article/1224043-overview [Accessed April, 2012].

888. MACULAR CORNEAL DYSTROPHY (GROENOUW DYSTROPHY TYPE II)

General

Autosomal recessive corneal dystrophy.

Clinical

None

Ocular

Diffuse clouding in central superficial stroma.

Laboratory

Diagnosis is made by clinical findings.

Treatment

Ocular—contact lens may "smooth" surface and improve vision. Surgical—phototherapeutic kera-tectomy (PTK) may help or penetrating corneal transplant or lamellar transplant may be necessary.

Bibliography

1. McKusick VA. Mendelian Inheritance in Man: A Catalog of Human Genes and Genetic Disorders, 12th edition. Baltimore: The Johns Hopkins University Press; 1998.
2. McKusick-Nathans Institute for Genetic Medicine, Johns Hopkins University and National Center for Biotechnology Information, National Library of Medicine. (2007). Online Mendelian Inheritance in Man (OMIM). [online] Available from http://www.ncbi.nlm.nih.gov/omim/ [Accessed April, 2012].

889. MACULAR DYSTROPHY

General

Sex-linked; macular dystrophy of fundus.

Ocular

Posterior pole changes; marked decrease in visual acuity; congenital stationary night blindness; color blindness; vitreotapetoretinal dystrophy; choroidal dystrophy; senile macular choroidal degeneration; retinoschisis; prognosis for retaining functional visual acuity is good.

Clinical

Lipidoses; neurologic disorders.

Laboratory

Diagnosis is made by clinical findings.

Treatment

None/Ocular.

Bibliography

1. Forsius H, Vainio-Mattila B, Eriksson A. X-linked hereditary retinoschisis. Br J Ophthalmol. 1962;46:678-81.
2. McKusick VA. Mendelian Inheritance in Man: A Catalog of Human Genes and Genetic Disorders, 12th edition. Baltimore: The Johns Hopkins University Press; 1998.

890. MACULAR DYSTROPHY, CONCENTRIC ANNULI (BULL'S-EYE MACULAR DYSTROPHY)

General

Autosomal dominant; no male-to-male transmission observed.

Ocular

Dyschromatopsia; foveal hyperpigmentation; perifoveal hyperpigmentation; perifoveal circular pigment epithelial atrophy.

Clinical

Lipidoses; neurologic disorders.

Laboratory

Diagnosis is made by clinical findings.

Treatment

None/Ocular.

Bibliography

1. Forsius H, Vainio-Mattila B, Eriksson A. X-linked hereditary retinoschisis. Br J Ophthalmol. 1962;46: 678-81.
2. McKusick VA. Mendelian Inheritance in Man: A Catalog of Human Genes and Genetic Disorders, 12th edition. Baltimore: The Johns Hopkins University Press; 1998.

891. MACULAR DYSTROPHY ECTODERMAL DYSPLASIA AND ECTRODACTYLY (EEM SYNDROME)

General

Associated with abetaloproteinemia.

Ocular

Macular dystrophy; hypotrichosis; vitreous hemorrhage; persistent hyloid artery.

Laboratory

Diagnosis is made by clinical findings.

Treatment

Vitreous hemorrhage: If possible the source of the bleeding needs to be isolated and treated with laser. Vitrectomy may be necessary.

Additional Resource

1. Afshari N (2010). Macular Dystrophy. [online] Available from http://www.emedicine.com/oph/TOPIC94.HTM [Accessed April, 2012].

892. MACULAR DYSTROPHY, FENESTRATED SHEEN TYPE

General

Autosomal dominant; progressive; onset in the sixth decade.

Ocular

Yellowish retractile sheen in sensory retina at the macula; red fenestrations present within sheen; hypopigmentation of retinal pigment epithelium.

Clinical

None

Laboratory

Diagnosis is made by clinical findings.

Treatment

None

Bibliography

1. McKusick VA. Mendelian Inheritance in Man: A Catalog of Human Genes and Genetic Disorders, 12th edition. Baltimore: The Johns Hopkins University Press; 1998.

2. McKusick-Nathans Institute for Genetic Medicine, Johns Hopkins University and National Center for Biotechnology Information, National Library of Medicine. (2007). Online Mendelian Inheritance in Man (OMIM). [online] Available from http://www.ncbi.nlm.nih.gov/omim [Accessed April, 2012].

3. Sneed SR, Sieving PA. Fenestrated sheen macular dystrophy. Am J Ophthalmol. 1991;112:1-7.

---

893. MACULAR EDEMA, CYSTOID

General

Autosomal dominant; edema due to leaking perimacular capillaries.

Ocular

Retinal capillary leakage all over posterior pole of the eye; whitish punctate deposits in vitreous; hyperopia; "beaten bronze" atrophy to macula; strabismus.

Clinical

Patients show cystoid macular edema (CME) at a young age with gradual progressive decrease in visual acuity starting between the first and fourth decades of life.

Laboratory

Optical coherence tomography (OCT) testing is used to identify CME.

Treatment

Treatment varies depending on the etiology causing CME. Avastin injections have shown some promise for the control of macular edema.

Additional Resource

1. Roth DB (2012). Nonpseudophakic Cystoid Macular Edema. [online] Available from http://www.emedicine.com/oph/TOPIC638.HTM [Accessed April, 2012].

---

894. MACULAR EDEMA, PSEUDOPHAKIC (IRVINE-GASS)

General

Painless loss of vision due to swelling or thickening of the macula; Frequently associated with cataract surgery (Irvine-Gass), age-related macular degeneration, uveitis, injury, diabetes and retinal vein occlusion.

Clinical

Diabetes; renal failure, following cataract surgery.

Ocular

Decreased visual acuity; uveitis; retinal vein occlusion; macular degeneration; macular pucker.

Laboratory

Fluorescein angiography and optical coherence tomography are helpful in determining the disease.

Treatment

Uses of corticosteroids, carbonic anhydrase inhibitors and NSAIDs are the mainstay of treatment. If traditional therapy is not effective, intraocular injections of Avastin may be helpful.

In cases that have vitreous strand tugging against the macula, pars plana vitrectomy may be necessary.

Additional Resource

1. Telander DG (2010). Macular Edema, Pseudophakic (Irvine-Gass). [online] Available from http://www.emedicine.medscape.com/article/1224224-overview [Accessed April, 2012].

895. MACULAR HALO SYNDROME

General

Probably variant of Niemann-Pick disease; major differences are the ocular lesion described as macular halo with a granular appearance instead of the classic cherry-red spot and the lack of major visual symptoms.

Ocular

Crystalloid opacities of foveolae; granular macula; macular halo.

Clinical

Hepatosplenomegaly; hyperlipidemia; histiocytes of bone marrow, spleen and liver.

Laboratory

Diagnosis is made by clinical findings.

Treatment

None/Ocular.

Bibliography

1. Cogan DG, Tedermann DD. Retinal involvement with reticuloendotheliosis of unclassified type. Arch Ophthalmol. 1964;71:489-91.

896. MACULAR HOLE

General

Full thickness defect in the neurosensory retina centered at the foveola resulting in a central scotoma.

Clinical

None

Ocular

Visual loss, distorted Amsler grid, metamorphopsia.

Laboratory

Diagnosis is made by clinical findings.

Treatment

Prophylactic vitrectomy.

Additional Resource

1. Oh KT (2011). Macular Hole. [online] Available from http://www.emedicine.com/oph/TOPIC401.HTM [Accessed April, 2012].

897. MAD HATTER SYNDROME

General

Chronic mercury intoxication; symptoms seldom improve regardless of treatment.

Ocular

Constricted visual fields; lens opacities.

Clinical

Anorexia; peripheral neuritis; ataxia; hearing impairment; hyperreflexia; progressive mental depression; tremor; insomnia; fatigue; irritability; lethargy; hallucinations; shyness; withdrawal; gingivitis; teeth loosening.

Laboratory

Magnetic resonance imaging (MRI), blood mercury levels, toenail mercury.

Treatment

Removal from the source of exposure, chelation therapy.

Additional Resource

1. Olson DA (2011). Mercury Toxicity. [online] Available from http://www.emedicine.com/neuro/TOPIC617.HTM [Accessed April, 2012].

898. MADAROSIS (LOSS OF LASHES)

General

Loss of eyelashes caused by systemic or topical infections and inflammation, eyelid tumors, the hysteric plucking of hairs, surgery and trauma.

Clinical

May have emotional problems in alopecia artefacta.

Ocular

Loss of lashes frequently in only one segment of lid.

Laboratory

Diagnosis is made by clinical findings.

Treatment

Lid hygiene, lid scrubs with baby shampoo and topical antibiotics, eyeliner and false eyelashes, transplantation of lashes to area missing lashes.

Bibliography

1. Roy FH, Fraunfelder FW, Fraunfelder FT. Roy and Fraunfelder's Current Ocular Therapy, 6th edition. Philadelphia: WB Saunders; 2008.

899. MAFFUCCI SYNDROME (KAST SYNDROME; MULTIPLE ENCHONDROMATOSIS; PROGRESSIVE DYSCHONDROPLASIA AND MULTIPLE HEMANGIOMAS; OSTEOCHONDROMATOSIS)

General

Rare; etiology unknown; no hereditary factor; manifest in ages 1–5 years; characterized by numerous cartilage tumors involving mainly small bones of hands and feet; malignant transformation common; no simple mendelian inheritance.

Ocular

Hemangiomas of lid and retina.

Clinical

Multiple enchondromas with secondary bony deformities (dyschondroplasia of Ollier); chondrosarcomas; multiple hemangiomas and phlebolithiasis; orthostatic hypotension (depending on extent and size of hemangiomas); frequent fractures following minimal trauma; precocious pseudopuberty.

Laboratory

None

Treatment

No medical care needed.

Additional Resource

1. Kuwahara RT (2012). Maffucci Syndrome. [online] Available from http://www.emedicine.com/derm/TOPIC256.HTM [Accessed April, 2012].

---

900. MAJEWSKI SYNDROME

General

Autosomal recessive; normal chromosomes; perinatal mortality; has been suggested to be related to Mohr syndrome.

Ocular

Cataract; optic disk edema; optic atrophy; hypertelorism; absent lashes and brows; persistent pupillary membrane.

Clinical

Short rib polydactyly; cleft lip; cleft palate; narrow thorax; short tibia; hypoplastic epiglottis; lung and visceral abnormalities.

Laboratory

Diagnosis is made by clinical findings.

Treatment

Optic atrophy: Intravenous steroids may be used with optic neuritis or ischemic neuropathy. Stem cell treatment may be the future treatment of choice.

Bibliography

1. Cherstvoy ED, Lurie IW, Shved IA, et al. Difficulties in classification of the short rib polydactyly syndromes. Eur J Pediatr. 1980;133:57-61.
2. Chess J, Albert DM. Ocular pathology of the Majewski syndrome. Br J Ophthalmol. 1982;66 :736-41.
3. Majewski F, Pfeiffer RA, Lenz W, et al. Polysyndaktylie, Verkuerzte Gliedmassen, und Genitalfehlbildungen. Z Kinderheilkd. 1971;111:118-38.
4. McKusick VA. Mendelian Inheritance in Man: A Catalog of Human Genes and Genetic Disorders, 12th edition. Baltimore: The Johns Hopkins University Press; 1998.
5. McKusick-Nathans Institute for Genetic Medicine, Johns Hopkins University and National Center for Biotechnology Information, National Library of Medicine. (2007). Online Mendelian Inheritance in Man (OMIM). [online] Available from http://www.ncbi.nlm.nih.gov/omim [Accessed April, 2012].
6. Silengo MC, Bell GL, Biagioli M, et al. Oro-facial-digital syndrome. II. Transitional type between the Mohr and the Majewski syndromes: report of two new cases. Clin Genet. 1987;31:331-6.

901. MALARIA

General

Caused by *Plasmodium*, which is transmitted by mosquito bite, blood transfusion or contaminated needles and syringes.

Ocular

Proliferative retinitis; vascular embolism; keratitis; ocular herpes simplex; blepharitis; optic atrophy; papilledema; papillitis; optic neuritis; anisocoria; Argyll Robertson pupil; vitreal hemorrhages and opacity; cataract; myopia; strabismus; uveitis; scleral icterus; scotoma; lagophthalmos; ptosis; subconjunctival hemorrhages; paralysis of third, fourth, or sixth nerve; epibulbar hemorrhage involving the conjunctiva, episclera and tendinous insertion of the medial rectus.

Clinical

Fever; anemia; splenomegaly; death.

Laboratory

Blood smear.

Treatment

Consult infectious disease specialist.

Additional Resource

1. Perez-Jorge EV (2012). Malaria. [online] Available from http://www.emedicine.com/med/TOPIC1385.HTM [Accessed April, 2012].

902. MALIGNANT GLAUCOMA (AQUEOUS MISDIRECTION; CILIARY BLOCK GLAUCOMA; CILOLENTICULAR/CILIOVITREAL BLOCK)

General

Rare, poor response to conventional treatment.

Clinical

None

Ocular

Shallow angle secondary glaucoma.

Laboratory

Ultrasound biomicroscopy.

Treatment

Argon laser treatment of ciliary processes, YAG laser hyaloidotomy and incisional surgery. Pars plana vitrectomy may be necessary sometimes with posterior capsulotomy and lensectomy.

Additional Resource

1. Pons ME (2012). Malignant Glaucoma. [online] Available from http://www.emedicine.com/oph/TOPIC134.HTM [Accessed April, 2012].

903. MALIGNANT HYPERPYREXIA SYNDROME (POSTCATARACT HYPERPYREXIA SYNDROME; POSTINDUCTION HYPERPYREXIA SYNDROME)

General

Etiology uncertain, but believed to be a secondary response to suxamethonium and halothane used with general anesthesia; high mortality rate of about 70%.

Ocular

Malignant hyperpyrexia following congenital cataract or strabismus surgery under general anesthesia.

Clinical

Rapid elevation of body temperature and vastly enhanced metabolic activity; hyperapnea; tachycardia.

Laboratory

Diagnosis is made by clinical findings.

Treatment

Early detection, if occurs, reduce temperature.

Bibliography

1. Geeraets WJ. Ocular Syndromes, 3rd edition. Philadelphia: Lea & Febiger; 1976.
2. Petersdorf RG. Malignant hyperthermia. In: Isselbacher KJ (Ed). Harrison's Principles of Internal Medicine, 13th edition. New York: McGraw-Hill; 1994. p. 2476.
3. Rosenberg H, Fletcher JE. An update on the malignant hyperthermia syndrome. Ann Acad Med Singapore. 1994;23(6 Suppl):84-97.
4. Snow JC, Keenan TJ. Malignant hyperpyrexia. Eye Ear Nose Throat Mon. 1970;49:427-30.

904. MALIGNANT HYPERTHERMIA SYNDROME

General

Pharmacogenetic disease with uninhibited flow of calcium ion into muscle substance; leads to combined metabolic and respiratory acidosis and liberation of heat; cellular death may result; autosomal dominant; more common in children and young adults; unusual disorder of skeletal and cardiac muscle triggered by anesthetic agents.

Ocular

Blepharoptosis; squint; pupils fixed and dilated.

Clinical

Hernias; kyphosis; clubfoot; excessive muscular bulk; muscle cramps; unstable blood pressure; rapid and deep respiration; mottled cyanosis; arrhythmias; muscle rigidity; oliguria; anuria; deep tendon reflexes absent.

Laboratory

Diagnosis is made by halothane contracture test.

Treatment

Cooling and early treatment of hyperkalemia are desirable. General administration of dantrolene is used.

Bibliography

1. Geeraets WJ. Ocular Syndromes, 3rd edition. Philadelphia: Lea & Febiger; 1976.
2. Snow JC, Keenan TJ. Malignant hyperpyrexia. Eye Ear Nose Throat Mon. 1970;49:427-30.

905. MALIGNANT MELANOMA OF THE POSTERIOR UVEA (CHOROIDAL MELANOMA, CILIARY BODY MELANOMA, INTRAOCULAR MELANOMA, UVEAL MELANOMA)

General

Most common primary intraocular tumor in adults.

Clinical

Metastic melanoma can appear in other parts of the body such as skin or liver.

Ocular

Intraocular tumors of the choroid, iris and ciliary body.

Laboratory

Ultrasonography, fluorescein angiography and indocyanine green angiography.

Treatment

Ocular therapy's goal is to eradicate the tumor before metastasis occurs. Diode laser, brachytherapy, stereotactic, local resection, enucleation and exenteration are all used to achieve this. Systemically intravenous therapy, intrahepatic chemoembolization has been used for isolated liver metastases. Proton beam is used to kill the tumor.

Additional Resource

1. Garcia-Valenzuela E (2011). Choroidal Melanoma. [online] Available from http://www.emedicine.com/oph/TOPIC403.HTM [Accessed April, 2012].

906. MANNOSIDOSIS

General

Rare; deficiency of alpha-mannosidase activity.

Ocular

Lens opacities; corneal opacities; strabismus; late onset retinal dystrophy.

Clinical

Coarse facial features; dysostosis multiplex; hearing defects; mental retardation; hepatosplenomegaly.

Laboratory

Complete blood count and CSF and blood chemistry test.

Treatment

No specific treatment available—systemic or ocular.

Strabismus: Equalized vision with correct refractive error; surgery may be helpful in patient with diplopia.

Cataract: Change in glasses can sometimes improve a patient's visual function temporarily; however, the most common treatment is cataract surgery.

Bibliography

1. Jolly RD, Shimada A, Dalefield RR, et al. Mannosidosis: ocular lesions in the bovine model. Curr Eye Res. 1987;6:1073-8.
2. Springer C, Gutschalk A, Meinck HM, et al. Late-onset retinal dystrophy in alpha-mannosidosis. Graefes Arch Clin Exp Ophthalmol. 2005;243:1277-9.

907. MARCHESANI SYNDROME (BRACHYMORPHY WITH SPHEROPHAKIA; DYSTROPHIA MESODERMALIS CONGENITA HYPERPLASTICA; INVERTED MARFAN SYNDROME; WEILL-MARCHESANI SYNDROME)

General

Pattern of inheritance uncertain; manifested between the ages of 9 months and 13 years.

Ocular

Lenticular myopia; secondary glaucoma (rare), caused by luxation of the lens; iridodonesis; ectopia lentis; spherophakia; optic atrophy; megalocornea; corneal opacity; acute pupillary block glaucoma.

Clinical

Brachydactyly; reduced growth; athletic build with abundant subcutaneous tissue; short neck and large thorax; short and clumsy hands and feet; decreased joint flexibility; hearing defects; inheritable connective tissue disorder, usually inherited as an autosomal recessive.

Laboratory

X-ray detects delayed carpal ossification.

Treatment/Glaucoma

Beta-blockers, carbonic anhydrase inhibitors and prostaglandin analogs. Surgery may be needed if IOP is uncontrolled.

Bibliography

1. Jensen AD, Cross HE, Paton D. Ocular complications in the Weill-Marchesani syndrome. Am J Ophthalmol. 1974;77:261-9.
2. Marchesani O. Brachydactylie und Angeborene Kugellinse als Systemerkrankung. Klin Monatsbl Augenheilkd. 1939;103:392.
3. McKusick-Nathans Institute for Genetic Medicine, Johns Hopkins University and National Center for Biotechnology Information, National Library of Medicine. (2007). Online Mendelian Inheritance in Man (OMIM). [online] Available from http://www.ncbi.nlm.nih.gov/omim/ [Accessed April, 2012].
4. McKusick VA. Mendelian Inheritance in Man: A Catalog of Human Genes and Genetic Disorders, 12th edition. Baltimore: The Johns Hopkins University Press; 1998.
5. Roy FH, Fraunfelder FW, Fruanfelder FT. Roy and Fraunfelder's Current Ocular Therapy, 6th edition. Philadelphia: WB Saunders; 2008.
6. Willi M, Kut L, Cotlier E. Pupillary-block glaucoma in the Marchesani syndrome. Arch Ophthalmol. 1973;90:504-8.
7. Young ID, Fielder AR, Casey TA. Weill-Marchesani syndrome in mother and son. Clin Genet. 1986;30:475-80.

908. MARCUS GUNN SYNDROME (CONGENITAL TRIGEMINO-OCULOMOTOR SYNKINESIS; JAW-WINKING SYNDROME)

General

Familial occurrence rare, although dominant inheritance has been reported; symptoms caused by abnormal connections between external pterygoid muscle and levator palpebrae, with supranuclear or supranuclear-nuclear involvement (see Marin Amat Syndrome).

Ocular

Unilateral congenital ptosis in more than 90% of cases; 10% have spontaneous onset, usually in older persons; lid elevates rapidly when mouth is opened or mandible is moved to one or the other side; left eye seems to be more frequently affected than right eye; high incidences of strabismus

(36%); amblyopia (34%); bilateral jaw-winking; decreased abduction.

Clinical

Stimulation of ipsilateral pterygoid with chewing, opening mouth, sucking or contralateral jaw thrusts.

Laboratory

Diagnosis is made by clinical findings.

Treatment

Treat amblyopia, if mild ptosis and mild jaw-winking, is considered Muller's muscle con-junctival resection; severe jaw-winking releases levator and performs a frontalis sling usually bilaterally; unilateral ptosis and mild jaw-winking are considered levator release and advance frontalis muscle to the superior tarsus.

Bibliography

1. Demirci H, Frueh BR, Nelson CC. Marcus Gunn jaw-winking sykinesis. Ophthalmology. 2010;117:1447-52.

Additional Resource

1. Blaydon SM (2011). Marcus Gunn Jaw-winking Syndrome. [online] Available from http://www.emedicine.com/oph/TOPIC608.HTM [Accessed April, 2012].

---

909. MARFAN SYNDROME (ARACHNODACTYLY; DOLICHOSTENOMELIA; DYSTROPHIA MESODERMALIS CONGENITA; HYPERCHONDROPLASIA)

General

Hypoplastic form of dystrophia mesodermalis congenita; autosomal dominant; affects both sexes; has been demonstrated that an abnormality of the gene coding for the connective tissue protein fibrillin is responsible for chronic Marfan syndrome.

Ocular

Exotropia; nystagmus; paralysis of accommodation; myopia (axial or lenticular); iridodonesis; miosis; persistent pupillary membrane; blue sclera; spherophakia; lens dislocation; cataract; megalocornea; retinal detachment (less frequently); pigmentary retinopathy; colobomata of macula, iris, optic nerve and uveal tract (less frequently); keratoconus; central retinal artery occlusion; rhegmatogenous retinal detachment; syringoma.

Clinical

Arachnodactyly; skeletal anomalies; asymmetric thorax; dolichocephaly and high-arched palate; dissecting aneurysm; mitral valve prolapse; prominent ears; kyphoscoliosis; pectus excavatum; flat feet; hammer toes; pulmonary and kidney defects.

Laboratory

Genetic testing, molecular studies.

Treatment

Keratoconus: Spectacle correction, hard contacts and avoid eye rubbing may be useful. If hydrops occurs discontinue contact lens, use NaCl drops and ointment, patching and short course of steroids. As the disease advances penetrating keratoplasty, deep anterior lamellar keratoplasty, intacs with laser grooves or collagen stabilization of cornea.

Cataract: Change in glasses can sometimes improve a patient's visual function temporarily; however, the most common treatment is cataract surgery.

Glaucoma: Its medication should be the first plan of action. If medication is unsuccessful, a filtering surgical procedure with or without antimetabolites may be beneficial.

Strabismus: Equalized vision with correct refractive error; surgery may be helpful in patient with diplopia.

Additional Resource

1. Chen H (2011). Genetics of Marfan Syndrome. [online] Available from http://www.emedicine.com/ped/TOPIC1372.HTM [Accessed April, 2012].

910. MARIN AMAT SYNDROME (INVERTED MARCUS GUNN PHENOMENON)

General

Intrafacial connection between the orbicularis oculi and external pterygoid muscles; occurs primarily after peripheral facial palsy.

Ocular

When mouth is opened and/or mandible is moved to side opposite ptosis, closure of the eye occurs; increased tearing during mastication.

Clinical

Signs of old facial palsy usually recognizable.

Laboratory

Diagnosis is made by clinical findings.

Treatment

If amblyopia is noted, occlusion therapy is needed.

Additional Resource

1. Blaydon SM (2011). Marcus Gunn Jaw-winking Syndrome. [online] Available from http://www.emedicine.com/oph/TOPIC608.HTM [Accessed April, 2012].

911. MARINESCO-SJÖGREN SYNDROME (CONGENITAL SPINOCEREBELLAR ATAXIA-CONGENITAL CATARACT-OLIGOPHRENIA SYNDROME)

General

Autosomal recessive trait; onset when child learns to walk; mitochondrial disease.

Ocular

Cataracts; aniridia; rotary and horizontal nystagmus; nystagmus; strabismus; optic atrophy.

Clinical

Cerebellar ataxia; oligophrenia; small stature; scoliosis; genu valgum; restricted extensibility of the knee; defects of fingers and toes; mental retardation; hair sparse; hypersalivation; sensorineural hearing loss.

Laboratory

Diagnosis is made by clinical findings.

Treatment

Cataract: Change in glasses can sometimes improve a patient's visual function temporarily; however, the most common treatment is cataract surgery.

Bibliography

1. Dotti MT, Bardelli AM, De Stefano N, et al. Optic atrophy in Marinesco-Sjögren syndrome: an additional ocular feature. Report of three cases in two families. Ophthalmic Paediatr Genet. 1993; 14:5-7.
2. Gillespie FD. Aniridia, cerebellar ataxia, and oligophrenia in siblings. Arch Ophthalmol. 1965;73: 338-41.
3. Lindal S, Lund I, Torbergsen T, et al. Mitochondrial diseases and myopathies: a series of muscle biopsy specimens with ultrastructural changes in the mitochondria. Ultrastruct Pathol. 1992;16: 263-75.
4. Marinesco G, Draganesco S, Vasiliu D. Nouvelle Maladie Familiale Caracterisee par une Cataracte Congenitale et un Arret du Developement Somato-Neuro-Psychique. Encephale. 1931;26: 97-109.
5. Sjögren T. Hereditary congenital spinocerebellar ataxia accompanied by congenital cataracts and oligophrenia; a genetic and clinical investigation. Confin Neurol. 1950;10:293-308.

912. MAROTEAUX-LAMY SYNDROME (MPS VI SYNDROME; MUCOPOLYSACCHARIDOSIS VI; SYSTEMIC MUCOPOLYSACCHARIDOSIS TYPE VI)

General

Onset in infancy; etiology unknown; autosomal recessive; excessive urinary excretion of chondroitin sulfate B; lysosomal storage disease; deficiency of the enzyme arylsulfatase B; multiple clinical phenotypes.

Ocular

Corneal haziness and opacities; pupillary membrane remnants.

Clinical

Skeleton deformities; restriction of articular movements; dyspnea; heart murmur; hearing impairment.

Laboratory

Urine—excessive glycosaminoglycan dermatan sulfate or chondroitin sulfate B.

Treatment

Enzyme replacement, bone marrow transplant and stem cell therapy are in the experimental.

Bibliography

1. Roy FH, Fraunfelder FW, Fraunfelder FT. Roy and Fraunfelder's Current Ocular Therapy, 6th edition. Philadelphia: WB Saunders; 2008.
2. Kenyon KR, Topping TM, Green WR, et al. Ocular pathology of the Maroteaux-Lamy syndrome. Am J Ophthalmol. 1972;73:718-41.
3. Matalon R, Arbogast B, Dorfman A. Deficiency of chondroitin sulfate N-acetylgalactosamine 4-sulfate sulfatase in Maroteaux-Lamy syndrome. Biochem Biophys Res Commun. 1974;61:1450-7.
4. Quigley HA, Kenyon KR. Ultrastructural and histochemical studies of a newly recognized form of systemic mucopolysaccharidosis. Am J Ophthalmol. 1974;77:809-18.
5. Voskoboeva E, Isbrandt D, von Figura K, et al. Four novel mutant alleles of the arylsulfatase B gene in two patients with intermediate form of mucopolysaccharidosis VI (Maroteaux-Lamy syndrome). Hum Genet. 1994;93:259-64.

913. MARQUARDT-LORIAUX SYNDROME (DIABETES INSIPIDUS-DIABETES MELLITUS-OPTIC ATROPHY-DEAFNESS SYNDROME; DIDMOAD SYNDROME; WOLFRAM SYNDROME)

General

Autosomal recessive; present from childhood; age of onset varies.

Ocular

Optic nerve atrophy; color blindness; visual field defects; anisocoria; diabetic retinopathy; nystagmus; cataract; pigmentation of retina.

Clinical

Juvenile diabetes mellitus; diabetes insipidus; neurosensory hearing loss; hypertension; cerebellar dysfunction; vertigo; atony of urinary tract; anosmia; peripheral neuropathy; mitochondrial abnormalities; moderate hearing loss.

Laboratory

Diagnosis is made by clinical findings.

Treatment

Optic nerve atrophy: Intravenous steroids may be used with optic neuritis or ischemic neuropathy.

Stem cell treatment may be the future treatment of choice.

Bibliography

1. Bundey S, Poulton K, Whitwell H, et al. Mitochondrial abnormalities in the DIDMOAD syndrome. J Inherit Metab Dis. 1992;15:315-9.
2. Higashi K. Otologic findings of DIDMOAD syndrome. Am J Otol. 1991;12:57-60.
3. Mtanda AT, Cruysberg JR, Pinckers AJ. Optic atrophy in Wolfram syndrome. Ophthalmic Paediatr Genet. 1986;7:159-65.
4. Niemeyer G, Marquardt JL. Retinal function in an unique syndrome of optic atrophy, juvenile diabetes mellitus, diabetes insipidus, neurosensory hearing loss, autonomic dysfunction, and hyperalanineuria. Invest Ophthalmol. 1972;11: 617-24.
5. Wolfram DJ, Wagner HP. Diabetes mellitus and simple optic atrophy among siblings: report of four cases. Mayo Clin Proc. 1938;13:715-8.

914. MARSHALL (D) SYNDROME (ATYPICAL ECTODERMAL DYSPLASIA)

General

Autosomal dominant; variant of ectodermal dysplasia; onset at birth.

Ocular

Myopia; congenital cataract (spontaneous absorption not uncommon); degenerative fluidvitreous; luxation of lens; cataract; shallow orbits.

Clinical

Facial malformation; saddle nose; hypohidrosis; partial deafness; flat or retracted midface.

Laboratory

Dilated examination, TORCH titers and venereal disease reaserch laboratory test.

Treatment

Cataract surgery is the treatment of choice.

Bibliography

1. Geeraets WJ. Ocular Syndromes, 3rd edition. Philadelphia: Lea & Febiger; 1976.
2. Marshall D. Ectodermal dysplasia: report of kindred with ocular abnormalities and hearing defect. Am J Ophthalmol. 1958;45:143-56.
3. McKusick VA. Mendelian Inheritance in Man: A Catalog of Human Genes and Genetic Disorders, 12th edition. Baltimore: The Johns Hopkins University Press; 1998.
4. McKusick-Nathans Institute for Genetic Medicine, Johns Hopkins University and National Center for Biotechnology Information, National Library of Medicine. (2007). Online Mendelian Inheritance in Man (OMIM). [online] Available from http://www.ncbi.nlm.nih.gov/omim [Accessed April, 2012].
5. Stratton RF, Lee B, Ramirez F. Marshall syndrome. Am J Med Genet. 1991;41:35-8.

915. MARSHALL (RE) SYNDROME

General

Present from birth; etiology unknown; death usually from pneumonia before age 20 months.

Ocular

Exophthalmos; blue sclera; megalocornea; thick eyebrows.

Clinical

Underweight for length; long cranium; prominent forehead; hyperextension; small mandible; small upturned nose; broad middle and proximal phalanges; repeated respiratory infections; failure to thrive; mental retardation; accelerated skeletal growth.

Laboratory

Thyroid function studies, imaging studies.

Treatment

Ocular lubricants.

Bibliography

1. Magalini SI, Scrascia E. Dictionary of Medical Syndromes, 2nd edition. Philadelphia: JB Lippincott; 1981.
2. Marshall RE, Graham CB, Scott CR, et al. Syndrome of accelerated skeletal maturation and relative failure to thrive: a newly recognized clinical growth disorder. J Pediatr. 1971;78: 95-101.

916. MARSHALL-SMITH SYNDROME

General

Rare congenital condition with advanced bone age, facial anomalies and relative failure to thrive.

Ocular

Hypertelorism, protuberant eyes with shallow orbits.

Clinical

Feeding and respiratory difficulties; developmental delay; advanced bone age; characteristic facies.

Laboratory

Diagnosis is made by clinical findings.

Treatment

Ocular lubricants.

Bibliography

1. Summers DA, Cooper HA, Butler MG. Marshall-Smith syndrome: case report of a newborn male and review of the literature. Clin Dysmorphol. 1999;8:207-10.
2. Williams DK, Carlton DR, Green SH, et al. Marshall-Smith syndrome: the expanding phenotype. J Med Genet. 1997;34:842-5.
3. Yoder CC, Wiswell T, Cornish JD, et al. Marshall-Smith syndrome: further delineation. South Med J. 1988;81:1297-300.

917. MARTSOLF SYNDROME

General

Autosomal recessive; rare; cardiac abnormalities.

Ocular

Cataracts

Clinical

Mental retardation; short stature; hypogonadism.

Laboratory

Diagnosis is made by clinical findings.

Treatment

Cataract: Change in glasses can sometimes improve a patient's visual function temporarily; however, the most common treatment is cataract surgery.

Bibliography

1. Harbord MG, Baraitser M, Wilson J. Microcephaly, mental retardation, cataracts, and hypogonadism in sibs: Martsolf's syndrome. J Med Genet. 1989;26:397-406.
2. Martsolf JT, Hunter AG, Haworth JC. Severe mental retardation, cataracts, short stature, and primary hypogonadism in two brothers. Am J Med Genet. 1978;1:291-9.
3. McKusick VA. Mendelian Inheritance in Man: A Catalog of Human Genes and Genetic Disorders, 12th edition. Baltimore: The Johns Hopkins University Press; 1998.
4. McKusick-Nathans Institute for Genetic Medicine, Johns Hopkins University and National Center for Biotechnology Information, National Library of Medicine. (2007). Online Mendelian Inheritance in Man (OMIM). [online] Available from http://www.ncbi.nlm.nih.gov/omim [Accessed April, 2012].
5. Sanchez JM, Barreiro C, Freilij H. Two brothers with Martsolf's syndrome. J Med Genet. 1985;22:308-10.

918. MASQUERADE SYNDROME

General

Chronic blepharoconjunctivitis due to an underlying conjunctival carcinoma.

Ocular

Squamous cell and sebaceous carcinomas that mimic chalazion or other eyelid lesions; lacrimal secretory and excretory systems; lymph node involvement; hematogenous spread (rare).

Clinical

Orbital or regional involvement; intracranial extension and dural invasion.

Laboratory/Ocular

Excisional biopsy.

Treatment

Excisional biopsy is the treatment of choice. Topical cytotoxic therapy.

Additional Resource

1. Monroe M (2011). Head and Neck Cutaneous Squamous Cell Carcinoma. [online] Available from http://www.emedicine.com/oph/TOPIC116. HTM [Accessed April, 2012].

919. MASTOCYTOSIS (URTICARIA; MAST CELL LEUKEMIA)

General

Increased mast cells found in tissues and organs; range from cutaneous to systemic condition.

Ocular

Conjunctival pigmentation; keratitis; pingueculae.

Clinical

Urticarial wheals; mast cells infiltrate into liver, spleen, gastrointestinal system and bones.

Laboratory

Complete blood count, plasma or urinary histamine, total tryptase levels, bone marrow biopsy.

Treatment

H1 and H2 antihistamines, oral disodium cromoglycate.

Additional Resource

1. Hogan DJ (2010). Mastocytosis. [online] Available from http://www.emedicine.com/derm/TOPIC258. HTM [Accessed April, 2012].

920. MATSOUKAS SYNDROME (OCULO-CEREBRO-ARTICULO-SKELETAL SYNDROME)

General

Autosomal dominant; some of the features are found in Larsen syndrome, Schwartz syndrome, Hallermann-Streiff syndrome, Mietens syndrome and Stickler syndrome; both sexes affected; onset at birth.

Ocular

Microphthalmia; myopia; increased pupillary distance; cataract; corneal sclerosis with vascular pericorneal net.

Clinical

Small stature; multiple joint dislocations; mental retardation; high palate; small mouth.

Laboratory/Ocular

Diagnosis is made by clinical findings.

Treatment

Cataract: Change in glasses can sometimes improve a patient's visual function temporarily; however, the most common treatment is cataract surgery.

Bibliography

1. Matsoukas J, Liarikos S, Giannikas A, et al. A newly recognized dominantly inherited syndrome: short stature, ocular and articular anomalies, mental retardation. Helv Paediatr Acta. 1973;28:383-6.
2. Schwartz O, Jumpel RS. Congenital blepharophimosis associated with a unique generalized myopathy. Arch Ophthalmol. 1962;68:52-7.

921. McFARLAND SYNDROME

General

Autosomal recessive; duplication of chromosome 16q22 has been proposed; prominent amniotic fluid leakage.

Ocular

Hypertelorism; dystropic canthi.

Clinical

Flat-appearing face; prominent forehead and frontal bossing; dislocation of joints (elbows, knees, hips most commonly); malformation of feet; short metacarpals; heart defects (usually ventricular septum); harelip; cleft palate; micrognathia.

Laboratory

Diagnosis is made by clinical findings.

Treatment

None/Ocular.

Bibliography

1. Geeraets WJ. Ocular Syndromes, 3rd edition. Philadelphia: Lea & Febiger; 1976.
2. Houlston RS, Renshaw RM, James RS, et al. Duplication of 16q22 qter confirmed by fluorescence in situ hybridization and molecular analysis. J Med Genet. 1994;31:884-7.
3. McFarland BL. Congenital dislocation of knee. J Bone Joint Surg. 1929;11:281-5.
4. Provenzano RW. Congenital dislocation of the knee: report of a case. N Engl J Med. 1947;236: 360-2.
5. Vedantam R, Douglas DL. Congenital dislocation of the knee as a consequence of persistent amniotic fluid leakage. Br J Clin Pract. 1994;48:342-3.

922. McKUSICK-WEIBLAECHER SYNDROME

General

Cataract; leg absence deformity; rare; two cases reported in Amish females whose parents share same ancestors; autosomal recessive.

Ocular

Congenital cataract; partial paralysis of oculomotor III nerve.

Clinical

Absence or deformity of leg; progressive scoliosis; partial duplication of foot; imperforate anus.

Laboratory

Congenital cataracts: Dilated examination, TORCH titers and venereal disease reaserch laboratory test.

Treatment

Congenital cataracts: Cataract surgery is the treatment of choice.

Bibliography

1. Magalini SI, Scrascia E. Dictionary of Medical Syndromes, 2nd edition. Philadelphia: JB Lippincott; 1981.
2. McKusick VA, Weiblaecher RG. Recessive inheritance of congenital malformation syndrome. JAMA. 1968;204:111-6.

923. MEASLES (MORBILLI; RUBEOLA)

General

Acute, extremely communicable disease that affects young school-aged children; caused by paramyxovirus.

Ocular

Hypopyon; uveitis; conjunctivitis; Koplik (Hirschberg) spots of conjunctiva; keratitis; corneal ulcer; cellulitis of lid; dacryocystitis; congenital cataract; optic atrophy; optic neuritis; strabismus; pigmentary retinopathy; iris prolapse; hemianopsia; secondary glaucoma; central retinal artery occlusion; orbital cellulitis; accommodative spasm; paralysis of sixth nerve; keratoconus.

Clinical

Maculopapular rash; fever.

Laboratory

Diagnosis is made by clinical findings.

Treatment

Good hydration.

Additional Resource

1. Chen SSP (2011). Measles. [online] Available from http://www.emedicine.com/derm/TOPIC259.HTM [Accessed April, 2012].

924. MEB DISEASE (MUSCLE-EYE-BRAIN DISEASE)

General

Autosomal recessive; possibly the same as Walker-Warburg syndrome.

Ocular

Severe congenital myopia; congenital glaucoma; pallor of optic disk; retinal hypoplasia.

Clinical

Congenital muscular dystrophy; mental retardation; hydrocephalus; myoclonic jerks; high serum creatine phosphokinase.

Laboratory

Congenital cataracts: Dilated examination, TORCH titers and venereal disease reaserch laboratory test.

Treatment

Congenital cataracts: Cataract surgery is the treatment of choice.

Bibliography

1. McKusick VA. Mendelian Inheritance in Man: A Catalog of Human Genes and Genetic Disorders, 12th edition. Baltimore: The Johns Hopkins University Press; 1998.
2. Santavuori P, Pihko H, Sainio K, et.al. Muscle-eye brain disease and Walker-Warburg syndrome. Am J Med Genet. 1990;36:371-4.

925. MECKEL SYNDROME (DYSENCEPHALIA SPLANCHNOCYSTIC SYNDROME; GRUBER SYNDROME)

General

Autosomal recessive; ocular manifestations are similar to those of trisomy 13–15 syndrome.

Ocular

Cryptophthalmos; clinical anophthalmos; microphthalmos; mongoloid slant of lid fissures; sclerocornea; microcornea; partial aniridia; cataract; retinal dysplasia; posterior staphyloma; optic nerve hypoplasia.

Clinical

Sloping forehead; posterior encephalocele; short neck; polydactyly and syndactyly (hands and feet); polycystic kidneys; cryptorchidism; cleft lip and palate; central nervous system abnormalities, including the Dandy-Walker malformation.

Laboratory

Chromosome analysis and MRI.

Treatment

Cardiac surgery may be warranted.

Additional Resource

1. Jayakar PB (2011). Meckel-Gruber Syndrome. [online] Available from http://www.emedicine. com/ped/TOPIC1390.HTM [Accessed April, 2012].

926. MEDULLOEPITHELIOMA (DIKTYOMA)

General

Rare embryonic ocular tumor which usually arises from the primitive nonpigmented medullary epithelium of the ciliary body and less commonly affects the optic nerve, iris and retina.

Clinical

None

Ocular

Decreased vision, leukocoria, rubeosis iridis, ectopia lentis, heterochromia, exophthalmos and hyphema.

Laboratory

Indirect ophthalmoscopy, slit lamp examination and echography aid in diagnosis. CT and MRI may also be helpful. Diagnosis is confirmed on histological examination.

Treatment

Iridocyclectomy is useful for small tumors in the ciliary body. Enucleation is recommended for large tumors.

Bibliography

1. Roy FH, Fraunfelder FW, Fraunfelder FT. Roy and Fraunfelder's Current Ocular Therapy, 6th edition. Philadelphia: WB Saunders; 2008.

927. MEGALOCORNEA

General

Nonprogressive enlargement of the cornea to 13 mm or greater; etiology unknown; X-linked recessive trait.

Ocular

Enlarged ciliary ring; stretching of zonules; phacodonesis; ectopia lentis; iridodonesis; pigment of the trabecular meshwork; glaucoma; cataract; iris hypoplasia and transillumination.

Laboratory

Corneal measurement; gonioscopy; A-scan ultrasound biometry and specular microscopy.

Treatment

Correction of refractive error. Surgery may be necessary for cataract and glaucoma if present.

Additional Resource

1. Oetting TA (2010). Megalocornea. [online] Available from http://www.emedicine.medscape.com/article/1196299-overview [Accessed April, 2012].

928. MELAS SYNDROME

General

Changing of threonine at amino acid 109 to an alanine; A3245G mitochondrial DNA point mutation cataracts; RPE abnormalities with age-related maculopathy.

Ocular

Ophthalmoplegia, blindness, optic atrophy, pigmentary retinopathy.

Clinical

Migraines; sensorineural hearing loss; grand mal seizures; stroke-like episodes; lactic acidosis; ragged-red muscle fibers.

Laboratory

Serum lactic acid, serum pyruvic acid, cerebrospinal fluid lactic acid and CSF pyruvic acid.

Treatment

No treatment available.

Additional Resource

1. Scaglia F (2010). MELAS Syndrome. [online] Available from http://www.emedicine.com/ped/TOPIC1406.HTM [Accessed April, 2012].

929. MELKERSSON-ROSENTHAL SYNDROME (MELKERSSON IDIOPATHIC FIBROEDEMA; MIESCHER CHEILITIS GRANULOMATOSIS)

General

Occurrence in childhood or youth; possible etiologies include viral infection, tuberculosis, sarcoidosis and allergic reactions (all affecting parasympathetic cells in geniculate ganglia); facial palsy resembles Bell palsy; possible localization of this disorder to the gene at 9p11 has been reported.

Ocular

Lagophthalmos; lid edema; lacrimation secondary to the "crocodile tear" phenomenon from aberrant seventh nerve regeneration; exposure keratitis and corneal ulcers; corneal opacities.

Clinical

Chronic edema of face and lips; peripheral facial palsy (may be bilateral), which may precede edema by weeks to years; furrowed tongue; granulomatous cheilitis and glossitis; lingua plicata.

Laboratory

Lip biopsy or facial tissues.

Treatment

Daily compressions may provide improvement.

Additional Resource

1. Scully C (2011). Cheilitis Granulomatosa (Miescher-Melkersson-Rosenthal Syndrome). [online] Available from http://www.emedicine.com/derm/TOPIC72.HTM [Accessed April, 2012].

930. MELNICK-NEEDLES SYNDROME (OSTEODYSPLASTY)

General

Bone dysplasia; fewer than 30 cases reported; familial congenital autosomal trait; affect both sexes; onset at birth.

Ocular

Exophthalmos; hypertelorism; bilateral sclerocornea; mild cornea plana; strabismus.

Clinical

Misaligned teeth; micrognathia; multiple symmetric bone deformities; large ears; broad nose; frontal bossing; rosy cheeks; short stature; recurrent respiratory and ear infections; pneumosinus dilatans; abnormalities of the distal phalanges.

Laboratory/Exophthalmos

Thyroid function studies, imaging studies.

Treatment/Exophthalmos

Ocular lubricants.

Bibliography

1. Melnick JC, Needles CF. An undiagnosed bone dysplasia. A 2 family study of 4 generations and 3 generations. Am J Roentgenol Radium Ther Nucl Med. 1966;97:39-48.

2. Memis A, Ustun EE, Sener RN. Case report 717. Osteodysplasty (Melnick-Needles syndrome). Skeletal Radiol. 1992;21:132-4.
3. Perry LD, Edwards WC, Bramson RT. Melnick-Needles syndrome. J Pediatr Ophthalmol Strabismus. 1978;15:226-30.
4. Stretch JR, Poole MD. Pneumosinus dilatans as the etiology of progressive bilateral blindness. Br J Plast Surg. 1992;45:469-73.

Additional Resource

1. Mercandetti M (2010). Exophthalmos. [online] Available from http://www.emedicine.com/oph/TOPIC616.HTM [Accessed April, 2012].

---

931. MÉNIÈRE SYNDROME

General

Etiology unknown; more common in males between the ages of 40 and 60 years.

Ocular

Nystagmus (rapid component toward the normal side), mainly during attacks; diplopia possible during and after attacks.

Clinical

Paroxysmal attacks of vertigo; tinnitus; gradually progressing deafness, although not prerequisite for diagnosis; during attacks, pallor, nausea, vomiting and fainting; allergy; giant cell arteritis; facial paralysis.

Laboratory

No specific laboratory test is available.

Treatment

Intravenous hydration, antihistamines.

Additional Resource

1. Li JC (2011). Meniere Disease (Idiopathic Endolymphatic Hydrops). [online] Available from http://www.emedicine.com/emerg/TOPIC308.HTM [Accessed April, 2012].

---

932. MENINGIOMA

General

Benign, slow-growing tumors that arise from the arachnoid matter, the middle layer of meninges that lies inside the dura mater and outside the pia mater; more common in females; peak incidence in the seventh decade of life.

Ocular

Exposure keratopathy; paralysis of extraocular muscles; proptosis; optic nerve atrophy; papilledema; choroidal folds; hyperopia; visual field defect; afferent pupil defect; optociliary shunt veins.

Clinical

Headache; intracranial pressure; vomiting.

Laboratory

Computed tomography (CT) or MRI will denote a well-circumscribed mass, extra-axial and adherent to dura. Due to location may compress brain, spinal cord or optic nerve.

Treatment

Total microsurgical intervention usually can be curative. Radiation therapy after surgery.

Additional Resource

1. Zachariah SB (2010). Meningioma, Sphenoid Wing. [online] Available from http://www.emedicine.com/oph/TOPIC670.HTM [Accessed April, 2012].

---

933. MENINGIOMA, OPTIC NERVE SHEATH

General

Primary arise from the cap cells of the arachnoid surrounding the intraorbital or, less frequently, the intracanalicular optic nerve. Secondary are extensions of intracranial meningioma into the orbit. Secondary are much more common than primary, but the unqualified term "optic nerve sheath meningioma" ordinarily refers to primary. May be caused by radiation; head trauma, hormonal factors and infectious agents.

Clinical

Headache; head trauma.

Ocular

Compressive optic neuropathy; transient visual obscurations; visual loss; proptosis; exophthalmos; ptosis; diplopia.

Laboratory

Computed tomography (CT) and MRI are the best imaging techniques.

Treatment

Radiotherapy following surgical removal. Chemotherapy is reserved for unresectable or recurrent meningiomas.

Additional Resource

1. Gossman MV (2010). Meningioma, Optic Nerve Sheath. [online] Available from http://www.emedicine.medscape.com/article/1217466-overview [Accessed April, 2012].

---

934. MENINGIOMA, SPHENOID WING

General

Arise from arachnoid cap cells which are attached to the dura at any location where meninges exist; may be associated with hyperostosis of the sphenoid ridge and be very invasive; may expand into the wall of the cavernous sinus and anteriorly into the orbit.

Clinical

Diffuse tumor infiltration; transient ischemic-attack; anosmia; mental changes; increased intracranial pressure.

Ocular

Unilateral exophthalmos; proptosis; oculomotor palsy; painful ophthalmoplegia; blindness; papilledema.

Laboratory

Endocrine testing; CT and MRI allow definitive diagnosis.

Treatment

Tumor resection without injury to the optic nerve if the bone has not been invaded; if resection is not complete radiation therapy will be necessary; antihormonal agents maybe useful in atypical and malignant meningiomas as an adjunct to surgery.

Additional Resource

1. Zachariah SB (2010). Meningioma, Sphenoid Wing. [online] Available from http://www. emedicine.medscape.com/article/1215752-overview [Accessed April, 2012].

935. MENINGOCOCCEMIA (MENINGITIS; NEISSERIA MENINGITIDIS)

General

Systemic bacterial infection caused by *Neisseria meningitidis*; can be present chronically in patients with immune deficiencies including deficient complement levels.

Ocular

Photophobia; conjunctivitis; chemosis; keratitis; uveitis; panophthalmitis; retinal endophlebitis; macular edema; papillitis; optic neuritis; paresis of sixth or seventh nerve; nystagmus; miosis; hippus; cortical blindness; papilledema (rare); conjunctival petechiae; strabismus.

Clinical

Meningitis; fever; malaise; joint pain; splenic enlargement.

Laboratory

Cultures from blood, spinal fluid or joint fluid.

Treatment

Treat with antibiotics promptly.

Additional Resource

1. Javid MH (2011). Meningococcemia. [online] Available from http://www.emedicine.com/med/TOPIC1445.HTM [Accessed April, 2012].

936. MENKES (2) SYNDROME (KINKY HAIR SYNDROME)

General

Etiology unknown; sex-linked recessive neurodegenerative disorder; focal cerebral and cerebellar degenerative changes involving the white and gray matter; affects only males; onset in early infancy.

Ocular

Decreasing visual function with progression of the disease.

Clinical

Spasticity; refractory motor seizures; retarded growth; dementia; abnormal pigmentation of hair with kinky, wiry texture; lack of facial expression; thick and dry skin; transient jaundice.

Laboratory

Copper levels, radiography, angiography.

Treatment

Treatment is mostly supportive.

Additional Resource

1. Imaeda S (2012). Dermatologic Manifestations of Menkes Kinky Hair Disease. [online] Available from http://www.emedicine.com/derm/TOPIC715.HTM [Accessed April, 2012].

937. MERCURY POISONING (MINAMATA SYNDROME)

General

Both sexes affected; onset several weeks or months after ingestion of fish from contaminated water or animals fed with contaminated grain; symptoms may be mild to severe.

Ocular

Constriction of visual fields; blindness.

Clinical

Paresthesia of mouth, tongue and extremity; hearing loss; asthenia; fatigue; inability to concentrate; dysarthria; tremors; persistent vegetative state; peripheral neuropathy; cerebella ataxia; gait disturbance; sensory impairment; anosmia; loss of taste; bladder disturbance; mental deterioration.

Laboratory

Mercury levels, CBC and serum chemistries, urine mercury levels.

Treatment

Oxygen, hemodialysis only on severe cases, chelating agents.

Additional Resource

1. Olson DA (2011). Mercury Toxicity. [online] Available from http://www.emedicine.com/emerg/TOPIC813.HTM [Accessed April, 2012].

938. MERETOJA SYNDROME (FINNISH TYPE, FAP IV)

General

Lattice corneal dystrophy type II with familial amyloid polyneuropathy type IV; also called primary hereditary systemic amyloidosis.

Ocular

Lattice corneal dystrophy; cranial nerve palsies.

Clinical

Multiple neurologic symptoms such as severe itching, various nerve palsies and diminished vibratory sensation; patients are said to develop a so-called bloodhound-like appearance due to skin and facial nerve degeneration.

Laboratory

Genetic analysis, corneal biopsy.

Treatment

Bandage contact lens or antibiotic ointment then patching the eye. If recurrent corneal erosion, treatment with excimer laser is an option.

Bibliography

1. Asaoka T, Amano S, Sunada Y, et al. Lattice corneal dystrophy type II with familial amyloid polyneuropathy type IV. Jpn J Ophthalmol. 1993; 37:426-31.
2. Purcell JJ, Rodrigues M, Chishti MI, et al. Lattice corneal dystrophy associated with familial systemic amyloidosis (Meretoja's syndrome). Ophthalmology. 1983;90:1512-7.
3. Rintala AE, Alanko A, Mäkinen J, et al. Primary hereditary systemic amyloidosis (Meretoja's syndrome): clinical features and treatment by plastic surgery. Scand J Plast Reconstr Surg Hand Surg. 1988;22:141-5.

939. MERRF SYNDROME

General

Associated with mitochondrial tRNA [Leu(UUR)] A3243G mutation.

Ocular

Optic neuropathy; pigmentary retinopathy, ophthalmoparesis; ptosis.

Clinical

Mitochondrial encephalomyopathy; lactic acidosis; strokelike episodes.

Laboratory/Ocular

Erythrocyte sedimentation rate, C-reactive protein.

Treatment/Ocular

Prednisone

Bibliography

1. Hwang JM, Park HW, Kim SJ. Optic neuropathy associated with mitochondrial tRNA[Leu(UUR)] A3243G mutation. Ophthalmic Genet. 1997;18: 101-5.

940. MESHERS MACRORETICULAR DYSTROPHY OF RETINAL PIGMENT EPITHELIUM (BUTTERFLY-SHAPED DYSTROPHY OF RETINAL PIGMENT EPITHELIUM)

General

Autosomal recessive; autosomal dominant inheritance has been reported.

Ocular

Butterfly-shaped dystrophies of retinal pigment epithelium; macular degeneration associated with fundus flavimaculatus; drusen of Bruch membrane; choroidal folds; bull's eye degeneration of macula; detachment of pigment epithelium.

Clinical

None

Laboratory

Diagnosis is made by clinical findings.

Treatment

Referral to a retinal specialist.

Bibliography

1. Bastiaensen LA, Hoefnagels KL. Patterned anomalies of the retinal pigment epithelium: dystrophy or syndrome? Doc Ophthalmol. 1983;55:17-29.
2. Girard P, Setbon G, Forest A, et al. Macroreticular and butterfly shaped dystrophies of the retinal pigment epithelium. J Fr Ophthalmol. 1980;3:101-8.
3. McKusick VA. Mendelian Inheritance in Man: A Catalog of Human Genes and Genetic Disorders, 12th edition. Baltimore: The Johns Hopkins University Press; 1998.
4. McKusick-Nathans Institute for Genetic Medicine, Johns Hopkins University and National Center for Biotechnology Information, National Library of Medicine. (2007). Online Mendelian Inheritance in Man (OMIM). [online] Available from http://www.ncbi.nlm.nih.gov/omim [Accessed April, 2012].
5. Nichols BE, Sheffield VC, Vandenburgh K, et al. Butterfly-shaped pigment dystrophy of the fovea caused by a point mutation in codon 167 of the RDS gene. Nat Genet. 1993;3:202-7.

941. MESODERMAL DYSGENESIS (ANTERIOR CHAMBER DYSGENESIS; ANTERIOR SEGMENT OCULAR DYSGENESIS SYNDROME; DYSEMBRYOGENESIS)

General

Mesodermal abnormalities, including oculocutaneous albinism; autosomal dominant.

Ocular

Capsular cataracts; external ophthalmoplegia; anterior chamber cleavage syndrome; atrophy of iris; ectropion; flat cornea; coloboma of iris and choroid; posterior embryotoxon; Axenfeld anomaly; Rieger anomaly; Peters anomaly; keratoconus; microphthalmos.

Clinical

None

Laboratory/Ocular

Diagnosis is made by clinical findings.

Treatment/Ocular

Cataract surgery, filtration surgery to control IOP, genetic counseling, keratoplasty.

Bibliography

1. Ferrell RE, Hittner HM, Kretzer FL, et al. Anterior segment mesenchymal dysgenesis: probable linkage to the MNS blood group on chromosome 4. Am J Hum Genet. 1982;34:245-9.
2. Ghose S, Singh NP, Kaur D, et al. Microphthalmos and anterior segment dysgenesis in a family. Ophthalmic Paediatr Genet. 1991;12:177-82.
3. Lubin JR. Oculocutaneous albinism associated with corneal mesodermal dysgenesis. Am J Ophthalmol. 1981;91:347-50.
4. Ricci B, Lacerra F. Oculocutaneous albinism and corneal mesodermal dysgenesis. Am J Ophthalmol. 1981;92:587.

942. METAPHYSEAL CHONDRODYSPLASIA WITH RETINITIS PIGMENTOSA

General

Autosomal recessive.

Ocular

Retinitis pigmentosa.

Clinical

Defective cartilage and growth of long bones, particularly the metacarpals and phalanges.

Laboratory/Ocular

Diagnosis is made by clinical findings.

Treatment/Ocular

Low vision clinic, vitamin A/beta-carotene.

Additional Resource

1. Telander DG (2012). Retinitis Pigmentosa. [online] Available from http://www.emedicine.com/oph/TOPIC704.HTM [Accessed April, 2012].

943. METASTATIC BACTERIAL ENDOPHTHALMITIS

General

Causative agent usually of low pathogenicity (e.g. *Staphylococcus albus*, *Staphylococcus epidermidis*); occasionally organisms of greater pathogenicity (e.g. *Pseudomonas aeruginosa*, *Diplococcus pneumoniae*); bilateral 45%; organisms originate in body or are introduced by drug addicts using nonsterile needles.

Ocular

Conjunctival hemorrhages; conjunctivitis; Roth spots; retinal arterial occlusion; uveitis; hypopyon; chorioretinitis; endophthalmitis; retinal hemorrhages.

Clinical

Manifestations are nonspecific.

Laboratory

Blood, sputum and urine cultures.

Treatment

Aggressive treatment with intravitreal and topical antibiotics, steroids and cycloplegics.

Additional Resource

1. Graham RH (2012). Bacterial Endophthalmitis. [online] Available from http://www.emedicine. com/oph/TOPIC393.HTM [Accessed April, 2012].

944. METASTATIC FUNGAL ENDOPHTHALMITIS

General

Usually occurs in immunosuppressed or immunocompromised patients; usually asymmetrical; *Candida albicans* frequent etiologic agent.

Ocular

Anterior uveitis; vitreitis; focal retinitis; Roth spots; chorioretinitis; Fusarium solani also has been isolated from immunocompromised patients with endogenous endophthalmitis.

Clinical

May be evidence of other monocular foci of metastatic fungal disease.

Laboratory

Blood, sputum and urine cultures. Examination of fungi with Gemsa, Gomori-methenamine-silver (GMS), and periodic-acid Schiff (PAS) stains should be done.

Treatment

Amphotericin B, fluconazole, ketoconazole, miconazole, flucytosine and itraconazole. Amphotericin is the treatment of choice. Vitrectomy may be needed.

Additional Resource

1. Wu L (2010). Endophthalmitis, Fungal. [online] Available from http://www.emedicine.com/oph/ TOPIC706.HTM [Accessed April, 2012].

945. METHEMOGLOBINEMIA

General

Deficiency of enzyme; inherited or acquired, with acquired most common; caused by contact with drugs and chemicals; disorder disappears when offending chemical is eliminated.

Ocular

Pigmentation of conjunctiva and retina.

Clinical

Cyanosis; mental retardation; central nervous system involvement.

Laboratory

Multiple wavelength co-oximeter, head CT scan.

Treatment

Supplemental oxygen, removal of oxidizing agent.

Additional Resource

1. Lee DC (2011). Methemoglobinemia in Emergency Medicine. [online] Available from http://www.emedicine.com/emerg/TOPIC313.HTM [Accessed April, 2012].

946. MEYER-SCHWICKERATH-WEYERS SYNDROME (MICROPHTHALMOS SYNDROME; OCULODENTODIGITAL DYSPLASIA)

General

Etiology unknown; two types recognized: (1) dysplasia oculodentodigitalis and (2) dyscraniopygophalangie; type I is characterized by microphthalmia with possible iris pathology and glaucoma, oligodontia and brown pigmentation of teeth, camptodactyly, and possible absence of middle phalanx of second to fifth toes; type II consists of severe microphthalmos to anophthalmos, polydactyly, and developmental anomalies of nose and oral cavity; both sexes affected; present from birth; abnormal cerebral white matter.

Ocular

Microphthalmos; hypotrichosis; glaucoma; iris anomalies (eccentric pupil; changes in normal iris texture; remnants of pupillary membrane along iris margins); microcornea; hypertelorism; myopia; hyperopia; keratoconus.

Clinical

Thin, small nose with anteverted nostrils and hypoplastic alae; syndactyly; camptodactyly (fourth and fifth fingers); anomalies of middle phalanx of fifth finger and toe; hypoplastic teeth; wide mandible; alveolar ridge; sparse hair growth; visceral malformations.

Laboratory

Diagnosis is made by clinical findings.

Treatment

Glaucoma: Its medication should be the first plan of action. If medication is unsuccessful, a filtering surgical procedure with or without antimetabolites may be beneficial.

Keratoconus: Spectacle correction, hard contacts and avoid eye rubbing may be useful. If hydrops occurs discontinue contact lens, use NaCl drops and ointment, patching and short course of steroids. As the disease advances penetrating keratoplasty, deep anterior lamellar keratoplasty, intacs with laser grooves or collagen stabilization of cornea.

Bibliography

1. Geeraets WJ. Ocular Syndromes, 3rd edition. Philadelphia: Lea & Febiger; 1976.

2. Gutmann DH, Zackai EH, McDonald-McGinn DM, et al. Oculodentodigital dysplasia syndrome associated with abnormal cerebral white matter. Am J Med Genet. 1991;41:18-20.
3. McKusick VA. Mendelian Inheritance in Man: A Catalog of Human Genes and Genetic Disorders, 12th edition. Baltimore: The Johns Hopkins University Press; 1998.

947. MICHEL SYNDROME

General

Autosomal dominant, characterized by agenesis of the inner ear.

Clinical

Profound but not total congenital deafness.

Ocular

Telecanthus

Laboratory

Diagnosis is made by clinical findings.

Treatment

Ocular/None.

Bibliography

1. Ghazli K, Merite-Drancy A, Marsot-Dupuch K, et al. A report of two familial cases of Michel syndrome (bilateral agenesis of the inner ear). Ann Otolaryngol Chir Cervicofac. 1998;115:29-34.

948. MICRO SYNDROME

General

Autosomal recessive microcephaly and microcornea; Muslim Pakistani inheritance; present at birth; consanguinity; autosomal recessive.

Ocular

Microcornea; congenital cataract; retinal dystrophy; optic nerve atrophy; ptosis; microphakia; microphthalmos; nuclear cataract; atonic pupils.

Clinical

Severe mental retardation; hypothalamic hypogenitalism; hypoplasia of the corpus callosum; short stature; cortical visual impairment; microcephaly; developmental delay.

Laboratory

Congenital cataracts: Dilated examination, TORCH titers and venereal disease reaserch laboratory test.

Treatment

Congenital cataracts: Cataract surgery is the treatment of choice.

Bibliography

1. Ainsworth JR, Morton JE, Good P, et al. Micro syndrome in Muslim Pakistan children. Ophthalmology. 2001;108:491-7.
2. Megarbane A, Choueiri R, Bleik J, et al. Microcephaly, microphthalmia, congenital cataract, optic atrophy, short stature, hypotonia, severe psychomotor retardation, and cerebral malformations: a second family with micro syndrome or a new syndrome? J Med Genet. 1999;36:637-40.
3. Rodriguez Criado G, Rufo M, Gomez de Terreros I. A second family with micro syndrome. Clin Dysmorphol. 1999;8:241-5.
4. Warburg M, Sjö O, Fledelius HC, et al. Autosomal recessive microcephaly, microcornea, congenital cataract, mental retardation, optic atrophy, and hypogenitalism. Micro syndrome. Am J Dis Child. 1993;147:1309-12.

949. MICROCEPHALY, MICROPHTHALMIA, CATARACTS, AND JOINT CONTRACTURES

General

Autosomal dominant; ocular features like Hagberg-Santavuori syndrome.

Ocular

Microphthalmia; cataracts; hypopigmented retinal degeneration.

Clinical

Microcephaly; shortening or wasting of muscle fibers, causing excess scar tissue over joints.

Laboratory

Diagnosis is made by clinical findings.

Treatment

Cataract: Change in glasses can sometimes improve a patient's visual function temporarily; however, the most common treatment is cataract surgery.

Bibliography

1. Bateman JB, Philippart M. Ocular features of the Hagberg-Santavuori syndrome. Am J Ophthalmol. 1986;102:262-71.
2. McKusick VA. Mendelian Inheritance in Man: A Catalog of Human Genes and Genetic Disorders, 12th edition. Baltimore: The Johns Hopkins University Press; 1998.

950. MICROCEPHALY WITH CHORIORETINOPATHY

General

Autosomal dominant; congenital infection; exposure to irradiation, chemical agents, mother's infection or injury.

Ocular

Chorioretinopathy usually inactive.

Clinical

Microcephaly; slow growth of brain; mild mental retardation.

Laboratory

None

Treatment

Laser photocoagulation, photodynamic therapy.

Additional Resource

1. Oh KT (2011). Central Serous Chorioretinopathy. [online] Available from http://www.emedicine. com/oph/TOPIC689.HTM [Accessed April, 2012].

951. MICROCORNEA, POSTERIOR MEGALOLENTICONUS, PERSISTENT FETAL VASCULATURE AND COLOBOMA

General

All patients found have microcornea with corneal diameters of less than 8 mm, lens found to be retrodisplaced with massive enlargement and a dramatic posterior lenticonus and ciliary processes frequently drawn to the lens capsule.

Clinical

Hydrocephus, craniosynostosis, absent anterior pituitary gland, tetralogy of Fallot, enlarged ventricles.

Ocular

Microcornea, persistent fetal vasculare, coloboma, posterior megalolenticonus, persistent vasculature, ciliary processes drawn to the lens capsule.

Laboratory

Clinical observation, examination under anesthesia, fluorescein angiography.

Treatment

Surgical intervention may be necessary if visual potential is revealed.

Bibliography

1. Ranchod TM, Quiram PA, Hathaway N, et al. Microcornea, posterior megalolenticonus, persistent fetal vasculature, and coloboma: a new syndrome. Ophthalmology. 2010;117:1843-7.

952. MICROPHTHALMIA AND MENTAL DEFICIENCY

General

Autosomal recessive.

Ocular

Microphthalmia; corneal opacities.

Clinical

Severe mental retardation; spastic cerebral palsy; glycinuria; abnormally small head.

Laboratory/Ocular

Computed tomography (CT) scan or MRI of head and orbits, ultrasound imaging.

Treatment/Ocular

Enlarge orbital cavity, slowly increase the size of conformers, inflatable expander, self-expanding hydrophilic, osmotic expander.

Bibliography

1. Balci S, Say B, Firat T. Corneal opacity, microphthalmos, mental retardation, microcephaly and generalized muscular spasticity associated with hyperglycinemia. Clin Genet. 1974;5:36-9.

953. MICROPHTHALMOS, MYOPIA AND CORECTOPIA

General

Autosomal dominant; characterized by microphthalmos, myopia and corectopia.

Ocular

Microphthalmos; myopia; corectopia; glaucoma; cataract; hypoplastic macula; spherophakia; microphakia.

Clinical

None

Laboratory

Congenital cataracts: Dilated examination, TORCH titers and venereal disease reaserch laboratory test.

Treatment

Congenital cataracts: Cataract surgery is the treatment of choice.

Bibliography

1. McKusick VA. Mendelian Inheritance in Man: A Catalog of Human Genes and Genetic Disorders, 12th edition. Baltimore: The Johns Hopkins University Press; 1998.
2. McKusick-Nathans Institute for Genetic Medicine, Johns Hopkins University and National Center for Biotechnology Information, National Library of Medicine. (2007). Online Mendelian Inheritance in Man (OMIM). [online] Available from http://www.ncbi.nlm.nih.gov/omim/ [Accessed April, 2012].
3. Scheie HG, Albert DM. Textbook of Ophthalmology, 10th edition. Philadelphia: WB Saunders; 1986.

954. MICROPHTHALMOS, PIGMENTARY RETINOPATHY, GLAUCOMA

General

Autosomal dominant; Three disorders combined of microphthalmos, pigmentary retinopathy, glaucoma.

Ocular

Microphthalmos; pigmentary retinopathy; glaucoma.

Clinical

None

Laboratory/Glaucoma

Chromosome analysis and genetic counseling.

Treatment/Glaucoma

Beta-blokers, carbonic anhydrase inhibitors and prostaglandin analogs. Surgery may be needed if IOP is uncontrolled.

Bibliography

1. Hermann P. Syndrome: microphthalmic-retinite pigmentaire-glaucoma. Arch Ophthalmol Rev Gen Ophtalmol. 1958;18:17-24.
2. McKusick VA. Mendelian Inheritance in Man: A Catalog of Human Genes and Genetic Disorders, 12th edition. Baltimore: The Johns Hopkins University Press; 1998.
3. McKusick-Nathans Institute for Genetic Medicine, Johns Hopkins University and National Center for Biotechnology Information, National Library of Medicine (2007). Online Mendelian Inheritance in Man (OMIM). [online] Available from http://www.ncbi.nlm.nih.gov/omim/ [Accessed April, 2012].

955. MICROPSIA SYNDROME (LILLIPUTIAN SYNDROME)

General

Psychosensory illusion produced by various mental derangements such as acute infections, alcoholism, toxic delirium, dementia or trauma.

Ocular

Illusions, with misjudging of distance, position and size of known objects (regarded as a psychovisual phenomenon).

Clinical

Fixed hallucinations or dreams are expressions of illusions and are misinterpreted by the patient.

Laboratory

Diagnosis is made by clinical findings.

Treatment

Identify cause.

Bibliography

1. Bender MB, Savitzky N. Micropsia and teleopsia limited to the temporal fields of vision. Arch Ophthalmol. 1943;29:904-8.
2. Savitzky N, Tarachow S. Lilliputian hallucinations during convalescence from scarlet fever in a child. J Nerv Ment Dis. 1941;93:310-2.

956. MICROSPHEROPHAKIA

General

Small and spheric lens, larger in the anteroposterior diameter, and the equatorial diameter is smaller than normal.

Clinical

Weill-Marchesani syndrome.

Ocular

Secondary glaucoma, peripheral anterior synechiae, myopia, lens dislocation.

Laboratory

Diagnosis is made by clinical findings.

Treatment

Glaucoma control is of primary concern, mydriatics to control pupillary block, laser iridectomy.

Bibliography

1. Roy FH, Fraunfelder FW, Fraunfelder FT. Roy and Fraunfelder's Current Ocular Therapy, 6th edition. Philadelphia: WB Saunders; 2008.

957. MICROSPHEROPHAKIA WITH HERNIA

General

Autosomal dominant.

Ocular

Microspherophakia; glaucoma.

Clinical

Inguinal hernia.

Laboratory/Glaucoma

Chromosome analysis and genetic counseling.

Treatment/Glaucoma

Beta-blokers, carbonic anhydrase inhibitors and prostaglandin analogs. Surgery may be needed if IOP is uncontrolled.

Bibliography

1. Johnson VP, Grayson M, Christian JC. Dominant microspherophakia. Arch Ophthalmol. 1971;85: 534-7.

2. McKusick VA. Mendelian Inheritance in Man: A Catalog of Human Genes and Genetic Disorders, 12th edition. Baltimore: The Johns Hopkins University Press; 1998.

3. McKusick-Nathans Institute for Genetic Medicine, Johns Hopkins University and National Center for Biotechnology Information, National Library of Medicine (2007). Online Mendelian Inheritance in Man (OMIM). [online] Available from http://www.ncbi.nlm.nih.gov/omim/ [Accessed April, 2012].

---

958. MICROSPORIDIAL INFECTION

General

Obligate intracellular, spore-forming, mitochondrial-lacking eukaryotic protozoan parasites.

Clinical

None

Ocular

Photophobia, blepharospasm, nonspecific or papillary conjunctival hyperemia.

Laboratory

Gram stain smears show Gram-positive, void spores in the cytoplasm of epithelial cells.

Treatment

Topical fumagillin which can be prepared from fumagillin bicylohexylammonium salt (Fumadil B).

Bibliography

1. Roy FH, Fraunfelder FW, Fraunfelder FT. Roy and Fraunfelder's Current Ocular Therapy, 6th edition. Philadelphia: WB Saunders; 2008.

---

959. MIDAS SYNDROME (DERMAL APLASIA AND SCLEROCORNEA, MICROPHTHALMIA)

General

X-linked phenotype; male-lethal trait.

Ocular

Bilateral microphthalmia; sclerocornea; blepharophimosis.

Clinical

Dermal aplasia; microcephaly; cardiomyopathy; ventricular fibrillation; congenital heart defect.

Laboratory/Sclerocornea

No laboratory needed.

Treatment/Sclerocornea

Surgical care, penetrating keratoplasty (PK) is recommended.

Bibliography

1. Cape CJ, Zaidman GW, Beck AD, et al. Phenotypic variation in ophthalmic manifestations of MIDAS syndrome (microphthalmia, dermal aplasia, and sclerocornea). Arch Ophthalmol. 2004;122: 1070-4.
2. Happle R, Daniels O, Koopman RJ. MIDAS syndrome (microphthalmia, dermal aplasia, and sclerocornea): an X-linked phenotype distinct from Goltz syndrome. Am J Med Genet. 1993;47: 710-3.

---

960. MIETENS SYNDROME (MIETENS-WEBER SYNDROME)

General

Etiology unknown; unclassifiable familial condition.

Ocular

Bilateral corneal opacities; horizontal and rotational nystagmus; strabismus; bushy eyebrows; ptosis.

Clinical

Growth failure; flexion contracture of the elbows; dislocation of the head of the radii; mental retardation; small pointed nose with a depressed root; low hairline; external ear defects; digital defects; hypertrichosis.

Laboratory

Diagnosis is made by clinical findings.

Treatment

Corneal opacity: Check for elevated intraocular pressure. Medical treatment includes the use of hyperosmotic drops, nonsteroidal and steroid eye drops. Corneal transplant may be necessary.

Ptosis: If visual acuity is affected most cases require surgical correction, and there are several procedures that may be used including levator resection, repair or advancement and Fasanella-Servat.

Bibliography

1. Magalini SI, Scrascia E. Dictionary of Medical Syndromes, 2nd edition. Philadelphia: JB Lippincott; 1981. p. 548.
2. Mietens C, Weber H. A syndrome characterized by corneal opacity, nystagmus, flexion contracture of the elbows, growth failure, and mental retardation. J Pediatr. 1966;69:624-9.
3. Waring GO, Rodrigues MM. Ultrastructural and successful keratoplasty of sclerocornea in Mietens' syndrome. Am J Ophthalmol. 1980;90:469-75.

---

961. MIGRAINE (VASCULAR HEADACHE)

General

Recurrent attacks of pain in the head; usually unilateral; often familial.

Ocular

Abnormal visual sensations; scotoma generally restricted to one half of the visual field; complete blindness; unilateral transient visual loss; photopsia; branch retinal artery occlusions; anisocoria.

Clinical

Nausea; vomiting; anorexia; sensory, motor and mood disturbances; fluid imbalance; headache.

Laboratory

Investigation studies. Rule out comorbid disease, exclude other causes of headaches such as structural and/or metabolic. Neurological examination. Lumbar puncture (LP) followed by CT scan or MRI.

Treatment

Treatment is based on the severity of the case.

Additional Resource

1. Chawla J (2011). Migraine Headache. [online] Available from http://www.emedicine.com/neuro/TOPIC218.HTM [Accessed April, 2012].

962. MIKULICZ-RADECKI SYNDROME (DACRYOSIALOADENOPATHY; MIKULICZ SYNDROME; MIKULICZ-SJÖGREN SYNDROME)

General

Not an individual disease but a manifestation of tuberculosis, syphilis, leukemia, lymphosarcoma, sarcoidosis, Hodgkin disease, mumps, Waldenström macroglobulinemia or lymphoma; exhibits a chronic course with frequent recurrences; milder form of Sjögren syndrome (see Schaumann Syndrome).

Ocular

Bilateral painless enlargement of lacrimal glands with bulging of upper lid; decreased or absent lacrimation; conjunctivitis; uveitis; optic atrophy; optic neuritis; phlyctenules; keratoconjunctivitis; dacryoadenitis; retinal candlewax spots; periphlebitis.

Clinical

Symmetrical, perhaps marked, enlargement of salivary glands; dryness of mouth and pharynx; hoarseness; neurologic complications.

Laboratory

Diagnosis is made by clinical findings.

Treatment

Identify cause.

Bibliography

1. Meyer D, Yanoff M, Hanno H. Differential diagnosis in Mikulicz's syndrome, Mikulicz's disease, and similar disease entities. Am J Ophthalmol. 1971; 71:516-24.

963. MILLARD-GUBLER SYNDROME (ABDUCENS-FACIAL HEMIPLEGIA ALTERNANS)

General

Vascular, infectious or tumorous lesion at the base of the pons affecting the nuclei of the sixth and seventh nerves and fibers of the pyramidal tract; demyelinating disease.

Ocular

Diplopia; esotropia; paralysis external rectus muscle (often bilateral); in unilateral cases, there is deviation of eyes to side opposite lesion and inability to move them toward side of lesion;

abduction of eye prevented by destruction of sixth nerve nucleus; opposite eye cannot be voluntarily adducted but can converge and move in this position by rotatory and caloric stimulation.

Clinical

Ipsilateral facial paralysis; contralateral hemiplegia of arm and leg from involvement of pyramidal tract.

Laboratory/Diplopia

None

Treatment/Diplopia

Occluding one eye, Fresnel prism, anticholinergic agent and corticosteroids may be needed in the treatment of myasthenia gravis.

Bibliography

1. Geeraets WJ. Ocular Syndromes, 3rd edition. Philadelphia: Lea & Febiger; 1976.
2. Gubler A. De l'Hemiplegie Alterne Envisagee Comme Signe de Lesion de la Protuberance Annulaire et Comme Preuve de la Decussation des Nerfs Faciaux. Gaz Hebd Med Chir. 1856;3:749, 789, 811.
3. Minderhoud JM. Diagnostic significance of symptomatology in brain stem ischaemic infarction. Eur Neurol. 1971;5:343-53.
4. Newman NJ. Third, fourth and sixth nerve lesions and the cavernous sinus. In: Albert DM, Jakobiec FA (Eds). Principles and Practice of Ophthalmology. Philadelphia: WB Saunders; 1994. p. 2458.

964. MILLER SYNDROME (GENEE-WIEDEMANN SYNDROME; POSTAXIAL ACROFACIAL DYSOSTOSIS)

General

Cause unknown; sporadic and familial cases known as Genee-Wiedemann Syndrome.

Ocular

Ectropion

Clinical

Malar hypoplasia; cleft palate and lip; postaxial limb deficiency; cup-shaped ears.

Laboratory

Diagnosis is made by clinical findings.

Treatment

Ectropion: Topical ocular lubricants. Congenital-full thickness skin graft with canthal tendon tightening. Involutional-tighten lid by resecting full thickness wedge-medial spindle procedure for punctal eversion. Paralytic may require a fascia lata sling procedure if does not resolve in 3–6 months.

Bibliography

1. Chrzanowska KH, Fryns JP, Krajewska-Walasek M, et al. Phenotype variability in the Miller acrofacial dysostosis syndrome. Report of two further patients. Clin Genet. 1989;35:157-60.

965. MILLER SYNDROME (WAGR SYNDROME; WILMS ANIRIDIA SYNDROME; WILMS TUMOR-ANIRIDIA-GENITOURINARY ABNORMALITIES-MENTAL RETARDATION SYNDROME)

General

Etiology unknown; manifests an association of aniridia, which is inherited as a dominant autosomal trait and Wilms tumor; this is one of the best studied continuous gene syndromes as defined by Schmickel.

Ocular

Glaucoma; bilateral aniridia (aniridia often not complete, with remnants of iris root present as rudimentary forms); cataract.

Clinical

Wilms tumor; mental retardation with microcephaly; genital malformations with cryptorchidism and hypospadias; hemihypertrophy; kidney anomalies (horseshoe kidney).

Laboratory/Glaucoma

Chromosome analysis and genetic counseling.

Treatment/Glaucoma

Beta-blokers, carbonic anhydrase inhibitors and prostaglandin analogs. Surgery may be needed if IOP is uncontrolled.

Bibliography

1. Fraumeni JF, Glass AG. Wilms' tumor and congenital aniridia. JAMA. 1968;206:825-8.
2. Mackintosh TF, Girdwood TG, Parker DJ, et al. Aniridia and Wilms' tumor (nephroblastoma). Br J Ophthalmol. 1968;52:846-8.
3. McKusick VA. Mendelian Inheritance in Man: A Catalog of Human Genes and Genetic Disorders, 12th edition. Baltimore: The Johns Hopkins University Press; 1998.
4. McKusick-Nathans Institute for Genetic Medicine, Johns Hopkins University and National Center for Biotechnology Information, National Library of Medicine. (2007). Online Mendelian Inheritance in Man (OMIM). [online] Available from http://www.ncbi.nlm.nih.gov/omim/ [Accessed April, 2012].
5. Miller RW, Fraumeni JF, Manning MD. Association of Wilms' tumor with aniridia, hemihypertrophy and other congenital malformations. N Engl J Med. 1964;270:922-7.
6. Schmickel RD. Chromosomal deletions and enzyme deficiencies. J Pediatr. 1986;108:244-6.

966. MIRROR IMAGE SYNDROME (AUTOSCOPIC SYNDROME; LUKIANOWICZ PHENOMENON)

General

Patient's delusion that he or she is seeing a double of himself or herself; seen in patients with schizophrenia, epilepsy, migraine, and even depression; the "double" usually appears suddenly and is of white or gray hue.

Ocular

Hallucination in the form of seeing a double of self.

Clinical

Migraine; schizophrenia; epilepsy; depression.

Laboratory

Diagnosis is made by clinical findings.

Treatment

Identify cause.

Bibliography

1. Lippman CW. Hallucinations of physical duality in migraine. J Nerv Ment Dis. 1953;117:345-50.
2. Lukianowicz N. Autoscopic phenomena. AMA Arch Neurol Psychiatry. 1958;80:199-220.
3. Magalini SI, Scrascia E. Dictionary of Medical Syndromes, 2nd edition. Philadelphia: JB Lippincott; 1981.

---

967. MISDIRECTED THIRD NERVE SYNDROME

General

May occur with a variety of inflammatory infections and parainfections, vascular lesions, tumors and degenerative and demyelinating diseases that may involve the nerve anywhere; may occur as primary aberrant regeneration without prior history of acute oculomotor nerve palsy.

Ocular

Bizarre eyelid movements that may accompany various eye movements; lid may rise as the medial rectus, the inferior rectus or the superior rectus muscle contracts; iridoplegia; ptosis.

Clinical

None

Laboratory

Diagnosis is made by clinical findings.

Treatment

Ptosis: If visual acuity is affected most cases require surgical correction, and there are several procedures that may be used including levator resection, repair or advancement and Fasanella-Servat.

Bibliography

1. Beard C. Misdirected third nerve syndrome. In: Mosby CV (Ed). Ptosis, 3rd edition. St. Louis: CV Mosby; 1981. p. 115.
2. Harley RD (Ed). Pediatric Ophthalmology, 4th edition. Philadelphia: WB Saunders; 1998.
3. Lepore FE, Glaser JS. Misdirection revisited: a critical appraisal of acquired oculomotor nerve synkinesis. Arch Ophthalmol. 1980;98:2206-9.
4. Roy FH:P Ocular Differential Diagnosis, 9th edition Jaypee Brothers Medical Publishers (P) Ltd. New Delhi (India).
5. Schatz NJ, Savino PJ, Corbett JJ. Primary aberrant oculomotor regeneration. A sign of intracavernous meningioma. Arch Neurol. 1977;34:29-32.

968. ML I (DYSMORPHIC SIALIDOSIS; LIPOMUCOPOLYSACCHARIDOSIS; MUCOLIPIDOSIS I; SPRANGER SYNDROME)

General

Rare storage disease; autosomal recessive; increased sialic acid and deficiency of the enzyme alpha-N-acetylneuraminidase in cultured mucolipidosis I fibroblasts.

Ocular

Variable corneal clouding; macular cherry-red spot; optic atrophy; lens opacity; pupillary reflexes anomaly; grayish area around cherry-red spot.

Clinical

Moderate progressive mental retardation; skeletal changes of dysostosis multiplex; peripheral neuropathy; myoclonic jerks; tremor; cerebellar signs; gait abnormalities.

Laboratory

Detecting deficiency of alpha-N-acetylneuraminidase activity.

Treatment

Limited only to supportive care and symptomatic relief.

Additional Resource

1. Roth KS (2010). Sialidosis (Mucolipidosis I). [online] Available from http://www.emedicine.com/ped/TOPIC2093.HTM [Accessed April, 2012].

969. ML II (I-CELL DISEASE; MUCOLIPIDOSIS II)

General

Autosomal recessive mucolipidosis is a Hurler-like disorder with some radiologic features, striking fibroblast inclusions and no excess mucopolysacchariduria; abnormal N-acetylglucosamine phosphotransferase.

Ocular

Minimal corneal clouding; glaucoma; megalocornea.

Clinical

Congenital dislocation of the hips; thoracic deformities; hernia; hyperplastic gums; retarded psychomotor development and restricted joint mobility; dysmorphic facies; skeletal deformities; organomegaly; short stature; mental retardation.

Laboratory

N-acetylglucosaminyl-1-phosphotransferase activity, various lysosomal enzymes activities.

Treatment

Treatment remains limited. Bone marrow transplantation.

Additional Resource

1. Roth KS (2009). I-Cell Disease (Mucolipidosis Type II). [online] Available from http://www.emedicine.com/ped/TOPIC1150.HTM [Accessed April, 2012].

970. ML III (MUCOLIPIDOSIS III; PSEUDO-HURLER POLYDYSTROPHY)

General

Autosomal recessive disorder, almost indistinguishable biochemically from mucolipidosis II; decreased levels of N-acetylglucosamine phosphotransferase.

Ocular

Increased corneal thickness; wrinkled maculopathy; granular pigmentary changes of fundus; papilledema; hyperopic astigmatism; corneal opacities; retinal vascular tortuosity; visual field defects.

Clinical

Joint stiffness; coarse facial feature; short stature; aortic valve disease; arm and hand deformities; self-mutilation of the distal phalanges; carpal tunnel syndrome.

Laboratory

Diagnosis is made by clinical findings.

Treatment

Corneal opacities: Medical treatment includes the use of hyperosmotic drops, nonsteroidal and steroid eye drops. Corneal transplant may be necessary.

Papilledema: Underlying cause should be determined and treated. Systemic acetazolamide is the medical therapy of choice.

Bibliography

1. Duane TD. Clinical Ophthalmology. Philadelphia: JB Lippincott; 1987.
2. Zammarchi E, Savelli A, Donati MA, et al. Self-mutilation in a patient with mucolipidosis III. Pediatr Neurol. 1994;11:68-70.

971. ML IV (BERMAN SYNDROME; MUCOLIPIDOSIS IV)

General

Storage disease in which corneal clouding is an early sign with no evidence of systemic involvement until age 1 year; autosomal recessive; cases seen in Ashkenazi Jews; abnormal neuraminidase.

Ocular

Corneal clouding; corneal opacities; epithelial edema; retinal atrophy; pale optic nerve; diffuse corneal clouding present at birth or in early infancy.

Clinical

Progressive psychomotor retardation; skeletal dysplasia; facial anomalies.

Laboratory

Diagnosis is made by clinical findings.

Treatment

Corneal opacities: Medical treatment includes the use of hyperosmotic drops, nonsteroidal and steroid eye drops. Corneal transplant may be necessary.

Additional Resource

1. Roy H (2011). Xanthelasma. [online] Available from http://www.emedicine.medscape.com article/1213423 -overview [Accessed April, 2012].

972. MMMM SYNDROME (MACROCEPHALY, MEGALOCORNEA, MENTAL AND MOTOR RETARDATION; NEUHAUSER SYNDROME)

General

Rare

Ocular

Megalocornea

Clinical

Mental retardation; hearing loss; sensorineural complications; hypoplasia; corpus callosum; macrocephaly.

Laboratory/Ocular

Gonioscopy, A-scan ultrasound biometry.

Treatment

Spectacles, glaucoma or cataract surgery if necessary.

Bibliography

1. Tominaga N, Kamimura N, Matsumoto T, et al. A case of megalocornea mental retardation syndrome complicated with bilateral sensorineural hearing impairment. Pediatr Int. 1999;41:392-4.
2. Balci S, Tekşam O, Gedik S. Megalocornea, macrocephaly, mental and motor retardation: MMMM syndrome (Neuhäuser syndrome) in two sisters with hypoplastic corpus callosum. Turk J Pediatr. 2002;44:274-7.

973. MÖBIUS I SYNDROME (HEMICRANIA, HEMIPLEGIC; HEMIPLEGIC-OPHTHALMOPLEGIC MIGRAINE; HEMIPLEGIC FAMILIAL MIGRAINE)

General

Etiology unknown; indirect indications of unilateral cerebral edema due to vasomotor phenomena; occurs in young adults; recovery usually follows after a few days; no clear etiology has been determined, including a vascular theory of embryopathogenesis, a chromosome translocation and exposure to teratogens.

Ocular

Extraocular palsy; permanent damage of oculomotor nerve III.

Clinical

Hemicrania; hemiparesis; aneurysm of internal carotid; neoplasia; headache.

Laboratory

None

Treatment

No definitive treatment available.

Additional Resource

1. Palmer CA (2012). Mobius Syndrome. [online] Available from http://www.emedicine.com/neuro/TOPIC612.HTM [Accessed April, 2012].

974. MÖBIUS II SYNDROME (CONGENITAL FACIAL DIPLEGIA; CONGENITAL PARALYSIS OF THE SIXTH AND SEVENTH NERVES; CONGENITAL OCULOFACIAL PARALYSIS; VON GRAEFES SYNDROME)

General

Congenital; possibly failure of development of facial nerve cells or primary defect of muscles deriving from first two brachial arches or both; recovery in a few weeks or nonprogressive permanent paralysis of face; asymmetrical; if incomplete, usually spares lower face and platysma.

Ocular

Proptosis; ptosis; weakness of abductor muscles; normal convergence; limitation to internal rotation in lateral movements; esotropia.

Clinical

Facial diplegia; deafness; loss of vestibular responses; webbed fingers or toes; clubfoot.

Laboratory

Diagnosis is made by clinical findings.

Treatment

Ptosis: If visual acuity is affected most cases require surgical correction, and there are several procedures that may be used including levator resection, repair or advancement and Fasanella-Servat.

Bibliography

1. Abbott RL, Metz HS, Weber AA. Saccadic velocity studies in Mobius syndrome. Ann Ophthalmol. 1978;10:619-23.
2. Fenichel GM. Congenital facial asymmetry (aplasia of facial muscles). In: Fenichel GM (Ed). Clinical Pediatric Neurology, 2nd edition. Philadelphia: WB Saunders; 1993. pp. 341-2.
3. Kawai M, Momoi T, Fujii T, et al. The syndrome of Mobius sequence, peripheral neuropathy, and hypogonadotropic hypogonadism. Am J Med Genet. 1990;37:578-82.
4. Menkes JH, Kenneth T. Mobius syndrome. In: Menkes JH (Ed). Textbook of Child Neurology, 5th edition. Baltimore: Williams & Wilkins; 1995. pp. 309-10.
5. Merz M, Wojtowicz S. The Mobius syndrome. Report of electromyographic examinations in two cases. Am J Ophthalmol. 1967;63:837-40.
6. Mobius PJ. Uber Angeborene Doppelseitige Abducens-Facialislahmung. Munch Med Wochenschr. 1888;35:91-4.
7. Puckett CL, Beg SA. Facial reanimation in Mobius syndrome. South Med J. 1978;71:1498-501.

975. MOHR-CLAUSSEN SYNDROME (OFD SYNDROME; ORAL-FACIAL-DIGITAL SYNDROME TYPE II; OROFACIODIGITAL SYNDROME II)

General

Rare; autosomal recessive; certain features similar to Papillon-Leage-Psaume, Carpenter, Laurence-Moon-Bardet-Biedl and Ellis-Van Creveld syndromes.

Ocular

Epicanthus; bridged chorioretinal colobomata.

Clinical

Clefts and fibroma of tongue; polydactylia; broad nasal bridge; narrow-arched palate; short humerus, femur, and tibia; irregular teeth; hypotonia; mental retardation; deafness; thin and fair hair; cerebellar atrophy.

Laboratory

Diagnosis is made by clinical findings.

Treatment

None/Ocular.

Bibliography

1. Anneren G, Gustavson KH, Jòzwiak S, et al. Abnormalities of the cerebellum in oro-facio-digital syndrome II (Mohr syndrome). Clin Genet. 1990;38:69-73.

976. MOLLER-BARLOW DISEASE

General

Vitamin C deficiency in children.

Ocular

Hemorrhages around and, in rare cases, in eyes; yellow-brown discoloration from hemosiderin may remain for sometime after resolution of a subconjunctival hemorrhage; hemorrhage in eyelids, conjunctiva, anterior chamber and retina; proptosis in infantile scurvy.

Clinical

Tenderness of the lower extremities; ecchymoses.

Laboratory

Vitamin C level.

Treatment

Resolve deficiency.

Bibliography

1. Gabay C, Voskuyl AE, Cadiot G, et al. A case of scurvy presenting with cutaneous and articular signs. Clin Rheumatol. 1993;12:278-80.
2. Goskowicz M, Eichenfield LF. Cutaneous findings of nutritional deficiencies in children. Curr Opin Pediatr. 1993;5:441-5.
3. Pau H. Differential Diagnosis of Eye Diseases. New York: Thieme; 1987.

977. MOLLUSCUM CONTAGIOSUM

General

Etiologic agent of this disease is a poxvirus that can cause proliferative skin lesions anywhere on the body; commonly found in patients who are immunosuppressed.

Ocular

Lesions of lid, lid margin, conjunctiva and cornea; conjunctivitis; keratitis; corneal ulcer.

Clinical

Well-defined, pearly appearing papules with umbilicated centers of varying size (3–10 mm); eczematization of the surrounding skin.

Laboratory

Craters have epithelial cells with large eosinophilic intracytoplasmic inclusion bodies (Molluscum or Henderson Patterson bodies) when virus particles migrate to the granular layer of the epidermis, the inclusion bodies become basophilic.

Treatment

Topical agents cantharidin, tretinoin, podophyllin, trichloroacetic acid, tincture of iodine, silver nitrate or phenol, potassium hydroxide. Systemic agents include griseofulvin, methisazone and cimetidine.

Additional Resource

1. Bhatia AC (2012). Molluscum Contagiosum. [online] Available from http://www.emedicine. com/oph/TOPIC500.HTM [Accessed April, 2012].

---

978. MONBRUN-BENISTY SYNDROME (OCULAR STUMP CAUSALGIA)

General

Sympathetic irritation of resected sympathetic fiber to the eye; occurs after trauma of eye.

Ocular

Severe refractory pain of orbital cavity.

Clinical

Pain of face and the corresponding hemicranium; congestion and hyperhidrosis of region involved.

Laboratory

Diagnosis is made by clinical findings.

Treatment

Treat pain.

Bibliography

1. Magalini SI, Scrascia E. Dictionary of Medical Syndromes, 2nd edition. Philadelphia: JB Lippincott; 1981.

---

979. MONOFIXATION SYNDROME (BLIND SPOT SYNDROME; PARKS SYNDROME, PRIMARY MONOFIXATION)

General

No hereditary factor; uncommon.

Ocular

Deviation of 8 prism diopters or less by simultaneous prism and cover test; central scotoma; stereopsis; good fusional vergences found in patients with congenital esotropia; unilateral syphilitic optic perineuritis (rare); congenital esotropia (inherited in a multifactorial fashion).

Clinical

Syphilis (rare).

Laboratory

Diagnosis is made by clinical findings.

Treatment

Orthoptics or surgery is of no benefit. Amblyopia treatment may be necessary.

Additional Resource

1. Gupta BK (2010). Monofixation Syndrome. [online] Available from http://www.emedicine. com/oph/TOPIC566.HTM [Accessed April, 2012].

980. MOOREN'S ULCER (CHRONIC SERPIGINOUS ULCER OF THE CORNEA, ULCUS RODENS)

General

Chronic and progressive disorder of cornea.

Clinical

None

Ocular

Ulcerative keratitis.

Laboratory

Diagnosis is made by clinical findings.

Treatment

Topical—cycloplegic agents, steroids, antibiotic drops. Bandage contact lens and cyanoacrylate glue over perforation may be useful. Surgical—conjunctival recession/resection, conjunctival excision and superficial lamellar keratectomy. Systemic if hepatitis C treat with interferon alpha and Roferon A; if HCV and not chronican immunosuppressive specialist should be consulted.

Additional Resource

1. Murillo-Lopez FH (2010). Ulcer, Corneal. [online] Available from http://www.emedicine.com/oph/TOPIC249.HTM [Accessed April, 2012].

981. MORAXELLA LACUNATA

General

Gram-negative rod; causes chronic angular blepharoconjunctivitis; without treatment, may persist for months or years; normally found in flora of respiratory tract; seen more frequently in alcoholics and those with poor sanitary habits; Moraxella organisms produce proteases, although those are not related directly to their pathogenetic mechanism.

Ocular

Catarrhal angular conjunctivitis; corneal ulcer; hypopyon, chronic blepharitis; eczema; lateral canthal skin erythema; iridocyclitis.

Clinical

Alcoholism; impaired nutrition; dermatitis.

Laboratory

Aerobic, oxidase positive, Gram-negative diplococci or coccobacilli morphologically indistinguishable from Neisseria.

Treatment

Artificial tears, cold compresses and antibiotics.

Bibliography

1. Baum J, Fedukowicz HB, Jordan A. A survey of Moraxella corneal ulcers in a derelict population. Am J Ophthalmol. 1980;90:476-80.
2. Burd EM. Bacterial keratitis and conjunctivitis. In: Smolin G, Thoft RA (Eds). The Cornea. Boston: Little, Brown and Company; 1994. pp. 20-1.
3. Roy FH, Fraunfelder FW, Fraunfelder FT. Roy and Fraunfelder's Current Ocular Therapy, 6th edition. Philadelphia: WB Saunders; 2008.
4. van Bijsterveld OP. The incidence of Moraxella on mucous membranes and the skin. Am J Ophthalmol. 1972;74:72-6.

982. MORGAGNI SYNDROME (HYPEROSTOSIS FRONTALIS INTERNA SYNDROME; INTRACRANIAL EXOSTOSIS; METABOLIC CRANIOPATHY)

General

Dominant inheritance; onset around age 45 years; occurs almost exclusively in females.

Ocular

Cataract; optic nerve injury within the optic canal by bony protrusions, with resulting blindness.

Clinical

Hyperostosis frontalis interna; obesity (mainly trunk and proximal portions of limbs); hirsutism; menstrual disorders; hypertension; arteriosclerosis; headache; hypertrichosis; no case of male-to-male transmission is known; hyperprolactinemia.

Laboratory

Computed tomography (CT) scan of orbit.

Treatment

Cataract: Change in glasses can sometimes improve a patient's visual function temporarily; however, the most common treatment is cataract surgery.

Bibliography

1. Falconer MA, Pierard BE. Failing vision caused by a bony spike compressing the optic nerve within the optic canal, report of two cases associated with Morgagni's syndrome benefited by operation. Br J Ophthalmol. 1950;34:265-81.
2. Geeraets WJ. Ocular Syndromes, 3rd edition. Philadelphia: Lea & Febiger; 1976.

983. MORNING GLORY SYNDROME (HEREDITARY CENTRAL GLIAL ANOMALY OF THE OPTIC DISK)

General

No hereditary factor; rare; anomaly of optic disk with deep excavation resembling the flower for which syndrome is named.

Ocular

Strabismus; abnormality of embryologic development of anterior chamber (anterior chamber cleavage syndrome); remnants of hyaloid system; chorioretinal pigment surrounding optic disk; narrow branches of retinal arteries at edge of optic disk; retinal exudates and detachment; subretinal hemorrhages and retinal neovascularization; enlarged pink optic disk, funnel-shaped with a central white fluffy dot; nerve head surrounded by elevated annulus of chorioretinal pigment, unilateral.

Clinical

Midline cranial facial defects such as hypertelorism, cleft lip/palate, basal encephalocele, agenesis of corpus callosum, sphenoid encephalocele defects in the floor of the sella turcica; cranial, facial and neurologic associations; pituitary dwarfism; association with the CHARGE syndrome.

Laboratory

Diagnosis is made by clinical findings.

Treatment

Glaucoma: Its medication should be the first plan of action. If medication is unsuccessful, a filtering surgical procedure with or without antimetabolites may be beneficial.

Retinal detachment: Scleral buckle, pneumatic retinopexy and vitrectomy may be used to close all the breaks.

Bibliography

1. Caprioli J, Lesser RL. Basal encephalocele and morning glory syndrome. Br J Ophthalmol. 1983;67:349-51.
2. Cennamo G, de Crecchio G, Iaccarino G, et al. Evaluation of morning lory syndrome with spectral optical coherence tomography and echography. Ophthalmology. 2010;117:1269-73.
3. Chang S, Haik BG, Ellsworth RM, et al. Treatment of total retinal detachment in morning glory syndrome. Am J Ophthalmol. 1984;97:596-600.
4. Eustis HS, Sanders MR, Zimmerman T. Morning glory syndrome in children. Association with endocrine and central nervous system anomalies. Arch Ophthalmol. 1994;112:204-7.
5. Handemann M. Erbliche, Vermutlich Angeborene Zentrale Gliose Entartung des Sehnerven mit Besonderer Beteiligung der Zentralgefasse. Klin Monatsbl Augenheilkd. 1929;83:145.
6. Itakura T, Miyamoto K, Uematsu Y, et al. Bilateral morning glory syndrome associated with sphenoid encephalocele. Case report. J Neurosurg. 1992;77:949-51.
7. Kindler P. Morning glory syndrome: unusual congenital optic disk anomaly. Am J Ophthalmol. 1970;69:376-84.

984. MORPHEA (CIRCUMSCRIBED SCLERODERMA; LOCALIZED SCLERODERMA)

General

Localized chronic connective tissue disease of unknown etiology; etiology remains unknown, although there is a possible association with *Borrelia burgdorferi* infection.

Ocular

Circumscribed plaque like lesions of the eyelid; prevalent in females; onset usually in the second to fourth decades of life; onset occasionally associated with trauma, pregnancy or menopause.

Clinical

Firm skin plaques over entire body, but most frequently on trunk, lower extremities, upper extremities, face and genitalia; abdominal pain; migraine; generalized joint pain; renal crisis; Raynaud phenomenon; systemic sclerosis; eosinophilia; positive antinuclear factor; increased immunoglobulin [immunoglobulin G (IgG)]; seizures; skin sclerosis; alterations in tryptophan metabolism.

Laboratory

Tests are limited and are on a case-by-case basis.

Treatment

No definite treatment is available.

Additional Resource

1. Nguyen JV (2010). Morphea. [online] Available from http://www.emedicine.com/derm/TOPIC272.HTM [Accessed April, 2012].

985. MORQUIO SYNDROME (ATYPICAL CHONDRODYSTROPHY; BRAILSFORD-MORQUIO DYSTROPHY; CHONDRODYSTROPHIA TARDA; CHONDRO-OSTEODYSTROPHY; DYSOSTOSIS ENCHONDRALIS METAEPIPHYSARIA; ECCENTRO-OSTEOCHONDRODYSPLASIA; FAMILIAL OSSEOUS DYSTROPHY; HEREDITARY OSTEOCHONDRODYSTROPHY; HEREDITARY POLYTOPIC ENCHONDRAL DYSOSTOSIS; INFANTILE HEREDITARY CHONDRODYSPLASIA; KERATOSULFATURIA; MORQUIO-BRAILSFORD SYNDROME; MORQUIO-ULLRICH SYNDROME; MPS IV; MUCOPOLYSACCHARIDOSIS IV; OSTEOCHONDRODYSTROPHIA DEFORMANS; SPONDYLOEPIPHYSEAL DYSPLASIA)

General

Autosomal recessive dystrophy of cartilage and bone; slight predilection for males; apparent between the ages of 4 and 10 years; excess production of keratosulfate (see Hurler Syndrome; Hunter Syndrome; Sanfilippo-Good Syndrome; Scheie Syndrome; Maroteaux-Lamy Syndrome); autosomal recessive; abnormal N-acetylgalactosamine-G-sulfate sulfatase.

Ocular

Enophthalmos; ptosis; excessive tear secretion; ocular hypotony; miosis; occasionally hazy cornea; bushy eyebrows; optic nerve atrophy; moderate-to-late corneal clouding.

Clinical

Dwarfism; skeletal deformities (progressive); delayed ossification of epiphyses; decreased muscle tone; deafness; weak extremities; waddling gait; coarse broad mouth; spaced teeth; aortic regurgitation; normal intelligence.

Laboratory

Blood—Reilly's granules in leukocytes; X-ray—flat vertebrae and odontoid hypoplasia.

Treatment

Treatment is limited to supportive care.

Additional Resource

1. Bittar T (2010). Mucopolysaccharidosis. [online] Available from http://www.emedicine.com/orthoped/TOPIC203.HTM [Accessed April, 2012].

986. MORT D'AMOUR SYNDROME (DEATH OF LOVE SYNDROME)

General

Sudden death during sexual intercourse.

Ocular

Pupillary dilation.

Clinical

Hypertension; arrhythmia; heart ischemia; rupture of cerebral aneurysm.

Laboratory

Diagnosis is made by clinical findings.

Treatment

Treat systemic manifestations.

Bibliography

1. Heggtveit HA. La mort d'amour. Am Heart J. 1965;69:287.
2. Magalini SI, Scrascia E. Dictionary of Medical Syndromes, 2nd edition. Philadelphia: JB Lippincott; 1981.

987. MOSSE SYNDROME (POLYCYTHEMIA-HEPATIC CIRRHOSIS SYNDROME)

General

Unknown etiology.

Ocular

Scleral icterus; marked retinal venous tortuosity and dilation; retinal artery occlusion (occasionally); papilledema.

Clinical

Thrombosis portal vein secondary to polycythemia; hepatosplenomegaly; ascites; clinical features of liver cirrhosis.

Laboratory

Diagnosis is made by clinical findings.

Treatment

Retinal artery occlusion: Intraocular pressure lowering medications, carbogen therapy, hyperbaric oxygen. Vitrectomy may be necessary.

Papilledema: Underlying cause should be determined and treated. Systemic acetazolamide is the medical therapy of choice.

Bibliography

1. Barabas AP. Surgical problems associated with polycythaemia. Br J Hosp Med. 1980;23:289-90, 292, 294.
2. Geeraets WJ. Ocular Syndromes, 3rd edition. Philadelphia: Lea & Febiger; 1976.
3. Mosse M. Uber Policythamie mit Urobilinikterus und Milztumor. Dtsch Med Wochenschr. 1907;33: 2175.

988. MOYAMOYA DISEASE (MULTIPLE PROGRESSIVE INTRACRANIAL ARTERIAL OCCLUSIONS)

General

Almost exclusively seen in Japanese infants and children; cerebrovascular disorder that results in occlusion of the large vessels at the base of the brain; slight female prevalence; collateral vascular networks (secondary to bilateral carotid occlusive disease) resembling puffs of smoke (Moyamoya in Japanese).

Ocular

Hemianopsia; nystagmus; papilledema; central retinal vein occlusion; visual field defects; amaurosis fugax; diplopia; optic pallor; ischemic chiasmal syndrome; bilateral renal artery stenosis.

Clinical

Loss of consciousness; seizures; hemiplegia; hemiparesis; intracranial hemorrhage; mental retardation; speech disturbances; unsteady gait; headache; psychiatric manifestations; focal epileptic attacks; chronic cerebrovascular disorder; intracerebral hemorrhage; pituitary adenoma (association).

Laboratory

Erythrocyte sedimentation rate, cerebral angiography.

Treatment

Treatment is directed to complications of the disease.

Nystagmus: See-saw nystagmus—visual field to consider neoplastic or vascular etiologies. Up-beat nystagmus—may indicate multiple sclerosis, cerebellar degeneration, tumors or infarcts. Treatment is directed toward identification and resolution of underlying cause. Downbeat nystagmus—affects the cerebellum or craniocervical junction including Arnold-Chiari malformation, multiple sclerosis, trauma, tumor, infarction and many toxic metabolic entities. MRI may indicate a surgically correctable lesion. Periodic alternating nystagmus is continuous horizontal nystagmus from stroke, tumor, multiple sclerosis, trauma, infection and drug intoxication. Can occur from cataract, vitreous hemorrhage or optic atrophy.

Amaurosis fugax: When the Doppler test is positive, carotid surgery may be indicated.

Central vein occlusion: Anticoagulation, surgical adventitial sheathotomy, radial optic neurotomy, intravitreal injection of triamcinolone acetonide for macular edema. Vitrectomy may be necessary.

Additional Resource

1. Sucholeiki R (2012). Moyamoya Disease. [online] Available from http://www.emedicine.com/neuro/TOPIC616.HTM [Accessed April, 2012].

---

989. MOYNAHAN SYNDROME (XTE; XERODERMA, TALIPES AND ENAMEL DEFECT)

General

Autosomal dominant inheritance; xeroderma, talipes and enamel defect.

Ocular

Absence of eyelashes of lower lid.

Clinical

Cleft palate; hypohidrosis; defective enamel; nail anomalies; coarse and dry hair; short-lasting skin bullae.

Laboratory

Diagnosis is made by clinical findings.

Treatment

None/Ocular.

Bibliography

1. Magalini SI, Scrascia E. Dictionary of Medical Syndromes, 2nd edition. Philadelphia: JB Lippincott; 1981.
2. Moynahan EJ. XTE syndrome (xeroderma, talipes and enamel defect): a new heredo-familial syndrome. Two cases. Homozygous inheritance of a dominant gene. Proc R Soc Med. 1970;63: 447-8.

990. MUCOCELE (PYOCELE)

General

Accumulation and retention of mucoid material within the sinus as a result of continuous or periodic obstruction of the sinus ostium.

Ocular

Paralysis of extraocular muscles; exophthalmos; lacrimation; erosion of bony walls of orbit; decreased visual acuity; diplopia; elevation of lower lid; ptosis; compression optic neuropathy; globe distortion; enophthalmos; epiphora; scleral indentation; choroidal folds; discharging lesion of the upper lid; pseudotelecanthus; spontaneous nontraumatic enophthalmos; local anesthesia.

Clinical

Headache; epidural abscess; subdural empyema; meningitis; brain abscess; occlusion of nasal passage; loosening of teeth.

Laboratory

Computed tomography (CT) scanning helps to outline bony changes, MRI helps to differentiate mucoceles from neoplasms in the paranasal sinuses.

Treatment

Gamma-linolenic acid.

Additional Resource

1. Flaitz CM (2012). Mucocele and Ranula. [online] Available from http://www.emedicine.com/derm/ TOPIC648.HTM [Accessed April, 2012].

991. MUCOCUTANEOUS LYMPH NODE SYNDROME (KAWASAKI DISEASE; MLN SYNDROME)

General

Multisystem syndrome with worldwide distribution; occurs between the ages of 2 months and 9 years; increased incidence in summer; etiology unknown, but allergic reactions to chemicals or abnormal reactions to numerous infections have been suggested.

Ocular

Severe conjunctival congestion and hyperemia (88%); uveitis; dacryocystitis; anterior uveitis (commonly bilateral); punctate keratitis.

Clinical

Fever (1–2 weeks; does not respond to antibiotics) "strawberry tongue"; red palms and soles; indurative edema; membranous desquamation from fingertips; polymorphous exanthema; arthritis; myocarditis; enlarged cervical lymph nodes.

Laboratory

White blood cell count, test for anemia, erythrocyte sedimentation rate and C-reactive protein.

Treatment

Intravenous immunoglobulin and acetylsalicylic acid.

Additional Resource

1. Jatla KK (2011). Ophthalmologic Manifestations of Kawasaki Disease. [online] Available from http://www.emedicine.com/oph/TOPIC438.HTM [Accessed April, 2012].

992. MUCORMYCOSIS (PHYCOMYCOSIS)

General

Acute, often fatal infection caused by saprophytic fungi; associated with diabetes mellitus and ketoacidosis.

Ocular

Corneal ulcer; striate keratopathy; ptosis; panophthalmitis; proptosis; cellulitis of orbit; immobile pupil; retinitis; optic neuritis; paralysis of extraocular muscles; central retinal artery thrombosis.

Clinical

Epistaxis; nasal discharge; facial pain; facial palsies; anhidrosis; cranial nerve or peripheral motor and sensory nerve deficits may occur.

Laboratory

Tissue biopsy and culture of paranasal sinuses demonstrate the presence of the fungi, which appear as broad, irregular, nonseptate and branching hyphae on hematoxylin and eosin (H&E) stain.

Treatment

Amhotericin B is the treatment of choice.

Additional Resource

1. Crum-Cianflone NF (2011). Mucormycosis. [online] Available from http://www.emedicine.com/oph/TOPIC225.HTM [Accessed April, 2012].

993. MUCOUS MEMBRANE PEMPHIGOID

General

Immune-mediated disease characterized by autoantibodies to the basement membrane zone at the subepithelial junction of mucous membranes.

Ocular

Progressive cicatrizing conjunctivitis; symblepharon; corneal clouding.

Clinical

Nasal and oral mucosa cicatrization; trachea and esophagus cicatrization.

Laboratory

Diagnosis is made by clinical findings.

Treatment

No topical agent is effective. Systemic corticosteroids can control the progression of the disease. Surgeries such as marginal rotation of the eyelid, mucous membrane grafting, retractor plication, fornix reconstruction.

Additional Resource

1. Foster CS (2011). Ophthalmologic Manifestations of Cicatricial Pemphigoid. [online] Available from http://www.emedicine.com/oph/TOPIC83.HTM [Accessed April, 2012].

994. MUCUS FISHING SYNDROME

General

Excessive mucus production created by mechanical damage of conjunctival epithelium; epithelial injury created by mechanical removal of excess mucus, which leads to further increased mucus production, causing a continuous cycle; initial mucus production may be associated with an underlying ocular disease, such as pterygium, keratoconus, blepharitis or keratoconjunctivitis.

Ocular

Excessive mucus production; blepharitis; pterygium; keratoconjunctivitis; keratoconus; corneal foreign body; floppy lid syndrome; map-dot fingerprint dystrophy; squamous cell cancer of conjunctiva.

Clinical

None

Laboratory

Diagnosis is made by clinical findings.

Treatment

Pterygium: Patients with pterygia can be observed unless the lesions exhibit growth toward the center of the cornea or the patient exhibits symptoms of significant redness, discomfort or alterations in visual function. Surgery for excision of pterygia is beneficial if visual function is disturbed.

Keratoconus: Spectacle correction, hard contacts and avoid eye rubbing may be useful. If hydrops occurs discontinue contact lens, use NaCl drops and ointment, patching and short course of steroids. As the disease advances penetrating keratoplasty, deep anterior lamellar keratoplasty, intacs with laser grooves or collagen stabilization of cornea.

Blepharitis: Oral tetracyclines, omega-3 fatty acids, flax seed oil or fish oil. Ocular therapy includes eyelid scrubs, warm compresses, bacitracin ointment to lid margins, topical cyclosporine A and preservative-free lubricants.

Bibliography

1. McCulley JP, Moore MB, Matoba AY. Mucus fishing syndrome. Ophthalmology. 1985;92:1262-5.
2. McCulley JP, Dougherty JM, Deneau DG. Classification of chronic blepharitis. Ophthalmology. 1982;89:1173-80.

995. MUIR-TORRE SYNDROME

General

Rare; autosomal dominant; characterized by sebaceous tumors and internal malignancies.

Ocular

Sebaceous tumor of the eyelids.

Clinical

Gastrointestinal, breast and genitourinary malignancies; sebaceous neoplasms.

Laboratory

Radiological imaging of facial and orbital bones.

Treatment

Radiation therapy, photodynamic therapy, cryo-surgery, electrodesiccation and curettage, surgical excision, Mohs micrographic surgery.

Bibliography

1. Font RL, Rishi K. Sebaceous gland adenoma of the tarsal conjunctiva in a patient with Muir-Torre syndrome. Ophthalmology. 2003;110:1833-6.

2. Mathiak M, Rutten A, Mangold E, et al. Loss of DNA mismatch repair proteins in skin tumors form patients with Muir-Torre syndrome and MSH2 or MLH1 germline mutations: establishment of immunohistochemical analysis as a screening test. Am J Surg Pathol. 2002;26:338-43.

---

996. MULIBREY NANISM SYNDROME (PERHEENTUPA SYNDROME)

General

Autosomal recessive inheritance; progressive growth failure; myocardial fibrosis.

Ocular

Alternating esotropia and exotropia; yellowish retinal dots and scattered pigment dispersion in clusters (especially in the midperiphery); drusen of Bruch membrane; hypoplasia of choriocapillaries (diagnostic sign).

Clinical

Triangular face with bulging forehead and low, broad nasal bridge; hypotonia; hepatomegaly; ascites; pulmonary congestion; cardiac enlargement with possible heart failure; pericardial constriction; dwarfism; immunoglobulin deficiency; isolated growth hormone deficiency.

Laboratory

Diagnosis is made by clinical findings.

Treatment

Strabismus: Equalized vision with correct refractive error; surgery may be helpful in patient with diplopia.

Bibliography

1. Haraldsson A, van der Burgt CJ, Weemaes CM, et al. Antibody deficiency and isolated growth hormone deficiency in a girl with Mulibrey nanism. Eur J Pediatr. 1993;152:509-12.

---

997. MULTIPLE ENDOCRINE NEOPLASIA 2B OR 3 (MEN 2B OR 3)

General

Autosomal dominant inheritance; multiple endocrine neoplasia type 3 (MEN 3) has been separated from MEN 2 because of low incidence of associated parathyroid disease in these cases; poor prognosis; several different point mutations in the RET proto-oncogene on chromosome 10 have been associated with the multiple endocrine neoplasia type 2 syndromes.

Ocular

Prominent corneal nerves in clear stroma; diffuse, nodular thickening of eyelids; nasal displacement of lacrimal puncta; rostral displacement of eyelashes; eversion of eyelids; subconjunctival neuromas; thickened conjunctival nerves; decreased tear formation; prominent eyebrows; impaired pupillary dilation; thickened iris nerves; increased intraocular pressure (rare); localized orbital neurofibromas (orbit, conjunctiva); lesions of the tongue resembling neuromas.

Clinical

May be present at birth or develop later; 50% show complete syndrome of multiple neuromas (lips, tongue, eyelids), bumpy lips, pheochromocytoma and medullary carcinoma; others exhibit variable combinations of the preceding, without the pheochromocytoma; diarrhea; marfanoid habitus.

Laboratory

Genetic screening, biochemical screening, CT scanning or MRI.

Treatment

Surgery is the treatment of choice. Hormone replacement therapy after total thyroidectomy.

Additional Resource

1. Richards ML (2010). Multiple Endocrine Neoplasia, Type 2. [online] Available from http://www.emedicine.com/med/TOPIC1520.HTM [Accessed April, 2012].

998. MULTIPLE EVANESCENT WHITE DOT SYNDROME (MEWDS)

General

Unilateral disease including multiple white dots at the level of the pigment epithelium; etiology unknown; recurrent; no systemic involvement.

Ocular

Retinal pigment granularity in the macula; reduced visual acuity; vitreitis; loss of retinal sensitivity; white dots of pigment epithelium; uveitis; blind spot enlargement; choroidal neovascularization.

Clinical

None

Laboratory

Diagnosis is made by clinical findings.

Treatment

Systemic corticosteroids, chlorambucil, azathioprine, cyclophosphamide, methotrexate, cyclosporine. Periocular corticosteroids are very effective. Cryotherapy is used on patients who are intolerant to corticosteroids.

Additional Resource

1. Tewari A (2012). White Dot Syndromes. [online] Available from http://www.emedicine.com/oph/TOPIC749.HTM [Accessed April, 2012].

999. MULTIPLE LENTIGINES SYNDROME (LEOPARD SYNDROME)

General

Familial occurrence; classic features include lentigines (small focal hyperpigmentation of skin), electrocardiographic conduction abnormalities, ocular hypertelorism, pulmonary stenosis, abnormal genitalia, retardation of growth, and deafness (LEOPARD).

Ocular

Hypertelorism; exophthalmos; epicanthal folds; strabismus; nystagmus; keratoconus.

Clinical

Lowset ears; receding chin; deafness; lentigines; pulmonary stenosis; genital abnormalities;

growth retardation; skeletal malformations (bony fusion involving cervical vertebrae, ossicles, carpal and tarsal bones, scoliosis); hyposmia; heart murmur; mental retardation; hypospadias; congenital heart defect; thoracic deformities; respiratory insufficiency.

Laboratory

Computed tomography (CT) scanning or MRI, skeletal radiography, echocardiography.

Treatment

Cryosurgery and laser treatment may be helpful, beta-adrenergic receptor or calcium channel blocking agents.

Additional Resource

1. Jozwiak S 2012). LEOPARD Syndrome. [online] Available from http://www.emedicine.com/derm/ TOPIC627.HTM [Accessed April, 2012].

1000. MULTIPLE MUCOSAL NEUROMATA WITH ENDOCRINE TUMORS SYNDROME (MULTIPLE MUCOSAL NEUROMAS, PHEOCHROMOCYTOMA, AND MEDULLARY THYROID CARCINOMA SYNDROME)

General

Pheochromocytoma can be inherited and found in combination with neurofibromatosis and other brain tumors (meningioma, spongioblastoma, ependymoma, astrocytoma, cerebellar hemangioblastoma), multiple mucosal neuromas and medullary carcinoma of the thyroid.

Ocular

Conjunctival neuromas; multiple, white and myelinated nerve fibers in corneal stroma arising at limbus with anastomoses in center of the cornea.

Clinical

Neuromas of lips or anterior portion of tongue or, more rarely, of buccal, gingival or laryngeal mucosa; hypertension; flushing; weakness; sweating; palpitations; headaches.

Laboratory

Plasma metanephrine testing.

Treatment

Tumor resection is the treatment of choice.

Additional Resource

1. Blake MA (2011). Pheochromocytoma. [online] Available from http://www.emedicine.com/med/ TOPIC1816.HTM [Accessed April, 2012].

1001. MULTIPLE PTERYGIUM SYNDROME, LETHAL TYPE (LETHAL TYPE, MULTIPLE, PTERYGIUM)

General

Autosomal recessive; nonconsanguineous parents; lethal.

Ocular

Hypertelorism; epicanthal folds.

Clinical

Multiple pterygia involving chin to sternum, cervical, axillary, antecubital and popliteal areas; flexion contracture of multiple joints; small chest; hydrops; markedly flattened nasal bridge with hypoplastic nasal alae; cleft palate;

micrognathia; lowset, malformed ears; short neck with a cystic hygroma on back of neck and head; pulmonary and cardiac hypoplasia; hypoplastic teeth; elongated clavicles; cryptorchidism; foot deformities; arthrogryposis; hypoplasia of the left arm, leg, pelvis and kidney.

Laboratory

Diagnosis is made by clinical findings.

Treatment

None/Ocular.

Bibliography

1. Chen H, Immken L, Lachman R, et al. Syndrome of multiple pterygia, camptodactyly, facial anomalies, hypoplastic lungs and heart, cystic hygroma, and skeletal anomalies: delineation of a new entity and review of lethal forms of multiple pterygium syndrome. Am J Med Genet. 1984;17:809-26.
2. McKusick VA. Mendelian Inheritance in Man: A Catalog of Human Genes and Genetic Disorders, 12th edition. Baltimore: The Johns Hopkins University Press; 1998.
3. McKusick-Nathans Institute for Genetic Medicine, Johns Hopkins University and National Center for Biotechnology Information, National Library of Medicine. (2007). Online Mendelian Inheritance in Man (OMIM). [online] Available from http://www.ncbi.nlm.nih.gov/omim [Accessed April, 2012].
4. Spearritt DJ, Tannenberg AE, Payton DJ. Lethal multiple pterygium syndrome: report of a case with neurological anomalies. Am J Med Genet. 1993;47:45-9.
5. Willems PJ, Colpaert C, Vaerenbergh M, et al. Multiple pterygium syndrome with body asymmetry. Am J Med Genet. 1993;47:106-11.

1002. MULTIPLE SCLEROSIS (DISSEMINATED SCLEROSIS)

General

Disseminated demyelination affecting white matter of the brain, spinal cord and optic nerves; etiology unknown.

Ocular

Nystagmus; ptosis; myokymia; optic atrophy; papillitis; optic neuritis; anisocoria; Argyll Robertson pupil; Marcus Gunn pupil; hippus, decreased or absent papillary reaction to light; periphlebitis; visual field defects; gaze palsy; paralysis of third or sixth nerve; uveitis; oscillopsia; Uhthoff symptom (reduction of visual acuity with exercise or ocular hyperthermia); pars planitis; retinal venous sheathing; retinitis; granulomatous uveitis.

Clinical

Incoordination; paresthesia; spasticity; tic douloureux; urinary frequency and infections; progressive disability; paralysis; death.

Laboratory

Magnetic resonance imaging (MRI), cerebrospinal fluid positive for oligoclonal band, albumin and IgG index; brainstem auditory evoked response (BAER) and somatosensory evoked potentials (SEPs).

Treatment

Patients with multiple sclerosis (MS) may require multiple consultations to rule out other causes for their symptoms. Drugs such as immunodulator, immunosuppressors, anti-Parkinson agent and CNS stimulants are all used in the management of the disease.

Additional Resource

1. Luzzio C (2012). Multiple Sclerosis. [online] Available from http://www.emedicine.com/neuro/topic228.htm [Accessed April, 2012].

1003. MULTIPLE SULFATASE DEFICIENCY

General

Autosomal recessive.

Ocular

Congenital peripheral cataract; retinal degeneration; cherry-red spot of macula.

Clinical

Progressive neurologic disease with death in the teenage years; ichthyosis.

Laboratory

Diagnosis is made by clinical findings.

Treatment

Cataract: Change in glasses can sometimes improve a patient's visual function temporarily; however, the most common treatment is cataract surgery.

Bibliography

1. Johnson JL. Prenatal diagnosis of molybdenum cofactor deficiency and isolated sulfite oxidase deficiency. Prenat Diagn. 2003;23:6-8.

1004. MULVIHILL-SMITH SYNDROME

General

Progeroid disorder.

Ocular

Keratoconus; conjunctivitis.

Clinical

Patients have short stature, microcephaly, unusual facies, numerous pigmented nevi, hypodontia, sensorineural hearing loss, immunodeficiency (low IgG) and a high-pitched voice.

Laboratory

Diagnosis is made by clinical findings.

Treatment

Keratoconus: Spectacle correction, hard contacts and avoid eye rubbing may be useful. If hydrops occurs discontinue contact lens, use NaCl drops and ointment, patching and short course of steroids. As the disease advances penetrating keratoplasty, deep anterior lamellar keratoplasty, intacs with laser grooves or collagen stabilization of cornea.

Conjunctivitis: Symptomatic control may include cold compresses and artificial tears; nonsteroidal and occasionally steroidal drops to relieve itching.

Bibliography

1. Bartsch O, Tympner KD, Schwinger E, et al. Mulvihill-Smith syndrome: case report and review. J Med Genet. 1994;31:707-11.
2. Ohashi H, Tsukahara M, Murano I, et al. Premature aging and immunodeficiency: Mulvihill-Smith syndrome? Am J Med Genet. 1993;45:597-600.
3. Rau S, Duncker GI. Keratoconus in Mulvihill-Smith syndrome. Klin Monbl Augenheilkd. 1994;205: 44-6.

1005. MUMPS

General

Viral infection.

Ocular

Conjunctivitis; keratitis; corneal ulcer; tenonitis; exophthalmos; microphthalmos; optic atrophy; optic neuritis; papillitis; scleritis; uveitis; cortical blindness; congenital punctal occlusion; paralysis of extraocular muscles; dacryoadenitis; iritis; paralysis of accommodation; internal and external ophthalmoparesis.

Clinical

Affects the parotid glands, but infection of other glandular tissue occurs, including the lacrimal gland and testicles; encephalitis; meningitis.

Laboratory

Mumps virus by acute serologic studies.

Treatment

Generous hydration and alimentation, analgesics for headaches. No antiviral agent is available.

Additional Resource

1. Defendi GL (2012). Mumps. [online] Available from http://www.emedicine.com/ped/TOPIC1503. HTM [Accessed April, 2012].

1006. MUSCULAR DYSTROPHY, CONGENITAL, WITH INFANTILE CATARACT AND HYPOGONADISM

General

Autosomal recessive; rare; reported in isolated Norwegian village.

Ocular

Infantile cataract.

Clinical

Ovarian agenesis in females; Klinefelter syndrome in males; congenital muscular dystrophy.

Laboratory/Ocular

Diagnosis is made by clinical findings.

Treatment/Ocular

Amblyopia therapy may be necessary in unilateral cataracts; cataract surgical intervention is the usual therapy of choice.

Bibliography

1. Bassoe HH. Familial congenital muscular dystrophy with gonadal dysgenesis. J Clin Endocrinol Metab. 1956;16:1614-21.
2. McKusick VA. Mendelian Inheritance in Man: A Catalog of Human Genes and Genetic Disorders, 12th edition. Baltimore: The Johns Hopkins University Press; 1998.

1007. MYASTHENIA GRAVIS, NEONATAL OR INFANTILE (INFANTILE MYASTHENIA GRAVIS; NEONATAL MYASTHENIA GRAVIS)

General

Occurs in newborn of myasthenic mother; caused by compound in circulation received through placenta (see Erb-Goldflam Syndrome).

Ocular

Transient diplopia; ptosis of upper eyelids; internuclear ophthalmoplegia.

Clinical

Excessive fatigue musculature; symptoms appear and increase as day progresses; expressionless face; sagging jaw; sucking, swallowing and respiratory difficulties.

Laboratory

"Ice test" crushed ice in a surgical glove over ptotic eyelid for 2 minutes and watch for brief elevation of eyelid. Tensilon test and Prostigmin test may result in elevation of ptotic eyelid or improved strabismus.

Treatment

Adrenal corticosteroids are frequently used. In some cases, mycophenolate, mofetil, cyclosporin and cyclophosphamide may be useful. Patching one eye or using prisms may be helpful.

Additional Resource

1. Awwad S (2011). Ophthalmologic Manifestations of Myasthenia Gravis. [online] Available from http://www.emedicine.com/oph/TOPIC263.HTM [Accessed April, 2012].

1008. MYCOSIS FUNGOIDES SYNDROME (MALIGNANT CUTANEOUS RETICULOSIS SYNDROME; SÉZARY SYNDROME)

General

Lymphoma characterized by abnormal lymphocytes having hyperchromatic, hyperconvoluted nuclei; malignant, cutaneous T-cell lymphoma, which initially presents as a nonspecific erythematous cutaneous eruption that progresses to form plaques and tumors.

Ocular

Thick and swollen eyelids; ectropion; blepharitis; loss of eyelashes; keratoconjunctivitis; uveitis; retinal edema and exudates; papilledema; exophthalmos; retinal hemorrhage; endophthalmitis; pupillary dilatation; scleritis; corneal opacity; optic disk swelling.

Clinical

Pruritus followed by thickening and edema of the skin; dermatitis exfoliativa; eczema; pyoderma; pigmentary changes of body and extremities (mottled appearance); hyperhidrosis.

Laboratory

Blood work and biopsy of eyelids.

Treatment

Ectropion: Topical ocular lubricants. Congenital-full thickness skin graft with canthal tendon tightening. Involutional-tighten lid by resecting full thickness wedge-medial spindle procedure for punctal eversion. Paralytic may require a fascia lata sling procedure if does not resolve in 3–6 months.

Blepharitis: Oral tetracyclines, omega-3 fatty acids, flax seed oil or fish oil. Ocular therapy includes eyelid scrubs, warm compresses, bacitracin ointment to lid margins, topical cyclosporine A and preservative-free lubricants.

Uveitis: Topical steroids and cycloplegic medication should be the initial treatment of choice. Oral steroids if not responsive to topical steroids, immunosuppressants if bilateral disease that does not respond to oral steroids, periocular steroids for unilateral or posterior uveitis. Vitrectomy can be used for severe vitreous opacification. Cryotherapy and laser photocoagulation may be used for localized pars plana exudates.

Papilledema: Underlying cause should be determined and treated. Systemic acetazolamide is the medical therapy of choice.

Exophthalmos: Reversing the problem, which is causing the exophthalmos, is the treatment of choice and will minimize the ocular complications. Ocular lubricants are beneficial for control of the corneal exposure.

Bibliography

1. Deutsch AR, Duckworth JK. Mycosis fungoides of upper lid. Am J Ophthalmol. 1968;65:884-8.
2. Foerster HC. Mycosis fungoides with intraocular involvement. Trans Am Acad Ophthalmol Otolaryngol. 1960;64:308-13.
3. Leitch RJ, Rennie IG, Parsons MA. Ocular involvement in mycosis fungoides. Br J Ophthalmol. 1993;77:126-7.
4. Meekins B, Proia AD, Klintworth GK. Cutaneous T-cell lymphoma presenting as a rapidly enlarging ocular adnexal tumor. Ophthalmology. 1985;92:1288-93.
5. Roy FH, Fraunfelder FW, Fraunfelder FT. Roy and Fraunfelder's Current Ocular Therapy, 6th edition. Philadelphia: WB Saunders; 2008.

1009. MYELINATED OPTIC NERVE FIBERS

General

Autosomal dominant; transmission has been reported as autosomal recessive.

Ocular

White area adjacent to the disk caused by myelin sheath; pseudopapilledema.

Clinical

None

Laboratory

Diagnosis is made by clinical findings.

Treatment

None/Ocular.

Bibliography

1. Francois J. Heredity in Ophthalmology. St. Louis: CV Mosby; 1961. p. 945.
2. Mann I. Developmental Abnormalities of the Eye, 2nd edition. Philadelphia: JB Lippincott; 1957.
3. McKusick VA. Mendelian Inheritance in Man: A Catalog of Human Genes and Genetic Disorders, 12th edition. Baltimore: The Johns Hopkins University Press; 1998.
4. McKusick-Nathans Institute for Genetic Medicine, Johns Hopkins University and National Center for Biotechnology Information, National Library of Medicine. (2007). Online Mendelian Inheritance in Man (OMIM). [online] Available from http://www.ncbi.nlm.nih.gov/omim/ [Accessed April, 2012].

1010. MYOPIA, CLEAR LENS EXTRACTION

General

Clear lens extraction, also called refractive lens exchange, is the removal of a noncataractous natural lens of the eye with or without intraocular lens placement as a refractive procedure.

Clinical

None

Ocular

High myopia or hyperopia.

Laboratory

Refractive history including contact lens wear, keratometry, uncorrected and best corrected vision, slit lamp examination, tonometry, manifest and cycloplegic refraction, dilated fundus examination.

Treatment

Glasses or contact lens can be used to correct myopia or hyperopia. If patient is unhappy with glasses or contact lens, clear lens extraction can be considered. Clear lens extraction should be performed as a traditional cataract surgery.

Additional Resource

1. Bashour M (2011). Clear Lens Extraction Myopia Treatment & Management. [online] Available from http://www.emedicine.medscape.com/article /1221340-treatment [Accessed April, 2012].

1011. MYOPIA, HYPEROPIA PRK

General

Nearsightedness or farsightedness corrected with a surgical procedure photorefractive keratectomy (PRK) which is the application of energy products by the excimer laser to the anterior corneal stroma to change its curvature and to allow correction of the refractive error.

Clinical

None

Ocular

Inability to see well at distance or near without correction. Possible complications include corneal perforation or unstability.

Laboratory

Refractive history including contact lens wear, keratometry, uncorrected and best corrected vision, slit lamp examination, tonometry, manifest and cycloplegic refraction, dilated fundus examination.

Treatment

Glasses or contact lens can be used to correct myopia. If patient is unhappy with glasses or contact lens, PRK can be considered.

Additional Resource

1. Murillo-Lopez FH (2010). Myopia, PRK. [online] Available from http://www.emedicine.medscape. com/article/1221828-overview [Accessed April, 2012].

1012. MYOPIA, INFANTILE SEVERE

General

Autosomal recessive; consanguineous parents.

Ocular

High myopia; optic disk cupping.

Clinical

None

Laboratory

Diagnosis is made by clinical findings.

Treatment

Myopic glasses or contact lens. Refractive surgery may also be beneficial.

Bibliography

1. Drack AV. Myopia. In: Wright KW (Ed). Pediatric Ophthalmology and Strabismus. St. Louis: CV Mosby; 1995. p. 55.
2. Karlsson JL. Evidence for recessive inheritance of myopia. Clin Genet. 1975;7:197-202.

1013. MYOPIA LASIK

General

Nearsightedness corrected with a surgical procedure LASIK which is done by cutting a corneal flap and using an excimer laser to flatten the cornea to correct the myopia.

Clinical

None

Ocular

Inability to see well at distance without correction. Possible complications include displaced flap, corneal perforation, interface debris and diffuse lamellar keratitis.

Laboratory

Refractive history including contact lens wear, keratometry, uncorrected and best corrected vision, slit lamp examination, tonometry, manifest and cycloplegic refraction, dilated fundus examination.

Treatment

Glasses or contact lens can be used to correct myopia. If patient is unhappy with glasses or contact lens, LASIK can be considered.

Additional Resource

1. Murillo-Lopez FH (2010). Myopia, PRK Treatment & Management. [online] Available from http://www.emedicine.medscape.com/article/1221828-treatment [Accessed April, 2012].

1014. MYOPIA-OPHTHALMOPLEGIA SYNDROME

General

Sex-linked; characteristics seen in males; carried by females.

Ocular

Ptosis; myopia; complete or partial ophthalmoplegia; abnormal pupil; progressive degeneration of retina and choroid.

Clinical

Patellar reflex absent; Achilles reflex absent; spina bifida; cardiac defects; absent deep tendon reflex in carriers only.

Laboratory

Diagnosis is made by clinical findings.

Treatment

Ptosis: If visual acuity is affected most cases require surgical correction, and there are several procedures that may be used including levator resection, repair or advancement and Fasanella-Servat.

Ophthalmoplegia: A complex disorder requiring the involvement of physicians from various spe-

cialties including neurology, cardiology, ophthalmology and endocrinology.

Bibliography

1. McKusick VA. Mendelian Inheritance in Man: A Catalog of Human Genes and Genetic Disorders, 12th edition. Baltimore: The Johns Hopkins University Press; 1998.
2. McKusick-Nathans Institute for Genetic Medicine, Johns Hopkins University and National Center for Biotechnology Information, National Library of Medicine. (2007). Online Mendelian Inheritance in Man (OMIM). [online] Available from http://www.ncbi.nlm.nih.gov/omim/ [Accessed April, 2012].
3. Ortiz de Zarate JC. Recessive sex-linked inheritance of congenital external ophthalmoplegia and myopia coincident with other dysplasias. A reappraisal after 15 years. Br J Ophthalmol. 1966;50:606-7.

1015. MYOPIA, PHAKIC IOL

General

Nearsightedness corrected with a surgical procedure, phakic IOL. Used more frequently in individuals with higher degree of myopia.

Clinical

None

Ocular

Inability to see well at distance without correction.

Laboratory

Corneal topography; corneal pachymetry; keratometry; cycloplegic refraction; slit lamp examination; IOL power calculation.

Treatment

Glasses or contact lens can be used to correct myopia. If patient is unhappy with glasses or contact lens, phakic IOL can be considered.

Additional Resource

1. Verma A (2011). Phakic IOL Myopia. [online] Available from http://www.emedicine.medscape.com/article/1221908-overview [Accessed April, 2012].

1016. MYOPIA, SEX-LINKED

General

Sex-linked; linkage to factor VIII gene; probable location Xq28.

Ocular

Myopia; hemeralopia; deuteranopia in males; hypoplasia of the optic nerve head.

Clinical

Short stature.

Laboratory

Diagnosis is made by clinical findings.

Treatment

Generally treated with glasses, contact lens and refractive surgery.

Bibliography

1. Bartsocas CS, Kastrantas AD. Sex-linked form of myopia. Hum Hered. 1981;31:199-200.
2. Haim M, Fledelius HC, Skarsholm. X-linked myopia in a Danish family. Acta Ophthalmol. 1988;66:450-6.
3. McKusick VA. Mendelian Inheritance in Man: A Catalog of Human Genes and Genetic Disorders, 12th edition. Baltimore: The Johns Hopkins University Press; 1998.
4. McKusick-Nathans Institute for Genetic Medicine, Johns Hopkins University and National Center for Biotechnology Information, National Library of Medicine. (2007). Online Mendelian Inheritance in Man (OMIM). [online] Available from http://www.ncbi.nlm.nih.gov/omim/ [Accessed April, 2012].
5. Schwartz M, Haim M, Skarsholm D. X-linked myopia: Bornholm eye disease. Linkage to DNA markers on the distal part of Xq. Clin Genet. 1990;38:281-6.

1017. MYOPIA, INTRACORNEAL RINGS

General

The intrastromal corneal ring is a device designed to correct mild-to-moderate myopia by flattening the anterior curvature of the cornea.

Clinical

None

Ocular

Inability to see well at distance; side effects of the surgery may include increased intraocular pressure, overcorrection, decreased corneal sensation, decrease in contrast sensitivity.

Laboratory

Refractive history including contact lens wear, keratometry, uncorrected and best corrected vision, slit lamp examination, tonometry, manifest and cycloplegic refraction, dilated fundus examination.

Treatment

Glasses or contact lens can be used to correct myopia. If patient is unhappy with glasses or contact lens, intracorneal rings can be considered.

Additional Resource

1. Roque MR (2011). Intracorneal Rings Myopia. [online] Available from http://www.emedicine.medscape.com/article/1221441-overview [Accessed April, 2012].

1018. MYOPIA, RADIAL KERATOTOMY

General

Nearsightedness corrected with a surgical procedure, radial keratotomy which is radial corneal incisions used to flatten the corneal curvature to correct the myopia.

Clinical

None

Ocular

Inability to see well at distance without correction. Possible complications include displaced flap, corneal perforation, interface debris and diffuse lamellar keratitis.

Laboratory

Refractive history including contact lens wear, keratometry, uncorrected and best correctedvision, slit lamp examination, tonometry, manifest and cycloplegic refraction, dilated fundus examination.

Treatment

Glasses or contact lens can be used to correct myopia. If patient is unhappy with glasses or contact lens, radial keratotomy can be considered.

Additional Resource

1. Bashour M (2012). Radial Keratotomy Myopia. [online] Available from http://www.emedicine. medscape.com/article/1222168-overview [Accessed April, 2012].

1019. MYOTONIC DYSTROPHY SYNDROME (CURSCHMANN-STEINERT SYNDROME; DYSTROPHIA MYOTONICA; MYOTONIA ATROPHICA SYNDROME)

General

Rare, autosomal dominant disease; onset age about 20 years; condition is worsened by administration of neostigmine (Prostigmin); associated with an unstable DNA sequence composed of varying numbers of CTG triplet repeats (which allows a specific molecular test for this disorder).

Ocular

Mild ptosis (occasionally); myotonic cataract with small, dotlike subcapsular cortical opacities during early stage, with polychromatic properties on biomicroscopic examination; corneal epithelial dystrophy; loss of corneal sensitivity; tapetoretinal degeneration; macular red spot; macular degeneration; chorioretinitis; pilomatrixomas; ocular hypotony; pattern pigmentary changes; abnormal saccades.

Clinical

Progressive muscular atrophy with selection of certain muscles (mainly sternocleidomastoid, temporalis, dorsiflexor muscles of the ankle, anterior oblique); myotonia; blank facial expression; speech disturbance due to involvement of vocal cords and palatal muscles; dysphagia; endocrine disturbances.

Laboratory

Diagnosis is made by clinical findings.

Treatment

Ptosis: If visual acuity is affected most cases require surgical correction, and there are several procedures that may be used including levator resection, repair or advancement and Fasanella-Servat.

Cataract: Change in glasses can sometimes improve a patient's visual function temporarily; however, the most common treatment is cataract surgery.

Corneal dystrophy: Mild cases can be observed and soft contact lenses are helpful, penetrating keratoplasty may be necessary, graft recurrences treated by superficial keratectomy, phototherapeutic keratectomy or repeat penetrating keratoplasty.

Macular degeneration: No treatment is available for non-neovascular age-related macular degeneration (AMD). Preventative therapy includes no smoking, control of hypertension, cholesterol, and blood sugar, exercise and vitamins. Neovascular AMD treatment consists of laser, Avastin and Lucentis.

Bibliography

1. Brooke NM, Cwik VE. Myotonic dystrophy. In: Bradley WG et al. (Eds). Neurology in Clinical Practice, 2nd edition. Boston: Butterworth-Heinemann; 1995. pp. 2020-2.

2. Gjertsen IK, Sandvig KU, Eide N, et al. Recurrence of secondary opacification and development of a dense posterior vitreous membrane in patients with myotonic dystrophy. J Cataract Refract Surg. 2003;29:213-6.

3. Kimizuka Y, Kiyosawa M, Tamai M, et al. Retinal changes in myotonic dystrophy. Clinical and follow-up evaluation. Retina. 1993;13:129-35.

4. Koca MR, Horn F, Korth M. Alterations of saccadic eye movements in myotonic dystrophy. Graefes Arch Clin Exp Ophthalmol. 1992;230:437-41.

5. Kuwabara T, Lessell S. Electron microscopic study of extraocular muscles in myotonic dystrophy. Am J Ophthalmol. 1976;82:303-9.

6. Mausolf FA, Burns CA, Burian HM. Morphologic and functional retinal changes in myotonic dystrophy unrelated to quinine therapy. Am J Ophthalmol. 1972;74:1141-3.

7. Meyer E, Navon D, Auslender L, et al. Myotonic dystrophy: pathological study of the eyes. Ophthalmologica. 1980;181:215-20.

8. Reardon W, MacMillan JC, Myring J, et al. Cataract and myotonic dystrophy: the role of molecular diagnosis. Br J Ophthalmol. 1993;77:579-83.

9. Rosa N, Lanza M, Borrelli M, et al. Low intraocular pressure resulting from ciliary body detachment in patients with myotonic dystrophy. Ophthalmology. 2011;118:260-4.

1020. MYXOMAS, SPOTTY PIGMENTATION, AND ENDOCRINE OVERACTIVITY SYNDROME (CARNEY COMPLEX)

General

Autosomal dominant.

Ocular

Eyelid myxomas; pigmented lesions of the caruncle or conjunctival semilunar fold.

Clinical

Cardiac, cutaneous or mammary myxomas; acromegaly; adrenal, pituitary and testicular neoplasms; Cushing syndrome; sexual precocity; spotty skin pigmentation.

Laboratory

Diagnosis is made by clinical findings.

Treatment

Excision of lid myxomas.

Bibliography

1. Danoff A, Jormark S, Lorber D, et al. Adrenocortical micronodular dysplasia, cardiac myxomas, lentigines and spindle cell tumors. Report of a kindred. Arch Intern Med. 1987;147:443-8.

2. Kennedy RH, Waller RR, Carney JA. Ocular pigmented spots and eyelid myxomas. Am J Ophthalmol. 1987;104:533-8.
3. Koopman RJ, Happle R. Autosomal dominant transmission of the NAME syndrome (nevi, atrial myxoma, mucinosis of the skin and endocrine overactivity). Hum Genet. 1991;86:300-4.
4. McKusick VA. Mendelian Inheritance in Man: A Catalog of Human Genes and Genetic Disorders, 12th edition. Baltimore: The Johns Hopkins University Press; 1998.
5. McKusick-Nathans Institute for Genetic Medicine, Johns Hopkins University and National Center for Biotechnology Information, National Library of Medicine. (2007). Online Mendelian Inheritance in Man (OMIM). [online] Available from http://www.ncbi.nlm.nih.gov/omim/ [Accessed April, 2012].

1021. NAEGELI SYNDROME (FRANCESCHETTI-JADASSOHN SYNDROME; MELANOPHORIC NEVUS SYNDROME; NAEGELI INCONTINENTIA PIGMENTI; RETICULAR PIGMENTED DERMATOSIS)

General

Autosomal dominant; separate entity from incontinentia pigmenti (Bloch-Sulzberger syndrome) based on mode of inheritance; blisters and inflammatory lesions of skin as seen in incontinentia pigmenti not present in Naegeli syndrome; skin pigmentation appears at age 2 years.

Ocular

Nystagmus; strabismus; pseudoglioma; papillitis; optic atrophy.

Clinical

Reticular pigmentary skin changes; hypohidrosis; defective teeth with yellow spotting; keratoderma of palms and soles; disturbed regulation of temperature by reduction of number of sweat glands.

Laboratory

None

Treatment

Nystagmus: See-saw nystagmus—visual field to consider neoplastic or vascular etiologies. Upbeat nystagmus—may indicate multiple sclerosis, cerebellar degeneration, tumors or infarcts. Treatment is directed toward identification and resolution of underlying cause. Downbeat nystagmus—affects the cerebellum or craniocervical junction including Arnold-Chiari malformation, multiple sclerosis, trauma, tumor, infarction and many toxic metabolic entities. MRI may indicate a surgically correctable lesion. Periodic alternating nystagmus is continuous horizontal nystagmus from stroke, tumor, multiple sclerosis, trauma, infection and drug intoxication. Can occur from cataract, vitreous hemorrhage or optic atrophy.

Strabismus: Equalized vision with correct refractive error; surgery may be helpful in patient with diplopia.

Optic atrophy: Intravenous steroids may be used with optic neuritis or ischemic neuropathy. Stem cell treatment may be the future treatment of choice.

Additional Resource

1. Clifford RH (2010). Naegeli-Franceschetti-Jadassohn Syndrome. [online] Available from http://www.emedicine.com/derm/TOPIC736.HTM [Accessed April, 2012].

1022. NAFFZIGER SYNDROME (SCALENUS ANTICUS SYNDROME)

General

Compression of brachial plexus and subclavian artery by scalenus anticus muscle; symptoms vary from mild, with remissions and exacerbations, to severe.

Ocular

Enophthalmos; ptosis (unilateral); small pupil.

Clinical

Weakness of ipsilateral hand grip; reduced ipsilateral biceps reflex; diminution of pulse volume on affected side; numbness and coldness in hand and fingers.

Laboratory

Diagnosis is made by clinical findings.

Treatment

Ptosis: If visual acuity is affected most cases require surgical correction, and there are several procedures that may be used including levator resection, repair or advancement and Fasanella-Servat.

Bibliography

1. Aligne C, Barral X. Rehabilitation of patients with thoracic outlet syndrome. Ann Vasc Surg. 1992;6:381-9.
2. Atasoy E. Thoracic outlet compression syndrome. Orthop Clin North Am. 1996;27:265-303.
3. Davies AH, Walton J, Stuart E, et al. Surgical management of the thoracic outlet compression syndrome. Br J Surg. 1991;78:1193-5.
4. Geeraets WJ. Ocular Syndromes, 3rd edition. Philadelphia: Lea & Febiger; 1976.
5. Karas SE. Thoracic outlet syndrome. Clin Sports Med. 1990;9:297-310.
6. Naffziger HD. Quoted in: Ochsner A, Gage M, DeBakey M. Scalenus anticus (Naffziger) syndrome. Am J Surg. 1935;28:669-95.
7. Pfaltz CR, Richter HR. Syndrome of vertebrobasilar insufficiency. Etiology and pathogenesis of the cochleovestibular symptoms in cerebral circulation disorders. Arch Klin Exp Ohren Nasen Kehlkopfheilkd. 1969;193:190-200.

1023. NAGER SYNDROME (NAGER ACROFACIAL DYOSTOSIS)

General

Rare congenital syndrome characterized by mandibulofacial dyostosis with associated radial defects.

Ocular

Downward slanting palpebral fissures; absent eyelashes in the medial third of the lower lids.

Clinical

Mandibular and malar hypoplasia; dysplastic ears with conductive deafness; variable degrees of palatal clefting; upper limb malformation (often bilateral hand deformities).

Laboratory

Diagnosis is made by clinical findings.

Treatment

None/Ocular.

Bibliography

1. Danziger I, Brodsky L, Perry R, et al. Nager's acrofacial dysostosis. Case report and review of the literature. Int J Pediatr Otorhinolaryngol. 1990;20:225-40.

2. Friedman RA, Wood E, Pransky SM, et al. Nager acrofacial dysostosis: management of a difficult airway. Int J Pediatr Otorhinolaryngol. 1996;35: 69-72.

3. Pfeiffer RA, Stoess H. Acrofacial dysostosis (Nager syndrome): synopsis and report of a new case. Am J Med Genet. 1983;15:255-60.

1024. NANCE-HORAN SYNDROME

General

Rare; X-linked oculodental trait; occurs in both sexes; present from birth.

Ocular

Posterior sutural cataracts in females; zonular cataracts in males; decreased visual acuity; nystagmus; microcornea; punctate opacities of cornea; affected males have dense nuclear cataracts and frequently microcorneas; carrier females may show posterior Y sutural cataracts with small corneas and only slightly reduced vision.

Clinical

Dental anomalies, including supernumerary central incisors; short fourth metacarpals; diastemata in females.

Laboratory

Diagnosis is made by clinical findings.

Treatment

Cataract: Change in glasses can sometimes improve a patient's visual function temporarily; however, the most common treatment is cataract surgery.

Bibliography

1. Bixler D, Higgins M, Hartsfield J. The Nance-Horan syndrome: a rare X-linked ocular-dental trait with expression in heterozygous females. Clin Genet. 1984;26:30-5.

2. Horan MB, Billson FA. X-linked cataract and Hutchinsonian teeth. Aust Paediatr J. 1974;10: 98-102.

3. McKusick VA. Mendelian Inheritance in Man: A Catalog of Human Genes and Genetic Disorders, 12th edition. Baltimore: The Johns Hopkins University Press; 1998.

4. McKusick-Nathans Institute for Genetic Medicine, Johns Hopkins University and National Center for Biotechnology Information, National Library of Medicine. (2007). Online Mendelian Inheritance in Man (OMIM). [online] Available from http://www.ncbi.nlm.nih.gov/omim [Accessed April, 2012].

5. Nance WE, Warburg M, Bixler D, et al. Congenital sex-linked cataract, dental anomalies, and brachymetacarpalia. Birth Defects Orig Artic Ser. 1974;10:285-91.

6. van Dorp DB, Delleman JW. A family with X-chromosomal recessive congenital cataract, microphthalmia, a peculiar form of the ear and dental anomalies. J Pediatr Ophthalmol Strabismus. 1979;16:166-71.

1025. NARP SYNDROME

General

Neurogenic weakness (N), ataxia (A) and retinitis pigmentosa (RP) syndrome.

Ocular

Retinitis pigmentosa; bull's-eye maculopathy; salt-and-pepper retinopathy.

Clinical

NARP syndrome patients develop ataxia, weakness, and have retinitis pigmentosa, causing gradual visual field constriction.

Laboratory/Ocular

Diagnosis is made by clinical findings.

Treatment

Retinitis pigmentosa: Vitamin A 15,000 IU/day is thought to slow the decline of retinal function, dark sunglasses for outdoor use, surgery for cataract, genetic counseling.

Bibliography

1. Chowers I, Lerman-Sagie T, Elpeleg ON, et al. Cone and rod dysfunction in the NARP syndrome. Br J Ophthalmol. 1999;83:190-3.
2. Holt IJ, Harding AE, Petty RK, et al. A new mitochondrial disease associated with mitochondrial DNA heteroplasmy. Am J Hum Genet. 1990;46: 428-33.

1026. NASAL RETINAL NERVE FIBER LAYER ATTENUATION

General

Associated with the use of the antiepileptic drug, vigabatrin.

Clinical

Epilepsy, seizures.

Ocular

Visual field loss—severe bilateral and symmetric, "concentric" constriction of sudden/rapid but variable onset; deep and steeply bordered bilateral nasal annulus with a relative sparing of the temporal field.

Laboratory

Visual field testing and optical coherence tomography (OCT) testing.

Treatment

Visual field and OCT testing should be done routinely. 3.4 RNFL thickness can be used as a biomarker of vigabatrin toxicity and when that is noted vigabatrin should be stopped.

Bibliography

1. Lawthom C, Smith PE, Wild JM. Nasal retinal nerve fiber layer attenuation: a biomarker for vigabatrin toxicity. Ophthalmology. 2009;116: 565-71.
2. Hardus P, Verduin W, Berendschot T, et al. Vigabatrin: long-term follow-up of electrophysiology and visual field examinations. Acta Ophthalmol Scand. 2003;81:459-65.

1027. NEGATIVE ACCELERATION SYNDROME (HYDROSTATIC PRESSURE SYNDROME; SUPERSONIC BAILOUT SYNDROME)

General

At rapid deceleration, blood volume is shifted to the brain and face of the individual due to rapid elevation of intravascular blood pressure; the abrupt rise in hydrostatic pressure simultaneous with the decelerative force results in the signs of cerebral concussion, confusion, retrograde amnesia and circulatory shock.

Ocular

Periorbital edema; ecchymosis of lids; transient visual loss; subconjunctival hemorrhages; retinal hemorrhages and exudates; retinal arteriolar spasm.

Clinical

Mental confusion; shock; possible perforation of internal organs.

Laboratory

Diagnosis is made by clinical findings.

Treatment

None/Ocular.

Bibliography

1. Geeraets WJ. Ocular Syndromes, 3rd edition. Philadelphia: Lea & Febiger; 1976.

1028. NELSON SYNDROME

General

Caused by elevated, incompletely suppressible or nonsuppressible levels of circulating adrenocorticotropic hormone (ACTH) and possibly melanocyte-stimulating hormone; originally reported as hyperpigmentation with associated pituitary inactivity following bilateral adrenalectomy for Cushing syndrome; appears that age at the time of adrenalectomy is an important predictive factor for development of this disorder.

Ocular

Progressive visual deterioration; recurrent visual field defects with bilateral hemianopsia caused by a pituitary mass diagnosed as chromophobe adenoma.

Clinical

Hyperpigmentation; intermittent headaches.

Laboratory

Adrenocorticotropic hormone (ACTH) measurement, thyroid function test, prolactin measurement, growth hormone measurement, gonadotropin measurement, visual field test.

Treatment

Dopamine receptor agonist, radiotherapy, and surgery is the treatment of choice.

Additional Resource

1. Wilson TA (2012). Nelson Syndrome. [online] Available from http://www.emedicine.com/ped/TOPIC1558.HTM [Accessed April, 2012].

1029. NEMATODE OPHTHALMIA SYNDROME (TOXOCARIASIS; VISCERAL LARVA MIGRANS SYNDROME)

General

Usually found in children; invasion by larvae of *Toxocara canis* and *T. cati* of viscera and eyes; pronounced eosinophilia; as many as 30% of asymptomatic children demonstrate serologic evidence of prior Toxocara infestations.

Ocular

Leukocoria; uveitis; cataract; marked vitreous reaction with large floaters; choroiditis; large, cystlike white masses extending into vitreous; optic neuritis; papillitis; strabismus; hemorrhagic, exudative or granulomatous retinitis; retinal detachment; endophthalmitis; larvae present in the cornea.

Clinical

Hepatosplenomegaly; pulmonary infiltration; fever; cough; lack of appetite.

Laboratory

Eosinophilia in patients with visceral disease. ELISA test is best to document systemic or ocular infection with *T. canis*.

Treatment

Treatment is by case-by-case basis; in most cases no treatment is needed. Systemic anthelmintic agents. Vitrectomy may be necessary.

Bibliography

1. Biglan AW, Glickman LT, Lobes LA. Serum and vitreous Toxocara antibody in nematode endophthalmitis. Am J Ophthalmol. 1979;88: 898-901.
2. Roy FH, Fraunfelder FW, Fraunfelder FT. Roy and Fraunfelder's Current Ocular Therapy, 6th edition. Philadelphia: WB Saunders; 2008.
3. Maguire AM, Green WR, Michels RG, et al. Recovery of intraocular Toxocara canis by pars plana vitrectomy. Ophthalmology. 1990;97:675-80.
4. Raistrick ER, Hart JC. Ocular toxocariasis in adults. Br J Ophthalmol. 1976;60:365-70.
5. Wilder HC. Nematode endophthalmitis. Trans Am Acad Ophthalmol Otolaryngol. 1950;55:99-109.
6. Wilkinson CP. Ocular toxocariasis. In: Ryan SJ (Ed). Retina, 2nd edition. St. Louis: CV Mosby; 1994. pp. 1545-52.

1030. NEONATAL HEMOLYTIC DISEASE OF HYPERBILIRUBINEMIA (BILIRUBIN ENCEPHALOPATHY; KERNICTERUS)

General

Condition with severe neural symptoms associated with high levels of bilirubin in the blood.

Ocular

Disturbance of supranuclear vertical gaze; mild ocular motility defects; involuntary levator palpebrae inhibition.

Clinical

Athetosis; hearing loss; possible central nervous system (CNS) damage, characterized by deep yellow staining of the basal nuclei, globus pallidus, putamen and caudate nucleus, cerebellar and bulbar nuclei, and gray substance of the cerebrum.

Laboratory

Bilirubin levels.

Treatment

Consult hematologist.

Additional Resource

1. Springer SC (2010). Kernicterus. [online] Available from http://www.emedicine.com/ped/TOPIC1247.HTM [Accessed April, 2012].

1031. NEOVASCULARIZATION, CORNEAL, CONTACT LENS-RELATED

General

Pathologic state in which new blood vessels extending in the corneal stroma from trauma, inflammation, infection, toxic insults secondary to contact lens usage.

Clinical

None

Ocular

Vessel ingrowth into the cornea, ocular irritation.

Laboratory

Diagnosis is made by clinical findings.

Treatment

Observation, eliminate cause, topical steroid drops, reduce time individual uses contact lens, corneal laser photocoagulation.

Additional Resource

1. Weissman BA (2011). Neovascularization, Corneal, CL-related. [online] Available from http://www.emedicine.medscape.com/article/1195886-overview [Accessed April, 2012].

1032. NEPHROTIC SYNDROME (EPSTEIN SYNDROME; IDIOPATHIC NEPHROTIC SYNDROME; LIPOID NEPHROSIS)

General

Unknown etiology, although some connection seems to exist between use of various drugs (penicillamine, heavy metals, trimethadione) and certain disease entities, such as intercapillary glomerulosclerosis, renal vein thrombosis, renal amyloidosis and congestive heart failure; age at onset usually 1–6 years.

Ocular

Diffuse periorbital swelling; lid edema (mainly upper lids) more pronounced in the morning; uveitis; retinal edema around optic disk.

Clinical

Impaired renal function (depending on severity of renal involvement); anasarca (generalized and changing with time).

Laboratory

Diagnosis is made by clinical findings.

Treatment

Corticosteroids are frequently used.

Additional Resource

1. Cohen EP (2011). Nephrotic Syndrome. [online] Available from http://www.emedicine.com/med/TOPIC1612.HTM [Accessed April, 2012].

1033. NEU SYNDROME

General

Characterized by microcephaly, growth retardation and flexion deformities; both sexes affected; autosomal recessive; early death.

Ocular

Hypertelorism; absent eyelids.

Clinical

Flexion deformities; overlapping fingers; rocker-bottom feet; protruding heels; toe syndactyly; microcephaly; short neck; tiny nose; brain atrophy.

Laboratory

Diagnosis is made by clinical findings.

Treatment

Hypertelorism: It is treated with surgical procedure that involves orbital reconstruction.

Bibliography

1. Magalini SI, Scrascia E. Dictionary of Medical Syndromes, 2nd edition. Philadelphia: JB Lippincott; 1981.

1034. NEURILEMOMA (NEURINOMA; SCHWANNOMA)

General

Slow-growing encapsulated neoplasm from the Schwann cells of nerves; seen most frequently with patients with von Recklinghausen disease.

Ocular

Ptosis; exophthalmos; visual loss; pupillary dilation; lacrimal sac mass.

Clinical

Facial numbness; retro-orbital headaches; intermittent pain radiating from the distribution of the appropriate sensory nerve branch.

Laboratory

Computed tomography (CT) scan can characterize the tumor's size and extent. MRI has high sensitivity to define nature and invasiveness of the tumor. Orbital and ocular echography shows sharply outlined capsule, a well-defined central cystic space, slight compressibility and blood flow.

Treatment

Ptosis: If visual acuity is affected most cases require surgical correction, and there are several procedures that may be used including levator resection, repair or advancement and Fasanella-Servat.

Exophthalmos: Reversing the problem, which is causing the exophthalmos, is the treatment of choice and will minimize the ocular complications. Ocular lubricants are beneficial for control of the corneal exposure.

Additional Resource

1. Kao GF (2012). Dermatologic Manifestations of Neurilemmoma. [online] Available from http://www.emedicine.com/derm/TOPIC285.HTM [Accessed April, 2012].

1035. NEUROBLASTOMA

General

Highly malignant solid tumor arising from undifferentiated sympathetic neuroblasts of the adrenal medulla, sympathetic ganglia, ectopic adrenal and theoretically the ciliary ganglion; autosomal dominant.

Ocular

Ptosis; exophthalmos; optic atrophy; optic neuritis; papilledema; metastatic tumor of orbit; retinal hemorrhage; convergent strabismus; paralysis of sixth or seventh nerve; nonreactive pupil; primary differentiated neuroblastoma of the orbit also has been reported; tonic pupils; microphthalmia; choroidal metastases (rare); iris metastases (rare).

Clinical

Skeletal metastasis to the cranium.

Laboratory

Serum lactate dehydrogenase (LDH), ferritin, CBC, serum creatinine, liver function test, CT and MRI test, echocardiogram.

Treatment

Treatment is provided by a multidisciplinary team.

Additional Resource

1. Lacayo NJ (2010). Pediatric Neuroblastoma. [online] Available from http://www.emedicine.com/ped/TOPIC1570.HTM [Accessed April, 2012].

1036. NEUROCUTANEOUS SYNDROME

General

Triad of linear nevus sebaceous; seizures; mental retardation.

Ocular

Colobomas of irides and choroid; nystagmus; keratoconus; corneal vascularization; optic glioma; epibulbar choristomas; connective tissue nevi of the eyelids.

Clinical

Multiple nevi; seizures; mental retardation; failure to thrive; hydrocephalus; deformities of skull; lipoma of the cranium; alopecia of the scalp.

Laboratory

Diagnosis is made by clinical findings.

Treatment

Keratoconus: Spectacle correction, hard contacts and avoid eye rubbing may be useful. If hydrops occurs discontinue contact lens, use NaCl drops and ointment, patching and short course of steroids. As the disease advances penetrating keratoplasty, deep anterior lamellar keratoplasty, intacs with laser grooves or collagen stabilization of cornea.

Bibliography

1. Kodsi SR, Bloom KE, Egbert JE, et al. Ocular and systemic manifestations of encephalocraniocutaneous lipomatosis. Am J Ophthalmol. 1994;118: 77-82.
2. Kucukoduk S, Ozsan H, Turanli AY, et al. A new neurocutaneous syndrome: nevus sebaceous syndrome. Cutis. 1993;51:437-41.
3. Marden PM, Venters HD. A new neurocutaneous syndrome. Am J Dis Child. 1966;112:79-81.
4. Sato K, Kubota T, Kitai R. Linear sebaceous nevus syndrome (sebaceous nevus of Jadassohn) associated with abnormal neuronal migration and optic glioma: case report. Neurosurgery. 1994;35: 318-20.

1037. NEURODERMATITIS (LICHEN SIMPLEX CHRONICUS)

General

Skin altered due to chronic rubbing or scratching.

Ocular

Keratoconjunctivitis; lid edema; lid pigmentation; lid lichenification; atopic cataracts; keratoconus.

Clinical

Pruritus; dermatitis; seborrheic dermatitis; contact dermatitis; lichenification of skin; skin hyperpigmentation.

Laboratory

Serum immunoglobulin E level, potassium hydroxide examination, skin biopsy.

Treatment

Topical steroids are the treatment of choice.

Additional Resource

1. Hogan DJ (2010). Lichen Simplex Chronicus. [online] Available from http://www.emedicine.com/derm/TOPIC236.HTM [Accessed April, 2012].

1038. NEURONAL CEROID LIPOFUSCINOSIS (NEURONAL INTRANUCLEAR INCLUSION DISEASE (NIID))

General

Probably autosomal recessive.

Ocular

Nystagmus; sluggish pupil reaction; restricted ocular movements; optic disk pallor; loss of nerve fiber around macula; loss of pigment; widespread loss of photoreceptor function with abnormal electroretinogram.

Clinical

Slurred speech; extrapyramidal and lower motor neuron abnormalities; atrophy of skeletal muscles; bronchopneumonia; cerebral deterioration.

Laboratory

Diagnosis is made by clinical findings.

Treatment

Nystagmus: See-saw nystagmus—visual field to consider neoplastic or vascular etiologies. Upbeat nystagmus—may indicate multiple sclerosis, cerebellar degeneration, tumors or infarcts. Treatment is directed toward identification and resolution of underlying cause. Downbeat nystagmus—affects the cerebellum or craniocervical junction including Arnold-Chiari malformation, multiple sclerosis, trauma, tumor, infarction and many toxic metabolic entities. MRI may indicate a surgically correctable lesion. Periodic alternating nystagmus is continuous horizontal nystagmus from stroke, tumor, multiple sclerosis, trauma, infection and drug intoxication. Can occur from cataract, vitreous hemorrhage or optic atrophy.

Bibliography

1. Haltia M, Tarkkanen A, Somer H, et al. Neuronal intranuclear inclusion disease. Clinical ophthalmological features and ophthalmic pathology. Acta Ophthalmol (Copenh). 1986;64:637-43.
2. Michaud J, Gilbert JJ. Multiple system atrophy with neuronal intranuclear hyaline inclusions. Report of a new case with light and electron microscopic studies. Acta Neuropathol. 1981;54:113-9.
3. Patel H, Norman MG, Perry TL, et al. Multiple system atrophy with neuronal intranuclear hyaline inclusions. Report of a case and review of the literature. J Neurol Sci. 1985;67:57-65.
4. Weleber RG. Retinitis pigmentosa and allied disorders. In: Ryan SJ (Ed). Retina, St. Louis: CV Mosby; 1989.

1039. NEUROPARALYTIC KERATITIS (NEUROTROPHIC KERATITIS, TRIGEMINAL NEUROPATHIC KERATOPATHY)

General

Numbness of the cornea from injury of trigeminal nerve. Causes include surgery of trigeminal neuralgias, surgery of acoustic neuroma and herpes zoster ophthalmicus and Riley-Day syndrome.

Clinical

None

Ocular

Abnormalities of the tear film and punctate corneal keratopathy, epithelial detachment, stromal lysis.

Laboratory

Diagnosis is made by clinical findings.

Treatment

Stage 1: Punctate keratopathy—treated with intermittent patching. Oral tetracyclines and discontinuing contact lens may be helpful.

Stage 2: Epithelial detachment—atropine, Blenderm or temporary tarsorrhaphy. Inject botulism toxin into levator palpebrae superioris.

Stage 3: Closure of lid—atropine, botulism toxin, local antibiotics and systemic antibiotics. Permanent tarsorrhaphy.

Additional Resource

1. Graham RH (2012). Neurotrophic Keratopathy. [online] Available from http://www.emedicine.com/oph/TOPIC106.HTM [Accessed April, 2012].

1040. NEWCASTLE DISEASE (FOWLPOX)

General

Acquired directly by people handling chickens (see Parinaud Oculoglandular Syndrome); self-limiting conjunctivitis caused by a paramyxovirus.

Ocular

Acute follicular conjunctivitis, unilateral; keratitic precipitates; lid edema; decreased accommodation and visual acuity.

Clinical

Fatigue; fever; headache; pulmonary complications; preauricular lymphadenopathy.

Laboratory

Diagnosis is made by clinical findings.

Treatment

Topical antibiotics, cold compresses and artificial tears.

Bibliography

1. Roy FH, Fraunfelder FW, Fraunfelder FT. Roy and Fraunfelder's Current Ocular Therapy, 6th edition. Philadelphia: WB Saunders; 2008.
2. Gordon S. Viral keratitis and conjunctivitis. Adenovirus and other non-herpetic viral diseases. In: Smolin G, Thoft RA (Eds). The Cornea. Boston: Little, Brown and Company; 1994.
3. Pau H. Differential Diagnosis of Eye Diseases. New York: Thieme; 1987.

1041. NIACIN OVERDOSE (NICOTINIC ACID OVERDOSE)

General

Vitamin B used in large doses to lower serum cholesterol and triglyceride levels or as a vasodilator.

Ocular

Cystoid maculopathy without leakage on fluorescein angiography, usually resolves when patient stops taking niacin.

Clinical

Facial flushing; gastric irritation; liver function impairment.

Laboratory

Perform LFTs, uric acid levels and glucose levels.

Treatment

Supportive treatment as needed.

Additional Resource

1. Rosenbloom M (2011). Vitamin Toxicity. [online] Available from http://www.emedicine.com/emerg/TOPIC638.HTM [Accessed April, 2012].

1042. NICOLAU SYNDROME (NICOLAU-HOIGNE SYNDROME)

General

First described as a nonallergic reaction following injection of bismuth; assumed to be caused by emboli of medication inadvertently introduced into an artery.

Ocular

Visual loss, depending on degree of involvement of retinal arteries.

Clinical

Tachycardia; acoustic sensations; somnolence; motoric irritation; sudden pain in extremities and abdomen; pallor, cyanosis and edema of extremities; shock; paresis-paralysis; arterial hypotension.

Laboratory

Diagnosis is made by clinical findings.

Treatment

Retinal artery occlusion: Intraocular pressure lowering medications, carbogen therapy, hyperbaric oxygen. Vitrectomy may be necessary.

Bibliography

1. Geeraets WJ. Ocular Syndromes, 3rd edition. Philadelphia: Lea & Febiger; 1976.
2. Hoigne R. Akute Nebenreaktionen auf Pencillinpraparate. Acta Med Scand. 1962;171:201-8.
3. Nicolau S. Dermite Livedoide et Gangreneuse de la Fesse, Consecutive aux Injections Intramusculaires, dans la Syphilis. A Propos d'un Cas d'Embolie Arterielle Bismuthique. Ann Mal Vener (Paris). 1925;20:321.

1043. NIEDEN SYNDROME (TELANGIECTASIA-CATARACT SYNDROME)

General

Etiology unknown; familial occurrence; onset from birth.

Ocular

Sparse eyebrows; glaucoma; dyscoria; defects of iris mesenchyme; bilateral cataract (cortical or mature).

Clinical

Telangiectasia of face and upper extremities; pigmentary changes of the neck; thick, atrophic skin; heart enlargement; congenital valvular defect.

Laboratory

Diagnosis is made by clinical findings.

Treatment

Glaucoma: Its medication should be the first plan of action. If medication is unsuccessful, a filtering surgical procedure with or without antimetabolites may be beneficial.

Bibliography

1. Geeraets WJ. Ocular Syndromes, 3rd edition. Philadelphia: Lea & Febiger; 1976.
2. Nieden A. Cataractbildung bei Teleangiectatischer Ausdehnung der Capillaren der Ganzen Gesichtshaut. Zentbl Parkt Augenheilkd. 1887;11:353.
3. Petersen HP. Telangiectasis and cataract. Acta Ophthalmol. 1954;32:565-71.

1044. NIELSEN SYNDROME (EXHAUSTIVE PSYCHOSIS SYNDROME; NEUROMUSCULAR EXHAUSTION SYNDROME)

General

Chronic infections; postoperative phases frequently are associated with extreme stress and fatigue; similar manifestations often have been reported during and after prolonged combat; develops subacutely after severe overexertion during a period of euphoria.

Ocular

Paralysis of extraocular muscles; diplopia.

Clinical

Physical exhaustion; extreme weakness; delirium; fascicular twitching; poor attention; restlessness; lack of concentration; irritability; depression; anxiety; pain in muscles; weight loss; muscle flaccidity; absence of deep reflexes.

Laboratory

Diagnosis is made by clinical findings.

Treatment

Strabismus: Equalized vision with correct refractive error; surgery may be helpful in patient with diplopia.

Bibliography

1. Nielsen JM. Subacute generalized neuromuscular exhaustion syndrome: a report of three cases. Calif Med. 1947;66:338-40.
2. Strassman HD, Thaler MB, Schein EH. A prisoner of war syndrome: apathy as a reaction of severe stress. Am J Psychiatry. 1956;112:998-1003.

1045. NIEMANN-PICK SYNDROME (ESSENTIAL LIPOID HISTIOCYTOSIS; SEA-BLUE HISTIOCYTOSIS; SPHINGOMYELINASE DEFICIENCY)

General

Phospholipidosis with degeneration of ganglion cells of CNS and lipid storage involving entire reticuloendothelial system and parenchymatous tissue; autosomal recessive; occurs during first few months of life; similar to Tay-Sachs syndrome; predisposition for Jews (*see Tay-Sachs Syndrome*); lysosomal storage disease resulting from diminished activity or deficiency of sphingomyelinase.

Ocular

Vision may be reduced but usually not complete blindness; cherry-red spot of macula, similar to that of *Tay-Sachs syndrome*; progressive optic atrophy; supranuclear ophthalmoplegia; periorbital fullness; macular halo syndrome; abnormal visual evoked potentials.

Clinical

Mental retardation; extensive hepatosplenomegaly; epileptic seizures; progressive physical deterioration; deafness; skin pigmentation; abdominal enlargement.

Laboratory

Acid sphingomyelinase (ASM) activity in white blood cells.

Treatment

No treatment exists.

Additional Resource

1. Schwartz RA (2011). Dermatologic Manifestations of Niemann-Pick Disease. [online] Available from http://www.emedicine.com/derm/TOPIC699. HTM [Accessed April, 2012].

1046. NOCARDIOSIS

General

Aerobic *Actinomycetaceae* that may cause a chronic suppurative process; aerobic Gram-positive filamentous bacteria with branching pattern which resemble fungi.

Ocular

Conjunctivitis; keratitis; corneal ulcer; uveitis; lid involvement; orbital cellulitis; endophthalmitis; glaucoma; external ophthalmoplegia; scleritis; canaliculitis; preseptal cellulitis.

Clinical

Granuloma; draining sinuses; brain abscess; meningitis.

Laboratory

Gram-positive filamentous structures with an intermittent or a beaded staining pattern, weakly acid-fast. Organism culture from the infection (i.e. respiratory secretion, skin biopsies or aspirates from abscesses).

Treatment

Antimicrobial therapy is the treatment of choice.

Additional Resource

1. Greenfield RA (2011). Nocardiosis. [online] Available from http://www.emedicine.com/med/TOPIC1644.HTM [Accessed April, 2012].

1047. NONNE-MILROY-MEIGE DISEASE (BLEPHAROSPASM-OROMANDIBULAR DYSTONIA; CHRONIC HEREDITARY EDEMA; CHRONIC HEREDITARY TROPHEDEMA; CHRONIC TROPHEDEMA; CHRONIC HEREDITARY LYMPHEDEMA; CONGENITAL TROPHEDEMA; ELEPHANTIASIS ARABUM CONGENITA; ELEPHANTIASIS CONGENITA HEREDITARIA; FAMILIAL HEREDITARY EDEMA; HEREDITARY EDEMA; IDIOPATHIC HEREDITARY LYMPHEDEMA; MEIGE DISEASE; MEIGE-MILROY SYNDROME; MILROY DISEASE; NONNE-MILROY SYNDROME; OROMANDIBULAR DYSTONIA; PSEUDOEDEMATOUS HYPODERMAL HYPERTROPHY; PSEUDOELEPHANTIASIS NEUROARTHRITICA; TROPHOLYMPHEDEMA; TROPHONEUROSIS)

General

Autosomal dominant; prevalent in females; two types: (1) praecox—at birth to 35 years and (2) tarda—after age 35 years.

Ocular

Lid and conjunctival edema; blepharoptosis; distichiasis; strabismus; buphthalmos; ectropion.

Clinical

Lymphedema; mandibulofacial dysostosis; unilateral or bilateral edema of ankle ascending to the knee and eventually above; rough, pigmented skin over swollen parts.

Laboratory

None

Treatment

Prevention of infection and control local complications.

Additional Resource

1. Kiel RJ (2010). Milroy Disease. [online] Available from http://www.emedicine.com/med/TOPIC1482.HTM [Accessed April, 2012].

1048. NOONAN SYNDROME (MALE TURNER SYNDROME)

General

Similar to *Turner syndrome*, but with normal chromosomal analysis; X-linked dominant inheritance; X-linked dominant phenotype.

Ocular

Hypertelorism; exophthalmos; ptosis (unilateral or bilateral); antimongoloid-slanting palpebral fissure; myopia; keratoconus; optic disk coloboma.

Clinical

Valvular pulmonary stenosis; short stature; webbed neck; low hairline in the back; cubitus valgus; deformed chest wall; micrognathia; low-set ears; mild mental retardation.

Laboratory

Factor Xl deficiency, bleeding diathesis, karyotyping test, cardiac examination.

Treatment

Growth hormone therapy.

Additional Resource

1. Ibrahim J (2011). Noonan Syndrome. [online] Available from http://www.emedicine.com/ped/TOPIC1616.HTM [Accessed April, 2012].

1049. NORMAL-TENSION GLAUCOMA (LOW TENSION GLAUCOMA)

General

Normal intraocular pressure with progressive optic nerve changes and visual field changes. Seen more frequently in patients over 50 years old.

Clinical

None

Ocular

Normal intraocular pressure with cup/disk or visual field changes.

Laboratory

Diagnosis is made by clinical findings.

Treatment

Medical—glaucoma medications. Surgical—argon laser trabeculectomy, selective laser trabeculoplasty, trabeculectomy with or without antimetabolites, tube-shunt surgery and cyclodestructive procedures.

Bibliography

1. Roy FH, Fraunfelder FW, Fraunfelder FT. Roy and Fraunfelder's Current Ocular Therapy, 6th edition. Philadelphia: WB Saunders; 2008.

1050. NOTHNAGEL SYNDROME (OPHTHALMOPLEGIA-CEREBELLAR ATAXIA SYNDROME)

General

Lesion of superior cerebellar peduncle, red nucleus, and emerging oculomotor fibers, such as pineal tumor, or tumor or vascular disturbance in corpora quadrigemina or vermis cerebelli (*see Bruns Syndrome*).

Ocular

Oculomotor paresis; gaze paralysis most frequently upward, combined with some degree of internal or external ophthalmoplegia.

Clinical

Cerebellar ataxia; poor upper extremity movements; neoplasia; infarction; midbrain lesion.

Laboratory

Computed tomography (CT) and MRI of brain.

Treatment

Consult neurologist.

Bibliography

1. Magalini SI, Scrascia E. Dictionary of Medical Syndromes, 2nd edition. Philadelphia: JB Lippincott; 1981.

1051. NYSTAGMUS

General

A repetitive involuntary eye movement that often indicates an underlying ocular or neurologic disorder.

Ocular

Oscillopsia, vertical and/or torsional diplopia, superior oblique myokymia.

Clinical

Vertigo

Laboratory

Diagnosis is made by clinical findings.

Treatment

Nystagmus: See-saw nystagmus—visual field to consider neoplastic or vascular etiologies. Upbeat nystagmus—may indicate multiple sclerosis, cerebellar degeneration, tumors or infarcts. Treatment is directed toward identification and resolution of underlying cause. Downbeat nystagmus—affects the cerebellum or craniocervical junction including Arnold-Chiari malformation, multiple sclerosis, trauma, tumor, infarction and many toxic metabolic entities. MRI may indicate a surgically correctable lesion. Periodic alternating nystagmus is continuous horizontal nystagmus from stroke, tumor, multiple sclerosis, trauma, infection and drug intoxication. Can occur from cataract, vitreous hemorrhage or optic atrophy.

Additional Resources

1. Bardorf CM (2012). Acquired Nystagmus. [online] Available from http://www.emedicine.com/oph/TOPIC339.HTM [Accessed April, 2012].
2. Curtis T (2010). Nystagmus, Congenital. [online] Available from http://www.emedicine.com/oph/TOPIC688.HTM [Accessed April, 2012].

1052. NYSTAGMUS BLOCKAGE SYNDROME (NBS)

General

Congenital (see Ethan Syndrome, Primary; Ethan Syndrome Secondary; Nystagmus Compensation Syndrome); convergence is used to diminish nystagmus.

Ocular

Esotropia; nystagmus; amblyopia; most patients with this syndrome prefer to fixate with one eye, but others show alternating fixation.

Clinical

Abnormal head position.

Laboratory

Diagnosis is made by clinical findings.

Treatment

Nystagmus: See-saw nystagmus—visual field to consider neoplastic or vascular etiologies. Up-beat nystagmus—may indicate multiple sclerosis, cerebellar degeneration, tumors or infarcts. Treatment is directed toward identification and resolution of underlying cause. Downbeat nystagmus—affects the cerebellum or craniocervical junction including Arnold-Chiari malformation, multiple sclerosis, trauma, tumor, infarction and many toxic metabolic entities. MRI may indicate a surgically correctable lesion. Periodic alternating nystagmus is continuous horizontal nystagmus from stroke, tumor, multiple sclerosis, trauma, infection and drug intoxication. Can occur from cataract, vitreous hemorrhage or optic atrophy.

Bibliography

1. Isenberg SJ, Yee RD. The Ethan syndrome. Ann Ophthalmol. 1986;18:358-61.
2. von Noorden GK, Avilla CW. Nystagmus blockage syndrome revisited. In: Reinecke RD (Ed). Strabismus II. New York: Grune & Stratton; 1984. pp. 75-82.
3. Miller NR (Ed). Walsh and Hoyt's Clinical Neuro-Ophthalmology, 4th edition. Baltimore: Williams & Wilkins; 1985. p. 897.

1053. NYSTAGMUS COMPENSATION SYNDROME (NCS)

General

Congenital *(see Ethan Syndrome, Primary; Ethan Syndrome, Secondary; Nystagmus Blockage Syndrome).*

Ocular

Esotropia; amblyopia; onset may be preceded by manifest nystagmus; abnormal head posture toward the adducted fixing eye; nystagmus reduced or absent, with the fixing eye adducted.

Clinical

Abnormal head position.

Laboratory

Diagnosis is made by clinical findings.

Treatment

Strabismus: Equalized vision with correct refractive error; surgery may be helpful in patient with diplopia.

Bibliography

1. Frank JW. Diagnostic signs in the nystagmus compensation syndrome. J Pediatr Ophthalmol Strabismus. 1979;16:317-20.
2. von Noorden GK. The nystagmus compensation (blockage) syndrome. Am J Ophthalmol. 1976;82: 283-90.

1054. NYSTAGMUS, CONGENITAL (CONGENITAL IDIOPATHIC NYSTAGMUS)

General

Autosomal dominant; pattern of inheritance in congenital nystagmus, whether of the "motor" or "sensory" type, may be autosomal dominant, recessive or sex-linked.

Ocular

Vertical and horizontal nystagmus; this nystagmus occasionally is vertical or torsional; in addition, periodic alternating, downbeat and see-saw nystagmus may be present at birth; normal electroretinogram.

Clinical

None

Laboratory

None

Treatment

Baclofen, gabapentin, retrobulbar injection of botulinum toxin.

Additional Resource

1. Curtis T (2010). Nystagmus, Congenital. [online] Available from http://www.emedicine.com/oph/ TOPIC688.HTM [Accessed April, 2012].

1055. NYSTAGMUS, HEREDITARY VERTICAL

General

Autosomal dominant.

Ocular

Motor type vertical and horizontal nystagmus; hyperactive vestibulo-ocular response; strabismus.

Clinical

Mild ataxia; poor line walking.

Laboratory

Diagnosis is made by clinical findings.

Treatment

Strabismus: Equalized vision with correct refractive error; surgery may be helpful in patient with diplopia.

Bibliography

1. Marmor MF. Hereditary vertical nystagmus. Arch Ophthalmol. 1973;90:107-11.
2. McKusick VA. Mendelian Inheritance in Man: A Catalog of Human Genes and Genetic Disorders, 12th edition. Baltimore: The Johns Hopkins University Press; 1998.
3. McKusick-Nathans Institute for Genetic Medicine, Johns Hopkins University and National Center for Biotechnology Information, National Library of Medicine. (2007). Online Mendelian Inheritance in Man (OMIM). [online] Available from http://www.ncbi.nlm.nih.gov/omim [Accessed April, 2012].

1056. NYSTAGMUS, PRIMARY HEREDITARY (CONGENITAL NYSTAGMUS)

General

Autosomal recessive, sex-linked or irregular dominant; may be associated with albinism.

Ocular

Horizontal nystagmus; myopia.

Clinical

Head spasms; carpopedal spasms (Trousseau sign); Chvostek sign.

Laboratory

Diagnosis is made by clinical findings.

Treatment

Nystagmus: See-saw nystagmus—visual field to consider neoplastic or vascular etiologies. Up-beat nystagmus—may indicate multiple sclerosis, cerebellar degeneration, tumors or infarcts. Treatment is directed toward identification and resolution of underlying cause. Downbeat nystagmus—affects the cerebellum or craniocervical junction including Arnold-Chiari malformation, multiple sclerosis, trauma, tumor, infarction and many toxic metabolic entities. MRI may indicate a surgically correctable lesion. Periodic alternating nystagmus is continuous horizontal nystagmus from stroke, tumor, multiple sclerosis, trauma, infection and drug intoxication. Can occur from cataract, vitreous hemorrhage or optic atrophy.

Bibliography

1. Allen M. Primary hereditary nystagmus: case study with genealogy. J Hered. 1942;33:454-6.
2. Gutmann DH, Brooks ML, Emanuel BS, et al. Congenital nystagmus in a (40,XX/45,X) mosaic woman from a family with X-linked congenital nystagmus. Am J Med Genet. 1991;39:167-9.
3. Lavin PJM. Congenital nystagmus. In: Bradley WG (Ed). Neurology in Clinical Practice, 2nd edition. Boston: Butterworth-Heinemann; 1995. p. 200.
4. McKusick VA. Mendelian Inheritance in Man: A Catalog of Human Genes and Genetic Disorders, 12th edition. Baltimore: The Johns Hopkins University Press; 1998.
5. McKusick-Nathans Institute for Genetic Medicine, Johns Hopkins University and National Center for Biotechnology Information, National Library of Medicine. (2007). Online Mendelian Inheritance in Man (OMIM). [online] Available from http://www.ncbi.nlm.nih.gov/omim [Accessed April, 2012].
6. Stromberg A, Pavan-Langston D. Extraocular muscles, strabismus, and nystagmus. In: Pavan-Langston D (Ed). Nystagmus: Manual of Ocular Diagnosis and Therapy, 4th edition. Boston: Little, Brown and Company; 1995. pp. 333-6.

Additional Resource

1. Curtis T (2010). Nystagmus, Congenital. [online] Available from http://www.emedicine.com/oph/TOPIC688.HTM [Accessed April, 2012].

1057. NYSTAGMUS, VOLUNTARY

General

Autosomal dominant; usually is purely horizontal, but it may be vertical or torsional.

Ocular

Voluntary rapid to-and-fro synchronous movements of eyes.

Clinical

Simultaneous head tremor has been associated with this condition.

Laboratory

Diagnosis is made by clinical findings.

Treatment

None/Ocular.

Bibliography

1. Keyes MJ. Voluntary nystagmus in two generations. Arch Neurol. 1973;29:63-4.
2. Lee J, Gresty M. A case of "voluntary nystagmus" and head tremor. J Neurol Neurosurg Psychiatry. 1993;56:1321-2.
3. McKusick VA. Mendelian Inheritance in Man: A Catalog of Human Genes and Genetic Disorders, 12th edition. Baltimore: The Johns Hopkins University Press; 1998.
4. McKusick-Nathans Institute for Genetic Medicine, Johns Hopkins University and National Center for Biotechnology Information, National Library of Medicine. (2007). Online Mendelian Inheritance in Man (OMIM). [online] Available from http://www.ncbi.nlm.nih.gov/omim [Accessed April, 2012].
5. Miller NR (Ed). Walsh and Hoyt's Clinical Neuro-Ophthalmology, 4th edition. Baltimore: Williams & Wilkins; 1985. p. 4554.

1058. OBESITY-CEREBRAL-OCULAR-SKELETAL ANOMALIES SYNDROME

General

Rare, autosomal recessive disease; similar to *Prader-Willi* and *Laurence-Moon-Bardet-Biedl* syndromes.

Ocular

Microphthalmia; antimongoloid slant of lid fissure; asymmetrical size of fissure; strabismus; myopia; iris and chorioretinal colobomata; mottled retina; prominent choroidal vessels.

Clinical

Obesity (mid-childhood onset); hypotonia; mental retardation; craniofacial anomalies with microcephaly; tapering extremities; hyperextensibility at elbows and proximal interphalangeal joints; cubitus valgus; genu valgum; simian creases; syndactyly.

Laboratory

Diagnosis is made by clinical findings.

Treatment

Strabismus: Equalized vision with correct refractive error; surgery may be helpful in patient with diplopia.

Bibliography

1. Cohen MM, Hall BD, Smith DW, et al. A new syndrome with hypotonia, obesity, mental deficiency, and facial, oral, ocular, and limb anomalies. J Pediatr. 1973;83:280-4.
2. Hall BD, Smith DW. Prader-Willi syndrome. A resumé of 32 cases including an instance of affected first cousins, one of whom is of normal stature and intelligence. J Pediatr. 1972;81:286-93.

1059. OCULAR DOMINANCE

General

Autosomal dominant; 97% of people with normal vision have a sighting-dominant eye; experimental data suggest a relationship between eye dominance and head tilt.

Ocular

Sighting-dominant eye.

Clinical

None

Laboratory

Diagnosis is made by clinical findings.

Treatment

None/Ocular.

Bibliography

1. McKusick VA. Mendelian Inheritance in Man: A Catalog of Human Genes and Genetic Disorders, 12th edition. Baltimore: The Johns Hopkins University Press; 1998.
2. McKusick-Nathans Institute for Genetic Medicine, Johns Hopkins University and National Center for Biotechnology Information, National Library of Medicine. (2007). Online Mendelian Inheritance in Man (OMIM). [online] Available from http://www.ncbi.nlm.nih.gov/omim [Accessed April, 2012].
3. Previc FH. The relationship between eye dominance and head tilt in humans. Neuropsychologia. 1994;32:1297-303.
4. Zoccolotti P. Inheritance of ocular dominance. Behav Genet. 1978;8:377-9.

1060. OCULAR HYPERTENSION

General

Elevated intraocular pressure without any evidence of glaucomatous optic neuropathy.

Clinical

None

Ocular

Normal eye examination with elevated intraocular pressure.

Laboratory

Diagnosis is made by clinical findings.

Treatment

If abnormalities occur in cup/disk ratio or visual field with serial examinations start on monotherapy as topical beta-blocker.

Additional Resource

1. Bell JA (2012). Ocular Hypertension. [online] Available from http://www.emedicine.com/oph/TOPIC578.HTM [Accessed April, 2012].

1061. OCULAR HYPOTONY

General

Low intraocular pressure resulting in anatomical or functional abnormalities to the eye.

Clinical

None

Ocular

Thin corneas, corneal striae, aqueous flare, choroidal folds, effusion, macular folds, low IOP.

Laboratory

Diagnosis is made by clinical findings.

Treatment

Topical corticosteroids and cycloplegic agents.

Bibliography

1. Roy FH, Fraunfelder FW, Fraunfelder FT. Roy and Fraunfelder's Current Ocular Therapy, 6th edition. Philadelphia: WB Saunders; 2008.

1062. OCULAR MYOPATHY WITH CURARE SENSITIVITY

General

Autosomal recessive.

Ocular

Static ophthalmoparesis.

Clinical

Limb weakness; sensitivity to tubocurarine.

Laboratory

Diagnosis is made by clinical findings.

Treatment

Omit curare.

Bibliography

1. Mathew NT, Jacob JC, Chandy J. Familial ocular myopathy with curare sensitivity. Arch Neurol. 1970;22:68-74.
2. McKusick VA. Mendelian Inheritance in Man: A Catalog of Human Genes and Genetic Disorders, 12th edition. Baltimore: The Johns Hopkins University Press; 1998.
3. McKusick-Nathans Institute for Genetic Medicine, Johns Hopkins University and National Center for Biotechnology Information, National Library of Medicine. (2007). Online Mendelian Inheritance in Man (OMIM). [online] Available from http://www.ncbi.nlm.nih.gov/omim [Accessed April, 2012].

1063. OCULAR TOXOPLASMOSIS
(TOXOPLASMIC RETINOCHOROIDITIS; TOXOPLASMOSIS)

General

Parasite infestation caused by *Toxoplasma gondii*; cell-mediated immunity is believed to be the major defense mechanism against *Toxoplasma* infection; ocular toxoplasmosis occurs in approximately 1% of patients with acquired immunodeficiency syndrome (AIDS); AIDS-related toxoplasma retinochoroiditis may have several atypical clinical manifestations.

Ocular

Keratitis; uveitis; optic atrophy; papillitis; anisocoria; persistent pupillary membrane; focal retinochoroiditis; scleritis; cataract; microphthalmos; myopia; nystagmus; esotropia.

Clinical

Cysts are seen in many organs, including brain and muscle; hydrocephalus; intracerebral calcification; various CNS complaints.

Laboratory

Serologic tests for anti-*T. gondii* antibiodies are common.

Treatment

Triple drug therapy pyrimethamine, sulfadiazine and prednisone. Pyrimethamine should be combined with folinic acid, surgical care including photocoagulation, cryotherapy or vitrectomy.

Bibliography

1. Lasave AF, Díaz-Llopis M, Muccioli C, et al. Intravitreal clindamycin and dexamethasone for zone 1 toxoplasmic retinochoroiditis at twenty-four months. Ophthalmology. 2010;117:1831-8.
2. Soheilian M, Ramezani A, Azimzadeh A, et al. Randomized trial of intravitreal clindamycin and dexamethasone versus pyrimethamine, sulfadiazine, and prednisolone in treatment of ocular toxoplasmosis. Ophthalmology. 2011;118:134-41.

Additional Resource

1. Wu L (2011). Ophthalmologic Manifestations of Toxoplasmosis. [online] Available from http://www.emedicine.com/oph/TOPIC707.HTM [Accessed April, 2012].

1064. OCULAR VACCINIA

General

Occurs from virus used for smallpox vaccination; transferred from vaccination site to eye.

Ocular

Chemosis; nonfollicular, catarrhal or purulent conjunctivitis; punctate epithelial keratitis; corneal vascularization; lid edema; vesicles of lid; uveitis; choroiditis; extraocular muscle palsies; optic neuritis; orbital cellulitis; ocular vaccinia may mimic signs of herpes simplex virus, varicella-zoster virus and acanthamoeba keratitis.

Clinical

Dermatitis; encephalitis.

Laboratory

Conjunctival scraping Gram stain, culture on blood agar for other bacteria.

Treatment

Treatment is determind by specific type of conjunctivitis.

Additional Resource

1. Lee JJ (2012). Vaccinia. [online] Available from http://www.emedicine.com/med/TOPIC2356.HTM [Accessed April, 2012].

1065. OCULO-OROGENITAL SYNDROME (GOPALAN II SYNDROME; JOLLIFFE SYNDROME; RIBOFLAVIN DEFICIENCY SYNDROME)

General

Vitamin B deficiency and possible vitamin A deficiency; prognosis good with diet therapy.

Ocular

Conjunctivitis, varying from mild to severe; keratitis; optic atrophy; corneal vascularization.

Clinical

Stomatitis; glossitis; scrotal dermatitis with pruritus, erythema, erythema of pharynx and soft palate; small sensitive ulcers of buccal membranes; diarrhea; fatigue; muscular weakness; painful feet with erythema, exfoliation and ulceration; burning; itching; mental depression; dizziness; oral mucosa becomes pale and macerated with fissuring of skin.

Laboratory

Red blood cell (RBC) glutathione reductase activity levels.

Treatment

Vitamin B2.

Additional Resource

1. Baker MZ (2011). Riboflavin Deficiency. [online] Available from http://www.emedicine.com/med/TOPIC2031.HTM [Accessed April, 2012].

1066. OCULO-OSTEOCUTANEOUS SYNDROME

General

Autosomal recessive.

Ocular

Strabismus; myopia; distichiasis; nystagmus; lenticular opacities.

Clinical

Short stature; brachydactyly; hypoplastic maxilla; scanty hair; hypopigmentation; mental retardation.

Laboratory/Ocular

Diagnosis is made by clinical findings.

Treatment

Cataract: Change in glasses can sometimes improve a patient's visual function temporarily; however, the most common treatment is cataract surgery.

Strabismus: Equalized vision with correct refractive error; surgery may be helpful in patient with diplopia.

Nystagmus: See-saw nystagmus—visual field to consider neoplastic or vascular etiologies. Upbeat nystagmus—may indicate multiple sclerosis, cerebellar degeneration, tumors or infarcts. Treatment is directed toward identification and resolution of underlying cause. Downbeat nystagmus—affects the cerebellum or craniocervical junction including Arnold-Chiari malformation, multiple sclerosis, trauma, tumor, infarction and many toxic metabolic entities. MRI may indicate a surgically correctable lesion. Periodic alternating nystagmus is continuous horizontal nystagmus from stroke, tumor, multiple sclerosis, trauma, infection and drug intoxication. Can occur from cataract, vitreous hemorrhage or optic atrophy.

Bibliography

1. McKusick VA. Mendelian Inheritance in Man: A Catalog of Human Genes and Genetic Disorders, 12th edition. Baltimore: The Johns Hopkins University Press; 1998.
2. McKusick-Nathans Institute for Genetic Medicine, Johns Hopkins University and National Center for Biotechnology Information, National Library of Medicine. (2007). Online Mendelian Inheritance in Man (OMIM). [online] Available from http://www.ncbi.nlm.nih.gov/omim [Accessed April, 2012].
3. Tuomaala P, Haapanen E. Three siblings with similar anomalies in the eyes, bones and skin. Acta Ophthalmol. 1968;46:365-71.

1067. OCULO-OTO-ORO-RENO-ERYTHROPOIETIC DISEASE

General

Etiology unknown; slowly progressive course; ocular lesions similar to those of tuberous sclerosis, but no other signs of that disorder.

Ocular

Exotropia; progressive visual loss to complete blindness; secondary glaucoma with iris bombe; iridocyclitis; chronic uveitis; vitreous opacities; cataract; retinal hemorrhages and exudates.

Clinical

Anemia; atypical development of periodontia and teeth with caries; high-arched palate; abdominal colic; genu valgum and pectus excavatum; dizziness.

Laboratory

Diagnosis is made by clinical findings.

Treatment

Glaucoma: Its medication should be the first plan of action. If medication is unsuccessful, a filtering surgical procedure with or without antimetabolites may be beneficial.

Uveitis: Topical steroids and cycloplegic medication should be the initial treatment of choice. Oral steroids if not responsive to topical steroids, immunosuppressants if bilateral disease that does not respond to oral steroids, periocular steroids for unilateral or posterior uveitis. Vitrectomy can be used for severe vitreous opacification. Cryotherapy and laser photocoagulation may be used for localized pars plana exudates.

Cataract: Change in glasses can sometimes improve a patient's visual function temporarily; however, the most common treatment is cataract surgery.

Bibliography

1. Jacobsen CD, Brodwall EK. A Clinical syndrome with inborn defect in erythropoiesis, dysplastic kidneys, eye lesions, malformation of the teeth and impaired hearing. A new syndrome in a 28-year-old woman. Acta Med Scand. 1974;195:230-5.
2. McCance RA, Matheson WJ, Gresham GA, et al. The cerebro-ocular-renal dystrophies: a new variant. Arch Dis Child. 1960;35:240-9.

1068. OCULOCEREBELLAR TEGMENTAL SYNDROME

General

Vascular lesion of mesencephalon with softening in peduncular area.

Ocular

Paralysis of associated ocular movements (internuclear anterior ophthalmoplegia).

Clinical

Sudden onset of hemiplegia with rapid recovery; bilateral cerebellar syndrome.

Laboratory

Diagnosis is made by clinical findings.

Treatment

Treat vascular lesion.

Bibliography

1. Fournier A, Ducoulombier H, Cousin J, et al. Oculo-cerebello-myoclonic syndrome and neuroblastoma. J Sci Med Lille. 1972;90:189-97.

2. Rodriquez B et al. A new type of peduncular syndrome: internuclear ophthalmoplegia and bilateral cerebellar syndrome from a tegmental lesion. Arch Urug Med. 1945;10:353, Am J Ophthalmol. 1946;29:511.

1069. OCULOCEREBRAL SYNDROME WITH HYPOPIGMENTATION (AMISH OCULOCEREBRAL SYNDROME; CROSS SYNDROME)

General

Autosomal recessive.

Ocular

Spastic ectropion; microphthalmos; enophthalmos; microcornea; corneal opacification; corneal vascularization; palpebral conjunctival injection; narrow lid fissures; aniridia; nystagmus; bilateral optic atrophy.

Clinical

Spastic diplegia; cutaneous hypopigmentation; mental retardation; hypogonadism; growth retardation; developmental defects of the CNS, such as cystic malformation of the posterior fossa of the Dandy-Walker type.

Laboratory

Diagnosis is made by clinical findings.

Treatment

There is no known treatment.

Bibliography

1. Cross HE, McKusick VA, Breen W. A new oculocerebral syndrome with hypopigmentation. J Pediatr. 1967;70:398-406.

2. De Jong G, Fryns JP. Oculocerebral syndrome with hypopigmentation (Cross syndrome): the mixed pattern of hair pigmentation as an important diagnostic sign. Genet Couns. 1991;2:151-5.

3. Lerone M, Pessagno A, Taccone A, et al. Oculocerebral syndrome with hypopigmentation (Cross syndrome): report of a new case. Clin Genet. 1992; 41:87-9.

4. Pinsky L, Digeorge AM, Harley RD, et al. Microphthalmos, corneal opacity, mental retardation, and spastic cerebral palsy: an oculocerebral syndrome. J Pediatr. 1965;67:387-98.

1070. OCULOCEREBROCUTANEOUS SYNDROME (DELLEMAN SYNDROME)

General

Congenital; possibly autosomal recessive or a result of an environmental problem; Dutch descent appears to be a predisposing factor; in most cases, involvement is unilateral, with left to right 2:1.

Ocular

Orbital cyst; absence of orbital structures; microphthalmos; anophthalmia.

Clinical

Cerebral malformations; focal dermal hypoplasia; aplasia; epilepsy; developmental delay; cranial skin appendages; cutaneous punched-out lesions.

Laboratory/Ocular

Diagnosis is made by clinical findings.

Treatment/Ocular

Orbital expansion with serial implants in the growing orbit, increase horizontal length of palpebral fissure, dermis fat graft, inflatable silicone expander.

Bibliography

1. Delleman JW, Oorthuys JW, Bleeker-Wagemakers EM, et al. Orbital cyst in addition to congenital cerebral and focal dermal malformations: a new entity. Clin Genet. 1984;25:470-2.
2. Hoo JJ, Kapp-Simon K, Rollnick B, et al. Oculocerebrocutaneous (Delleman) syndrome: a pleiotropic disorder affecting ectodermal tissues with unilateral predominance. Am J Med Genet. 1991;40:290-3.

1071. OCULODENTAL SYNDROME (PETERS SYNDROME; RUTHERFORD SYNDROME)

General

Similar to *Rieger syndrome* and *Meyer-Schwickerath-Weyer syndrome*; Peters syndrome inherited as autosomal recessive with defect of corneogenetic mesoderm characterized by incomplete separation of lens vesicle, causing central opacities of cornea, shallow anterior chamber, synechiae and remnants of pupillary membrane; anterior pole cataract; Rutherford syndrome inherited as autosomal dominant; exhibits iris and dental anomalies and mental retardation.

Ocular

High myopia; corneoscleral staphyloma; aniridia; macrocornea; opacities of the corneal margin; ectopia lentis with deposits of pigment; macular pigmentation; large excavation of optic nerve with atrophy.

Clinical

Oligodontia; microdontia; hypoplasia of enamel; abnormal tooth positions; hypertrophy of gums; failure of tooth eruption.

Treatment

Consult an oral health specialist.

Bibliography

1. Houston IB. Rutherford's syndrome: a familial oculo-dental disorder and electrophysiological study. Acta Paediatr Scand. 1966;55:233-8.
2. McKusick VA. Mendelian Inheritance in Man: A Catalog of Human Genes and Genetic Disorders, 12th edition. Baltimore: The Johns Hopkins University Press; 1998.
3. McKusick-Nathans Institute for Genetic Medicine, Johns Hopkins University and National Center for Biotechnology Information, National Library of Medicine. (2007). Online Mendelian Inheritance in Man (OMIM). [online] Available from http://www.ncbi.nlm.nih.gov/omim [Accessed April, 2012].
4. Peters A. Uber Angeborene Defektbildung der Descemetschen Membran. Klin Monatsbl Augenheilkd. 1906;44:27-40.
5. Reisner SH, Kott E, Bornstein B, et al. Oculodentodigital dysplasia. Am J Dis Child. 1969;118:600-7.
6. Rutherford ME. Three generations of inherited dental defects. Br Med J. 1931;2:9-11.

1072. OCULOGASTROINTESTINAL MUSCULAR DYSTROPHY

General

Autosomal recessive; visceral myopathy with external ophthalmoplegia; intestinal pseudo-obstruction with external ophthalmoplegia.

Ocular

Ptosis; ophthalmoplegia.

Clinical

Chronic diarrhea; abdominal distention; diffuse abdominal pain; impaired motility of the lower esophagus; demyelinating and axonal neuropathy with focal spongiform degeneration of the posterior columns; proximal muscle weakness and atrophy; primary myopathy of the smooth muscles of the stomach and intestine; dilated duodenum and jejunum; recurrent intestinal obstruction in childhood or adolescence.

Laboratory/Ocular

Diagnosis is made by clinical findings.

Treatment

Ptosis: If visual acuity is affected most cases require surgical correction, and there are several procedures that may be used including levator resection, repair or advancement and Fasanella-Servat.

Bibliography

1. Alstead EM, Murphy MN, Flanagan AM, et al. Familial autonomic visceral myopathy with degeneration of muscularis mucosae. J Clin Pathol. 1988;41:424-9.
2. Ionasescu V. Oculogastrointestinal muscular dystrophy. Am J Med Genet. 1983;15:103-12.
3. McKusick VA. Mendelian Inheritance in Man: A Catalog of Human Genes and Genetic Disorders, 12th edition. Baltimore: The Johns Hopkins University Press; 1998.
4. McKusick-Nathans Institute for Genetic Medicine, Johns Hopkins University and National Center for Biotechnology Information, National Library of Medicine. (2007). Online Mendelian Inheritance in Man (OMIM). [online] Available from http://www.ncbi.nlm.nih.gov/omim [Accessed April, 2012].

1073. OCULOMOTOR PARALYSIS (THIRD NERVE PALSY)

General

Congenital or acquired may occur in association with trochlear nerve palsy.

Clinical

Diabetes, neurological.

Ocular

Exotropia, hypotropia, diplopia, paralysis of the ciliary muscles and iris sphincter, dilated pupil, blepharoptosis, pseudoptosis.

Laboratory

Diagnosis is made by clinical findings.

Treatment

Prism therapy, surgical—muscle surgery on the affected muscle, occlusion of the involved eye to relieve diplopia.

Additional Resource

1. Goodwin J (2012). Oculomotor Nerve Palsy. [online] Available from http://www.emedicine.com/oph/TOPIC183.HTM [Accessed April, 2012].

1074. OCULOPALATOCEREBRAL DWARFISM (OPC DWARFISM)

General

Autosomal recessive; persistent hyperplastic primary vitreous.

Ocular

Persistent hypertrophic primary vitreous; microphthalmos; leukocoria; retrolental fibrovascular membrane.

Clinical

Microcephaly; mental retardation; spasticity; cleft palate; short stature.

Laboratory

Diagnosis is made by clinical findings.

Treatment

Persistent hyperplastic primary vitreous: Monocular congenital cataract surgery and amblyopia therapy. Posterior transciliary for pars plana vitrectomy and removal of tissue.

Bibliography

1. Frydman M, Kauschansky A, Leshem I, et al. Oculo-palato-cerebral dwarfism: a new syndrome. Clin Genet. 1985;27:414-9.
2. McKusick VA. Mendelian Inheritance in Man: A Catalog of Human Genes and Genetic Disorders, 12th edition. Baltimore: The Johns Hopkins University Press; 1998.
3. McKusick-Nathans Institute for Genetic Medicine, Johns Hopkins University and National Center for Biotechnology Information, National Library of Medicine. (2007). Online Mendelian Inheritance in Man (OMIM). [online] Available from http://www.ncbi.nlm.nih.gov/omim [Accessed April, 2012].

1075. OCULOPHARYNGEAL SYNDROME (OCULOPHARYNGEAL MUSCULAR DYSTROPHY; PROGRESSIVE MUSCULAR DYSTROPHY WITH PTOSIS AND DYSPHAGIA)

General

Etiology unknown; autosomal dominant inheritance; no CNS pathology; muscles of pharynx, hypopharynx and proximal third of esophagus involved with myopathy; onset late in life; progressive hereditary myopathy in which the levator palpebrae and pharyngeal muscles are selectively involved; progressive usually symmetrical blepharoptosis with or without dysphagia appears in the fifth decade of life.

Ocular

Ptosis

Clinical

Dysphagia; occasionally, weakness of facial muscles.

Laboratory/Ocular

Diagnosis is made by clinical findings.

Treatment

Ptosis: If visual acuity is affected most cases require surgical correction, and there are several procedures that may be used including levator resection, repair or advancement and Fasanella-Servat.

Bibliography

1. Codere F. Oculopharyngeal muscular dystrophy. Can J Ophthalmol. 1993;28:1-2.
2. Duranceau A, Forand MD, Fauteux JP. Surgery in oculopharyngeal muscular dystrophy. Am J Surg. 1980;139:33-9.
3. Jordan DR, Addison DJ. Surgical results and pathological findings in the oculopharyngeal dystrophy syndrome. Can J Ophthalmol. 1993;28:15-8.
4. Molgat YM, Rodrigue D. Correction of blepharoptosis in oculopharyngeal muscular dystrophy: review of 91 cases. Can J Ophthalmol. 1993; 28:11-4.
5. Murphy SF, Drachman DB. The oculopharyngeal syndrome. JAMA. 1968;203:1003-8.
6. Taylor EW. Progressive glossopharyngeal paralysis with ptosis: contribution to a group of family diseases. J Nerv Ment Dis. 1915;42:129-39.

1076. OCULORENOCEREBELLAR SYNDROME (ORC SYNDROME)

General

Autosomal recessive.

Ocular

Progressive tapetoretinal degeneration with loss of retinal vessels.

Clinical

Mental retardation; continuous jerky movements; spastic diplegia; glomerulopathy with most renal glomeruli completely sclerosed.

Laboratory

Diagnosis is made by clinical findings.

Treatment

None/Ocular.

Bibliography

1. Hunter AG, Jurenka S, Thompson D, et al. Absence of the cerebellar granular layer, mental retardation, tapetoretinal degeneration and progressive glomerulopathy: an autosomal recessive oculorenal-cerebellar syndrome. Am J Med Genet. 1982;11:383-95.
2. McKusick VA. Mendelian Inheritance in Man: A Catalog of Human Genes and Genetic Disorders, 12th edition. Baltimore: The Johns Hopkins University Press; 1998.
3. McKusick-Nathans Institute for Genetic Medicine, Johns Hopkins University and National Center for Biotechnology Information, National Library of Medicine. (2007). Online Mendelian Inheritance in Man (OMIM). [online] Available from http://www.ncbi.nlm.nih.gov/omim [Accessed April, 2012].

1077. OGUCHI DISEASE

General

Autosomal recessive; usually Japanese; form of congenital hemeralopia; one form of essential, congenital night blindness.

Ocular

Fundus has white-gray coloration, especially around the optic disk and in macular region after light exposure (30 minutes to 1 hour); color sometimes is more brown; after 2–3 hours in the dark (Mizuo-Nakamura phenomenon), the posterior pole appears normal; the pathogenesis of Mizuo phenomenon has been postulated to be secondary to an excess of extracellular potassium in the retina as a result of a decreased potassium scavenging capacity of retinal Muller cells; central visual acuity and visual fields normal; night blindness always present.

Clinical

None

Laboratory

Diagnosis is made by clinical findings.

Treatment

No available treatment.

Bibliography

1. de Jong PT, Zrenner E, van Meel GJ, et al. Mizuo phenomenon in X-linked retinoschisis. Pathogenesis of the Mizuo phenomenon. Arch Ophthalmol. 1991;109:1104-8.
2. Magalini SI, Scrascia E. Dictionary of Medical Syndromes, 2nd edition. Philadelphia: JB Lippincott; 1981.
3. Pau H. Differential Diagnosis of Eye Diseases. New York: Thieme; 1987.

1078. OHAHA SYNDROME (ATAXIA, ATHETOSIS, HYPOACUSIS, HYPOTONIA, OPHTHALMOPLEGIA)

General

Ophthalmoplegia, hypotonia, ataxia, hypoacusis, athetosis (OHAHA) are distinguishing symptoms; sudden onset of deafness at an age after patient has learned to speak.

Ocular

Kernicterus; strabismus; nystagmus; ocular migraine; ophthalmoplegia; vascular spasm in branches of the ophthalmic artery; intact convergence.

Clinical

Hemiplegia; athetosis; choreoathetosis; tremor; hypoxia; corticospinal tract disease; diabetes mellitus; ataxia; medulloblastoma; asynergia; dysdiadochokinesia; Holmes rebound phenomenon; acute cerebellar lesion; dysmetria; dysarthria; Fox syndrome; vascular occlusion; congenital athetosis.

Laboratory

Diagnosis is made by clinical findings.

Treatment

Strabismus: Equalized vision with correct refractive error; surgery may be helpful in patient with diplopia. Local-ocular lubrication (drops or ointment) may be useful for exposure.

Bibliography

1. Kallis AK et al. A new syndrome of ophthalmoplegia, hypoacusis, ataxia, hypotonia, and athetosis (OMAHA). Adv Audiol. 1985;3:84-90.
2. McKusick VA. Mendelian Inheritance in Man: A Catalog of Human Genes and Genetic Disorders, 12th edition. Baltimore: The Johns Hopkins University Press; 1998.
3. McKusick-Nathans Institute for Genetic Medicine, Johns Hopkins University and National Center for Biotechnology Information, National Library of Medicine. (2007). Online Mendelian Inheritance in Man (OMIM). [online] Available from http://www.ncbi.nlm.nih.gov/omim [Accessed April, 2012].
4. Woody RC, Blaw ME. Ophthalmoplegic migraine in infancy. Clin Pediatr (Phila). 1986;25:82-4.

1079. OKIHIRO SYNDROME

General

Autosomal recessive syndrome of *Duane syndrome* (retraction syndrome).

Ocular

Narrowing of palpebral fissures on adduction, widening on abduction; primary global retraction.

Clinical

May be associated with craniofacial abnormalities and various associated syndromes, such as Duane syndrome, cervico-oculo-acoustic syndrome, acro-renal-ocular syndrome, cat's-eye syndrome; association with cardiac defects, urinary tract anomalies, Duane anomaly associated with mental retardation, thenar hypoplasia and radial ray abnormalities.

Laboratory

Diagnosis is made by clinical findings.

Treatment

Indications for surgery include anomalous head position, strabismus in primary gaze, significant upshoot or downshoot in adduction and cosmetically significant palpebral fissure. Type 1 Duane retraction syndrome (DRS)—(absent abduction, esotropia in primary position and head turn toward the affected side to fuse) medial rectus recession of the affected eye, DRS with exotropia—recess lateral rectus of involved side. Retraction of the globe—recess medial and lateral rectus of involved eye. Upshoots and downshoots—recess the lateral rectus.

Bibliography

1. Collins A, Baraitser M, Pembrey M. Okihiro syndrome: thenar hypoplasia and Duane anomaly in three generations. Clin Dysmorphol. 1993;2:237-40.
2. McGowan KF, Pagon RA. Okihiro syndrome. Am J Med Genet. 1994;51:89.
3. Stoll C, Alembik Y, Dott B. Association of Duane anomaly with mental retardation, cardiac and urinary tract abnormalities: a new autosomal recessive condition? Ann Genet. 1994;37:207-9.

1080. OLIVER-McFARLANE SYNDROME (TRICHOMEGALY SYNDROME)

General

Rare syndrome.

Ocular

Trichomegaly; pigmentary retinal degeneration.

Clinical

Prenatal onset growth failure; anterior pituitary deficiencies; peripheral neuropathy; mental retardation, sparse scalp hair, endocrinologic deficiencies, and koilonychia may be found.

Laboratory

Diagnosis is made by clinical findings.

Treatment

None/Ocular.

Bibliography

1. Sampson JR, Tolmie JL, Cant JS. Oliver McFarlane syndrome: a 25-year follow-up. Am J Med Genet. 1989;34:199-201.
2. Shaker AG, Fleming R, Jamieson ME, et al. Ovarian stimulation in an infertile patient with growth hormone-deficient Oliver-McFarlane syndrome. Hum Reprod. 1994;9:1997-8.
3. Zaun H, Stenger D, Zabransky S, et al. The long-eyelash syndrome (trichomegaly syndrome, Oliver-McFarlane). Hautarzt. 1984;35:162-5.

1081. OLIVOPONTOCEREBELLAR ATROPHY III (OPCA III; OPCA WITH RETINAL DEGENERATION)

General

Autosomal dominant; neurologic lesion; dominant with variable penetration.

Ocular

Retinopathy variable: peripheral, macular and circumpapillary; retinal degeneration; blindness; external ophthalmoplegia; variable electroretinogram function.

Clinical

Ataxia

Laboratory

Anti-Purkinje cell antibodies, MRI.

Treatment

Treatment is directed to symptoms.

Additional Resource

1. Azevedo CJ (2010). Olivopontocerebellar Atrophy. [online] Available from http://www.emedicine.com/neuro/TOPIC282.HTM [Accessed April, 2012].

1082. ONCHOCERCIASIS SYNDROME (ONCHOCERCA VOLVULUS INFESTATION; RIVER BLINDNESS)

General

Nematode infestation; positive diagnosis made with microfilariae from a skin biopsy and the presence of microfilariae in anterior chamber; infection results from the bite of the blackfly genus *Simulium*; recent findings suggest an autoimmune etiology for the occurrence of chorioretinopathy.

Ocular

Punctate keratitis (fluffy opacities); sclerosing keratitis; chronic iritis; pear-shaped pupil deformation; chorioretinitis; optic atrophy; uveitis; iris atrophy; papillitis; glaucoma; retinal degeneration; perivascular sheathing; microfilariae present in the anterior chamber, cornea and vitreous; pannus; synechiae; cataracts; secondary glaucoma.

Clinical

Subcutaneous nodules; pruritus; atrophic skin changes; pretibial pigmentation; dermatitis; lymphadenitis.

Laboratory

Skin biopsy, oncho-dipstick assay.

Treatment

Ivermectin (mectizan, stromectol).

Additional Resource

1. Eezzuduemhoi DR (2010). Ophthalmologic Manifestations of Onchocerciasis. [online] Available from http://www.emedicine.com/oph/TOPIC709.HTM [Accessed April, 2012].

1083. ONE-AND-A-HALF SYNDROME

General

Lesions in medial longitudinal fasciculus and paramedian pontine reticular formation; lateral gaze palsy on the side of the lesion and contralateral internuclear ophthalmoplegia; most common etiologies are ischemic infarction, demyelinating lesions, compressive lesion and infections.

Ocular

Paralysis of abduction; lateral gaze palsy; nystagmus; ocular bobbing; exotropia; esotropia.

Clinical

Dysarthria; dysphagia; hemiparesis; multiple sclerosis frequently associated in young patients with this condition.

Laboratory

Diagnosis is made by clinical findings.

Treatment

Strabismus: Equalized vision with correct refractive error; surgery may be helpful in patient with diplopia.

Bibliography

1. Bogousslavsky J, Miklossy J, Regli F, et al. One-and-a-half syndrome in ischaemic locked-in state: a clinico-pathological study. J Neurol Neurosurg Psychiatry. 1984;47:927-35.
2. Hommel M, Gato JM, Pollack P, et al. Magnetic resonance imaging and the "one-and-a-half" syndrome: a case report. J Clin Neuroophthalmol. 1987;7:161-4.
3. Wall M, Wray SH. The one-and-a-half syndrome: a unilateral disorder of the pontine tegmentum: a study of 20 cases and review of the literature. Neurology. 1983;33:971-80.

1084. OPEN-ANGLE GLAUCOMA

General

Chronic, bilateral ocular disease characterized by optic nerve damage and visual field defects.

Clinical

Diabetes mellitus, systemic hypertension, migraine headaches.

Ocular

Visual field defects, optic nerve cupping, arcuate scotoma, thin central cornea, high myopia, elevated intraocular pressure.

Laboratory

Diagnosis is made by clinical findings.

Treatment

Topical antiglaucoma agents, laser trabeculoplasty and surgical interventions—tube-shunt and cyclodestructive procedures.

Additional Resource

1. Bell JA (2012). Primary Open-Angle Glaucoma. [online] Available from http://www.emedicine.com/oph/TOPIC139.HTM [Accessed April, 2012].

1085. OPHTHALMIA NEONATORUM (NEONATAL CONJUNCTIVITIS)

General

Conjunctivitis of newborns which may be viral or bacterial in nature. Maternal infection may be a factor.

Clinical

None

Ocular

Purulent discharge in the first few days of life, can be sight threatening if untreated.

Laboratory

Gram stain intracellular, Gram-negative gonococcus, Gram-negative coccobacilli-*Haemophilus influenzae*, Gram-positive staphylococcus or streptococcus. Giemsa stain or polymerase chain reaction—chlamydia intracytoplasmic inclusion bodies.

Treatment

Prevention—2% silver nitrate or topical erythromycin or povidone-iodide drops. Oral and topical antibiotics may be necessary.

Additional Resource

1. Enzenauer RW (2011). Neonatal Conjunctivitis. [online] Available from http://www.emedicine.com/oph/TOPIC325.HTM [Accessed April, 2012].

1086. OPHTHALMODYNIA HYPERTONICA COPULATIONIS SYNDROME

General

Provocation of a diagnosed and otherwise controlled angle-closure glaucoma by prolonged sexual intercourse in the prone position.

Ocular

Acute attacks of angle-closure glaucoma during copulation in prone position.

Clinical

Nausea; vomiting.

Laboratory

Diagnosis is made by clinical findings.

Treatment

Glaucoma: Its medication should be the first plan of action. If medication is unsuccessful, a filtering surgical procedure with or without antimetabolites may be beneficial.

Bibliography

1. Hyams SW, Friedman Z, Neumann E. Elevated intraocular pressure in the prone position. A new provocative test for angle-closure glaucoma. Am J Ophthalmol. 1968;66:661-72.

2. Markovits AS. Ophthalmodynia hypertonica copulationis: a new syndrome? Can J Ophthalmol. 1974;9:484-5.

1087. OPHTHALMOPATHIC SYNDROME (THYROHYPOPHYSIAL SYNDROME)

General

Exophthalmos, usually bilateral; pituitary hypersecretion or enhanced tissue sensitivity to exophthalmos-producing factor that has been separated from thyroid-stimulating hormone (TSH).

Ocular

Exophthalmos; paralysis of ocular muscles.

Clinical

Thyroid disorders.

Laboratory

Thyroid-stimulating hormone (thyrotropin), T4 (thyroxine), orbital ultrasound, CT scan or MRI.

Treatment/Ocular

There is no immediate cure available. Artificial tears and/or punctal plugs; topical steroids are used in patients with severe inflammation or compressive optic neuropathy.

Additional Resource

1. Ing E (2012). Thyroid-Associated Orbitopathy. [online] Available from http://www.emedicine. com/oph/topic237.htm [Accessed April, 2012].

1088. OPHTHALMOPLEGIA, FAMILIAL STATIC

General

Autosomal dominant; forms include internal, external and total ophthalmoplegia.

Ocular

Ptosis; almost completely fixed eyes; nystagmoid movements; unequal pupils; pupil paralysis.

Clinical

None

Laboratory

Diagnosis is made by clinical findings.

Treatment

Ptosis: If visual acuity is affected most cases require surgical correction, and there are several procedures that may be used including levator resection, repair or advancement and Fasanella-Servat.

Bibliography

1. Lees F. Congenital, static familial ophthalmoplegia. J Neurol Neurosurg Psychiatry. 1960;23: 44-51.

1089. OPHTHALMOPLEGIA, PROGRESSIVE EXTERNAL

General

Autosomal recessive; progressive limitation of ocular motility with clinical sparing of pupillary function; underlying pathogenesis is secondary to a mitochondrial cytopathy; appearance of ragged red fibers in the abnormal muscles is primarily caused by mitochondrial accumulations beneath the plasma membrane and between the myofibrils.

Ocular

Oculopharyngeal muscular dystrophy; retinitis pigmentosa; progressive external ophthalmoplegia; some patients show only ptosis and ophthalmoplegia; most patients have multisystem involvement.

Clinical

Heart block; ataxia.

Laboratory

Thyroid studies, acetylcholine receptor antibody, MRI, CT, and ultrasound may show enlarged extraocular muscles.

Treatment

If ptosis is present, lid crutches may be helpful or ptosis surgery. Strabismus surgery may be helpful in patients with diplopia.

Additional Resource

1. Roy H (2011). Chronic Progressive External Ophthalmoplegia. [online] Available from http://www.emedicine.com/oph/TOPIC510.HTM [Accessed April, 2012].

1090. OPHTHALMOPLEGIA, PROGRESSIVE EXTERNAL, WITH RAGGED RED FIBERS

General

Autosomal dominant.

Ocular

Progressive ophthalmoplegia.

Clinical

Ragged red fibers in skeletal muscle from the extremities; subsarcolemmal clusters of mitochondria containing paracrystalline inclusions.

Laboratory

Thyroid studies, acetylcholine receptor antibody, MRI, CT, and ultrasound may show enlarged extraocular muscles.

Treatment

If ptosis is present, lid crutches may be helpful or ptosis surgery. Strabismus surgery may be helpful in patients with diplopia.

Additional Resource

1. Roy H (2011). Chronic Progressive External Ophthalmoplegia. [online] Available from http://www.emedicine.com/oph/TOPIC510.HTM [Accessed April, 2012].

1091. OPHTHALMOPLEGIA, PROGRESSIVE EXTERNAL, WITH SCROTAL TONGUE AND MENTAL DEFICIENCY

General

Autosomal dominant.

Ocular

Progressive external ophthalmoplegia; progressive chorioretinal sclerosis; bilateral ptosis; convergence paresis; myopia; optic atrophy; retinitis pigmentosa.

Clinical

Bilateral facial weakness; lingua scrotalis; mental retardation; cerebellar ataxia; weakness and spasticity of the limbs.

Laboratory

Thyroid studies, acetylcholine receptor antibody, MRI, CT, and ultrasound may show enlarged extraocular muscles.

Treatment

If ptosis is present, lid crutches may be helpful or ptosis surgery. Strabismus surgery may be helpful in patients with diplopia.

Additional Resource

1. Roy H (2011). Chronic Progressive External Ophthalmoplegia. [online] Available from http://www.emedicine.com/oph/TOPIC510.HTM [Accessed April, 2012].

1092. OPHTHALMOPLEGIC MIGRAINE SYNDROME

General

Symptoms produced by ipsilateral herniation of hippocampal gyrus of temporal lobe through incisura tentorii; dependent upon unilateral cerebral edema due to vascular or vasomotor phenomena, intracranial aneurysm or tumor; incidence may be greater in women with the initial attack in the first decade of life; pathogenesis is unclear, but it is likely secondary to ischemia of the ocular motor nerve.

Ocular

Severe unilateral supraorbital pain; ptosis; transitory partial or complete homolateral oculomotor paralysis; fourth or sixth nerve occasionally involved; retinal hemorrhages; papilledema (may be bilateral); moderate to severe headache with partial to complete cranial nerve III paresis including the pupil; more than one ocular nerve may be affected.

Clinical

Migraine headache, not present in all instances; dizziness; diminution in sense of smell; hypalgesia contralateral side of face; nausea/vomiting may be present; recurrent sinus arrest.

Laboratory

Diagnosis is made by clinical findings.

Treatment

Ptosis: If visual acuity is affected then most cases require surgical correction, and there are several procedures that may be used including levator resection, repair or advancement and Fasanella-Servat.

Bibliography

1. Bazak I, Margulis T, Shnaider H, et al. Ophthalmoplegic migraine and recurrent sinus arrest. J Neurol Neurosurg Psychiatry. 1991;54:935.

2. Ehlers H. On pathogenesis of ophthalmoplegic migraine. Acta Psychiatr Neurol (Scand). 1928;3: 219-25.
3. Geeraets WJ. Ocular Syndromes, 3rd edition. Philadelphia: Lea & Febiger; 1976.
4. Gulkilik G, Cagatay HH, Oba EM, et al. Ophthalmoplegic migraine associated with recurrent isolated ptosis. Ann Ophthalmol (Skokie). 2009;41:206-7.
5. Raskin NH. Migraine and other headaches. In: Rowland LP (Ed). Merritt's Textbook of Neurology,
9th edition. Baltimore: Williams & Wilkins; 1995. pp. 837-45.
6. Stommel EW, Ward TN, Harris RD. Ophthalmoplegic migraine or Tolosa-Hunt syndrome? Headache. 1994;34:177.
7. Vanpelt W. On the early onset of ophthalmoplegic migraine. Am J Dis Child. 1964;107:628-31.
8. Vijayan N. Ophthalmoplegic migraine: ischemic or compressive neuropathy? Headache. 1980;20: 300-4.

1093. OPHTHALMOPLEGIC NEUROMUSCULAR DISORDER WITH ABNORMAL MITOCHONDRIA

General

Autosomal recessive.

Ocular

Ptosis; external ophthalmoplegia.

Clinical

Involvement of cranial nerves and skeletal muscles; morphologic alterations of mitochondria; diffuse low-density deep cerebral white matter; weak limbs.

Laboratory

Diagnosis is made by clinical findings.

Treatment

Ptosis: If visual acuity is affected then most cases require surgical correction, and there are several procedures that may be used including levator resection, repair or advancement and Fasanella-Servat.

Bibliography

1. Okamoto T, Mizuno K, Iida M, et al. Ophthalmoplegia plus. Its occurrence with periventricular diffuse low density on computed tomography scan. Arch Neurol. 1981;38:423-6.
2. McKusick VA. Mendelian Inheritance in Man: A Catalog of Human Genes and Genetic Disorders, 12th edition. Baltimore: The Johns Hopkins University Press; 1998.
3. McKusick-Nathans Institute for Genetic Medicine, Johns Hopkins University and National Center for Biotechnology Information, National Library of Medicine. (2007). Online Mendelian Inheritance in Man (OMIM). [online] Available from http://www.ncbi.nlm.nih.gov/omim [Accessed April, 2012].

1094. OPHTHALMOPLEGIC RETINAL DEGENERATION SYNDROME (BARNARD-SCHOLZ SYNDROME)

General

Onset at all ages (see Kearns-Sayre Syndrome).

Ocular

Unilateral or bilateral progressive weakness of muscles of eyelids, up to severe ptosis; progressive ocular myopathy up to complete ophthalmoplegia; retinitis pigmentosa.

Clinical

Facial, neck and shoulder muscle weakness; hearing defects; heart block.

Laboratory

Diagnosis is made by clinical findings.

Treatment

Ptosis: If visual acuity is affected then most cases require surgical correction, and there are several procedures that may be used including levator resection, repair or advancement and Fasanella-Servat.

Bibliography

1. Barnard RI, Scholz RO. Ophthalmoplegia and retinal degeneration. Am J Ophthalmol. 1944;27:621-4.
2. Geeraets WJ. Ocular Syndromes, 3rd edition. Philadelphia: Lea & Febiger; 1976.
3. Kiloh LG, Nevin S. Progressive dystrophy of the external ocular muscles (ocular myopathy). Brain. 1951;74:115-43.

1095. OPTIC ATROPHY

General

Axon degeneration in the retinogeniculate pathway; causes vary from hereditary, circulatory, metabolic, postinflammatory, traumatic and consecutive.

Clinical

Multiple sclerosis; orbit tumors.

Ocular

Axial myopia; myelinated nerve fibers; optic nerve pit; tilted disk; optic nerve hypoplasia; scleral crescent areas; optic disk drusen; papilledema.

Laboratory

Magnetic resonance imaging (MRI) to look for solid lesions; B-scan ultrasonography to look for sheath dilatation; CT if associated with trauma; contrast sensitivity, color vision and pupillary evaluation are also useful.

Treatment

Intravenous steroids may be used with optic neuritis or ischemic neuropathy. Stem cell treatment may be the future treatment of choice.

Additional Resource

1. Gandhi R (2010). Optic Atrophy Treatment & Management. [online] Available from http://www.emedicine.medscape.com/article/1217760-treatment [Accessed April, 2012].

1096. OPTIC ATROPHY, CATARACT AND NEUROLOGIC DISORDER

General

Autosomal dominant; similar to syndromes of Behr, Marinesco, Sjögren and Friedreich which are autosomal recessive.

Ocular

Cataract; optic atrophy.

Clinical

Neurologic disorder.

Laboratory

Diagnosis is made by clinical findings.

Treatment

Intravenous steroids may be used with optic neuritis or ischemic neuropathy. Stem cell treatment may be the future treatment of choice.

Additional Resource

1. Gandhi R (2010). Optic Atrophy. [online] Available from http://www.emedicine.com/oph/TOPIC777. HTM [Accessed April, 2012].

1097. OPTIC ATROPHY, JUVENILE [KJER-TYPE OPTIC ATROPHY; OPTIC ATROPHY, CONGENITAL; OPTIC ATROPHY, KJER-TYPE; OAK SYNDROME (OPTIC ATROPHY, KJER TYPE)]

General

Autosomal dominant; dominant pattern distinguishes it from Leber optic atrophy; insidious onset; onset in childhood; pathogenetic mechanism may be primary degeneration of retinal ganglion cells.

Ocular

Central scotoma; color defects; choroidal sclerosis; optic neuritis; temporal optic atrophy; aggregation of retinal pigment epithelium; tortuosity of retinal arteries and veins; reduced central vision; retinal lesions; may present with mild-to-moderate reduction of visual acuity with 50% of patients having vision between 20/60 and 20/200; visual field defect associated may be a central, paracentral or cecocentral scotoma.

Clinical

Keratosis pilaris on the extremities; approximately 10% of patients present with mental abnormalities and approximately 80% of patients with neural hearing loss.

Laboratory

Study depends on the disease process.

Treatment

No treatment available.

Additional Resource

1. Gandhi R (2010). Optic Atrophy. [online] Available from http://www.emedicine.com/oph/TOPIC777. HTM [Accessed April, 2012].

1098. OPTIC ATROPHY, NERVE DEAFNESS

General

Autosomal recessive.

Ocular

Degeneration of optic nerves.

Clinical

Degeneration of the acoustic nerves; progressive polyneuropathy, distally.

Laboratory

Study depends on the disease process.

Treatment

No treatment available.

Additional Resource

1. Gandhi R (2010). Optic Atrophy. [online] Available from http://www.emedicine.com/oph/TOPIC777. HTM [Accessed April, 2012].

1099. OPTIC ATROPHY, NON-LEBER-TYPE, WITH EARLY ONSET

General

Sex-linked; onset early in life.

Ocular

Optic atrophy.

Clinical

Mental retardation; hyperactive knee jerks; absent ankle jerks, extensor plantar reflexes; dysarthria; tremor; dysdiadochokinesia; difficulty with tandem gait.

Laboratory

Study depends on the disease process.

Treatment

No treatment is available.

Additional Resource

1. Gandhi R (2010). Optic Atrophy. [online] Available from http://www.emedicine.com/oph/TOPIC777. HTM [Accessed April, 2012].

1100. OPTIC ATROPHY-SPASTIC PARAPLEGIA SYNDROME

General

Degenerative disorder of CNS associated with optic atrophy; sex-linked.

Ocular

Optic atrophy.

Clinical

Neurologic spastic paraplegia.

Laboratory

Study depends on the disease process.

Treatment

No treatment available.

Additional Resource

1. Gandhi R (2010). Optic Atrophy. [online] Available from http://www.emedicine.com/oph/TOPIC777. HTM [Accessed April, 2012].

1101. OPTIC ATROPHY WITH DEMYELINATING DISEASE OF CNS

General

Autosomal dominant; demyelinated optic nerves appear smaller than normal and are pale-white or gray in color; blood vessels may seem to be less prominent than normal.

Ocular

Optic neuritis; Leber optic atrophy.

Clinical

Ataxia; leg weakness; dysarthria; hemiparesis.

Laboratory/Ocular

Lumbar puncture, cerebrospinal fluid studies, MRI of brain and orbits.

Treatment/Ocular

Prednisolone, methylprednisolone.

Additional Resource

1. Gandhi R (2010). Optic Atrophy. [online] Available from http://www.emedicine.com/oph/TOPIC777. HTM [Accessed April, 2012].

1102. OPTIC CANAL SYNDROME

General

Caused by severe blow to the head, usually the face or occiput.

Ocular

Unilateral blindness (rarely bilateral); amaurotic pupillary paralysis; pathogenesis is a shearing or tearing injury to the nerve at the transition point from where it is fixed in the optic canal and the free intracranial portion.

Clinical

None

Laboratory

Diagnosis is made by clinical findings.

Treatment

None/Ocular.

Bibliography

1. Snebold NG. Neuroophthalmic manifestations of trauma. In: Albert DM, Jakobiec FA (Eds). Principles and Practice of Ophthalmology. Philadelphia: WB Saunders; 1994. pp. 3463-77.

1103. OPTIC DISK TRACTION SYNDROME

General

Optic disk traction with elevation associated with posterior vitreous detachment or vitreopapillary fibrous membrane may be associated with retinal surgery.

Ocular

Central retinal vein occlusion; optic disk traction (vitreopapillary); localized retinal detachment.

Clinical

None

Laboratory

None

Treatment

Posterior vitreous detachment: No treatment is necessary, but the patient needs to advised to look for the warning signs for retinal detachment (flashing lights, swarms of vitreous floaters and a cut in visual field).

Bibliography

1. Rumelt S, Karatas M, Pikkel J, et al. Optic disc traction syndrome associated with central retinal vein occlusion. Arch Ophthalmol. 2003;121:1093-7.

1104. OPTIC FORAMEN FRACTURES

General

Caused by nonpenetrating blow to the head with subsequent transfer of force to the optic canal and its contents or with basilar skull fractures.

Clinical

Loss of consciousness, cerebrospinal fluid leak.

Ocular

Traumatic optic neuropathy hematoma, ischemic necrosis.

Laboratory

Computed tomography (CT) to identify bony anomaly.

Treatment

Intravenous steroids alone or in conjunction with optic canal decompression.

Additional Resource

1. Patel B (2012). Apex Orbital Fracture. [online] Available from http://www.emedicine.com/oph/ TOPIC228.HTM [Accessed April, 2012].

1105. OPTIC GLIOMAS

General

Juvenile pilocytic astrocytomas type I tumors intrinsic to the optic nerve, chiasm or tracts are termed optic gliomas.

Clinical

None

Ocular

Proptosis, afferent pupil defect, hypotropia.

Laboratory

Magnetic resonance imaging (MRI) with gadolinium contrast is essential.

Treatment

Observation: No proven efficacy has shown for excision of tumor to prevent contralateral eye involvement.

Additional Resource

1. Woodcock RJ (2011). Optic Nerve Glioma Imaging. [online] Available from http://www.emedicine. com/radio/TOPIC486.HTM [Accessed April, 2012].

1106. OPTIC NERVE DECOMPRESSION FOR TRAUMATIC NEUROPATHY

General

A complication of closed head injury; can be temporary or permanent.

Clinical

Closed head injury.

Ocular

Afferent pupillary defect; decreased visual function; subnormal color vision; visual field loss; optic nerve sheath hematoma; optic nerve impingement.

Laboratory

Thin slice CT provides the best imaging of orbital soft tissue.

Treatment

Contemporary treatments for traumatic optic neuropathy have included observation, steroids and surgical decompression.

Additional Resource

1. O'Brien EK (2011). Optic Nerve Decompression for Traumatic Optic Neuropathy. [online] Available from http://www.emedicine.medscape.com article/868252-overview [Accessed April, 2012].

1107. OPTIC NERVE HYPOPLASIA, FAMILIAL (BILATERAL, UNILATERAL)

General

Autosomal dominant; congenital defect of optic nerve and retina that occurs in both unilateral and bilateral forms; onset at birth; majority of cases are sporadic, although there are reports of familial cases; association of this condition with maternal ingestion of various substances, including quinine, lysergic acid diethylamide (LSD) and anticonvulsants.

Ocular

Optic nerve hypoplasia; diameter of optic disk is one-third of normal size; nystagmus; peripapillary halos; situs inversus of disk; strabismus; choroidal atrophy; microphthalmos; coloboma of choroid and/or optic disk; blepharophimosis; ptosis; aniridia; ocular motor nerve palsy.

Clinical

Central nervous system (CNS) defects; chromosomal abnormalities; cerebral malformations; vascular hypertension.

Laboratory

Diagnosis is made by clinical findings.

Treatment

No treatment available.

Bibliography

1. Hackenbruch Y, Meerhoff E, Besio R, et al. Familial bilateral optic nerve hypoplasia. Am J Ophthalmol. 1975;79:314-20.

1108. OPTIC NEURITIS

General

Inflammatory demyelinating condition of the optic nerve that usually presents as a subacute painful unilateral impairment of vision, although bilateral visual loss can occur.

Clinical

Multiple sclerosis.

Ocular

Retro-ocular pain, visual loss, decreased color vision, central scotoma.

Laboratory

Orbital MRI, cerebrospinal fluid examination to rule out infectious or other inflammatory optic neuropathy.

Treatment

Systemic corticosteroids.

Additional Resources

1. Ergene E (2012). Adult Optic Neuritis. [online] Available from http://www.emedicine.com/oph/ TOPIC186.HTM [Accessed April, 2012].
2. Schatz MP (2011). Childhood Optic Neuritis. [online] Available from http://www.emedicine. com/oph/TOPIC343.HTM [Accessed April, 2012].

1109. OPTIC NEURITIS, ADULT

General

Demyelinating inflammation of the optic nerve; can be associated with multiple sclerosis, neuromyelitis optica, infectious process of orbits or sinuses or be idiopathic.

Clinical

Multiple sclerosis; neuromyelitis optica; infectious or viral process of orbits or sinuses.

Ocular

Decreased visual acuity; changes in color perception; pupillary light reaction decreased; papillitis; altitudinal swelling of the disk; arterial attenuation; pallor of disk.

Laboratory

Magnetic resonance imaging (MRI); visually evoked potentials testing.

Treatment

Oral and intravenous steroids are used, but there is controversy over its effectiveness.

Additional Resource

1. Ergene E (2012). Adult Optic Neuritis. [online] Available from http://www.emedicine.medscape. com/article/1217083-overview [Accessed April, 2012].

1110. OPTIC NEURITIS, CHILDHOOD

General

Inflammatory process of the optic nerve. In children, most cases of optic neuritis are due to a viral or other infection or with immunization.

Clinical

Multiple sclerosis; acute disseminated encephalomyelitis; neuromyelitis; injections of sinuses or orbital structures; Lyme disease; syphilis; leukemia; wasp stings; cat scratch disease; toxoplasmosis; toxocariasis; helminths.

Ocular

Visual loss; change in color perception; loss of visual field change in brightness sense; afferent pupil defect; disk edema.

Laboratory

Magnetic resonance imaging (MRI) and lumbar puncture help to determine the cause.

Treatment

Some propose no treatment. Some give intravenous steroids for initial therapy. Plasma exchange and intravenous immunoglobulin have also been used.

Additional Resource

1. Schatz MP (2011). Childhood Optic Neuritis. [online] Available from http://www.emedicine.medscape.com/article/1217290-overview [Acessed April, 2012].

1111. OPTIC NEUROPATHIES, COMPRESSIVE

General

Disease of the optic nerve that leads to visual loss secondary to pressure on the optic nerve, either within the orbit, inside the optic canal or intracranially.

Clinical

None

Ocular

Progressive visual loss, enlarged extraocular muscles.

Laboratory

Computed tomography (CT) with contrast imaging with gadolinium enhancement and fat suppression techniques; orbital ultrasonography.

Treatment

Oral or intravenous steroids, radiation therapy.

Additional Resource

1. Kim JW (2011). Compressive Optic Neuropathy. [online] Available from http://www.emedicine.com/oph/TOPIC167.HTM [Accessed April, 2012].

1112. OPTIC NEUROPATHY, ANTERIOR ISCHEMIC

General

Ischemic process affecting the posterior circulation of the globe; may be arteritic or nonarteritic; usually occurs in individuals over the age of 50 years.

Clinical

Hypertension; myocardial infarction; atherosclerosis; giant cell arteritis; malaise; headache; scalp tenderness; jaw pain; diabetes mellitus; migraine; Takayasu disease; polycythemia vera; sickle cell disease; hypotension; syphilis; lupus; Buerger disease; postimmunization; radiation necrosis; sleep apnea.

Ocular

Visual loss; ocular palsies; temporal pain.

Laboratory

Erythrocyte sedimentation rate is the most important test to determine if it is elevated; temporal artery biopsy is used to diagnose giant cell arteritis.

Treatment

Comanagement with an internist is recommended; large doses of systemic prednisone on a tapered scale is the usual treatment.

Additional Resource

1. Younge BR (2012). Anterior Ischemic Optic Neuropathy. [online] Available from http://www.emedicine.medscape.com/article/1216891-overview [Accessed April, 2012].

1113. OPTIC PIT SYNDROME

General

Congenital

Ocular

Serous detachment of macula; situs inversus; peripapillary chorioretinal changes; cilioretinal vessels; large optic disk; tortuous retinal vessels; retinoschisis.

Clinical

None

Laboratory

Diagnosis is made by clinical findings.

Treatment

Retinal detachment: Scleral buckle, pneumatic retinopexy and vitrectomy may be used to close all the breaks.

Bibliography

1. Gass JD. Serous detachment of the macula. Secondary to congenital pit of the optic nerve head. Am J Ophthalmol. 1969;67:821-41.
2. Giuffre G. Optic pit syndrome. Doc Ophthalmol. 1986;64:187-99.
3. Lincoff H, Lopez R, Kreissig I, et al. Retinoschisis associated with optic nerve pits. Arch Ophthalmol. 1988;106:61-7.

1114. ORAL-FACIAL-DIGITAL SYNDROME (OFDS)

General

Group of syndromes characterized by congenital anomalies of the oral cavity, face and digits; see-saw walking; hypertelorism; strabismus.

Ocular

Chorioretinal coloboma; optic nerve coloboma; retinal hamartoma.

Clinical

Patients with OFDS have been known to have various congenital anomalies, including cleft palate, tongue hamartomas, bifid tongue, multiple hyperplastic frenula, hypoplastic nasal cartilage, syndactyly, polydactyly, brachydactyly, clinodactyly and the ocular ophthalmologic findings; nine distinct types of OFDS have been described.

Laboratory

Diagnosis is made by clinical findings.

Treatment

None

Bibliography

1. Gurrieri F, Sammito V, Ricci B, et al. Possible new type of oral-facial-digital syndrome with retinal abnormalities: OFDS type (VIII). Am J Med Genet. 1992;42:789-92.

1115. ORBITAL CELLULITIS AND ABSCESS

General

Potentially life threatening, requires prompt evaluation and treatment.

Clinical

Sinusitis, ear infection, diabetes, dental disease.

Ocular

Orbital pain, proptosis, diplopia, decreased ocular motility, eyelid swelling and erythema, vision loss.

Laboratory

Diagnosis is made by clinical findings.

Treatment

Intravenous and oral antibiotics.

Additional Resource

1. Harrington JN (2012). Orbital Cellulitis. [online] Available from http://www.emedicine.com/oph/TOPIC205.HTM [Accessed April, 2012].

1116. ORBITAL FAT HERNIATION (ADIPOSE PALPEBRAL BAGS, BAGGY EYELIDS, EYELID FAT PROLAPSE, ORBITAL FAT PROLAPSE)

General

Upper or lower eyelid fat herniation through orbital septum. Hereditary, thyroid-related orbitopathy and orbital steroid injection may accelerate the process.

Clinical

None

Ocular

Lid fullness.

Laboratory

Diagnosis is made by clinical findings.

Treatment

Surgical removal of tissue of the upper and lower eyelids.

Bibliography

1. Roy FH, Fraunfelder FW, Fraunfelder FT. Roy and Fraunfelder's Current Ocular Therapy, 6th edition. Philadelphia: WB Saunders; 2008.

1117. ORBITAL FRACTURE, APEX

General

Affects the most posterior portion of the pyramidal-shaped orbit, positioned at the craniofacial junction. Usually associated with blunt or penetrating trauma to the face or skull.

Clinical

Intracranial or Facial trauma.

Ocular

Visual loss; optic neuropathy; optic nerve sheath hematoma; optic nerve impingement; optic nerve compression; retrobulbar hemorrhage; extraocular muscle nerve palsy; diplopia; afferent pupil defect; periocular ecchymosis; proptosis.

Laboratory

Computed tomography (CT) scan is the most appropriate to make diagnosis.

Treatment

In cases that involve decreased vision and optic nerve injury, medical or surgical nerve decompression should be considered. Corticosteroids should be the initial treatment, and if it is not effective surgical intervention is necessary.

Additional Resource

1. Patel B (2012). Apex Orbital Fracture. [online] Available from http://www.emedicine.medscape.com/article/1218196-overview [Accessed April, 2012].

1118. ORBITAL FRACTURE, ZYGOMATIC

General

Zygoma is the main buttress between the maxilla and the skull, this fracture usually involves a blow to the side of the face from a fist, a motor vehicle accidents, etc.

Clinical

Facial trauma; difficult with movement of the mandible.

Ocular

Visual loss; diplopia; periocular ecchymosis; proptosis; orbital hematoma.

Laboratory

Computed tomography (CT) scan is the most appropriate to make diagnosis.

Treatment

Many require no treatment. If surgery is required then most are done by closed-reduction techniques.

Additional Resource

1. Seiff S (2012). Zygomatic Orbital Fracture. [online] Available from http://www.emedicine.medscape.com/article/1218360-overview [Accessed April, 2012].

1119. ORBITAL HEMORRHAGES

General

Occurs acutely, substantial hemorrhage behind the orbit septum will raise intraorbital and intraocular pressure.

Clinical

None

Ocular

Elevated intraocular pressure, orbital pain, diplopia, vision loss, ptosis, lid retraction, immobile globe, cloudy cornea, hemorrhagic conjunctiva, disk pallor, hyperemia of the disk, disk edema, choroidal folds.

Laboratory

Diagnosis is made by clinical findings.

Treatment

Topical medication to lower intraocular pressure, lateral canthotomy and inferior cantholysis.

Bibliography

1. Roy FH, Fraunfelder FW, Fraunfelder FT. Roy and Fraunfelder's Current Ocular Therapy, 6th edition. Philadelphia: WB Saunders; 2008.

1120. ORBITAL IMPLANT EXTRUSION

General

Involves the displacement of implants use in enucleations to replace volume loss.

Clinical

None

Ocular

Superior tarsal sulcus deformity, defect in conjunctiva and Tenon's capsule.

Laboratory

Diagnosis is made by clinical findings.

Treatment

Immediate replacement with a fascia-enveloped sphere. If socket is infected, systemic and topical antibiotics are recommended.

Bibliography

1. Roy FH, Fraunfelder FW, Fraunfelder FT. Roy and Fraunfelder's Current Ocular Therapy, 6th edition. Philadelphia: WB Saunders; 2008.

1121. ORBITAL INFLAMMATORY SYNDROMES

General

Traditionally these syndromes are clumped together under the genetic term inflammatory pseudotumor, defined loosely as a non-neoplastic orbital inflammatory mass. Cause is unknown.

Clinical

Multifocal fibrosclerosis including retroperitoneal fibrosis and sclerosing cholangitis.

Ocular

Anterior myositis; dacryoadenitis.

Laboratory

Computed tomography (CT); histology to identify acute polymorphous, sclerosing, granulomatous and vasculitic orbital inflammatory syndromes.

Treatment

Oral corticosteroids are tapered over 4–8 weeks.

Bibliography

1. Roy FH, Fraunfelder FW, Fraunfelder FT. Roy and Fraunfelder's Current Ocular Therapy, 6th edition. Philadelphia: WB Saunders; 2008.

1122. ORBITAL LYMPHOMA

General

Localized form of systemic lymphoma affecting the orbit, lacrimal gland, eyelid and conjunctiva.

Clinical

Systemic lymphoma.

Ocular

Diplopia; exophthalmos; ocular pain; salmon-colored mass of the conjunctiva or eyelid.

Laboratory

Open biopsy and MRI or CT of the orbit.

Treatment

Radiation is the most frequently used treatment. Chemotherapy may be indicated for large diffuse B-cell lymphoma or with systemic treatment. Excision of localized lesions. Cryotherapy may be beneficial.

Additional Resource

1. Miguel Gonzalez-Candial, LuzMaria Vasquez (2010). Orbital Lymphoma. [online] Available from http://www.eyewiki.aao.org/Orbital_Lymphoma [Accessed April, 2012].

1123. ORBITAL RHABDOMYOSARCOMA

General

Embryonal or Alveolar varieties of this tumor have a tendency to affect the orbit and adjacent structures.

Clinical

Skeletal, muscles and renal tumors.

Ocular

Rapid onset of painless proptosis, ptosis, ocular congestion, decreased extraocular motility.

Laboratory

Complete blood count, liver function test, renal function and CT of lung and orbit.

Treatment

Local debulking of the orbital mass, adjunctive radiotherapy and chemotherapy.

Bibliography

1. Roy FH, Fraunfelder FW, Fraunfelder FT. Roy and Fraunfelder's Current Ocular Therapy, 6th edition. Philadelphia: WB Saunders; 2008.

1124. ORF SYNDROME (ECTHYMA INFECTIOSUM)

General

Infectious disease; transmitted between animals; worldwide distribution; human infection from sheep.

Ocular

Pigmentation of lids.

Clinical

Single or multiple lesions of hands and other parts of body; itching; fever; concurrent aseptic meningitis caused by enterovirus.

Laboratory

Confirmation of the clinical diagnosis is performed by electron microscopy with negative staining of the crust or a small biopsy.

Treatment

If it is a self-limited disease, symptomatic treatment with moist dressings, local antiseptics, and finger immobilization is helpful. Secondary bacterial infection is not uncommon and must be treated with topical or systemic antibiotics.

Additional Resource

1. Hawayek LH (2011). Orf. [online] Available from http://www.emedicine.com/derm/TOPIC605. HTM [Accessed April, 2012].

1125. ORMOND SYNDROME (RETROPERITONEAL FIBROSIS)

General

Periureteral fibrosis that constricts ureter; most frequent in males; average age at onset is 46 years in males and 32 years in females; etiology possibly is a fasciculitis of collagen disease; clinical variant of multiple fibrosclerosis.

Ocular

Exophthalmos; orbital pseudotumor; nongranulomatous panuveitis.

Clinical

Pain in back progressing to ureteral colic or abdominal pain without specific localization; vomiting; nausea; anorexia; malaise; fatigue; weight loss; constipation; diarrhea; pyelonephritis.

Laboratory

Intravenous urography, lymphangiography, retrograde pyelography, CT, MRI and positron emission tomography.

Treatment

The aims of management are to preserve renal function, to prevent other organ involvement, to exclude malignancy and to relieve symptoms. Empirical therapy includes corticosteroids, tamoxifen and azathioprine.

Additional Resource

1. Biyani CS (2012). Retroperitoneal Fibrosis. [online] Available from http://www.emedicine.com/med/TOPIC3664.HTM [Accessed April, 2012].

1126. ORZECHOWSKI SYNDROME (ENCEPHALITIS-OPSOCLONIA-TREMULOUSNESS; TRUNCAL ATAXIA-OPSOCLONIA)

General

Etiology unknown; follows a benign upper respiratory infection; spontaneous resolution; opsoclonus has been described in patients with encephalitis with Epstein-Barr virus, mumps and coxsackievirus infections.

Ocular

Opsoclonia; excessive blinking.

Clinical

Incapacitating postural tremulousness of the body; fever; headache.

Laboratory

Diagnosis is made by clinical observation.

Treatment

Therapy for the causative agent such as encephalitis, Epstein-Barr or other infections.

Bibliography

1. Magalini SI, Scrascia E. Dictionary of Medical Syndromes, 2nd edition. Philadelphia: JB Lippincott; 1981.
2. Orzechowski K. De l'Ataxie Dysmetrique des Yeux; Remarques sur l'Ataxie des Yeux Dite Myoclonique. J Psychol Neurol. 1927;35:1-18.

1127. OSTEOGENESIS IMPERFECTA CONGENITA, MICROCEPHALY, AND CATARACTS

General

Autosomal recessive.

Ocular

Cataracts; blue sclera; keratoconus.

Clinical

Brain abnormally small; multiple prenatal bone fractures; calvaria soft; shortening and bowing of lower limbs.

Laboratory

Diagnosis is made by clinical findings.

Treatment

Keratoconus: Spectacle correction, hard contacts and avoid eye rubbing may be useful. If hydrops occurs discontinue contact lens, use NaCl drops and ointment, patching and short course of steroids. As the disease advances penetrating keratoplasty, deep anterior lamellar keratoplasty, intacs with laser grooves or collagen stabilization of cornea.

Cataract: Change in glasses can sometimes improve a patient's visual function temporarily; however, the most common treatment is cataract surgery.

Additional Resource

1. Plotkin H (2012). Genetics of Osteogenesis Imperfecta. [online] Available from http://www.emedicine.com/ped/TOPIC1674.HTM [Accessed April, 2012].

1128. OTA SYNDROME (NEVUS OF OTA; NEVUS FUSCOCERULEUS-OPHTHALMOMAXILLARIS SYNDROME; OCULODERMAL MELANOCYTOSIS)

General

Affects mainly black and Japanese populations; female preponderance (4:1); mode of transmission unknown; most frequently unilateral; pigmentary changes frequently spread during puberty, but no malignant transformation occurs; malignant transformation to melanoma in the uvea and orbit has been reported.

Ocular

Congenital benign periorbital pigmentation of brown, slate to bluish-black coloration, involving area of first and second (rarely third) division of trigeminal nerve; unilateral hyperchromic heterochromia iridis; possible scleral and conjunctival pigmentation; trabeculae heavily pigmented; slate-gray hyperpigmentation of fundus; optic disk pigmentation (occasionally).

Clinical

Pigmentation of temples, nose, forehead and malar region; "Mongolian spot" in sacral area (present at birth but usually disappears after puberty).

Laboratory

Diagnosis is made by clinical findings.

Treatment

Observation

Additional Resource

1. Lui H (2011). Nevi of Ota and Ito. [online] Available from http://www.emedicine.com/derm/TOPIC290.HTM [Accessed April, 2012].

1129. OTOCEPHALY

General

Birth defect; extreme malformation of first brachial arch characterized by almost complete aplasia of its parts.

Ocular

Bilateral anophthalmos.

Clinical

Mouth deformities; absence of lower jaw; joining of ears on the neck.

Laboratory

Diagnosis is made by clinical findings.

Treatment

Expansion of orbit and lid formation.

Bibliography

1. Duke-Elder S, MacFaul PA. System of Ophthalmology. St. Louis: CV Mosby; 1974.

2. Glange WD (Ed). The Mosby Medical Encyclopedia. St. Louis: CV Mosby; 1985.

1130. OUTER RETINAL ISCHEMIC INFARCTION SYNDROME

General

Complication that may occur during the course of cataract extraction or closed vitrectomy due to obstruction of choroidal circulation.

Ocular

Acute loss of central and paracentral vision; whitening of the outer retinal layers in posterior fundus; mottled changes in the pigment epithelium.

Clinical

None

Laboratory

Diagnosis is made by clinical findings.

Treatment

None/Ocular.

Additional Resource

1. Leibovitch I (2011). Ocular Ischemic Syndrome. [online] Available from http://www.emedicine.com/oph/TOPIC487.HTM [Accessed April, 2012].

1131. OXALOSIS (LEPOUTRE SYNDROME; PRIMARY HYPEROXALURIA)

General

Autosomal recessive and acquired forms; metabolic disorders with accumulation of oxalic acid in tissues; type I: glycolic aciduria, defect of 2-oxoglutarate/glyoxylate carboligase; type II: glyceric aciduria, defect of D-glyceric dehydrogenase.

Ocular

Calcium oxalate deposits may be found in the retina; retinitis punctate albescens; macular degeneration of Stargardt; pigmentary retinopathy; black, geographic central macular subretinal patches; oxalate may deposit in the retinal pigment epithelium, outer plexiform layer and nuclear layers of the retina.

Clinical

Recurrent calcium oxalate nephrolithiasis and nephrocalcinosis; progressive renal insufficiency; continuous excessive synthesis and excretion of oxalic acid; nausea; vomiting; abdominal pain; renal colic; calculi in urine; tetany.

Laboratory

Urinary oxalate level in excess of 100 mg/d. Spiral CT scanning without intravenous contrast is rapidly replacing intravenous pyelography (IVP) as the preferred method for evaluating patients with acute flank pain who may have a urinary stone.

Treatment

Early medical treatment is required to decrease the oxalate level and to prevent deterioration of renal function. Early liver-kidney transplantation is often required for definitive cure. Dietary oxalate restrictions are of no substantial benefit in this type of hyperoxaluric disease. Several medications have been useful.

Additional Resource

1. Shekarriz B (2011). Hyperoxaluria. [online] Available from http://www.emedicine.com/med/TOPIC3027.HTM [Accessed April, 2012].

1132. 18p- SYNDROME (18p DELETION SYNDROME)

General

Chromosome 18p deletion syndrome.

Ocular

Hypertelorism, epicanthus, horizontal palpebral fissures.

Clinical

Microcephaly, round face, broad-based nose, "carp mouth," microretrognathic; pterygium colli; dysplastic and low-set ears; clinodactyly; failure to grow; muscular hypotony; mental retardation; hypoplastic male genitalia.

Laboratory

Diagnosis is made by clinical findings.

Treatment

Hypertelorism: Minor degrees of deformity (referred to as telecanthus) can be corrected by removing a small amount of bone in the midline. A limited frontal craniotomy is performed in the midline osteotomy.

Epicanthus: Epicanthus tarsalis, palpebralis and supraculiarus will decrease with age. Skin resection such as Verwey's Y to V operation, double Z-plasty, Mustard's technique or five-flap procedure works.

Bibliography

1. Gocke H, Muradow I, Stein W. The fetal phenotype of the 18p- syndrome. Report of a male fetus at twenty-one weeks. Ann Genet. 1988;31:60-4.
2. Zumel RM, Darnaude MT, Delicado A, et al. The 18p- syndrome. Report of five cases. Ann Genet. 1989;32:160-3.

1133. 3p- SYNDROME (3p DELETION SYNDROME)

General

Chromosome 3p deletion syndrome.

Ocular

Blepharoptosis; telecanthus; mongoloid (down-slanting) palpebral fissures.

Clinical

Mental retardation; profound growth failure; characteristic facies; low-birth-weight; trigonocephaly; psychomotor delay; micrognathia.

Laboratory/Ocular

Diagnosis is made by clinical findings.

Treatment/Ocular

Ptosis: If visual acuity is affected most cases require surgical correction, and there are several procedures that may be used including levator resection, repair or advancement and Fasanella-Servat.

Bibliography

1. Drumheller T, McGillivray BC, Behrner D, et al. Precise localisation of 3p25 breakpoints in four patients with the 3p- syndrome. J Med Genet. 1996;33:842-7.
2. Higgins JJ, Rosen DR, Loveless JM, et al. A gene for nonsyndromic mental retardation maps to chromosome 3p25-pter. Neurology. 2000;55: 335-40.

1134. 9p- SYNDROME (9p DELETION SYNDROME)

General

Congenital mental retardation syndrome due to a 9p deletion.

Ocular

Mongoloid (down-slanting) eyes; usually glaucoma.

Clinical

Mental retardation; sociable personality; trigonocephaly; wide, flat nasal bridge; anteverted nostrils; long upper lip; short neck; long digits; predominance of finger whorls; choanal atresia; usually seizures.

Laboratory/Ocular

Diagnosis is made by clinical findings.

Treatment/Ocular

Glaucoma: Its medication should be the first plan of action. If medication is unsuccessful, a filtering surgical procedure with or without antimetabolites may be beneficial.

Bibliography

1. Alfi OS, Donnell GN, Allderdice PW, et al. The 9p-syndrome. Ann Genet. 1976;19:11-6.
2. Chaves-Carballo E, Frank LM, Rary J, et al. Neurologic aspects of the 9p- syndrome. Pediatr Neurol. 1985;1:57-9.
3. Shashi V, Golden WL, Fryburg JS. Choanal atresia in a patient with the deletion (9p) syndrome. Am J Med Genet. 1994;49:88-90.

1135. PAGE SYNDROME (HYPERTENSIVE DIENCEPHALIC SYNDROME)

General

Irritation of parasympathetic and sympathetic centers in diencephalon; intradermal histamine 0.25 mg reproduces syndrome; prognosis unpredictable; more frequent in women; onset age 18–30 years; spontaneous attacks lasting several minutes.

Ocular

Excessive lacrimation; arteriosclerotic and hypertensive fundus changes.

Clinical

Vasomotor blush over face, neck and trunk, followed by perspiration; tachycardia; palpitations; elevated baseline blood pressure with additional 20–30 mm Hg rise during attacks; reduced respiration, perhaps labored; increased bowel sounds; salivation; sexual frigidity; tremor of hands and generalized Paget tremulousness.

Laboratory

Diagnosis is made by clinical findings.

Treatment

Medical care involves evaluation of secondary causes and appropriate medical management involving life style changes and pharmacotherapy.

Bibliography

1. Page IH. A syndrome simulating diencephalic stimulation occurring in patients with essential hypertension. Am J Med Sci. 1935;190:9-14.

2. Schroeder HA, Goldman ML. Test for the presence of the hypertensive diencephalic syndrome using histamine. Am J Med. 1949;6:162-7.

1136. PAGET DISEASE (CHRONIC CONGENITAL IDIOPATHIC HYPERPHOSPHATEMIA; CONGENITAL HYPERPHOSPHATEMIA; FAMILIAL OSTEOECTASIA; HYPEROSTOSIS CORTICALIS DEFORMANS; OSTEITIS DEFORMANS; OSTEOCHALASIS DESMALIS FAMILIARIS; POZZI SYNDROME)

General

Autosomal dominant; more frequent in men, but more severe in women; onset after age 40 years; characterized by diffuse cortical thickening of involved bones with osteoporosis, bowing deformities and shortening of stature; osteogenic sarcoma not infrequent.

Ocular

Shallow orbits with progressive unilateral or bilateral proptosis palsy of extraocular muscles; corneal ring opacities; cataract; retinal hemorrhages; pigmentary retinopathy; macular changes resembling Kuhnt-Junius degeneration; angioid streaks; papilledema; optic nerve atrophy; blue sclera; exophthalmos.

Clinical

Skull deformities; kyphoscoliosis; hypertension and arteriosclerosis; muscle weakness; waddling gait; hearing impairment; osteoarthritis.

Laboratory

Bone-specific alkaline phosphatase (BSAP) levels. Radiographs may demonstrate both osteolysis and excessive bone formation. Bone biopsies may be necessary for diagnostic purposes in rare cases.

Treatment

Medical therapy for Paget disease should include bisphosphonate treatment with serial monitoring of bone markers. Nonsteroidal anti-inflammatory drugs and acetaminophen may be effective for pain management. Chemotherapy, radiation or both may be used to treat neoplasms arising from pagetic bone.

Additional Resource

1. Lohr KM (2011). Paget Disease. [online] Available from http://www.emedicine.com/med/TOPIC2998.HTM [Accessed April, 2012].

1137. PAINE SYNDROME

General

Microcephaly-spastic diplegia; occurs only in males; onset from birth; sex-linked inheritance; poor prognosis, death usually within first year of life.

Ocular

Optic atrophy.

Clinical

Microcephaly; poor swallowing; retarded physical and mental development; seizures; lack of interest in environment; hyperreflexia; cerebellar hypoplasia; myoclonic fits; elevated level of amino acids in the cerebrospinal fluid; hypoplasia of cerebellar inferior olives and pons.

Laboratory

Diagnosis is made by clinical findings.

Treatment

Optic atrophy: Intravenous steroids may be used with optic neuritis or ischemic neuropathy. Stem cell treatment may be the future treatment of choice.

Bibliography

1. Magalini SI, Scrascia E. Dictionary of Medical Syndromes, 2nd edition. Philadelphia: JB Lippincott; 1981.
2. McKusick VA. Mendelian Inheritance in Man: A Catalog of Human Genes and Genetic Disorders, 12th edition. Baltimore: The Johns Hopkins University Press; 1998.
3. McKusick-Nathans Institute for Genetic Medicine, Johns Hopkins University and National Center for Biotechnology Information, National Library of Medicine. (2007). Online Mendelian Inheritance in Man (OMIM). [online] Available from http://www.ncbi.nlm.nih.gov/omim [Accessed April, 2012].
4. Paine RS. Evaluation of familial biochemically determined mental retardation in children, with special reference to aminoaciduria. N Engl J Med. 1960;262:658-65.

1138. PALATAL MYOCLONUS SYNDROME

General

Vascular disorders of brainstem that involve inferior olive and olivo-dentate connection; continuous rhythmic contractions of the palate that occur 100–180 times per minute.

Ocular

Opsoclonia; ocular bobbing; nystagmus; torsional, pendular nystagmus; gaze-evoked nystagmus.

Clinical

Contraction of pharynx, larynx, tongue, floor of the mouth, neck and diaphragm; nodding of head; tremor of hand; sleep apnea; multiple sclerosis.

Laboratory

Computed tomography (CT), MRI and transcranial Doppler.

Treatment

Anticoagulation therapy, angioplasty. In addition, physical, occupational and speech therapists consultations may be necessary.

Bibliography

1. Magalini SI, Scrascia E. Dictionary of Medical Syndromes, 2nd edition. Philadelphia: JB Lippincott; 1981.

2. Miller NR (Ed). Walsh and Hoyt's Clinical Neuro-Ophthalmology, 4th edition. Baltimore: Williams & Wilkins; 1995. p. 4371.

3. Sakurai N, Koike Y, Kaneoke Y, et al. Sleep apnea and palatal myoclonus in a patient with neuro-Behçet syndrome. Intern Med. 1993;32:336-9.

4. Yap CB, Barron K, Mayo C. "Ocular bobbing" in palatal myoclonus. Arch Neurol. 1968;18:304-10.

1139. PALLIDAL DEGENERATION, PROGRESSIVE, WITH RETINITIS PIGMENTOSA (HYPOPREBETALIPOPROTEINEMIA, ACANTHOCYTOSIS, RETINITIS PIGMENTOSA, AND PALLIDAL DEGENERATION; HARP SYNDROME)

General

Autosomal recessive; destruction of global pallida and reticular portions of substantia nigra; also may be associated with hypoprebetalipoproteinemia and acanthocytosis; various combinations of components of HARP syndrome may be caused by several distinct genetic diseases or may represent variable manifestations of a contiguous gene defect.

Ocular

Retinitis pigmentosa.

Clinical

Progressive extrapyramidal rigidity; dysarthria.

Laboratory

Diagnosis is made by clinical findings and visual fields.

Treatment

Maximize the vision they do have with refraction and low-vision evaluation. Vitamin A 15,000 IU/day is thought to slow the decline of retinal function, dark sunglasses for outdoor use, surgery for cataract, genetic counseling.

Additional Resource

1. Telander DG (2012). Retinitis Pigmentosa. [online] Available from http://www.emedicine.com/oph/TOPIC704.HTM [Accessed April, 2012].

1140. PALLISTER-KILLIAN SYNDROME (MOSAIC TETRASOMY; PKS)

General

Variable condition caused by a mosaic tetrasomy of chromosome 12p.

Ocular

Reported manifestations include hypertelorism, narrow palpebral fissures, prominent epicanthal folds, lower eyelid entropion, ptosis, sparse eyebrows, sparse eyelashes, hypoplastic supraorbital ridge, miotic pupils, sluggish pupils, iris atrophy/hypoplasia, iris heterochromia, cataracts, nystagmus, esotropia, exotropia, optic nerve atrophy, oval optic disks, fundus hypopigmentation, amblyopia and retinal pigmentary mosaicism.

Clinical

Patients have "coarse" facial features, midface malformations, psychomotor delay, hypotonia, scalp hair sparsity and variegated lightly and darkly pigmented skin.

Laboratory

Diagnosis is made by clinical findings which include visual fields, electroretinogram and dark adaptation studies.

Treatment

Maximize the vision they do have with proper refraction and low-vision evaluation. Vitamin A/beta-carotene may also be useful.

Bibliography

1. Bielanska MM, Khalifa MM, Duncan AM. Pallister-Killian syndrome: a mild case diagnosed by fluorescence in situ hybridization. Review of the literature and expansion of the phenotype. Am J Med Genet. 1996;65:104-8.

2. Birch M, Patterson A, Fryer A. Hypopigmentation of the fundi associated with Pallister-Killian syndrome. J Pediatr Ophthalmol Strabismus. 1995;32:128-31.

3. Graham W, Brown SM, Shah F, et al. Retinal pigment mosaicism in Pallister-Killian syndrome (mosaic tetrasomy 12p). Arch Ophthalmol. 1999;117:1648-9.

4. Horn D, Majewski F, Hildebrandt B, et al. Pallister-Killian syndrome: normal karyotype in prenatal chorionic villi, in postnatal lymphocytes, and in slowly growing epidermal cells, but mosaic tetrasomy 12p in skin fibroblasts. J Med Genet. 1995;32:68-71.

5. Horneff G, Majewski F, Hildebrand B, et al. Pallister-Killian syndrome in older children and adolescents. Pediatr Neurol. 1993;9:312-5.

6. Pallister PD, Meisner LF, Elejalde BR, et al. The Pallister mosaic syndrome. Birth Defects Orig Artic Ser. 1977;13:103-10.

7. Reynolds JF, Daniel A, Kelly TE, et al. Isochromosome 12p mosaicism (Pallister mosaic aneuploidy or Pallister-Killian syndrome): report of 11 cases. Am J Med Genet. 1987;7:257-74.

8. Schaefer GB, Jochar A, Muneer R, et al. Clinical variability of tetrasomy 12p. Clin Genet. 1997;51:102-8.

9. Teschler-Nicola M, Killian W. Case report 72: mental retardation, unusual facial appearance, abnormal hair. Synd Ident. 1981;7:6-7.

10. Warburton D, Anyane-Yeboa K, Francke U. Mosaic tetrasomy 12p: four new cases, and confirmation of the chromosomal origin of the supernumerary chromosome in one of the original Pallister-Mosaic syndrome cases. Am J Med Genet. 1987;27:275-83.

1141. PALPEBRAL COLOBOMA-LIPOMA SYNDROME (NASOPALPEBRAL LIPOMA-COLOBOMA)

General

Autosomal dominant; described in a Venezuelan family.

Ocular

Coloboma of upper and lower eyelids at junction between their middle and inner thirds; fat deposits of both upper eyelids; malposition of lacrimal puncta; hypertelorism; telecanthus.

Clinical

Broad nasal bridge; fatty accumulations on nasal bridge and nasolabial area; maxillary hypoplasia.

Laboratory

Diagnosis is made by clinical findings.

Treatment

Corneal protection is the primary goal in the medical treatment of eyelid colobomas. The eyelid coloboma is large, immediate surgical closure is usually needed to prevent corneal compromise.

Additional Resource

1. Bashour M (2010). Eyelid Coloboma. [online] Available from http://www.emedicine.com/oph/TOPIC673.HTM [Accessed April, 2012].

1142. PANCOAST SYNDROME (HARE SYNDROME; SUPERIOR PULMONARY SULCUS SYNDROME)

General

Mass occupying lesion in pulmonary apex; erosion of first three ribs frequent; primary bronchogenic carcinoma most frequent cause; symptomatology similar to lower radicular (Dejerine-Klumpke) syndrome and scalenus anticus (Naffziger) syndrome; Horner syndrome—caused by involvement of sympathetic chain (also can be caused by locally invasive fungus such as *Cryptococcus neoformans*) or lymphomatoid granulomatosis.

Ocular

Mild enophthalmos; ptosis; narrowing of the palpebral fissure; miosis.

Clinical

Pulmonary apical tumor; severe shoulder pain; paresthesia, pain and paresis of the homolateral arm with atrophy of arm and hand muscles.

Laboratory

Imaging and biopsy are the cornerstones of diagnosis.

Treatment

Radiation and chemotherapy, surgical treatment of choice is complete removal of the tumor by en bloc chest wall resection combined with lobectomy and node staging.

Additional Resource

1. D'Silva KJ (2011). Pancoast Syndrome. [online] Available from http://www.emedicine.com/med/TOPIC3418.HTM [Accessed April, 2012].

1143. PANCREATITIS

General

Inflammation of pancreas.

Ocular

Xerosis; night blindness; multiple branch retinal artery occlusions; cotton-wool patches; retinal edema; striate and blot hemorrhages; retinopathy of pancreatitis has been considered to indicate multiple-organ failure and poor prognosis in severe acute pancreatitis; mechanism may be secondary to granulocyte aggregation and leukoembolization due to activated complement.

Clinical

Chronic pancreatitis; lipid emboli; malabsorption; vitamin A deficiency.

Laboratory

Pancreatic function tests, diagnosis of chronic pancreatitis requires morphologic abnormalities to appear on imaging procedures.

Treatment

The goals of medical treatment are to modify behaviors that may exacerbate the disease, to enable the pancreas to heal itself, to determine the cause of abdominal pain and alleviate it, to detect pancreatic exocrine insufficiency and restore digestion and absorption to normal, and to diagnose and treat endocrine insufficiency. Cessation of alcohol consumption and tobacco smoking are important. Endoscopic treatment is sometimes necessary.

Additional Resource

1. Huffman JL (2012). Chronic Pancreatitis. [online] Available from http://www.emedicine.com/med/TOPIC1721.HTM [Accessed April, 2012].

1144. PAPILLEDEMA

General

Swelling of the optic disk due to increased intracranial pressure.

Clinical

Holocranial headaches, neck and back pain, pulsatile tinnitus, nausea and vomiting.

Ocular

Visual loss, nerve fiber loss, intermittent or constant diplopia.

Laboratory

Lumbar puncture to determine if intracranial pressure is elevated.

Treatment

Underlying cause should be determined and treated. Systemic acetazolamide is the medical therapy of choice.

Additional Resource

1. Gossman MV (2012). Papilledema. [online] Available from http://www.emedicine.com/oph/TOPIC187.HTM [Accessed April, 2012].

1145. PAPILLOMA (VERRUCA; WART)

General

Cutaneous or mucosal tumor of proliferating epithelial and fibrovascular tissues; viral etiology or noninfectious.

Ocular

Papillary conjunctivitis; pseudopterygium; corneal opacity; epithelial keratitis; corneal vascularization; lid ulcers; lacrimal system obstruction; hemorrhages of conjunctiva, lids and lacrimal system.

Clinical

Mulberry- or cauliflower-like tumors that may occur on any cutaneous or mucosal surface.

Laboratory

Histologic evaluation is diagnostic.

Treatment

Salicylic acid is a first-line therapy used to treat warts. Intralesional immunotherapy using injections, cryosurgery, carbon dioxide lasers, electrodesiccation and curettage or surgical excision.

Additional Resource

1. Shenefelt PD (2011). Nongenital Warts. [online] Available from http://www.emedicine.com/derm/TOPIC457.HTM [Accessed April, 2012].

1146. PAPILLON-LEAGE-PSAUME SYNDROME (DYSPLASIA LINGUOFACIALIS; GORLIN SYNDROME; GROB LINGUOFACIAL DYSPLASIA; LINGUOFACIAL DYSPLASIA OF GROB; ORO-DIGITAL-FACIAL SYNDROME; OFD SYNDROME; ORO-DIGITAL-FACIAL DYSOSTOSIS)

General

Familial with strong female preponderance; transmitted as a dominant; partial trisomy has been suggested for the 6-12 (C) chromosome.

Ocular

Hypertelorism; displaced medial and lateral canthi; antimongoloid slanting of palpebral fissures; exotropia; see-saw winking.

Clinical

Clefts of jaws and tongue due to abnormalities in development of frenulum; syndactyly; polydactyly; alopecia; white, hamartomatous patches of midline of tongue; mental retardation; bradydactyly; hypoplastic nasal cartilages; seborrheic changes; dystopia canthus; pseudocleft of upper lip; alopecia; missing mandibular lateral incisors.

Laboratory

Patients with suspected Gorlin syndrome undergo biopsy with samples obtained from several suspicious skin lesions.

Treatment

Wide range of congenital anomalies may need to be treated by a wide range of specialists, including dermatologists, dentists, cardiologists, oncologists and orthopedic surgeons. Patients most commonly present to a dermatologist because of skin nodules.

Additional Resource

1. Berg D (2011). Nevoid Basal Cell Carcinoma Syndrome. [online] Available from http://www.emedicine.com/ped/TOPIC890.HTM [Accessed April, 2012].

1147. PAPILLON-LEFEVRE SYNDROME (HYPERKERATOSIS PALMOPLANTARIS WITH PERIODONTOSIS)

General

Autosomal recessive; onset between the ages of 1 and 4 years.

Ocular

Nystagmus

Clinical

Hyperkeratosis of the palms and soles associated with destruction of the periodontal ligament and premature exfoliation of the teeth; bad breath; loose teeth; loss of teeth.

Laboratory

Diagnosis is made by clinical findings.

Treatment

Treatment is symptomatic and includes topical keratolytics, topical retinoids, potent topical steroids and oral retinoids.

Additional Resource

1. Lee RA (2011). Keratosis Palmaris et Plantaris. [online] Available from http://www.emedicine. com/derm/TOPIC589.HTM [Accessed April, 2012].

1148. PAPILLORENAL SYNDROME (RENAL-COLOBOMA SYNDROME)

General

Inherited condition often characterized by the association of bilateral centrally excavated optic disks with multiple cilioretinal vessels and dysplastic kidneys.

Clinical

Dysplastic kidneys, glomerulonephropathy and proteinuria.

Ocular

Retinal detachment; disk abnormalities.

Laboratory

Ultrasound of the kidneys, elevated blood urea nitrogen (BUN) and creatinine levels, urinalysis to show proteinuria and blood for Paz2 mutation analysis.

Treatment

Retinal detachment: Scleral buckle, pneumatic retinopexy and vitrectomy may be used to close all the breaks.

Bibliography

1. Roy FH, Fraunfelder FW, Fraunfelder FT. Roy and Fraunfelder's Current Ocular Therapy, 6th edition. Philadelphia: WB Saunders; 2008.

1149. PAPPATACI FEVER (PHLEBOTOMUS FEVER; SANDFLY FEVER)

General

Viral etiology; transmitted by the sandfly *Phlebotomus papatasii.*

Ocular

Pick sign of conjunctiva (conjunctival injection limited to the exposed portion of the conjunctiva);

uveitis; optic neuritis; papilledema; papillitis; blepharospasm; retinal venous engorgement; vitreal exudates.

Clinical

Fever; headache; myalgia; pain; stiffness of the neck and back.

Laboratory

Parasite can be detected through direct evidence from peripheral blood, bone marrow or splenic aspirates.

Treatment

Sodium stibogluconate, a pentavalent antimonial compound (Sbv), is the drug of choice.

Additional Resource

1. Vidyashankar C (2011). Pediatric Leishmaniasis. [online] Available from http://www.emedicine. com/ped/TOPIC1292.HTM [Accessed April, 2012].

1150. PARAGONIMIASIS (DISTOMIASIS; ENDEMIC HEMOPTYSIS)

General

Chronic lung infection; causative agent is *Paragonimus* (a trematode); transmitted by eating undercooked crabs or crayfish and drinking contaminated water; affects all ages; most severe in children.

Ocular

Convergence paralysis; optic atrophy; lid cysts; dacryocystitis; papilledema; homonymous hemianopsia.

Clinical

Hemoptysis; dyspnea; fever; anorexia; weight loss; pleural effusion; pneumothorax; diarrhea; epileptic seizures; hemiplegia; leukocytosis; eosinophilia; anemia; cystic bronchiectasis; encephalitis; chronic bronchitis; intestinal or peritoneal infections; central nervous system— paragonimiasis occurs predominantly in persons under age 30 years.

Laboratory

Chest radiography reveals abnormalities in approximately 80–90% of patients. Lumbar puncture: examination of infected CSF reveals bloody or turbid fluid containing numerous eosinophils.

Treatment

Antiparasitic therapy is the mainstay of paragonimiasis treatment. Therapy may also be required for seizures caused by an inflammatory reaction to dying worms in the setting of cerebral. After penicillin therapy, lesions become noninfectious in 24 hours.

Additional Resource

1. Rosenbaum SD (2012). Paragonimiasis. [online] Available from http://www.emedicine.com/ped/ TOPIC1729.HTM [Accessed April, 2012].

1151. PARINAUD OCULOGLANDULAR SYNDROME (BARTONELLA HENSELAE; CAT SCRATCH DISEASE; CAT SCRATCH OCULOGLANDULAR SYNDROME; PARINAUD CONJUNCTIVA-ADENITIS SYNDROME)

General

Most frequently seen in children; incubation time 7–10 days; caused by small pleomorphic Gram-negative bacillus; good prognosis; affects both sexes; about 90% of patients with this condition have serologic evidence of infection by *Rochalimaea henselae.*

Ocular

Conjunctivitis; retrotarsal conjunctival granulations; formation of granulomata in anterior segment about 3 mm high and 2–6 mm in diameter; inferior fornix usually affected; ulceration common; neuroretinitis; optic neuritis.

Clinical

Tender, red papule at the site of a cat scratch; regional preauricular and cervical lymphadenitis (often only one gland involved); irregular fever for 4–5 days and malaise; fever; parotid gland swelling.

Laboratory

Histopathology of biopsied lymph node of Warthin-Starry silver stain.

Treatment

Symptomatic treatment includes warm compresses, analgesics and antipyretics. Aspiration of lymph node if distention causes pain. Antibiotics may be necessary in severe cases.

Additional Resource

1. Nervi SJ (2011). Catscratch Disease. [online] Available from http://www.emedicine.com/med/TOPIC304.HTM [Accessed April, 2012].

1152. PARINAUD SYNDROME (DIVERGENCE PARALYSIS; PARALYSIS OF VERTICAL MOVEMENTS; PRETECTAL SYNDROME; SUBTHALAMIC SYNDROME)

General

Various causes including pineal tumor, supranuclear lesions, vascular lesions, inflammation, hemorrhages, midbrain lesions, lesion of posterior white commissure of pons, red nucleus or superior cerebellar peduncle; combination of Parinaud and von Monakow syndromes is known as Gruner-Bertolotti syndrome, which consists of paralysis in upward gaze, tremors, hemiplegia and sensory disturbances.

Ocular

Retraction of lids with lesion in mesencephalic gray matter and ptosis with lesions more anteriorly; paralysis of conjugate upward movement of the eye without paralysis of convergence; occasionally paralysis of upward and downward movement; spasm with convergence insufficiency; contralateral hemianopsia occurs when the lateral geniculate body becomes involved in case of infiltrating tumor; wide pupils that fail to react to light but sometimes react during accommodation (Holmes); papilledema (usually severe).

Clinical

Vertigo; contralateral cerebellar ataxia and choreoathetoid movement if lesion involves superior cerebellar peduncle after decussation.

Laboratory

Diagnosis is made by clinical findings. CT and MRI may also be helpful.

Treatment

Papilledema: Underlying cause should be determined and treated. Systemic acetazolamide is the medical therapy of choice.

Additional Resource

1. Chi-Shing Zee (2011). Imaging in Pineal Germinoma. [online] Available from http://www.emedicine.com/radio/TOPIC554.HTM [Accessed April, 2012].

1153. PARKINSON SYNDROME (PARALYSIS AGITANS; SHAKING PALSY)

General

Late stages of epidemic encephalitis; present with arteriosclerosis and with manganese and carbon monoxide poisoning; widespread destruction of pigmented cells in substantia nigra.

Ocular

Decreased blinking; lid fluttering; blepharospasm; oculogyric crises; ocular hypotony; blepharoplegia; ptosis; nystagmus; paralysis of convergence; paralysis of lateral rectus muscle; absent or sluggish pupillary reactions to light or convergence; mydriasis or anisocoria; optic neuritis; papilledema; abnormal saccades.

Clinical

Slowness of movements; loss of facial expression; "cogwheel" rigidity of the arms; rhythmical tremors; drooling; shuffling gait; stooping; monotonous voice.

Laboratory

Magnetic resonance imaging (MRI) and CT scan reveal calcium and ceruloplasmin to exclude other conditions.

Treatment

The goal of medical management is to provide control of signs and symptoms for as long as possible while minimizing adverse effects. Medications usually provide good symptomatic control.

Additional Resource

1. Hauser RA (2012). Parkinson Disease. [online] Available from http://www.emedicine.com/neuro/TOPIC304.HTM [Accessed April, 2012].

1154. PAROTID APLASIA OR HYPOPLASIA (LACRIMAL PUNCTA ABSENCE; SALIVARY GLAND ABSENCE)

General

Autosomal dominant.

Ocular

Lacrimal gland aplasia; absence or severe dysfunction of lacrimal glands.

Clinical

Aplasia of parotid salivary glands; hemifacial microsomia; mandibulofacial dysostoses; xerostomia; rampant caries; edentulous, salivary gland dysfunction; parotid agenesis or hypoplasia; impalpable parotid gland; absence of the orifice of Stensen duct; bilateral parotid gland aplasia.

Laboratory

Diagnosis is made by clinical findings.

Treatment

Ocular lubrication with topical drops and ointments. Bandage contact lens may sometimes be necessary.

Additional Resource

1. DeAngelis DD (2010). Alacrima. [online] Available from http://www.emedicine.com/oph/TOPIC693.HTM [Accessed April, 2012].

1155. PARS PLANITIS (ANGIOHYALITIS, CHRONIC CYCLITIS, PERIPHERAL UVEITIS, PERIPHERAL UVEORETINITIS, VITREITIS)

General

Idiopathic inflammatory condition.

Clinical

Sarcoidosis, multiple sclerosis, Lyme disease, toxocariasis, HTLV1.

Ocular

Cells and debris in the vitreous, vitreitis, vascular sheathing, neovascularization, cystoid macular edema, vitreous hemorrhage, cataracts, glaucoma, retinal detachment, retinoschisis.

Laboratory

Diagnosis is made by clinical findings.

Treatment

Systemic corticosteroids, chlorambucil, azathioprine, cyclophosphamide, methotrexate, cyclosporine. Periocular corticosteroids are very effective. Cryotherapy is used on patients who are intolerant to corticosteroids.

Bibliography

1. Roy FH, Fraunfelder FW, Fraunfelder FT. Roy and Fraunfelder's Current Ocular Therapy, 6th edition. Philadelphia: WB Saunders; 2008.

1156. PARTIAL TRISOMY 16q SYNDROME

General

Partial trisomy 16q with chromosome banding; rare.

Ocular

Narrow palpebral fissures; antimongoloid lid slant; hypertelorism; strabismus; epicanthus; congenital glaucoma; corneal edema; shallow anterior chamber; Rieger anomaly.

Clinical

Dry skin; periorbital edema; hydrocele; general hypotonia; low-set ears; micrognathia; hypoplastic lower lip; long philtrum; stumpy hands with short fingers; pectus excavatum.

Laboratory

Diagnosis is made by clinical findings.

Treatment

Congenital glaucoma: Primary congenital glaucoma almost always is managed surgically, both goniotomy and trabeculectomy may be useful. When multiple goniotomies and/or trabeculectomies fail, the surgeon usually resorts to a filtering procedure.

Corneal edema: Control IOP, hypertonic salt solution or ointment, soft contact lens, anterior stromal puncture or conjunctival flap, PTK, hairdryer held at arms length and posterior lamellar keratoplasty.

Bibliography

1. Balestrazzi P, Giovannelli G, Landucci Rubini L, et al. Partial trisomy 16q resulting from maternal translocation. Hum Genet. 1979;49:229-35.
2. Ferguson JG, Hicks EL. Rieger's anomaly and glaucoma associated with partial trisomy 16q. Case report. Arch Ophthalmol. 1987;105:323.

1157. PASSOW SYNDROME (BREMER STATUS DYSRAPHICUS; STATUS DYSRAPHICUS SYNDROME; SYRINGOBULBIA; SYRINGOMYELIA)

General

Congenital nonclosure of the neural tube; familial occurrence or may be sporadic; insidious onset in the second to third decade of life.

Ocular

Enophthalmos; ptosis; rotatory nystagmus; heterochromia iridis; anterior uveitis; corneal anesthesia; neuroparalytic keratitis; paralysis of III, V, VI and VII cranial nerves; Horner syndrome; anisocoria; papilledema; optic atrophy; zonular cataract (see Horner Syndrome).

Clinical

Anesthesia over area of first division of trigeminal nerve; facial hemiatrophy; facial nerve paralysis; muscular weakness; cervical ribs; kyphoscoliosis; spina bifida; unilateral numbness of fingers; loss of deep reflexes; insensitivity to pain and temperature in affected areas; neurogenic bladder.

Laboratory

Magnetic resonance imaging (MRI) and computed tomography (CT).

Treatment

Suboccipital and cervical decompression, laminectomy and syringotomy, shunt, fourth ventriculostomy, terminal ventriculostomy, and neuroendoscopic surgery may be considered.

Additional Resource

1. Al-Shatoury HAH (2012). Syringomyelia. [online] Available from http://www.emedicine.com/neuro/TOPIC359.HTM [Accessed April, 2012].

1158. PATTERNED DYSTROPHY OF RETINAL PIGMENT EPITHELIUM

General

Autosomal dominant; probably there is a migration of pigment granules in the pigment epithelium, resulting in a specific configuration.

Ocular

Reticular fishnet-like dystrophy; macroreticular (spider-shaped); butterfly-shaped pigment dystrophy of fovea.

Clinical

None

Laboratory

Optical coherence tomography; multifocal electroretinography; fluoroscein angiography.

Treatment

Laser photocoagulation.

Bibliography

1. Deutman AF. Macular dystrophies. In: Ryan SJ (Ed). Retina, 2nd edition. St. Louis: CV Mosby; 1994.
2. Hsieh RC, Fine BS, Lyons JS. Patterned dystrophies of the retinal pigment epithelium. Arch Ophthalmol. 1977;95:429-35.

1159. PEDIATRIC CONGENITAL GLAUCOMA (BUPHTHALMOS; PRIMARY INFANTILE GLAUCOMA)

General

Rare, found in infants who have aqueous outflow obstruction.

Clinical

None

Ocular

Open-angle glaucoma, photophobia, cloudy cornea, blepharospasm and lacrimation.

Laboratory

Diagnosis is made by clinical findings.

Treatment

Prompt surgical intervention for intraocular pressure control which includes angle surgery, goniotomy and trabeculectomy, correction of ametropia, rigorous amblyopia treatment.

Additional Resource

1. Cibis GW (2011). Primary Congenital Glaucoma. [online] Available from http://www.emedicine.com/oph/TOPIC138.HTM [Accessed April, 2012].

1160. PEDICULOSIS AND PHTHIRIASIS

General

Infestation of lice on head, body or pubic area.

Ocular

Conjunctivitis; keratitis; infestation of lice or nits glued to shafts of eyelashes and eyebrow.

Clinical

Pruritus; skin excoriation; impetigo; pyoderma with lymphadenitis and febrile episodes.

Laboratory

Removal from hair shaft and examination under microscope.

Treatment

Treatments involve spreading an ointment at the base of the eyelashes at night to trap mites as they emerge from their burrow and/or move from one follicle to another.

Additional Resource

1. Guenther L (2012). Pediculosis (Lice). [online] Available from http://www.emedicine.com/med/TOPIC1769.HTM [Accessed April, 2012].

1161. PELIZAEUS-MERZBACHER DISEASE (APLASIA AXIALIS EXTRACORTICALIS CONGENITA; SUDANOPHILIC LEUKODYSTROPHY)

General

Rare; subdivision of diffuse cerebral sclerosis predominantly involving the white matter of CNS; onset in infancy or childhood; X-linked recessive; male members affected through normal-appearing carrier mothers; abnormal myelin/myelin sheath structure secondary to abnormal gene on the X chromosome.

Ocular

Lateral, rotatory or vertical nystagmus or nonrhythmic wandering eye movements; visual impairment from occipital lobe involvement; tapetoretinal degeneration characteristic of retinitis pigmentosa; attenuated arterioles; optic atrophy; papilledema.

Clinical

Retarded development; gait instability and ataxia; intention tremor and athetosis; hearing and speech disturbances; atrophic disturbances; spastic paralysis; weight gain.

Laboratory

Magnetic resonance imaging (MRI) is the most useful imaging study and demonstrates symmetric and widespread abnormality of the white matter of cerebrum, brainstem and cerebellum.

Treatment

Severe spasticity may benefit from intrathecal baclofen. Surgical release of contractures and other orthopedic procedures.

Additional Resource

1. Chawla J (2012). Pelizaeus-Merzbacher Disease. [online] Available from http://www.emedicine.com/neuro/TOPIC520.HTM [Accessed April, 2012].

1162. PELLUCID MARGINAL DEGENERATION

General

Progressive, rare, noninflammatory peripheral corneal thinning disorder.

Clinical

None

Ocular

Inferior corneal thinning.

Laboratory

Videokeratography detects small amount of change.

Treatment

Contact lens, peripheral lamellar crescentic keratoplasty followed in a few months by a central penetrating keratopathy.

Additional Resource

1. Rasheed K (2010). Pellucid Marginal Degeneration. [online] Available from http://www.emedicine.com/oph/TOPIC551.HTM [Accessed April, 2012].

1163. PEMPHIGUS FOLIACEUS (CAZENAVE DISEASE)

General

Attacks on individuals of any race, age or sex; high incidence in Brazil; characterized by bullous skin lesions resulting in generalized exfoliation.

Ocular

Exfoliative or bullous lesions of lid and conjunctiva; pannus; infiltration of cornea and iris; cataract.

Clinical

Cutaneous manifestations that progress to scaling, crusted patches; simulates lupus erythematosus and exfoliative erythroderma.

Laboratory

Diagnosis is confirmed by direct immunofluorescence.

Treatment

Topical glucocorticosteroids. In more extensive cases adjuvant immunosuppressants, including systemic corticosteroids, azathioprine, mycophenolate mofetil, cyclophosphamide and cyclosporine A, may be necessary.

Additional Resource

1. Schwartz RA (2011). Pemphigus Foliaceus. [online] Available from http://www.emedicine.com/derm/TOPIC318.HTM [Accessed April, 2012].

1164. PEMPHIGUS VULGARIS

General

Primarily in middle-aged people; prognosis varies from poor to chronic; generalized bullous eruption; blistering autoimmune disease that affects the skin and mucous membranes; association between particular HLA-DR4 and pemphigus vulgaris has been reported.

Ocular

Conjunctival bullae; catarrhal conjunctivitis; scarring and adhesions of conjunctiva.

Clinical

Cutaneous blisters which may be clear, pustular or hemorrhagic.

Laboratory

Histopathology from the edge of a blister; indirect immunofluorescence (IDIF) using the patient's serum if direct immunofluorescence (DIF) is positive.

Treatment

Corticosteroids and immunosuppressive drugs are useful.

Additional Resource

1. Zeina B (2011). Pemphigus Vulgaris. [online] Available from http://www.emedicine.com/derm/TOPIC319.HTM [Accessed April, 2012].

1165. PENDRED SYNDROME (SPORADIC GOITER WITH DEAFNESS)

General

Autosomal recessive; defect in thyroxine biosynthesis.

Ocular

Retinal pigmentary degenerative changes; pendular nystagmus; bull's-eye-type macular degeneration.

Clinical

Thyroid enlargement; sensorineural hearing loss; mental retardation; thyroid carcinoma.

Laboratory

Diagnosis is confirmed by demonstrating decreased levels of serum thyroid hormone.

Treatment

The mainstay in the treatment is early diagnosis and thyroid hormone replacement.

Additional Resource

1. Postellon DC (2011). Congenital Hypothyroidism. [online] Available from http://www.emedicine.com/ped/TOPIC501.HTM [Accessed April, 2012].

1166. PERICENTRIC SYNDROME (PERICENTRIC INVERSION OF CHROMOSOME 11)

General

Etiology unknown; leukocyte chromosomes show a pericentric inversion of chromosome 11.

Ocular

Strabismus; hypertelorism; congenital glaucoma; aniridia; corneal disease; epicanthal folds.

Clinical

Microcephaly; broad nasal bridge; arched palate; hyperextensibility of elbows; left hand shows single transverse crease and right hand shows three palmar creases radiating from radial border.

Laboratory

Diagnosis is made by clinical findings.

Treatment

Congenital glaucoma: Primary congenital glaucoma almost always is managed surgically, both goniotomy and trabeculectomy may be useful. When multiple goniotomies and/or trabeculectomies fail, the surgeon usually resorts to a filtering procedure.

Anirida: Systemic or Topical antiglaucoma therapy.

Bibliography

1. Broughton WL, Rosenbaum KN, Beauchamp GR. Congenital glaucoma and other ocular abnormalities associated with pericentric inversion of chromosome 11. Arch Ophthalmol. 1983;101: 594-7.

1167. PERIOCULAR MERKEL CELL CARCINOMA

General

Aggressive primary cutaneous neoplasm that frequently involves the eyelids and periocular region.

Clinical

Skin cancer.

Ocular

Uvea, eyelid tumors.

Laboratory

Diagnosis is usually made on the basis of histologic findings.

Treatment

Chemotherapy, radiation, full-thickness resection of lid tumor.

Bibliography

1. Roy FH, Fraunfelder FW, Fraunfelder FT. Roy and Fraunfelder's Current Ocular Therapy, 6th edition. Philadelphia: WB Saunders; 2008.

1168. PERIOCULAR METASTATIC TUMORS (OCULAR METASTATIC TUMORS)

General

Neoplasms that develop from malignant cells and are carried from a primary site of malignancy.

Ocular

Retinal detachment; retinal hemorrhages; enophthalmos; exophthalmos; proptosis; rubeosis iridis; uveitis; papilledema; orbital hemorrhages; hyphema; paralysis of extraocular muscles; secondary glaucoma.

Clinical

Metastasis in the bloodstream and lymphatic system common; tumors of the lung or breast metastasize to globe; neoplasms that most commonly metastasize to the orbit are neuroblastomas of suprarenal medulla and retroperitoneal ganglia; Wilms tumor may involve the orbit.

Laboratory

Systemic studies include blood cell count, erythrocyte sedimentation rate and liver function tests. Ultrasound is useful with intraocular tumors.

Treatment

Chemotherapy or radiation with teletherapy if orbital tumor is nonresponsive to radiation, debulking is an option.

Additional Resource

1. Mercandetti M (2011). Orbital Tumors. [online] Available from http://www.emedicine.com/oph/TOPIC758.HTM [Accessed April, 2012].

1169. PERIPHERAL ULCERATIVE KERATITIS

General

Ulceration in the peripheral cornea; relatively uncommon; may be presenting characteristic of a systemic disease.

Clinical

Connective and vasculitic disease; herpes simplex, varicella; HIV; syphilis; hepatitis; bacillary dysentery; salmonella.

Ocular

Pain; foreign body sensation; tearing; photophobia; decreased visual acuity.

Laboratory

Testing should be focused on the suspected systemic disease.

Treatment

Local treatment is used for prevention and reduction of corneal damage. Systemic therapy is used for controlling the underlying disease. Tissue adhesives may be necessary for impending perforation. Keratectomy, conjunctival resection, amniotic membrane transplantation and keratoplasty may necessary.

Additional Resource

1. Yu EN (2012). Peripheral Ulcerative Keratitis. [online] Available from http://www.emedicine. medscape.com/article/1195980-overview [Accessed April, 2012].

1170. PERIPHERAL RETINAL BREAKS AND DEGENERATION

General

Causes are related to the development of rhegmatogenous retinal detachment.

Clinical

None

Ocular

Lattice lesions of the retina, tractional horseshoe breaks in the retina.

Laboratory

Diagnosis is made by clinical findings.

Treatment

Cryotherapy and laser use prophylacticly.

Additional Resources

1. Song MK (2010). Retinoschisis, Juvenile. [online] Available from http://www.emedicine.com/oph/ TOPIC639.HTM [Accessed April, 2012].
2. Sarraf D (2010). Lattice Degeneration. [online] Available from http://www.emedicine.com/oph/ TOPIC397.HTM [Accessed April, 2012].

1171. PERONEAL MUSCULAR ATROPHY (PMA; NEUROPATHY, HEREDITARY SENSORIMOTOR, WITH UPPER MOTOR NEURON, VISUAL PATHWAY, AND AUTONOMIC DISTURBANCE)

General

Peroneal muscular atrophy with involvement of other parts of nervous system; autosomal dominant; upper motor neuron and visual pathway lesions.

Ocular

Visual pathway lesions; ptosis; irregular pupils; iris atrophy; lack of response to light or near vision.

Clinical

Distal weakness and muscle atrophy; absent ankle jerks; foot drop; stocking-type sensory loss; diminished sweating in distal limbs.

Laboratory

Diagnosis is made by clinical findings.

Treatment

Iris atrophy: There is no treatment for this.

Ptosis: If visual acuity is affected most cases require surgical correction, and there are several procedures that may be used including levator resection, repair or advancement and Fasanella-Servat.

Bibliography

1. McKusick VA. Mendelian Inheritance in Man: A Catalog of Human Genes and Genetic Disorders, 12th edition. Baltimore: The Johns Hopkins University Press; 1998.
2. McKusick-Nathans Institute for Genetic Medicine, Johns Hopkins University and National Center for Biotechnology Information, National Library of Medicine. (2007). Online Mendelian Inheritance in Man (OMIM). [online] Available from http://www.ncbi.nlm.nih.gov/omim/ [Accessed April, 2012].
3. Rechthand E, Reife R, Kaplan JG. Hereditary neuropathy with upper motor-neuron, visual pathway, and autonomic disorders. Neurology. 1983;33:1495-7.

1172. PERSISTENT FETAL VASCULATURE

General

Spectrum of conditions caused by failure of apoptosis of the primary hyaloidal vasculature system, incomplete ocular neurovascular development.

Ocular

Amblyopia, persistent hyaloid stalk; persistent hyperplastic primary vitreous; cataract; progressive retinal detachment; vitreous hemorrhage; ciliary body detachment; decreased visual acuity.

Laboratory

Diagnosis is made based on clinical findings.

Treatment

Surgical procedure may be necessary to eliminate media opacities and relieve tractional forces.

Bibliography

1. Sisk RA, Berrocal AM, Feuer WJ, et al. Visual and anatomic outcomes with or without surgery in persistent fetal vasculature. Ophthalmology. 2010;117:2178-83.

1173. PERSISTENT HYPERPLASTIC PRIMARY VITREOUS (PERSISTENT FETAL VASCULATURE, PHPV)

General

Congenital ocular disorder with the potential to affect the eye's anterior and posterior anatomy. Usually only affects one eye.

Clinical

Systemic abnormalities may include polydactyly, microcephaly, and cleft palate and lip as well as central nervous system abnormalities.

Ocular

Anterior PHPV includes engorged radial iris vessels, microcornea, Mittendorf dot, elongated ciliary processes, microphthalmia and cataract.

Laboratory

Diagnosis is made by clinical findings.

Treatment

Monocular congenital cataract surgery and amblyopia therapy. Posterior transciliary for pars plana vitrectomy and removal of tissue.

Bibliography

1. Roy FH, Fraunfelder FW, Fraunfelder FT. Roy and Fraunfelder's Current Ocular Therapy, 6th edition. Philadelphia: WB Saunders; 2008.

1174. PERTUSSIS (WHOOPING COUGH)

General

Causative agent is *Haemophilus pertussis (Bordetella pertussis)*; not all patients who develop pertussis encephalopathy are children.

Ocular

Conjunctivitis; severe cortical blindness; papilledema; choroiditis; retinal ischemia; ocular muscle palsies; hemorrhages of eyelids, conjunctiva, orbit, anterior chamber and retina; chronic papilledema; optic neuritis; retinal and vitreous hemorrhages, and even intracranial and subarachnoid hemorrhage associated with increased intrathoracic and intra-abdominal pressures during coughing.

Clinical

Respiratory tract infection; nasal discharge; cough ending with a loud crowing; inspiratory noise (the "whoop"); thick mucoid sputum; soreness over trachea; ulcer of glottis; vomiting; tetany; encephalopathy; cortical blindness.

Laboratory

The criterion standard for diagnosis of pertussis is isolation of *B. pertussis* in culture.

Treatment

The goals of therapy include limiting the number of paroxysms, observing the severity of cough, providing assistance when necessary, and maximizing nutrition, rest and recovery. Antimicrobial agents help to prevent the spread of the infection.

Additional Resource

1. Guinto-Ocampo H (2012). Pediatric Pertussis. [online] Available from http://www.emedicine.com/ped/TOPIC1778.HTM [Accessed April, 2012].

1175. PETERS ANOMALY

General

Autosomal recessive; may be morphologic entity with several eye syndromes, including Rieger syndrome, Mietens syndrome and fetal alcohol syndrome; may be due to a developmental field defect, a contiguous gene syndrome or a defective homeotic gene controlling development of the eye and other body structures.

Ocular

Corneal opacification; lenticulocorneal adherence; iris adhesions; glaucoma; cataract; narrow lid fissures; colobomatous microphthalmia; persistent hyperplastic primary vitreous; retinal detachment; iris nodules.

Clinical

Short-limbed dwarfism; broad face; thin upper lip; hypoplastic columella; hypospadias; cleft lip and palate; craniofacial abnormalities; congenital heart disease; horseshoe kidney; polycystic kidneys; Wilms tumor; mental retardation; external ear anomalies; camptodactyly.

Laboratory

Diagnosis is made by clinical findings.

Treatment

Glaucoma therapy—peripheral optical iridectomy, filtration surgery, cryoablation, or a tube shunt may be necessary if medications do not control the pressure. Corneal transplantation may be necessary if visual acuity is decreased.

Additional Resource

1. Giri G (2012). Peters Anomaly. [online] Available from http://www.emedicine.com/oph/TOPIC112.HTM [Accessed April, 2012].

1176. PETZETAKIS-TAKOS SYNDROME (PHLYCTENULAR KERATOCONJUNCTIVITIS)

General

Malnutrition; lack of hygiene.

Ocular

Superficial keratitis; palpebral edema; corneal hyperesthesia; photophobia; blepharospasm; decreased pupillary response; xerophthalmia.

Clinical

Lymph node hypertrophy.

Laboratory

Diagnosis is made by clinical findings.

Treatment

Topical antihistamines, nonsteroidal anti-inflammatory drugs and corticosteroids may be useful.

Bibliography

1. Magalini SI, Scrascia E. Dictionary of Medical Syndromes, 2nd edition. Philadelphia: JB Lippincott; 1981.
2. Petzetakis M. Les Troubles Oculaires Pendant la Trophopenie et l'Epidemic de la Pellagre. La Keratopathie Superficielle Trophopenique. Presse Med. 1950;58:1082-4.

1177. PEUTZ-TOURAINE SYNDROME (PEUTZ-JEGHERS SYNDROME)

General

Recognized in infants; autosomal dominant; gastrointestinal polyps; jejunal polyps are consistent feature; these lesions are benign, melanin spots of the lips; buccal mucosa and digits represent second part of syndrome.

Ocular

Brownish speckled dots along border of skin and mucosa of eyelids; freckles similar to those seen on eyelids may appear on conjunctiva, primarily adjacent to limbus and along area of lid fissure;

pigment speckles of sclera and iris; brown-pigmented corneal spot.

Clinical

Brownish to black dotlike pigmentation similar to that seen on eyelids is present in the perinasal, perioral and periorbital regions, fewer on fingers and toes at birth; polyposis of gastrointestinal tract (primarily small intestine) with associated bleeding; potential for malignant transformation in the second decade of life.

Laboratory

Diagnosis is made by clinical findings.

Treatment

The benign pigmented lesions of the eyelids do not require any medical therapy. However, any benign lesion that affects vision should be excised with primary reconstruction.

Additional Resource

1. Bashour M (2011). Pigmented Lesions of the Eyelid. [online] Available from http://www.emedicine.com/oph/TOPIC715.HTM [Accessed April, 2012].

1178. PFEIFFER SYNDROME

General

Congenital craniosynostotic syndrome with a high rate of mortality shortly after birth.

Ocular

Severe proptosis (also described as extreme exophthalmic midface hyperplasia).

Clinical

Cloverleaf skull, elbow ankylosis, broad thumbs and/or broad halluces; variable additional abnormalities including pulmonary problems, brain abnormalities and prematurity that frequently lead to early death.

Laboratory

Diagnosis is made by clinical findings which include craniosynostosis and broadening of the great toes and thumbs.

Treatment

Limited medical treatment is available for abnormalities of the skin, hair, eyes or ears that result from a paucity or absence of melanocytes. The use of sunscreens and clothing is recommended to protect against ultraviolet light-induced skin damage.

Additional Resource

1. Boissy RE (2012). Congenital Patterned Leukodermas. [online] Available from http://www.emedicine.com/derm/TOPIC325.HTM [Accessed April, 2012].

1179. PHACOANAPHYLACTIC ENDOPHTHALMITIS (ENDOPHTHALMITIS PHACOANAPHYLACTICA, PHACOANAPHYLACTIC UVEITIS, PHACOANTIGENIC UVEITIS)

General

Inflammatory disease caused by immunologic sensitization of the individual to lens protein released from the sequestered capsular bag by a lens injury—surgical, traumatic or spontaneous

Clinical

None

Ocular

Lid edema, flare and cell of the anterior chamber, hypopyon, corneal edema, mutton-fat precipitates, conjunctival chemosis, anterior and posterior synechiae, papillary membranes, decreased visual acuity, retinal detachment, secondary glaucoma.

Laboratory

Diagnosis is made by clinical findings.

Treatment

Vitrectomy to remove lens material, systemic and topical corticosteroids.

Additional Resource

1. Graham RH (2012). Phacoanaphylaxis. [online] Available from http://www.emedicine.com/oph/TOPIC600.HTM [Accessed April, 2012].

1180. PHACOMORPHIC GLAUCOMA

General

Secondary angle-closure glaucoma due to lens swelling. Pupillary block is caused by the change in size and the position of the anterior lens surface. Causes can include traumatic cataract, intumescent cataract and rapidly developing senile cataract.

Clinical

Nausea; vomiting.

Ocular

Acute pain; blurred vision; rainbow-colored halos; elevated intraocular pressure; irregular pupil; corneal edema; shallow central anterior chamber; lens enlargement; weakened zonules.

Laboratory

Optical coherence tomography (OCT) and gonioscopy are useful in visualization of the anterior chamber angle.

Treatment

Beta-blockers and carbonic anhydrase inhibitors are used to initially lower the intraocular pressure. Argon iridoplasty can be then used to rapidly reduce the pressure and finally cataract extraction for a definitive treatment.

Additional Resource

1. Gill H (2010). Glaucoma, Phacomorphic. [online] Available from http://www.emedicine.medscape.com/article/1204917-overview [Accessed April, 2012].

1181. PHLYCTENULOSIS

General

Inflammation of cornea and conjunctiva that is induced by microbial antigens. It can be unilateral or bilateral.

Clinical

Tuberculosis

Ocular

Photophobia, tearing, conjunctival lesions single or multiple, corneal lesions unilateral or bilateral.

Laboratory

Culture lid for staphylococcus, tuberculin skin test, corneal scraping for mononuclear cells.

Treatment

Systemic—doxycycline for staphylococcal, appropriate systemic therapy for tuberculosis, topical—lid scrubs, antibiotic/steroid ointment and cycloplegics.

Bibliography

1. Roy FH, Fraunfelder FW, Fraunfelder FT. Roy and Fraunfelder's Current Ocular Therapy, 6th edition. Philadelphia: WB Saunders; 2008.

1182. PHOTOSENSITIVITY AND SUNBURN

General

Enhanced responsiveness to natural or artificial nonionizing electromagnetic radiation; photosensitivity induced by exogenous agents accounts for an increasing portion of the total undesirable effects caused by environmental chemicals.

Ocular

Photokeratoconjunctivitis; conjunctivitis; erythema of periorbital skin; photophobia; lacrimation; blepharospasm.

Clinical

Erythema of skin; edema; vesiculation of skin; fever; nausea; chills; delirium; irregular pigmentation of skin.

Laboratory

Diagnosis is made by history and clinical findings.

Treatment

Aspirin and other nonsteroidal anti-inflammatory drugs for pain, fluid replacement and systemic steroids are sometimes used to shorten the course and to reduce the pain.

Additional Resource

1. McStay CM (2010). Sunburn. [online] Available from http://www.emedicine.com/emerg/TOPIC798.HTM [Accessed April, 2012].

1183. PHTHISIS BULBI

General

Shrunken, not functional eye secondary to trauma, infection, radiation or other ocular abnormalities.

Clinical

Small shrunken globe; no light perception

Ocular

Scared swollen cornea; low intraocular pressure; distorted globe; cataract; ocular pain; blindness.

Laboratory

Diagnosis is made by clinical observation.

Treatment

No treatment is available to improve. Alcohol injection can sometimes be used to reduce pain. Enucleation may also be necessary to eliminate the pain.

Additional Resource

1. http://www.emedicine.medscape.com/article/ 1208794 -overview

1184. PIERRE ROBIN SYNDROME (MICROGNATHIA-GLOSSOPTOSIS SYNDROME; ROBIN SYNDROME)

General

Etiology unknown; manifestations at birth; pathogenesis based on arrested fetal development; history of intrauterine disturbance in early pregnancy (25% of cases); also increased incidence in offspring of mothers age 35 years or older; pathogenesis is thought to be incomplete development of the first brachial arch, which forms the maxilla and mandible.

Ocular

Microphthalmos; proptosis; ptosis; high myopia; glaucoma; cataract (rare); retinal disinsertion; megalocornea; iris atrophy; blue sclera; esotropia; conjunctivitis; distichiasis; vitreoretinal degeneration; retinal detachments.

Clinical

Micrognathia; cleft palate; glossoptosis; cyanosis; facial expression birdlike with flat base of nose and high-arched deformed palate with or without cleft; difficulty breathing.

Laboratory

Diagnosis is made by clinical findings.

Treatment

Multidisciplinary approach is required to manage the complex features involved in the care of these children and their families.

Additional Resource

1. Tewfik TL (2012). Pierre Robin Syndrome. [online] Available from http://www.emedicine.com/ent/ TOPIC150.HTM [Accessed April, 2012].

1185. PIERSON SYNDROME

General

Autosomal recessive; LAMB2, NPHS1 or NPHS2 association with renal dysfunction and severe posterior ocular segment findings traced through old order Mennonite generations.

Clinical

Chronic kidney disease; hypertension; neurodevelopmental deficits; infantile onset of nephrotic syndrome.

Ocular

Retinal detachment; microcornea; cataract; glaucoma; retinitis pigmentosa.

Laboratory

Urinalysis; ophthalmic examination; kidney biospy; serum DNA.

Treatment

Traditional retinal detachment surgery; management of hypertension and kidney disease.

Bibliography

1. Mohney BG, Pulido JS, Lindor NM, et al. A novel mutation of LAMB2 in a multigenerational Mennonite family reveals a new phenotypic variant of Pierson syndrome. Ophthalmology. 2011;118:1137-44.
2. Pierson M, Cordier J, Hervouuet F, et al. An unusual congential and familial congenital malformative combination involving the eye and kidney. J Genet Hum. 1963;12:184-213.

1186. PIGMENTARY DISPERSION SYNDROME AND PIGMENTARY GLAUCOMA

General

Shedding of pigment that is evident as midperipheral radial iris transillumination defects. Characterized by pigmentary deposits on the structures of the anterior and posterior chambers.

Clinical

Siderosis, hemosiderosis and diabetes mellitus.

Ocular

Krukenberg spindles, heterochromia, optic nerve damage, visual field defects Adie's pupil, chronic open-angle glaucoma; concave peripheral iris.

Laboratory

Diagnosis is made by clinical findings.

Treatment

Pilopine HS gel or Ocusert, laser therapy such as trabeculoplasty, iridectomy, iridoplasty and/or filtration surgery are useful.

Additional Resource

1. Ritch R (2010). Glaucoma, Pigmentary. [online] Available from http://www.emedicine.com/oph/TOPIC136.HTM [Accessed April, 2012].

1187. PIGMENTARY OCULAR DISPERSION SYNDROME (PIGMENTARY GLAUCOMA)

General

Polygenic inheritance; average age at onset is 52 years; distribution of pigment in chamber angle; atrophy of posterior iris epithelium; most commonly affects young Caucasian males with myopia; mechanism is likely to be mechanical rubbing between iris pigment epithelium and packets of lens zonules, resulting in aqueous flow obstruction secondary to accumulation of pigment granules in the trabecular meshwork.

Ocular

Myopia; glaucomatous field changes; ocular hypertension; iris translucency; abnormal number of iris processes; insertion of iris anterior to scleral spur; pigmentation of posterior trabecular meshwork, grades 3–4; Krukenberg spindles; presence of pigmentation on equatorial border of lens capsule; glaucomatous cupping and myopic optic nerve changes.

Clinical

None

Laboratory

Diagnosis is made by clinical findings.

Treatment

Topical glaucoma agents, laser trabeculoplasty, laser iridectomy, filtering surgery.

Additional Resource

1. Ritch R (2010). Glaucoma, Pigmentary. [online] Available from http://www.emedicine.com/oph/TOPIC136.HTM [Accessed April, 2012].

1188. PILLAY SYNDROME (OPHTHALMOMANDIBULOMELIC DYSPLASIA)

General

Autosomal dominant; both sexes affected.

Ocular

Corneal opacities.

Clinical

Temporomandibular fusion; obtuse mandibular angle; short forearms.

Laboratory

Diagnosis is made by clinical findings.

Treatment

Check for elevated intraocular pressure. Medical treatment includes the use of hyperosmotic drops, nonsteroidal and steroid eye drops. Corneal transplant may be necessary.

Bibliography

1. Magalini SI, Scrascia E. Dictionary of Medical Syndromes. 2nd edition. Philadelphia: JB Lippincott; 1981.
2. Pillay VK, Orth MC. Ophthalmo-mandibulo-melic dysplasia. An hereditary syndrome. J Bone Joint Surg Am. 1964;46:858-62.

1189. PILODENTAL DYSPLASIA WITH REFRACTIVE ERRORS (EUHIDROTIC ECTODERMAL DYSPLASIA; TRICHODENTAL DYSPLASIA WITH HYPEROPIA)

General

Autosomal recessive; damage to structures arising from the ectoderm.

Ocular

Hyperopia; astigmatism.

Clinical

Hypodontia; abnormally shaped teeth; scalp hypotrichosis; disorders of pigmentation of the hair; follicular hyperkeratosis on the trunk and limbs; intensified delineation and reticular hyperpigmentation of the skin of the nape; broadening of bridge and dorsum of the nose.

Laboratory

Diagnosis is made by clinical findings.

Treatment

Hyperopic glasses or contacts. Refractive surgery may also be beneficial.

Bibliography

1. Kopysc Z, Barczyk K, Król E. A new syndrome in the group of euhidrotic ectodermal dysplasia. Pilodental dysplasia with refractive errors. Hum genet. 1985;70:376-8.

1190. PINTA (NONVENEREAL TREPONEMATOSIS)

General

Caused by the spirochete *Treponema carateum*; infectious; contagious; found in Mexico, Central America, West Indies and the Northern countries of South America; caused by an organism that is morphologically and antigenically identical to the causative agent of venereal syphilis.

Ocular

Hypopigmentation of eyelid.

Clinical

Cutaneous lesions with marked pigmentary changes; chronic relapsing course.

Laboratory

The nontreponemal and treponemal serologic tests used in diagnosing venereal syphilis are used for serodiagnosis of pinta.

Treatment

After penicillin therapy, lesions become noninfectious in 24 hours.

Additional Resource

1. Klein NC (2011). Pinta. [online] Available from http://www.emedicine.com/med/TOPIC1836.HTM [Accessed April, 2012].

1191. PRESSURE-INDUCED INTERLAMELLAR STROMAL KERATITIS (PISK)

General

Associated with LASIK postoperative patients.

Ocular

Elevated intraocular pressure (IOP); ocular discomfort; blurred vision; stromal keratitis.

Clinical

None

Laboratory

Diagnosis is made by clinical findings.

Treatment

Topical glaucoma therapy, nonsteroidal anti-inflammatory agents.

Bibliography

1. Belin MW, Hannush SB, Yau CW, et al. Elevated intraocular pressure-induced interlamellar stromal keratitis. Ophthalmology. 2002;109:1929-33.
2. Caceres V. Post-LASIK iop measurements may help dect PISK. EyeWorld. March 2005;72-3.

1192. PITUITARY APOPLEXY

General

Acute expansion of a pituitary adenoma which causes sudden neurologic impairment due to a vascular process; occurs about 10% in individuals with adenoma; seen more frequently in males and usually in the third to fifth decade of life.

Clinical

Headache, nausea and vomiting; may occur following head trauma, endocrine stimulation testing, pituitary irradiation, cardiac bypass surgery or during pregnancy.

Ocular

Diplopia; changes in the visual field; decreased vision; ptosis.

Laboratory

Evaluate electrolytes, glucose and pituitary hormones. MRI and CT scan may be useful to evaluate the pituitary gland.

Treatment

Corticosteroids, endocrinologic replacement therapy and evacuation of the tumor may be necessary.

Additional Resource

1. Vaphiades MS (2011). Pituitary Apoplexy. [online] Available from http://www.emedicine.medscape.com/article/1198279-overview [Accessed April, 2012].

1193. PITUITARY DYSFUNCTION AND CHORIORETINOPATHY (CHORIORETINOPATHY AND PITUITARY DYSFUNCTION; CPD SYNDROME)

General

Rare, characterized by chorioretinopathy, trichosis and pituitary dysfunction.

Ocular

Long eyelashes; bushy eyebrows; severe early-onset chorioretinopathy.

Clinical

Growth retardation; sexual infantilism; hypothyroidism; mental retardation; low-birth-weight; cerebellar ataxia.

Laboratory

Evaluate electrolytes, glucose and pituitary hormones. MRI is the most sensitive imaging study for evaluating the pituitary gland.

Treatment

The goals of pharmacotherapy are to correct the corticosteroid deficiency, to reduce morbidity and to prevent complications.

Additional Resource

1. Vaphiades MS (2011). Pituitary Apoplexy. [online] Available from http://www.emedicine.com/oph/TOPIC471.HTM [Accessed April, 2012].

1194. PITUITARY GIGANTISM SYNDROME (GIGANTISM SYNDROME; LAUNOIS SYNDROME)

General

Increased production of growth hormone due to hyperplasia of the eosinophilic cells and chromophobe adenoma of the anterior pituitary gland; onset age 8–10 years; pituitary adenomas represent 10–15% of intracranial neoplasms; 40% of nonfunctioning tumors are prolactinomas; growth hormone-secreting tumors are the next most common type.

Ocular

Field defects according to extent and situation of the pituitary adenoma; optic nerve atrophy (partial).

Clinical

Gigantism; enlarged skull with prominent chin and forehead; retarded skeletal growth; delayed puberty; muscle weakness; headache; perspiration; joint pain; mental retardation; pallor; smooth skin; scanty facial and body hair; small penis and testes; high-pitched voice; large limbs, hands and feet.

Laboratory

Laboratory findings suggest growth hormone excess, obtain an MRI to confirm the presence of a pituitary adenoma.

Treatment

Somatostatin analogs and dopamine agonists may be useful. Transsphenoidal surgery to completely remove the tumor is the treatment of choice, and it may be curative.

Additional Resource

1. Ferry RJ (2010). Gigantism and Acromegaly. [online] Available from http://www.emedicine.com/ped/TOPIC2634.HTM [Accessed April, 2012].

1195. PITUITARY NECROSIS SYNDROME (POSTPARTUM HYPOPITUITARISM SYNDROME; SHEEHAN SYNDROME; SIMMONDS-SHEEHAN SYNDROME)

General

Etiology unknown; vascular occlusion of one of the vessels supplying the anterior lobe of the pituitary during childbirth; characterized by various degrees of anterior and/or posterior pituitary dysfunction due to pituitary necrosis after obstetric shock or hemorrhage.

Ocular

Hypotrichosis of eyebrows; loss of eyelashes; dry and scaly skin of the lids; visual loss due to vascular insufficiency; uveal depigmentation.

Clinical

Reduced sweating with dry skin; listlessness and lethargy; stupor; myxedema; premature aging; cutaneous hypopigmentation; reduced and sparse axillary and pubic hair; genital atrophy; menstrual irregularity; amenorrhea; thyroiditis.

Laboratory

Evaluate electrolytes, glucose and pituitary hormones. CT scan and MRI are radiologic tests used to evaluate the pituitary gland.

Treatment

Evaluation endocrinologist should be planned once the patient is medically stable.

Bibliography

1. Hoyt WF. Transient bilateral blurring of vision. Considerations of an episodic ischemic symptom of vertebral-basilar insufficiency. Arch Ophthalmol. 1963;70:746-51.
2. Sasaki H, Shijyo H, Cugini P, et al. Simultaneous occurrence of postpartum hypopituitarism (Sheehan's syndrome) and transient resolving thyrotoxicosis due to postpartum painless thyroiditis. South Med J. 1992;85:660-2.
3. Sheehan HL. Atypical hypopituitarism. Proc R Soc Med. 1961;54:43-8.
4. Simmonds M. Uber Hypophysisschwund mit Todlichem Ausgang. Dtsch Med Wochenschr. 1914;40:322.

1196. PITYRIASIS RUBRA PILARIS [DEVERGIE DISEASE; HEBRA DISEASE; KAPOSI DISEASE (2); LICHEN RUBER; LICHEN RUBER ACUMINATUS; PITYRIASIS PILARIS; TARRAL-BESNIER DISEASE]

General

Abnormal keratinization of unknown etiology; hereditary and acquired forms have been described in the literature; hereditary form tends to be less severe and more limited in extent.

Ocular

Papules on bulbar conjunctiva; keratitis; ectropion; pannus; corneal ulceration.

Clinical

Cutaneous manifestations; erythema; follicular papules.

Laboratory

The diagnosis is usually made on the basis of a correlation between clinical findings and histologic findings.

Treatment

Topical medications, calcipotriol is a vitamin D analog, emollients, extracorporeal photochemotherapy.

Additional Resource

1. Shenefelt PD (2010). Pityriasis Rubra Pilaris. [online] Available from http://www.emedicine.com/derm/TOPIC337.HTM [Accessed April, 2012].

1197. PLAGUE (BUBONIC PLAGUE; PNEUMONIC PLAGUE)

General

Infectious disease of animals (principally wild animals and rodents) that is transmitted through the bite of infected ectoparasites; causative agent is *Yersinia pestis*.

Ocular

Inflammatory infiltrate of lids; subconjunctival hemorrhages; chemosis; staphyloma of sclera; keratitis; corneal abscess; iridocyclitis; choroiditis.

Clinical

Abrupt onset; chills; fever; rapid, thready pulse; painful, enlarged lymph nodes in bubonic plague; headache and productive cough in pneumonic plague; meningitis; occasional patients infected with *Y. pestis* become septic and die with bacteremia without developing any detectable lymphadenitis (septicemic plague).

Laboratory

Laboratory diagnosis can be very slow. Any patient with suspected plague based on clinical or epidemiological reasons should be empirically treated. Associated laboratory findings include leukocytosis, elevated liver function enzymes and evidence of disseminated intravascular coagulopathy.

Treatment

Isolation should be continued until 48 hours of appropriate antibiotic treatment. Incision and drainage of buboes may be indicated.

Additional Resource

1. Dhawan VK (2010). Plague. [online] Available from http://www.emedicine.com/ped/TOPIC1819. HTM [Accessed April, 2012].

1198. PLASMA LECITHIN DEFICIENCY (CHOLESTEROL ACYLTRANSFERASE DEFICIENCY)

General

Autosomal recessive.

Ocular

Corneal stromal opacities comprising small gray dots in central and peripheral areas; retinal hemorrhages; disk protrusion; dilated veins.

Clinical

Storage of lipid materials in various tissues.

Laboratory

Definitive diagnosis requires mutational analysis of the LCAT gene and a functional analysis of the mutated gene product.

Treatment

Symptomatic treatment for anemia, renal insufficiency and atherosclerosis is indicated. Kidney transplantation is indicated in patients with renal failure.

Additional Resource

1. Raghavan VA (2011). Lecithin-Cholesterol Acyl-transferase Deficiency. [online] Available from http://www.emedicine.com/med/TOPIC1270. HTM [Accessed April, 2012].

1199. PLATEAU IRIS SYNDROME

General

Rare; occurs in younger age group; presumably due in part to an anterior insertion of the iris; pupillary block is not a significant part of the mechanism leading to angle closure.

Ocular

Spontaneous or mydriasis-induced angle closure despite a patent iridectomy; anterior chamber is of normal depth axially and the iris plane is flat, but a peripheral roll of iris can close the angle either when the pupil dilates spontaneously or after mydriatic drugs are administered.

Clinical

Nausea; vomiting.

Laboratory

Indentation gonioscopy.

Treatment

Iridotomy

Additional Resource

1. Wang JC (2010). Glaucoma, Plateau Iris. [online] Available from http://www.emedicine.com/oph/ TOPIC574.HTM [Accessed April, 2012].

1200. PLUMMER-VINSON SYNDROME (PATERSON-BROWN-KELLY SYNDROME; SIDEROPENIC DYSPHAGIA SYNDROME; WALDENSTROM-KJELLBERG SYNDROME)

General

Deficiency of vitamin B complex and iron; more common in females; onset in middle age; pathogenic mechanism may be related to a frameshift mutation in the human apolipoprotein mutation in the human apolipoprotein A-I gene.

Ocular

Reduced tear formation; pale conjunctiva; dry eyes; retinal hemorrhages; papilledema.

Clinical

Dysphagia for solid food with main difficulties originating in the upper portion of the esophagus;

glossitis and gastritis; anemia; atrophy of mucous membranes; dystrophy of the fingernails (koilonychia); fatigue.

Laboratory

Barium esophagram and videofluoroscopy. They are the most sensitive methods and diagnostic tests of choice to detect esophageal webs.

Treatment

Iron replacement and diet modification.

Additional Resource

1. http://www.emedicine.medscape.com/article/ 187341-overview

1201. PNEUMOCOCCAL INFECTIONS (STREPTOCOCCUS PNEUMONIAE INFECTIONS)

General

Gram-positive diplococcus *Streptococcus pneumoniae*; some strains are encapsulated while others are not; ocular infections usually are caused by the encapsulated strains; conjunctivitis and corneal scarring produced in an animal model have been attributed to a hemolytic cytolytic exopeptidase.

Ocular

Hypopyon; conjunctivitis; keratitis; corneal ulcer; endophthalmitis; dacryocystitis; uveitis; orbital cellulitis; secondary glaucoma; ophthalmia neonatorum.

Clinical

Upper respiratory infection; chills; sharp pain in hemithorax; cough with sputum production; fever; headache; gastrointestinal symptoms.

Laboratory

Gram stain demonstrates Gram-positive cocci in pairs. The unattached end of each cocci is slightly pointed outward.

Treatment

Impetigo—oral antibiotics and topical antibiotic ointment, preseptal cellulitis—oral antibiotics, orbital cellulitis—need team of infectious diseases, otolaryngology and ophthalmology to develop plan of therapy, dacryocystitis—oral and topical antibiotics, dacryocystorhinostomy may be necessary, conjunctivitis—topical antibiotic, keratitis—topical antibiotics, poststreptococcal reactive arthritis can occur with uveitis—topical steroids and cycloplegics, endophthalmitis—prompt and aggressive therapy with topical, intravitreal and sometimes systemic antibiotics and pars plana vitrectomy, postrefractive surgery keratitis—flap raised, cultured and treated. Occasionally the flap should be amputated.

Additional Resource

1. Muench DF (2010). Pneumococcal Infections. [online] Available from http://www.emedicine.com/med/TOPIC1848.HTM [Accessed April, 2012].

1202. POEMS SYNDROME (ENDOCRINOPATHY, MONOCLONAL GAMMOPATHY AND SKIN CHANGES; ORGANOMEGALY, POLYNEUROPATHY)

General

Rare, multisystemic, may be linked to changes in the levels of cytokine or a growth factor.

Clinical

Hyperpigmentaion and lower extremity edema; hypertrichosis; angiomas; motor deficiency; deep tendon reflexes are diminished; endocrinopathy; hypogonadism; pulmonary hypertension; hepatomegaly; splenomegaly and lymphadenopathy.

Ocular

Bilateral optic disk edema and bilateral cystoid macular edema.

Laboratory

Diagnosis is generally made from clinical observation. Once suspected a range of laboratory studies are needed to define the extent of involvement and to determine what organs are involved.

Treatment

Mainstay of treatment includes combination of corticosteroids, low-dose alkylators and peripheral blood stem cell transplantation followed by high-dose chemotherapy.

Bibliography

1. Kaushik M, Pulido JS, Abreu R, et al. Ocular findings in patients with polyneuropathy, organo-megaly, endocrinopathy, monoclonal gammopathy and skin changes syndrome. Ophthalmology. 2011;118:778-82.

Additional Resource

1. Chan JL (2011). POEMS Syndrome. [online] Available from http://www.emedicine.medscape. com/article/1097031-overview [Accessed April, 2012].

1203. POISON IVY DERMATITIS (POISON OAK DERMATITIS; POISON SUMAC DERMATITIS; RHUS DERMATITIS)

General

Direct contact or airborne contact from burning of plant.

Ocular

Keratitis; chemosis; blepharospasm; pustules of eyelids.

Clinical

Dermatitis; linear lesions; erythema; pruritus.

Laboratory

Diagnosis is made by clinical findings.

Treatment

Removal of the offending agent from the patient's environment. Oral antihistamines and corticosteroids are useful.

Additional Resource

1. Hogan DJ (2011). Allergic Contact Dermatitis. [online] Available from http://www.emedicine. com/oph/TOPIC480.HTM [Accessed April, 2012].

1204. POLAND-MÖBIUS SYNDROME

General

Rare congenital disorder that is a combination of Möbius syndrome and Poland anomaly; has been proposed that Möbius syndrome, the Poland anomaly and the Klippel-Feil defect all result from a transient interruption during the 6th week of gestation in the development of the subclavian artery and its branches.

Ocular

Bilateral sixth nerve paralysis; no movement of upper lid in horizontal gaze; no globe retraction during adduction; vertical nystagmus; diplopia; chronic keratitis; corneal ulcer.

Clinical

Paresis of the VI and VII cranial nerves; bilateral absence of pectoralis muscle and ipsilateral hand and digit anomalies; chronic drooling; speech difficulties; mask-like facial expression.

Laboratory

Chest wall abnormalities and determining the presence of the latissimus muscle may require evaluation with CT scan.

Treatment

Breast reconstruction surgery may be beneficial.

Additional Resource

1. Wilhelmi BJ (2012). Poland Syndrome. [online] Available from http://www.emedicine.com/plastic/TOPIC132.HTM [Accessed April, 2012].

1205. POLIOMYELITIS (INFANTILE PARALYSIS)

General

Acute viral infection characterized by varying degrees of neuronal injury, with special localization in the anterior horns and motor nuclei of the brainstem.

Ocular

Diplopia; nystagmus; paralysis of third, fourth and sixth nerves; paresis of seventh nerve; papilledema; visual agnosia; Horner syndrome; pupillary paralysis; optic neuritis; ophthalmoparesis; transient visual loss; internuclear ophthalmoplegia; papillary disturbances, spasm of near reflex.

Clinical

Flaccid paralysis of many muscle groups; death from asphyxia and involvement of vital centers in the brainstem.

Laboratory

Obtain specimens from the CSF, stool and throat for viral cultures.

Treatment

No antivirals are effective against polioviruses. The treatment of poliomyelitis is mainly supportive and will involve physical therapist and rehabilitation therapist, pulmonologist, neurologist, immunologist and infectious diseases specialist.

Additional Resource

1. Estrada B (2009). Pediatric Poliomyelitis. [online] Available from http://www.emedicine.com/ped/TOPIC1843.HTM [Accessed April, 2012].

1206. POLYCYTHEMIA VERA (CRYPTOGENIC POLYCYTHEMIA; ERYTHEMA; ERYTHROCYTOSIS MEGALOSPLENICA; MYELOPATHIC POLYCYTHEMIA; POLYCYTHEMIA RUBRA; SPLENOMEGALIC POLYCYTHEMIA VAQUEZ DISEASE; VAQUEZ-OSLER SYNDROME)

General

Increased number of red blood cells; myeloproliferative disorder.

Ocular

Conjunctival vascular engorgement; dilated tortuous retinal veins; retinal hemorrhages; optic disk edema; central retinal vein occlusion; visual field defects; visual hallucinations; diplopia.

Clinical

Elevated red blood cells; systemic vascular congestion; leukocytosis; thrombocytosis; central nervous system involvement; splenomegaly;

hepatomegaly; bleeding diathesis; gingival/mucosal bleeding; ecchymosis; epistaxis; neurologic abnormal dizziness; vertigo; ataxia.

Laboratory

The serum Epo level should be decreased in nearly all patients with polycythemia vera (PV) and no recent hemorrhage.

Treatment

Phlebotomy or bloodletting has been the mainstay of therapy.

Additional Resource

1. Besa EC (2012). Polycythemia Vera. [online] Available from http://www.emedicine.com/med/TOPIC1864.HTM [Accessed April, 2012].

1207. POLYMYALGIA RHEUMATICA

General

Affects older patients; usually Caucasian women; relationship between polymyalgia and temporal arteritis remains uncertain; in polymyalgia rheumatica alone there is no arteritis per se, and this syndrome is not associated with blindness or other neurologic or cardiovascular sequelae; many patients with temporal arteritis have polymyalgia rheumatica as part of their symptoms or as the presenting symptom.

Ocular

Amaurosis fugax; acute unilateral or bilateral visual loss; ischemic optic neuritis; optic atrophy; papilledema; retinal hemorrhages; cotton-wool spots; central retinal artery occlusion; palsy of extraocular muscles.

Clinical

Pain and stiffness in the neck, shoulders and hips; rapid erythrocyte sedimentation rate (ESR); prompt response to corticosteroids; weakness.

Laboratory

The erythrocyte sedimentation rate is the most sensitive diagnostic study for polymyalgia rheumatica.

Treatment

The therapeutic goals are to control painful myalgia, to improve muscle stiffness and to resolve constitutional features of the disease. Corticosteroids are considered the treatment of choice. Nonsteroidal anti-inflammatory drugs, methotrexate, azathioprine and other immunosuppressive drugs may also be useful.

Additional Resource

1. Papadopoulos PJ (2012). Polymyalgia Rheumatica. [online] Available from http://www.emedicine.com/med/TOPIC1871.HTM [Accessed April, 2012].

1208. POLYMYOSITIS-DERMATOMYOSITIS (DERMATOMUCOMYOSITIS; NEUROMYOSITIS; POLYMYOSITIS GREGARINA; WAGNER-UNVERRICHT SYNDROME)

General

Autoimmune disease; etiology unknown; variable symptoms according to prevalence of skin (dermatomyositis) or muscular (polymyositis) involvement; association with neoplastic disease; prevalent in females; onset in childhood before age 10 years and in adults predominant in the fourth to sixth decade; both children and adults are affected by this disease, but the prognosis is better for the childhood forms of disease.

Ocular

Violescent discoloration of eyelids; conjunctivitis; episcleritis; anterior uveitis; nystagmus; exophthalmos; cotton-wool spots; retinal edema; retinal hemorrhage; venous engorgement.

Clinical

Erythema involving face, forearms and upper back; muscle weakness, especially shoulder and pelvic girdles; dysphagia; respiratory difficulty; malaise; fever; tachycardia.

Laboratory

Serum creatine kinase (CK) levels are usually elevated from 5 to 50 times the normal value, MRI and ultrasonography may be useful to document and localize the extent of muscle involvement.

Treatment

Prednisone is the first-line treatment of choice. Immunosuppressive agents are indicated if patients do not show improvement with steroids.

Additional Resource

1. Pappu R (2011). Polymyositis. [online] Available from http://www.emedicine.com/med/TOPIC3441.HTM [Accessed April, 2012].

1209. POMPE DISEASE (GENERALIZED GLYCOGENOSIS)

General

Absence of acid maltase; type II glycogen storage disease with decreased acid maltase resulting in elevated levels of lysosomal glycogen; inheritance is autosomal recessive.

Ocular

Cortical blindness.

Clinical

Anorexia; retardation of growth; cyanosis; dyspnea; convulsions; death; enlarged tongue; large heart; hypotonicity.

Laboratory

Definitive diagnosis requires the measurement of acid alpha-glucosidase activity in cultured skin fibroblasts or peripheral blood lymphocytes.

Treatment

Enzyme replacement therapy. Consultation with a neurologist and a pediatric cardiologist are usually necessary.

Additional Resource

1. Ibrahim J (2011). Genetics of Glycogen-Storage Disease Type II (Pompe Disease). [online] Available from http://www.emedicine.com/ped/TOPIC1866.HTM [Accessed April, 2012].

1210. POPLITEAL PTERYGIUM SYNDROME (PPS)

General

Rare; autosomal dominant disorder.

Ocular

None

Clinical

Popliteal webbing; cleft lip; cleft palate, lower lip pits; syndactyly; genital and nail abnormalities; severe flexure contract at the knee; equinus foot; velar pterygium.

Laboratory

Although diagnosis is primarily clinical, chromosomal analysis may be appropriate.

Treatment

Surgical repair of cleft lip and cleft palate or other anomalies may be required.

Additional Resource

1. Conners GP (2011). van der Woude Syndrome. [online] Available from http://www.emedicine.com/ped/TOPIC2753.HTM [Accessed April, 2012].

1211. POROKERATOSIS

General

Autosomal dominant; prominent in males; onset in early childhood; characterized by scaly papules that enlarge to form gyrate lesions.

Ocular

Conjunctivitis; lesions of cornea.

Clinical

Squamous cell carcinoma within lesions; lesions may occur on oral mucosa, palms or soles.

Laboratory

The cornoid lamella is the histopathologic hallmark.

Treatment

The approach to treatment must be individualized, based on the size of the lesion and the anatomical location. Protection from the sun, use of emollients and watchful observation for signs of malignant degeneration are important.

Additional Resource

1. Spencer LV (2010). Porokeratosis. [online] Available from http://www.emedicine.com/derm/TOPIC343.HTM [Accessed April, 2012].

1212. PORPHYRIA CUTANEA TARDA

General

Disorder of porphyria metabolism; highest incidence in Bantu population; both sexes affected; onset between the ages of 40 and 60 years; insidious onset; autosomal dominant; light-sensitive dermatitis in later adult life; associated with excretion of large amounts of uroporphyrin in urine.

Ocular

Synophrys; keratitis; palsies of III and VII cranial nerves; scleromalacia perforans; optic atrophy; retinal hemorrhages and cotton-wool spots; macular edema; pinguecula; pterygium; brownish pigmentation in conjunctiva and lid margin.

Clinical

Cutaneous manifestations are solar hypersensitivity, vesiculobullous lesions, ulcerations, severe scarring and hypertrichosis; erythrodontia.

Laboratory

Urinary porphyrin levels are abnormally high, with several hundred to several thousand micrograms excreted in a 24-hour period. Direct immunofluorescence examination can help differentiate PCT from immunobullous diseases with dermoepidermal junction cleavage (epidermolysis bullosa acquisita, lupus erythematosus) in which the perivascular immunoglobulin deposition found in PCT is not observed.

Treatment

Sunlight avoidance, therapeutic phlebotomy to reduce iron stores, chelation with desferrioxamine, iron-rich foods should be consumed in moderation.

Additional Resource

1. Poh-Fitzpatrick MB (2010). Porphyria Cutanea Tarda. [online] Available from http://www.emedicine.com/derm/TOPIC344.HTM [Accessed April, 2012].

1213. POSNER-SCHLOSSMAN SYNDROME (GLAUCOMATOCYCLITIC CRISIS)

General

High intraocular tension lasting from hours to several weeks and recurring at varying frequencies; low-grade, intermittent, nongranulomatous inflammation; in one series of patients, HLA-BW54 was present in 41% of patients.

Ocular

Slight blurring of vision and colored halos during episodes of high intraocular tension; high intraocular pressure (unilateral); glaucomatocyclitic crisis (benign and usually unilateral); enlarged pupil; anisocoria; absence of ciliary or conjunctival injection; only trace of aqueous flare; no posterior synechiae; chamber angle open; heterochromia iridis; keratitic precipitates may be present.

Clinical

Allergy; associated with gastrointestinal disease (peptic ulcers).

Laboratory

Diagnosis is made by clinical findings.

Treatment

Ocular hypertension: Timolol and prostaglandin agents, inflammation—topical steroids and cycloplegics.

Additional Resource

1. Oakman JH (2012). Posner-Schlossman Syndrome. [online] Available from http://www.emedicine.com/oph/TOPIC137.HTM [Accessed April, 2012].

1214. POSTERIOR IRIS CHAFING SYNDROME

General

Complication following intraocular lens implantation attributed to sulcus-fixed posterior chamber lenses, decentration of the lens, traumatic insertion, movement of the lens during dilation and constriction of the pupil or difficulty with positioning of the lens.

Ocular

Iris transillumination defects; recurrent microhyphemas; pigment dispersion glaucoma; pigment deposition in trabecular meshwork; iris pigment atrophy.

Clinical

None

Laboratory

Diagnosis is made by clinical findings.

Treatment

Glaucoma therapy, repositioning of intraocular lens (IOL), suturing of the IOL.

Bibliography

1. Jaffe NS. Current concepts in posterior chamber lens technology. J Am Intraocul Implant Soc. 1985;11:456-60.
2. Johnson SH, Kratz RP, Olson PF. Iris transillumination defect and microhyphema syndrome. J Am Intraocul Implant Soc. 1984;10:425-8.
3. Smiddy WE, Ibanez GV, Alfonso E, et al. Surgical management of dislocated intraocular lenses. J Cataract Refract Surg. 1995;21:64-9.
4. Smith SG, Lindstrom RL. Malpositioned posterior chamber lenses: etiology, prevention, and management. J Am Intraocul Implant Soc. 1985;11:584-91.
5. Woodhams JT, Lester JC. Pigmentary dispersion glaucoma secondary to posterior chamber intraocular lenses. Ann Ophthalmol. 1984;16:852-5.

1215. POSTERIOR POLYMORPHOUS DYSTROPHY

General

Rare, bilateral corneal disorder of Descemet's membrane. Autosomal dominant associated with Alport's syndrome and keratoconus.

Clinical

None

Ocular

Corneal edema which usually develops in midlife, open- or closed-angle glaucoma.

Laboratory

Specular microscopy shows dark rings with scalloped-edges around a light center.

Treatment

Sodium chloride drops or ointment, glaucoma therapy (medical or surgical) and penetrating keratoplasty may be necessary.

Bibliography

1. Roy FH, Fraunfelder FW, Fraunfelder FT. Roy and Fraunfelder's Current Ocular Therapy, 6th edition. Philadelphia: WB Saunders; 2008.

1216. POSTERIOR UVEAL BLEEDING SYNDROME

General

Most commonly affects middle-aged black females; also observed in white or Asian people.

Ocular

Multiple recurrent pigment epithelial detachments; posterior uveal bleeding; polyps in the peripapillary macula and extramacular areas.

Clinical

Hypertension

Laboratory

Indocyanine green angiogram.

Treatment

Consult retinal specialist.

Bibliography

1. Ahuja RM, Stanga PE, Vingerling JR. Polypoidal choroidal vasculopathy in exudative and haemorrhagic pigment epithelial detachments. Br J Ophthalmol. 2000;84:479-84.
2. Stanga PE, Lim JI, Hamilton P. Indocyanine green angiography in chorioretinal diseases: indications and interpretation: an evidence-based update. Ophthalmology. 2003;110:15-21.

1217. POSTHYPOXIC ENCEPHALOPATHY SYNDROME (PARIETO-OCCIPITAL SYNDROME; POSTHYPOXIC SYNDROME)

General

Hypoxia secondary to carbon monoxide poisoning, high altitude, complication during anesthesia, hypoglycemia or cardiac failure, causing widespread demyelination in the parietal lobes, including the optic radiations.

Ocular

Nystagmus; nuclear ophthalmoplegia; visual hallucinations; partial cerebral blindness (predominant defects in the sphere of psychic elaboration rather than in primary visual perception); complete cortical blindness; central scotomata; pupillary paresis; retinal atrophy; optic atrophy.

Clinical

Confusion; irritability and agitation; alexia; disorientation (mainly spatial); muscle spasm.

Laboratory

HbCO analysis requires direct spectrophotometric measurement in specific blood gas analyzers. X-ray, CT and MRI may be beneficial.

Treatment

Promptly remove from continued exposure and immediately institute oxygen therapy with a nonrebreather mask. Hyperbaric oxygen therapy is useful.

Additional Resource

1. Shochat GN (2011). Carbon Monoxide Toxicity in Emergency Medicine. [online] Available from http://www.emedicine.com/emerg/TOPIC817.HTM [Accessed April, 2012].

1218. POSTOPERATIVE FLAT ANTERIOR CHAMBER

General

Flat anterior chamber following intraocular surgery.

Clinical

None

Ocular

Corneal decompensation, cataract, intractable glaucoma.

Laboratory

Seidel test to demonstrate wound leak.

Treatment

Wound leaks usually require surgical repairs.

Additional Resource

1. Aquavella JV (2010). Postoperative Flat Anterior Chamber. [online] Available from http://www.emedicine.com/oph/TOPIC531.HTM [Accessed April, 2012].

1219. POSTSTREPTOCOCCAL UVEITIS SYNDROME

General

Associated with bilateral nongranulomatous ocular inflammation; seen in individuals over 40 years of age.

Ocular

Vitreitis; focal retinitis; optic disk swelling; multifocal choroiditis.

Clinical

None

Laboratory

Chest radiography and a rapid plasma reagin (RPR) test with a fluorescent treponemal antibody absorption (FTA-ABS) test should be ordered.

Treatment

Cycloplegic drops, topical corticosteroids and topical aqueous suppressant if IOP is elevated.

Bibliography

1. Cokingtin CD, Han DP. Bilateral nongranulomatous uveitis and a poststreptococcal syndrome. Am J Ophthalmol. 1991;112:595-6.
2. Ur Rehman S, Anand S, Reddy A, et al. Poststreptococcal syndrome uveitis: a descriptive case series and literature review. Ophthalmology. 2006;113:701-6.

1220. POSTVACCINAL OCULAR SYNDROME

General

Immediate contamination and inoculation or as a delayed reaction; incubation time 3 days.

Ocular

Orbital cellulitis; pustules and vesicles on the eyelids (vesicles appear grayish with purulent discharge); lids swollen and red with swelling of preauricular and postauricular lymph nodes; ophthalmoplegia; mild anterior uveitis; conjunctival and corneal vesicles similar to the lid lesions; corneal marginal ulcers (eventually may lead to corneal perforation and loss of the eye); chorioretinitis (occasionally); central serous retinopathy; central retinal vein thrombosis; panophthalmitis; neuritis; ocular vaccinia may mimic signs of herpes simplex virus, varicella-zoster virus and acanthamoeba keratitis.

Clinical

Postvaccinal encephalitis; severe local purulent skin reaction; severe headache; fever; malaise.

Laboratory

Diagnosis is made by clinical findings which include consideration of postvaccinal encephalitis in any patient with neurologic symptoms developing 1–2 weeks after exposure to live vaccinia virus.

Treatment

Vaccinia immunoglobulin (VIG) and cidofovir may be helpful.

Additional Resource

1. Lee JJ (2012). Vaccinia. [online] Available from http://www.emedicine.com/med/TOPIC2356.HTM [Accessed April, 2012].

1221. POTTER SYNDROME (RENAL AGENESIS SYNDROME; RENOFACIAL SYNDROME)

General

Unknown etiology; may be severe form of the trisomy 18 syndrome; results from prolonged oligohydramnios of any cause.

Ocular

Hypertelorism; pronounced epicanthal folds extending down the cheeks; antimongoloid slant of palpebral fissure.

Clinical

Flat bridge of the nose; low-set ears; facial deformities; micrognathia; pulmonary hypoplasia; cystic dysplasia of kidney to agenesis; oligohydramnios; clubbing of hands and feet; spina bifida; prominent infracanthal folds; flattened beaked nose; creased skin; positional deformities of the limbs.

Laboratory

Serum electrolyte tests to evaluate electrolyte problems,1241 such as hyponatremia, hypernatremia, hyperkalemia, hypocalcemia, hyperphosphatemia and/or metabolic acidosis, which may be present in neonates with renal failure, Doppler ultrasonography.

Treatment

The renal function and respiratory status of neonates born with Potter syndrome must be assessed. Associated anomalies of the gastrointestinal, cardiovascular and musculoskeletal systems should also be evaluated. Once the long-term prognosis o f survival is determined, resuscitation and management plans should be addressed.

Additional Resource

1. Gupta S (2010). Potter Syndrome. [online] Available from http://www.emedicine.com/ped/TOPIC1878.HTM [Accessed April, 2012].

1222. PRADER-WILLI SYNDROME (H20 SYNDROME; HYPOGENITAL DYSTROPHY WITH DIABETIC TENDENCY; HYPOTONIA-HYPOMENTIA-HYPOGONADISM-OBESITY [HHHO] SYNDROME; PRADER-LABHART-WILLI-FANCONI SYNDROME; ROYER SYNDROME)

General

Etiology unknown; dominant inheritance is suspected; predominantly seen in males; Royer syndrome is Prader-Willi syndrome (PWS) associated with diabetes mellitus; nongenetic condition characterized by infantile hypotonia, hypogonadism and obesity.

Ocular

Strabismus; ocular hypertelorism; myopia; exotropia; glaucoma; cataracts; congenital ocular fibrosis syndrome; diabetic retinopathy.

Clinical

Mental retardation; short stature; muscular hypotonia; small hands and feet; obesity; cryptorchidism; hypogonadism; dental caries; clinodactyly; partial syndactyly of toes and fingers.

Laboratory

Chromosomal analysis and assessment for methylation patterns in the PWS region.

Treatment

Patients may require surgical care for treatment of complications of obesity, treatment of cryptorchidism and scoliosis intervention.

Additional Resource

1. Scheimann A (2011). Prader-Willi Syndrome. [online] Available from http://www.emedicine.com/ped/TOPIC1880.HTM [Accessed April, 2012].

1223. PREGNANCY

General

Pregnancy results in hormonal changes that produce ocular effects; symptoms resolve at end of pregnancy term.

Ocular

Myopia; visual field defects; corneal edema; acute ischemic optic neuropathy; central serous retinopathy; glaucoma; ptosis; diabetic retinop-athy; Krukenberg spindles; transient blindness; serous retinal detachment; retinal artery occlusion; retinal vein occlusion; disseminated intra-vascular coagulopathy; uveal melanoma.

Clinical

Nausea; headaches; hypertension; benign intracranial hypertension; preeclampsia; toxemia; fluid retention.

Laboratory

Home pregnancy tests that utilize the modern immunometric assay. Transvaginal ultrasound and transabdominal ultrasound are also useful.

Treatment

Most ocular symptoms resolve at the end of pregnancy. Obstetrician should be consulted before topical medications are prescribed.

Additional Resource

1. Somani S (2011). Pregnancy Special Considerations. [online] Available from http://www.emedicine.com/oph/TOPIC747.HTM [Accessed April, 2012].

1224. PRIMARY ANGLE-CLOSURE GLAUCOMA (PRIMARY CLOSED-ANGLE GLAUCOMA)

General

Obstruction of aqueous humor outflow form the anterior chamber which results form closure of the angle by the peripheral root of the iris.

Clinical

Pain, nausea.

Ocular

Flare in the anterior chamber, conjunctival chemosis, hyperemia, corneal epithelial edema, folds in Descemet's membrane, peripheral anterior synechiae, increased intraocular pressure (IOP), visual field defect.

Laboratory

Diagnosis is made by clinical findings.

Treatment

Systemic hyperosmotic agents, topical pilocarpine every 5 minutes, laser iridotomy and if IOP does not respond filtering surgery may be necessary.

Additional Resources

1. Noecker RJ (2011). Glaucoma, Angle Closure, Acute. [online] Available from http://www.emedicine.com/oph/TOPIC255.HTM [Accessed April, 2012].
2. Tham CC (2010). Glaucoma, Angle Closure, Chronic. [online] Available from http://www.emedicine.com/oph/TOPIC122.HTM [Accessed April, 2012].

1225. PRIMARY ANTIPHOSPHOLIPID SYNDROME (PAS)

General

Thrombophilic disorder characterized by the presence of autoantibodies and CNS involvement, venous thrombosis and ocular manifestations.

Ocular

Visual disturbances (visual obscurations, amaurosis fugax, diplopia, homonymous field defects and scintillating scotoma due to migraine); two forms of retinopathy: (1) cotton-wool spots with or without hemorrhages and (2) vaso-occlusive ocular disease.

Clinical

Many patients will experience CNS involvement in the form of either a stroke or a transient ischemic attack; visual disturbances are largely due to CNS rather than ocular ischemia.

Laboratory

Hallmark result from laboratory tests that defines antiphospholipid syndrome is the presence of antiphospholipid antibodies or abnormalities in phospholipid-dependent tests of coagulation.

Treatment

Treatment regimens must be individualized according to the patient's current clinical status and history of thrombotic events.

Additional Resource

1. Belilos E (2012). Antiphospholipid Syndrome. [online] Available from http://www.emedicine. com/med/TOPIC2923.HTM [Accessed April, 2012].

1226. PROGRESSIVE EXTERNAL OPHTHALMOPLEGIA AND SCOLIOSIS

General

Rare; isolated muscle dystrophic involvement of extraocular muscles; onset in childhood or early adulthood; slowly progressive.

Ocular

Horizontal gaze paralysis; pendular nystagmus; ptosis; orbicularis oculi weakness.

Clinical

Scoliosis; facial myokymia; contracture of facial muscles.

Laboratory

Diagnosis is made by clinical findings.

Treatment

Nystagmus: See-saw nystagmus—visual field to consider neoplastic or vascular etiologies. Upbeat nystagmus—may indicate multiple sclerosis, cerebellar degeneration, tumors or infarcts. Treatment is directed toward identification and resolution of underlying cause. Downbeat nystagmus—affects the cerebellum or craniocervical junction including Arnold-Chiari malformation, multiple sclerosis, trauma, tumor, infarction and many toxic metabolic entities. MRI may indicate a surgically correctable lesion. Periodic alternating nystagmus is continuous horizontal nystagmus from stroke, tumor, multiple sclerosis, trauma, infection and drug intoxication. Can occur from cataract, vitreous hemorrhage or optic atrophy.

Ptosis: If visual acuity is affected most cases require surgical correction, and there are several procedures that may be used including levator resection, repair or advancement and Fasanella-Servat.

Bibliography

1. Roddi R, Riggio E, Gilbert PM, et al. Clinical evaluation of techniques used in the surgical treatment of progressive hemifacial atrophy. J Craniomaxillofac Surg. 1994;22:23-32.
2. Moore MH, Wong KS, Proudman TW, et al. Progressive hemifacial atrophy (Romberg's disease): skeletal involvement and treatment. Br J Plast Surg. 1993;46:39-44.

1227. PROGRESSIVE FOVEAL DYSTROPHY (CENTRAL RETINAL PIGMENT EPITHELIAL DYSTROPHY)

General

Autosomal dominant; onset late in the first decade of life.

Ocular

Progressive foveal dystrophy; pigmentary changes and drusen of the macula; normal electroretinogram; subnormal electro-oculogram.

Clinical

Generalized aminoaciduria; increased glycine levels.

Laboratory

Fluorescein angiogram; electro-oculogram.

Treatment

No treatment exists. Secondary choroidal neovascularization can be managed with direct laser treatment.

Bibliography

1. Deutman AF. Macular dystrophies. In: Ryan SJ (Ed). Retina. St Louis: CV Mosby; 1994. pp. 1214-5.
2. McKusick VA. Mendelian Inheritance in Man: A Catalog of Human Genes and Genetic Disorders, 12th edition. Baltimore: The Johns Hopkins University Press; 1998.

1228. PROGRESSIVE INHERITED RETINAL ARTERIOLAR TORTUOSITY WITH RETINAL HEMORRHAGES (FAMILIAL RETINAL ARTERIOLAR TORTUOSITY WITH RETINAL HEMORRHAGES)

General

Autosomal dominant; tortuosity increases most dramatically during adolescence and progresses throughout adulthood.

Ocular

Tortuosity of the retinal arterioles; spontaneous retinal hemorrhages.

Clinical

None

Laboratory

Ocular B-scan ultrasonography is used when the media is opacified enough to preclude a complete and clear (including view of the ora serrata) funduscopic examination.

Treatment

Retinal breaks are closed by laser photocoagulation or cryotherapy. Vitrectomy may be necessary if vision decreased, or the physician is unable to see well enough to treat the retina.

Bibliography

1. Kayazawa F, Machida T. Retinal arteriolar tortuosity with macular hemorrhage. Ann Ophthalmol. 1983;15:42-3.
2. Wells CG, Kalina RE. Progressive inherited retinal arteriolar tortuosity with spontaneous retinal hemorrhages. Ophthalmology. 1985;92:1015-24.

1229. PROGRESSIVE INTRACRANIAL ARTERIAL OCCLUSION SYNDROME (TAVERAS SYNDROME)

General

Children and young adults; caused by previous trauma and atheroma; occlusive endarteritis; predilection for the circle of Willis; occurs mostly in Japanese and Caucasians.

Ocular

Unilateral ptosis; defective optokinetic nystagmus; visual agnosia; amaurosis fugax.

Clinical

Progressive intracranial arterial occlusion with both internal carotid arteries involved; memory loss; muteness; localized numbness; crying spells; catatonic states and episodes, staring; seizures.

Laboratory

Abnormally high ophthalmodynamometric readings may be the first correct diagnostic sign even before arteriography reveals the vascular pathologic condition.

Treatment

Nystagmus: See-saw nystagmus—visual field to consider neoplastic or vascular etiologies. Upbeat nystagmus—may indicate multiple sclerosis, cerebellar degeneration, tumors or infarcts.

Treatment is directed toward identification and resolution of underlying cause. Downbeat nystagmus—affects the cerebellum or craniocervical junction including Arnold-Chiari malformation, multiple sclerosis, trauma, tumor, infarction and many toxic metabolic entities. MRI may indicate a surgically correctable lesion. Periodic alternating nystagmus is continuous horizontal nystagmus from stroke, tumor, multiple sclerosis, trauma, infection and drug intoxication. Can occur from cataract, vitreous hemorrhage or optic atrophy.

Ptosis: If visual acuity is affected most cases require surgical correction, and there are several procedures that may be used including levator resection, repair or advancement and Fasanella-Servat.

Bibliography

1. Taveras JM. Multiple progressive intracranial arterial occlusions: a syndrome of children and young adults. Am J Roentgenol Radium Ther Nucl Med. 1969;106:235-68.
2. Zappia RJ, Winkelman JZ, Roberson GH, et al. Progressive intracranial arterial occlusion syndrome. Report of a case with unusually high ophthalmodynamometry (ODM) values. Arch Ophthalmol. 1971;86:455-8.

1230. PROGRESSIVE SYSTEMIC SCLEROSIS (SCLERODERMA; SYSTEMIC SCLERODERMA)

General

Chronic connective tissue disease of unknown etiology; chronic and usually progressive disorder; typical onset is in the third to fifth decade of life; ratio of women to men is 4:l; primary sites of pathology are the arterioles and capillaries of affected organs.

Ocular

Marginal corneal ulcers; shortened fornices of the conjunctiva; ptosis; cotton-wool patches of retina; papilledema; retinal hemorrhages; cicatrization of conjunctiva and cornea; blepharitis; blepharospasm; thready, tenacious yellow-white conjunctival discharge; hypertrophy of lacrimal gland; episcleritis; ocular myositis; Sjögren syndrome; uveitis; vitreal haze; keratitis sicca; decreased corneal sensation; iritis; ischemic choroidopathy; iris sectorial atrophy; blepharophimosis; heterochromia; keratoconus; central retinal vein occlusion; branch retinal vein occlusion.

Clinical

Vascular insufficiency; Raynaud phenomenon; malaise; weight loss; stiffness; fever; polyarticular arthritis; diffuse edema of the hands; calcinosis; esophageal involvement; sclerodactyly; telangiectasis; esophageal stricture; renal failure; diffuse interstitial fibrosis.

Laboratory

No specific test establishes diagnosis. Hypergammaglobulinemia (50% of cases), antinuclear antibody (ANA) increased in 40–70% of cases.

Treatment

Skin thickening can be treated with D-penicillamine and other experimental drugs. Pruritus can be treated with moisturizers and histamine. Raynaud phenomenon can be treated with calcium channel blockers. Renal crisis episodes are best prevented and treated with the aggressive use of angiotensin-converting enzyme (ACE) inhibitors. Myositis may be treated cautiously with steroids.

Additional Resource

1. Jimenez SA (2012). Scleroderma. [online] Available from http://www.emedicine.com/med/TOPIC2076.HTM [Accessed April, 2012].

1231. PROPIONIBACTERIUM ACNES

General

Gram-positive, pleomorphic, nonspore-forming bacillus that is considered part of the normal eyelid and conjunctival anaerobic flora. Pathogenic if introduced intraocular.

Clinical

None

Ocular

Chronic keratitis, endophthalmitis, vitreitis.

Laboratory

Aerobic and anaerobic cultures must be incubated for 14 days. Capsular biopsy may demonstrate Gram-positive, plemorphic, nonspore-forming bacillus or Gram stain.

Treatment

Vancomycin intravitreal or systemic; total capsulotomy with intraocular lens (IOL) exchange.

Bibliography

1. Roy FH, Fraunfelder FW, Fraunfelder FT. Roy and Fraunfelder's Current Ocular Therapy, 6th edition. Philadelphia: WB Saunders; 2008.

1232. PROTEIN C DEFICIENCY

General

Autosomal recessive; congenital; heterozygous individuals predisposed to recurrent venous thrombosis; homozygous individuals may develop widespread thrombotic complications in neonatal period; reduced clotting ability; neonatal protein C deficiency also may be acquired and transient in ill preterm babies.

Ocular

Vitreous opacities; vitreous hemorrhages; retinal detachment; cataract; shallow anterior chamber; leukocoria; prominent iris vessels; iris synechiae to lens; bilateral involvement; retinal hemorrhages; cavernous sinus thrombosis.

Clinical

Hematomas; epistaxis; prolonged bleeding; hydrocephalus; Candida sepsis; subarachnoid hemorrhage; pulmonary embolism; thrombotic hemorrhagic gastrointestinal and genitourinary mucosal infarcts.

Laboratory

Decreased protein C activity level is required to make the laboratory diagnosis of protein C deficiency.

Treatment

Medical care for patients with protein C deficiency depends largely on a particular patient's disease manifestations. Thrombotic episode should be treated with anticoagulant therapy.

Additional Resource

1. Cuker A (2011). Protein C Deficiency. [online] Available from http://www.emedicine.com/med/TOPIC1923.HTM [Accessed April, 2012].

1233. PROTEUS INFECTIONS

General

Gram-negative bacilli found in water, soil and decaying organic substances.

Ocular

Conjunctivitis; keratitis; corneal ulcers; endophthalmitis; panophthalmitis; dacryocystitis; gangrene of eyelid; uveitis; hypopyon; paralysis of seventh nerve.

Clinical

Cutaneous infection after surgery; usually occurs as a secondary infection of the skin, ears, mastoid sinuses, eyes, peritoneal cavity, bone, urinary tract, meninges, lung or bloodstream; meningitis; intracranial subdural and epidural empyema; brain abscess; intracranial septic thrombophlebitis affecting cavernous/lateral sinuses.

Laboratory

Proteus organisms are easily recovered through routine laboratory cultures. An ultrasound of the kidneys or a CT scan should be considered as part of a workup.

Treatment

Traditional treatment includes oral quinolone for 3 days or trimethoprim/sulfamethoxazole.

Additional Resource

1. Struble K (2011). Proteus Infections. [online] Available from http://www.emedicine.com/med/TOPIC1929.HTM [Accessed April, 2012].

1234. PROTEUS SYNDROME

General

A harmarteo neoplastic disorder with variable clinical manifestations.

Ocular

Myopia; band keratopathy; cataract; vitreous hemorrhage; chorioretinal mass; serous retinal detachment.

Clinical

Thickening of the bones of the external auditory meatus and cranial fossa; enlargement of the left internal auditory meatus; deformities of the feet and toes.

Laboratory

Proteus organisms are easily recovered through routine laboratory cultures. An ultrasound of the kidneys or a CT scan should be considered as part of a workup.

Treatment

Traditional treatment includes oral quinolone for 3 days or trimethoprim/sulfamethoxazole.

Additional Resource

1. Struble K (2011). Proteus Infections. [online] Available from http://www.emedicine.com/med/TOPIC1929.HTM [Accessed April, 2012].

1235. PROXIMAL AND DISTAL CLICK SYNDROME OF THE SUPERIOR OBLIQUE TENDON (SIMULATED SUPERIOR OBLIQUE TENDON SYNDROME)

General

Produced by quick head movements; caused by adhesions (secondary to trauma and inflammation) or frontal sinus surgery; proximal click adhesions in front to trochlea; distal click adhesions behind trochlea; associated with Brown syndrome.

Ocular

Decreased elevation in adduction; downshoot of the affected eye on adduction; overaction of the tethered inferior oblique after cutting superior oblique tendon; widening of palpebral fissure on adduction; diplopia.

Clinical

Rheumatoid arthritis.

Laboratory

Diagnosis is made by clinical findings.

Treatment

Superior oblique split tendon lengthening technique, tenotomy, superior oblique recession may be useful procedures.

Bibliography

1. Brown HW. True and simulated superior oblique tendon sheath syndromes. Doc Ophthalmol. 1973;34:123-36.
2. Pittke EC. The proximal and distal click syndrome of the superior oblique tendon. Graefes Arch Clin Exp Ophthalmol. 1987;225:28-32.

1236. PRURITUS

General

Unpleasant sensation perceived in the skin that elicits the response of scratching; causes may be physiologic or pathologic.

Ocular

Vesicles, urticaria and eczematization of lid.

Clinical

Urticaria; hives; macular erythema; vesicles; eczematization of lid; skin excoriations; secondary infection; lichenification.

Laboratory

When a primary dermatologic condition is excluded and a systemic cause is suspected, certain laboratory tests may aid diagnosis.

Treatment

Oilated soap for bathing, emollients for after the bath and oral antihistamines are usually initial therapy.

Additional Resource

1. Butler DF (2010). Pruritus and Systemic Disease. [online] Available from http://www.emedicine. com/derm/TOPIC946.HTM [Accessed April, 2012].

1237. PSEUDO-FOSTER KENNEDY SYNDROME

General

Mimic disease of Foster Kennedy syndrome consisting of ischemic optic neuropathy and glioma.

Ocular

Optic disk pallor; visual field defects.

Clinical

Slow, progressive, decreased vision.

Laboratory

B-scan ultrasonography, fluorescein angiography.

Treatment

Steroid treatment may be useful in some cases.

Bibliography

1. Lepore FE, Yarian DL. A mimic of the "exact diagnostic sign" of Foster Kennedy. Ann Ophthalmol. 1985;17:411-2.
2. Limaye SR, Adler J. Pseudo-Foster Kennedy syndrome in a patient with anterior ischemic optic neuropathy and a nonbasal glioma. J Clin Neuro-ophthalmol. 1990;10:188-92.

1238. PSEUDO-GRAEFE SYNDROME (FUCHS SIGN)

General

Misdirection of regenerating oculomotor nerve (cranial nerve III) fibers to other muscles after injury, aneurysm, tumor, exophthalmic goiter, tabes, anterior poliomyelitis or vascular lesions of the brainstem.

Ocular

Elevation of the upper lid in downward gaze; lagging in upper lid movement on downward gaze (Graefe sign).

Clinical

None

Laboratory

Diagnosis is made by clinical findings.

Treatment

Lid retraction or ptosis surgery may be necessary.

Bibliography

1. Bender MB. The nerve supply to the orbicularis muscle and the physiology of movements of the upper eyelid, with particular reference to the pseudo-Graefe phenomenon. Arch Ophthalmol. 1936;15:21.

1239. PSEUDOMALIGNANT GLAUCOMA SYNDROME

General

Related to obstruction of aqueous flow either by residual anterior hyaloid or by fibrin and other inflammatory debris at the level of the ciliary body/zonular apparatus following vitrectomy.

Ocular

Forward movement of lens-iris diaphragm; elevation of intraocular pressure; axial shallowing of anterior chamber; hydration of vitreous cavity.

Clinical

None

Laboratory

Diagnosis is made by clinical findings.

Treatment

Glaucoma: Its medication should be the first plan of action. If medication is unsuccessful, a filtering surgical procedure with or without antimetabolites may be beneficial.

Bibliography

1. Massicotte EC, Schuman JS. A malignant glaucoma-like syndrome following pars plana vitrectomy. Ophthalmology. 1999;106:1375-9.
2. Stern WH. Complications of vitrectomy. Int Ophthalmol Clin. 1992;32:205-12.

1240. PSEUDO-PSEUDO-FOSTER KENNEDY SYNDROME

General

Mimic disease of Pseudo-Foster Kennedy Syndrome consisting of ischemic optic neuropathy and meningioma.

Ocular

Optic disk pallor, visual field defects.

Clinical

Slow, progressive, decreased view.

Laboratory

B-scan ultrasonography, fluorescein angiography.

Treatment

Steroid treatment may be useful in some cases.

Bibliography

1. Gelwan MJ, Seidman M, Kupersmith MJ. Pseudo-Pseudo-Foster Kennedy syndrome. J Clin Neuroophthalmol. 1988;8:49-52.

1241. PSEUDOEXFOLIATION SYNDROME

General

Prevalent over age of 70 years; rare before age 40 years; unilateral involvement in 40–50% of cases; asymmetry of severity in bilateral cases; most common in Caucasians, especially from Iceland and Scandinavian countries; pseudoexfoliation fibers were identified in autopsy tissue specimens of skin, heart, lungs, liver and cerebral meninges; consistently associated with connective tissue components, i.e. fibroblasts, collagen and elastic fibers, myocardial tissue and heart muscle cell.

Ocular

Gray or white fluffy material deposited in particles, flakes or sheets on anterior surface of iris, ciliary body, posterior surface of cornea, pupillary margin, lens and trabecular meshwork; increased pigmentation of trabecular meshwork; zonular dialysis; displaced or dislocated lens; anterior chamber depth asymmetry; preoperative phacodonesis; glaucoma; cataract.

Clinical

None

Laboratory

Diagnosis is made by clinical findings.

Treatment

Annual eye examinations for early detection of glaucoma. Glaucoma in pseudoexfoliation is more resistant to medical therapy which is unsuccessful to control the glaucoma. Argon laser trabeculoplasty or trabeculectomy may be beneficial.

Additional Resource

1. Pons ME (2011). Pseudoexfoliation Glaucoma. [online] Available from http://www.emedicine.com/oph/TOPIC140.HTM [Accessed April, 2012].

1242. PSEUDOHYPOPARATHYROIDISM SYNDROME (ALBRIGHT HEREDITARY OSTEODYSTROPHY; CHRONIC RENAL TUBULAR INSUFFICIENCY SYNDROME; SEABRIGHT-BANTAM SYNDROME)

General

Etiology unknown; autosomal dominant; more common in females (2:1); present from birth; kidney and skeleton fail to respond to parahormone; if patients receive parathyroid extract, their kidneys fail to respond with phosphate diuresis; genetic form of hypoparathyroidism resulting from end-organ resistance to parathyroid hormone; resulting hypocalcemia is responsible for many of the clinical features of this syndrome.

Ocular

Strabismus; blue sclera; punctate cataracts (white opacities and polychromatic cortex); papill-edema; hypertelorism; keratitis; scleral and choroidal calcifications; blepharospasm; cataracts.

Clinical

Short stature; short metacarpals; short limbs; round face with short neck; decalcification of teeth; obesity; fat, stubby hands; tetany with positive Chvostek and Trousseau signs; atypical seizure disorder.

Laboratory

Hypocalcemia, hyperphosphatemia and low parathyroid hormone levels in the absence of renal failure or intestinal malabsorption.

Treatment

Papilledema: Underlying cause should be determined and treated. Systemic acetazolamide is the medical therapy of choice.

Cataract: Change in glasses can sometimes improve a patient's visual function temporarily; however, the most common treatment is cataract surgery.

Additional Resource

1. Gliwa A (2012). Hypoparathyroidism in Emergency Medicine. [online] Available from http://www.emedicine.com/emerg/TOPIC276.HTM [Accessed April, 2012].

1243. PSEUDOMONAS AERUGINOSA

General

Gram-negative rod that is ubiquitous in water, soil and plants. Commonly found in hospital environment.

Clinical

None

Ocular

Foreign body sensation, conjunctival injection, photophobia and corneal ulceration.

Laboratory

Gram-negative rod on Gram stain and Giemsa stain from corneal ulcer. Culturing contact lens and lens solutions may help to grow organisms.

Treatment

Fortified tobramycin and fortified cefazolin are drugs of choice.

Bibliography

1. Roy FH, Fraunfelder FW, Fraunfelder FT. Roy and Fraunfelder's Current Ocular Therapy, 6th edition. Philadelphia: WB Saunders; 2008.

1244. PSEUDO-OPHTHALMOPLEGIA SYNDROME (ROTH-BIELSCHOWSKY SYNDROME)

General

Supranuclear lesion in the temporal lobe.

Ocular

Paralysis of lateral gaze in one direction; vestibular nystagmus in which the fast phase is absent on the ipsilateral side but the slow phase is present.

Clinical

Basal ganglia or tectum lesion.

Laboratory

Diagnosis is made by clinical findings.

Treatment

Consult neurologist.

Bibliography

1. Bielschowsky A. Das Klinische Bild der Assoziierten Blicklahmung und Seine Bedeutung fur die Topische Diagnostik. Munchen Med Wochenschr. 1903;40:1666.
2. Cogan DG, Adams RD. A type of paralysis of conjugate gaze (ocular motor apraxia). AMA Arch Ophthalmol. 1953;50:434-42.
3. Geeraets WJ. Ocular Syndromes, 3rd edition. Philadelphia: Lea & Febiger; 1976.
4. Roth WC. Demonstration von Kranken mit Ophthalmoplegie. Neurol Zentbl. 1901;20:921.

1245. PSEUDOPAPILLEDEMA (OPTIC NERVE HEAD DRUSEN)

General

Autosomal dominant; incidence in males and females is approximately the same; two-thirds of cases are bilateral; visual acuity usually unaffected; may cause slowly progressive visual field defect.

Ocular

Elevation of optic disk; drusen; injected conjunctiva; associated with retinitis pigmentosa, subretinal and subretinal pigment epithelium hemorrhages (rare).

Clinical

None

Laboratory

B-scan ultrasonography, fluorescein angiography.

Treatment

No treatment is needed for most causes of pseudopapilledema because they represent normal physiologic variants.

Additional Resource

1. Gossman MV (2011). Pseudopapilledema. [online] Available from http://www.emedicine.com/oph/TOPIC615.HTM [Accessed April, 2012].

1246. PSEUDOPHAKIC PIGMENT DISPERSION SYNDROME

General

Caused by rubbing of peripheral iris on lens zonules with iris plane and posterior chamber lenses.

Ocular

Transillumination of iris defects; pigment granules in aqueous humor; pigment dusting of anterior iris surface; band of pigment in filtration portion of trabecular meshwork; glaucoma.

Clinical

None

Laboratory

Diagnosis is made by clinical findings.

Treatment

Topical glaucoma medications, laser trabeculoplasty, laser iridectomy, filtering surgery.

Additional Resource

1. Ritch R (2010). Glaucoma, Pigmentary. [online] Available from http://www.emedicine.com/oph/TOPIC136.HTM [Accessed April, 2012].

1247. PSEUDOPROGERIA SYNDROME

General

Rare; autosomal recessive; absent eyebrows and eyelashes with mental retardation.

Ocular

Glaucoma; absence of eyelashes and eyebrows.

Clinical

Progressive spastic quadriplegia; microcephaly; small, beaked nose; cervical spinal cyst; occipital cranium bifidum occultum; mental retardation.

Laboratory

Diagnosis is made by clinical findings.

Treatment

Glaucoma medications are used first. If medication does not control intraocular pressure (IOP), a surgical filtering procedure may be necessary.

Bibliography

1. Hall BD, Berg BO, Rudolph RS, et al. Pseudoprogeria-Hallermann-Streiff (PHS) syndrome. Birth Defects Orig Artic Ser. 1974;10:137-46.
2. McKusick VA. Mendelian Inheritance in Man: A Catalog of Human Genes and Genetic Disorders, 12th edition. Baltimore: The Johns Hopkins University Press; 1998.
3. McKusick-Nathans Institute for Genetic Medicine, Johns Hopkins University and National Center for Biotechnology Information, National Library of Medicine. (2007). Online Mendelian Inheritance in Man (OMIM). [online] Available from http://www.ncbi.nlm.nih.gov/omim [Accessed April, 2012].

1248. PSITTACOSIS (ORNITHOSIS)

General

Infectious disease transmitted from birds to man; causative agent is *Chlamydia psittaci*; poultry, pigeons, and parrots prominent carriers.

Ocular

Lid edema; corneal ulcers; scleritis; ophthalmoplegia; uveitis; acute focal retinitis; stellate retinopathy; cataract.

Clinical

Fever, malaise; headache; wheezing; intracranial hypertension.

Laboratory

The most common finding is unilateral, lower-lobe dense infiltrate/consolidation. Psittacosis may present in a bilateral, nodular, miliary or interstitial pattern. Serologic tests are the mainstays of diagnosis; however, because of the delayed appearance of specific antibodies, these tests are not helpful in emergent clinical management.

Treatment

Consider the diagnosis of psittacosis in patients with community-acquired pneumonia who have been exposed to birds. The mainstay of medical care is antibiotic therapy. Consultation with an infectious disease specialist.

Additional Resource

1. Lessnau KD (2011). Psittacosis. [online] Available from http://www.emedicine.com/med/TOPIC1951.HTM [Accessed April, 2012].

1249. PSORIASIS (PSORIASIS VULGARIS)

General

Chronic skin disease of unknown etiology; both sexes affected; onset at any age; disease peaks at puberty; strong human leukocyte antigen (HLA) association resulting in heritable disease susceptibility.

Ocular

Desquamative psoriatic plaques of lids resulting in madarosis, trichiasis or ectropion; corneal plaques; xerosis, symblepharon; keratitis; chronic corneal ulceration; phthisis bulbi; iritis.

Clinical

Thick, dry, elevated red patches of skin covered with coarse silvery scales that usually affect areas of skin not exposed to sun, such as scalp, sacrum, elbows and knees; positive association with Sjögren syndrome and keratitis sicca.

Laboratory

Diagnosis is made by clinical findings.

Treatment

The simplest treatment of psoriasis is daily sun exposure, sea bathing, topical moisturizers, and relaxation. Moisturizers, such as petrolatum jelly, are helpful. Anthralin, coal or wood tar, corticosteroids, salicylic acid, phenolic compounds and calcipotriene (a vitamin D analog) also may be effective. Ocular lubricants and punctal occlusion, oral and topical corticosteroids are sometimes beneficial.

Additional Resource

1. Meffert J (2012). Psoriasis. [online] Available from http://www.emedicine.com/oph/TOPIC483.HTM [Accessed April, 2012].

1250. PSORIATIC ARTHRITIS

General

Chronic skin disease of unknown etiology; both sexes affected; onset at any age; disease peaks at puberty.

Ocular

Conjunctivitis; iritis; keratitis; uveitis.

Clinical

Rash; spondylitis; inflammatory bowel disease; diarrhea; degenerative disease of spine.

Laboratory

The differentiation of psoriatic arthritis from rheumatoid arthritis and gout can be facilitated by the absence of the typical laboratory findings of those conditions. Joint X-rays can facilitate the diagnosis of psoriatic arthritis.

Treatment

The simplest treatment of psoriasis is daily sun exposure, sea bathing, topical moisturizers, and relaxation. Moisturizers, such as petrolatum jelly, are helpful. Anthralin, coal or wood tar, corticosteroids, salicylic acid, phenolic compounds and calcipotriene (a vitamin D analog) also may be effective. Ocular lubricants and punctal occlusion, oral and topical corticosteroids are sometimes beneficial.

Bibliography

1. Lambert JR, Wright V. Eye inflammation in psoriatic arthritis. Ann Rheum Dis. 1976;35:354-6.

1251. PTERYGIUM AND PSEUDOPTERYGIUM

General

Cause is hereditary or environmental. Exposure to sunlight, wind, dust and airborne allergen increase incidence.

Clinical

None

Ocular

Triangular elevated mass of thickened bulbar conjunctiva extending to the cornea which if approaches the pupil can threaten vision. Pseudopterygium is similar in appearance, but usually bridges the limbus.

Laboratory

Diagnosis is made by clinical findings.

Treatment

Corticosteroids; surgical removal if threatens visual axis.

Additional Resource

1. Fisher JP (2011). Pterygium. [online] Available from http://www.emedicine.com/oph/TOPIC542. HTM [Accessed April, 2012].

1252. PTERYGIUM OF CONJUNCTIVA AND CORNEA

General

Autosomal dominant; more frequent in people who work outdoors; occurs late in life.

Ocular

Wing-shaped thickening in the conjunctiva, usually nasal, in the interpalpebral fissure area; alterations in corneal topography can cause a reduction in visual acuity.

Clinical

None

Laboratory

Diagnosis is made by clinical findings.

Treatment

Patients with pterygia can be observed unless the lesions exhibit growth toward the center of the cornea or the patient exhibits symptoms of significant redness, discomfort or alterations in visual function. Surgery for excision of pterygia is beneficial if visual function is disturbed.

Additional Resource

1. Fisher JP (2011). Pterygium. [online] Available from http://www.emedicine.com/oph/TOPIC542. HTM [Accessed April, 2012].

1253. PTOSIS (ADULT PTOSIS, BLEPHAROPTOSIS)

General

Abnormal low-lying or droopy upper eyelid margin. Etiology includes myogenic, aponeurotic, neurogenic, mechanical, traumatic and pseudo-ptotic. This conditions can be acquired or congenital. Acquired can be secondary to diseases such as myasthenia gravis, multiple sclerosis and thyroid disease.

Clinical

Myasthenia gravis, multiple sclerosis, abnormal thyroid.

Ocular

Droopy upper lid, amblyopia, chronic progressive external ophthalmoplegia.

Laboratory

Diagnosis is made by clinical findings; however, testing should be done to confirm a systemic diagnosis in acquired cases. These tests would include cerebrospinal fluid (CSF) analysis, Tensilon test, CT and MRI.

Treatment

If myasthenia gravis is diagnosed, Mestinon may be beneficial. Most cases require surgical correction and there are several procedures that may be used including levator resection, repair or advancement and Fasanella-Servat.

Additional Resource

1. Cohen AJ (2011). Adult Ptosis. [online] Available from http://www.emedicine.com/oph/TOPIC201. HTM [Accessed April, 2012].

1254. PTOSIS, CONGENITAL

General

Drooping lid, upper lid falls to a position lower than normal. Drooping lid can cover the pupil resulting in amblyopia. Present at birth or develops in the first year of life is considered congenital. Can affect one or both eyes. Generally results form a localized myogenic dysgenesis rather than normal muscle fibers, fibrous and adipose tissues are present in the muscle belly, diminishing the ability of the levator to contract and relax. Cause is usually idiopathic. If autosomal dominant the ptosis can be associated with other disease or syndromes.

Clinical

Marcus Gunn syndrome; Duane syndrome; Kearns-Sayre syndrome; birth trauma; myasthenia gravis; pseudotumor of the orbit; myotonic dystrophy; Horner syndrome; blepharophimosis syndrome; III cranial nerve palsy.

Ocular

Unilateral or bilateral drooping of the upper lid; amblyopia; obstructed visual field; strabismus; abnormal head position.

Laboratory

Diagnosis is generally made by clinical findings; however, if associated disease or syndromes are suspected, additional lab and imaging studies may be necessary to determine the associated disease.

Treatment

Only observation is necessary in mild cases. Early surgical intervention is necessary in patients with significant amblyopia or ocular torticollis.

Additional Resource

1. Suh DW (2012). Congenital Ptosis. [online] Available from http://www.emedicine.medscape. com/article/1212815-overview [Accessed April, 2012].

1255. PUCKERING SYNDROME

General

Disturbance of vitreous with vitreous retraction.

Ocular

Epiretinal membrane formation following vitreous bleed, total retinal detachment, detachment of the macula, multiple retinal operations, multiple perforations, loss of formed vitreous at operation or posterior vitreous separation from trauma to the eye or whiplash injury.

Clinical

Neck injury with whiplash.

Laboratory

Diagnosis is made by clinical findings.

Treatment

Retinal detachment: Scleral buckle, pneumatic retinopexy and vitrectomy may be used to close all the breaks.

Vitreous hemorrhage: If possible the source of the bleeding needs to be isolated and treated with laser. Vitrectomy may be necessary.

Bibliography

1. Pau H. Differential Diagnosis of Eye Diseases. New York: Thieme; 1987.
2. Tanenbaum HL, Schepens CL, Elzeneiny I, et al. Macular pucker following retinal detachment surgery. Arch Ophthalmol. 1970;83:286-93.

1256. PUGH SYNDROME

General

May be misdiagnosed as UGH (uveitis, glaucoma, hyphema) syndrome; unrelated to the presence of an intraocular lens.

Ocular

Pseudouveitis; glaucoma; hyphema as in UGH syndrome, but also neovascular membrane covering the iris; central retinal vein occlusion.

Clinical

None

Laboratory

Diagnosis is made by clinical findings.

Treatment

Uveitis: Topical steroids and cycloplegic medication should be the initial treatment of choice.

Oral steroids if not responsive to topical steroids, immunosuppressants if bilateral disease that does not respond to oral steroids, periocular steroids for unilateral or posterior uveitis. Vitrectomy can be used for severe vitreous opacification. Cryotherapy and laser photocoagulation may be used for localized pars plana exudates.

Hyphema: Cycloplegia decreased the inflammation and discomfort associated with traumatic iritis. Topical beta-adrenergic antagonists are the therapy of choice for elevated intraocular pressures; laser may be used to cauterize the bleeding vessel.

Bibliography

1. Epstein E. UGH syndrome and contact lenses. J Cataract Refract Surg. 1987;13:216-7.
2. Hagan JC. Complications while removing the IOLAB 91Z lens for the UGH-UGH+syndrome. J Am Intraocul Implant Soc. 1984;10:209-13.

1257. PULMONARY INSUFFICIENCY

General

Elevated CO_2 levels.

Ocular

Tortuosity of conjunctival and retinal vasculature; retinal hemorrhages; papilledema; retinal edema.

Clinical

Vascular decompensation; elevation of cerebrospinal fluid pressure; polycythemia; chronic respiratory disease.

Laboratory

The arterial blood gas (ABG) is diagnostic.

Treatment

The goals of therapy are to remove the underlying cause and return the $PaCO_2$ level to baseline.

Additional Resource

1. Lal MK (2012). Pediatric Respiratory Acidosis. [online] Available from http://www.emedicine.com/ped/TOPIC16.HTM [Accessed April, 2012].

1258. PUPIL, EGG-SHAPED

General

Autosomal dominant; rare.

Ocular

Oval pupils; enlarged pupils; pupils react poorly to constricting stimuli.

Clinical

None

Laboratory

Diagnosis is made by clinical findings.

Treatment

None/Ocular.

Bibliography

1. McKusick VA. Mendelian Inheritance in Man: A Catalog of Human Genes and Genetic Disorders, 12th edition. Baltimore: The Johns Hopkins University Press; 1998.

1259. PUPILLARY BLOCK GLAUCOMA

General

Condition can occur following cataract surgery with or without an intraocular lens implant. Block is caused by mechanical closure of the pupil by the intraocular lens, by developing synechiae or by lens capsule.

Clinical

Pain in the eye, unilateral headache, nausea, vomiting.

Ocular

Elevated intraocular pressure, iris synechiae, anterior pupillary block, posterior pupillary block, postoperative iritis, photophobia, blurred vision, halos around lights.

Laboratory

B-scan ultrasonography to identify retained lens material, lens nucleus, choroidal hemorrhage or aqueous misdirection.

Treatment

Surgically, a peripheral iridectomy to break the block is the treatment of choice. Surgical breaking of the synechiae may be necessary. Vitrectomy may be needed. Filtration surgery may be indicated if the anterior chamber fails to open following the iridectomy. Transciliary filtration can be performed with a Fugo blade to relieve iris bombe. Medically, analgesics and antiemetics may be beneficial. Dilatation and topical steroids may be useful to relieve inflammation following the episode.

Additional Resources

1. Eezzuduemhoi DR (2010). Pupillary Block, Aphakic. [online] Available from http://www.emedicine.medscape.com/article/1220164-overview [Accessed April, 2012].
2. Singh D (2010). Pseudophakic Pupillary Block. [online] Available from http://www.emedicine.medscape.com/article/1220263-overview [Accessed April, 2012].

1260. PUPILLARY MEMBRANE, PERSISTENT

General

Autosomal dominant.

Ocular

Remnants of pupillary membrane persist as strands and other irregular tissue in pupil; congenital cataract; corneal edema; Rieger syndrome; keratoconus.

Clinical

None

Laboratory

Diagnosis is made by clinical findings.

Treatment

Cataract surgery may be necessary if vision is effected; steroids and Muro 128 may be used for corneal edema; keratoconus may be treated with spectacle correction, hard contacts, avoid eye rubbing. If hydrops occurs discontinue contact lens, use NaCl drops and ointment, patching and short course of steroids. As the disease advances penetrating keratoplasty, deep anterior lamellar keratoplasty, intacs with laser grooves or collagen stabilization of cornea.

Bibliography

1. Duane TD. Clinical Ophthalmology. Philadelphia: JB Lippincott; 1987.
2. McKusick VA. Mendelian Inheritance in Man: A Catalog of Human Genes and Genetic Disorders, 12th edition. Baltimore: The Johns Hopkins University Press; 1998.

1261. PURTSCHER SYNDROME (DUANE RETINOPATHY; FAT EMBOLISM SYNDROME; TRAUMATIC RETINAL ANGIOPATHY; TRAUMATIC LIPORRHAGIA; VALSALVA RETINOPATHY OF DUANE)

General

Most frequently seen in accidents associated with sudden rise in blood pressure and congestion in the head and chest; presence of fat embolism may be the causative factor; neurovascular changes in retina referred to as traumatic retinal angiopathy; several mechanisms have been proposed, including compressive trauma and post-traumatic fat embolism; most likely mechanism appears to be leukocyte aggregation by activated complement factor 5 (C5a), which can occur in diverse conditions such as trauma, acute pancreatitis and connective tissue disease.

Ocular

Retinal and preretinal hemorrhages over entire fundus; cotton-wool exudates, mainly posterior aspect; retinal edema; posterior and macular serous detachment; venous congestion and engorgement; papilledema; usually bilateral, although unilateral causes have been reported.

Clinical

Multiple fractures (mainly extensive crushing); lung congestion; dyspnea; lymphorrhagia; pancreatitis; scleroderma; dermatomyositis; lupus erythematosus; childbirth.

Laboratory

Amylase level: Purtscher-like retinopathy is associated with acute pancreatitis; thus, an elevated amylase level may be diagnostic of this condition.

Treatment

In patients with retinopathy due to systemic vasculitis, steroid therapy is beneficial. Surgical care may be required for traumatic chest and head injuries.

Additional Resource

1. Chaum E (2010). Retinopathy, Purtscher. [online] Available from http://www.emedicine.com/oph/TOPIC419.HTM [Accessed April, 2012].

1262. PYODERMA VEGETANS (DERMATITIS VEGETANS)

General

Occurs in both sexes and all ages; frequently seen with pre-existing eczema or infective dermatitis; nonspecific skin reaction; chronic; malnutrition and alcoholism are contributing factors.

Ocular

Lid lesions; keratitis.

Clinical

Chronic granulomatous growth with epithelial hyperplasia often with pustules, ulcers, multiple abscesses and fistulas; lesions of mouth and nose.

Laboratory

Cultures should also be taken for fungi and mycobacteria.

Treatment

Antibiotic treatment has often been used with variable results, copper sulfate or aluminum subacetate dressings and topical aluminum acetate soaks with intravenous ceftriaxone had moderate success.

Additional Resource

1. Schwartz RA (2011). Pyoderma Vegetans. [online] Available from http://www.emedicine.com/derm/TOPIC910.HTM [Accessed April, 2012].

1263. PYOSTOMATITIS

General

Reaction of chronic inflamed skin due to secondary infection; body resistance leads to folding of mucous membrane and development of a verrucous surface.

Ocular

Conjunctivitis; blepharitis.

Clinical

Early lesions are small pustules that can develop to large, weeping inflammatory plaques with foul odors; massive crust may form granulations of buccal mucosa, hand, soft palate, lips and gingiva.

Laboratory

Cultures of the ulcer/erosion for bacteria, fungi, atypical mycobacteria and viruses are needed.

Treatment

Topical therapies include local wound care and dressings, superpotent topical corticosteroids, cromolyn sodium 2% solution, nitrogen mustard and 5-aminosalicylic acid. Systemic therapies include corticosteroids, cyclosporine, mycophenolate mofetil, azathioprine, dapsone, tacrolimus, cyclophosphamide, chlorambucil, thalidomide, tumor necrosis factor-alpha (TNF-alpha) inhibitors and nicotine. Intravenous therapies include pulsed methylprednisolone, pulsed cyclophosphamide, infliximab and intravenous immunoglobulin, and hyperbaric oxygen.

Additional Resource

1. Jackson JM (2012). Pyoderma Gangrenosum. [online] Available from http://www.emedicine. com/derm/TOPIC367.HTM [Accessed April, 2012].

1264. Q FEVER (COXIELLA BURNETII)

General

Acute rickettsial infection caused by *Coxiella burnetii*; at least 11 serotypes of this organism are capable of causing human infection; elevated inflammatory response results in granulomatous formation.

Ocular

Conjunctivitis; gangrene of eyelids; retinal hemorrhages; perivasculitis; episcleritis; optic neuritis; uveitis; papilledema; nystagmus; ocular motor nerve pareses; Miller-Fisher syndrome.

Clinical

Fever; severe headache; tissue necrosis; pneumonia; self-limited fever; endocarditis; hepatitis.

Laboratory

Small Gram-negative rod which grows inside eukaryotic cells. Serologic test compliment fixation is specific but lacks sensitivity and indirect immunofluorescence is Q Fever highly specific and sensitive.

Treatment

Adequate antibiotic therapy initiated early in the first week of illness is highly effective and is associated with the best outcome. Doxycycline is the drug of choice.

Additional Resource

1. Rathore MH (2011). Rickettsial Infection. [online] Available from http://www.emedicine.com/ped/ TOPIC2015.HTM [Accessed April, 2012].

1265. 10q- SYNDROME (10q DELETION SYNDROME)

General

Chromosome 10q deletion syndrome.

Ocular

Microphthalmia

Clinical

Intrauterine growth retardation; microcephaly; truncus arteriosus type I; respiratory distress; craniofacial dysmorphism.

Laboratory/Ocular

Diagnosis is made by clinical findings.

Treatment/Ocular

None

Bibliography

1. Glanz A, Forse A, Polomeno RC, et al. Lenz microphthalmia: a malformation syndrome with variable expression of multiple congenital anomalies. Can J Ophthalmol. 1983;18:41-4.
2. Lewandowski RC, Kukolich MK, Sears JW, et al. Partial deletion 10q. Hum Genet. 1978;42:339-43.
3. Taysi K, Strauss AW, Yang V, et al. Terminal deletion of the long arm of chromosome 10: q26 to qter. Case report and review of literature. Ann Genet. 1982;25:141-4.

1266. 13q- SYNDROME (13q DELETION SYNDROME)

General

Chromosome 13q deletion syndrome.

Ocular

Retinoblastoma; telecanthus; hypertelorism; optic nerve hypoplasia; retinal dysplasia.

Clinical

Holoprosencephaly; abnormal lower extremity configuration; atrial septal defect; microcephaly; ambiguous genitalia; hypotonia; low-set ears; growth retardation; mild mental retardation; intestinal atresia.

Laboratory/Ocular

Diagnosis is made by clinical findings.

Treatment

Retinoblastoma: External beam radiation therapy is recommended on patients with significant vitreous seeding. Radioactive isotope plaques and chemotherapy are also an option. Removal of the tumor is the standard management for retinoblastoma.

Bibliography

1. Nishikawa A, Mitomori T, Matsuura A, et al. A 13q- syndrome with extensive intestinal atresia. Acta Paediatr Scand. 1985;74:305-8.
2. Santolaya J, McCorquodale MM, Torres W, et al. Ultrasonographic prenatal diagnosis of the 13q-syndrome. Fetal Diagn Ther. 1993;8:261-7.
3. Stoll C, Alembik Y. A patient with 13q- syndrome with mild mental retardation and with growth retardation. Ann Genet. 1998;41:209-12.
4. Weichselbaum RR, Zakov ZN, Albert DM, et al. New findings in the chromosome 13 long-arm deletion syndrome and retinoblastoma. Ophthalmology. 1979;86:1191-201.

1267. 18q- SYNDROME (18q DELETION SYNDROME)

General

Chromosome 18q deletion syndrome.

Ocular

Macular "fibrosis"; optic disk abnormalities with tractional retinal detachment, retinal degeneration and tilting of the optic disk.

Clinical

Microcephaly; short stature; hypotonia; hypothyroidism; diabetes mellitus; short neck; sensorineural hearing loss; sensorimotor axonal neuropathy; mild-to-moderate mental retardation; chronic arthritis; seizures.

Laboratory

Diagnosis is made by clinical findings.

Treatment

Retinal detachment: Scleral buckle, pneumatic retinopexy and vitrectomy may be used to close all the breaks.

Bibliography

1. Gordon MF, Bressman S, Brin MF, et al. Dystonia in a patient with deletion of 18q. Mov Disord. 1995;10:496-9.
2. Hansen US, Herlin T. Chronic arthritis in a boy with 18q- syndrome. J Rheumatol. 1994;21:1958-9.
3. Smith A, Caradus V, Henry JG. Translocation 46XY t (17;18) (q25;q21) in a mentally retarded boy with progressive eye abnormalities. Clin Genet. 1979;16:156-62.

1268. 4q- SYNDROME (4q DELETION SYNDROME)

General

Chromosome 4q deletion syndrome.

Ocular

Hypertelorism; epicanthal folds.

Clinical

Depressed nasal bridge; short nasal septum with upturned nose, cleft lip and palate; micrognathia; low-set malformed ears; short neck; distally placed nipples; sacral dimple; hypospadias; dysplastic nails; overriding toes; simian creases; hypoplasia of gallbladder; cardiac defects; mental retardation.

Laboratory

Diagnosis is made by clinical findings.

Treatment

Hypertelorism: The primary correction involves orbital reconstruction and the nasal deformity correction that is universally associated with this deformity.

Bibliography

1. Robertson SP, O'Day K, Bankier A. The 4q- syndrome: delineation of the minimal critical region to within band 4q31. Clin Genet. 1998;53:70-3.
2. Townes PL, White M, Di Marzo SV. 4q-syndrome. Am J Dis Child. 1979;133:383-5.
3. Yu CW, Chen H, Baucum RW, et al. Terminal deletion of the long arm of chromosome 4. Report of a case of 46, XY, del(4)(q31) and review of 4q- syndrome. Ann Genet. 1981;24:158-61.

1269. 11q- SYNDROME

General

Chromosome 11q deletion syndrome.

Ocular

Telecanthus/Hypertelorism; rarely, congenital glaucoma, cyclopia.

Clinical

Psychomotor retardation; trigonocephaly; broad depressed nasal bridge; micrognathia; low-set abnormal ears; cardiac anomalies; hand and foot anomalies; renal agenesis; anal atresia; supratentorial white matter abnormality on CT or MRI; microphallus; holoprosencephaly; female preponderance.

Treatment

Hypertelorism: The primary correction involves orbital reconstruction and the nasal deformity correction that is universally associated with this deformity.

Congenital cataract: Primary congenital glaucoma almost always is managed surgically, both goniotomy and trabeculectomy may be useful. When multiple goniotomies and/or trabeculectomies fail, the surgeon usually resorts to a filtering procedure.

Bibliography

1. Helmuth RA, Weaver DD, Wills ER. Holoprosencephaly, ear abnormalities, congenital heart defect, and microphallus in a patient with 11q-mosaicism. Am J Med Genet. 1989;32:178-81.
2. Ishida Y, Watanabe N, Ishihara Y, et al. The 11q-syndrome with mosaic partial deletion of 11q. Acta Paediatr Jpn. 1992;34:592-6.
3. Leegte B, Kerstjens-Frederikse WS, Deelstra K, et al. 11q- syndrome: three cases and a review of the literature. Genet Couns. 1999;10:305-13.

1270. RADIATION INJURY (GAMMA RAYS; INFRARED RAYS; MICROWAVES; RADIOWAVES; X-RAYS)

General

Electromagnetic radiation can cause ionization in biologic tissues.

Ocular

Hyperemia of conjunctiva; corneal ulcer; punctate keratitis; keratoconjunctivitis sicca; blepharitis; ectropion; entropion; madarosis; poliosis; depigmentation of eyelids; uveitis; atrophy of lacrimal gland; cataracts; true exfoliation of lens capsule; orbital necrosis; retinal hemorrhage; macular degeneration; macular holes; neovascularization of retina; glaucoma; macular edema; retinal microvascular changes; optic nerve edema and hemorrhage; atrophy.

Clinical

Thermal burns of any part of the body; necrosis; carcinomas; edema.

Laboratory

Diagnosis is made by clinical findings.

Treatment

Corneal ulcer: Corneal cultures may be taken and treatment initiated. Treatment includes a broad spectrum of antibiotics and cycloplegic drops.

Cataract: Change in glasses can sometimes improve a patient's visual function temporarily; however, the most common treatment is cataract surgery.

Glaucoma: Its medication should be the first plan of action. If medication is unsuccessful, a filtering surgical procedure with or without antimetabolites may be beneficial.

Ectropion: Topical ocular lubricants. Congenital-full thickness skin graft with canthal tendon tightening. Involutional-tighten lid by resecting full thickness wedge-medial spindle procedure for punctal eversion. Paralytic may require a fascia lata sling procedure if does not resolve in 3–6 months.

Entropion: Topical antibiotics and lubricants, temporary sutures to evert the eyelid, lateral cantholysis with subconjunctival incision just inferior to the tarsus. Inferior retractors are isolated and reattached to anteroinferior portion of tarsus with multiple interrupted sutures.

Additional Resource

1. Pae JS (2011). CBRNE - Radiation Emergencies. [online] Available from http://www.emedicine.com/emerg/TOPIC934.HTM [Accessed April, 2012].

1271. RAEDER SYNDROME (CLUSTER HEADACHE; CILIARY NEURALGIA; HISTAMINE CEPHALALGIA; HORTON HEADACHE; PARATRIGEMINAL PARALYSIS; PERIODIC MIGRAINOUS NEURALGIA)

General

Interruption of sympathetic fibers about the carotid artery and involvement of the fifth nerve; meningioma and aneurysm of the internal carotid artery most frequent causes; prominent in males; possible pathogenetic mechanism of this condition is an ischemic injury of the Gasserian ganglion.

Ocular

Mild enophthalmos; mild ptosis (unilateral); epiphora; scotoma possible; hypotonia; unilateral miosis; increased tear secretion; periocular pain; Horner syndrome.

Clinical

Facial pain; occasionally weakness of the jaw muscles; headaches (V-region); hypertension; associated inflammatory processes are not infrequent.

Laboratory

Brain scan to rule out meningioma and basilar artery aneurysm.

Treatment

Oxygen inhalation and subcutaneous Sumatriptan are useful in acute attacks.

Additional Resource

1. Bardorf CM (2012). Horner Syndrome. [online] Available from http://www.emedicine.com/oph/TOPIC336.HTM [Accessed April, 2012].

1272. RAYMOND SYNDROME [CESTAN (2) SYNDROME; DISASSOCIATION OF LATERAL GAZE SYNDROME; PONTINE SYNDROME; RAYMOND-CESTAN SYNDROME]

General

Lesion involving the pyramidal tracts as they traverse the pons; posterior longitudinal bundle and medial lemniscus may be involved; tumor and vascular thromboses are common causes; can be caused iatrogenically after neurosurgical procedures.

Ocular

Ipsilateral abducens palsy; paralysis of lateral conjugate gaze.

Clinical

Contralateral hemiplegia; anesthesia of the face, limbs and trunk.

Laboratory

Computed tomography (CT) scan of the head.

Treatment

Tape or base-out prism on one eyeglass may be useful, botulinum toxin type A into the antagonist medial rectus muscle, if no improvement after 6–12 months—recess/resect of medial and lateral rectus.

Bibliography

1. Isobe I, Fujita T, Yoshida K, et al. Rare case of Raymond-Cestan syndrome. Naika. 1970;26: 388-92.
2. Raymond F, Cestan R. Trois Observations de Paralysie des Mouvements Associes des Globes Oculaires. Rev Neurol (Paris). 1901;9:70-7.
3. Seyer H, Honegger J, Schott W, et al. Raymond's syndrome following petrosal sinus sampling. Acta Neurochir (Wien). 1994;131:157-9.

1273. RAYNAUD DISEASE (SYMMETRICAL ASPHYXIA; SYMMETRICAL GANGRENE)

General

Primary or Idiopathic form of paroxysmal digital cyanosis; possible abnormality of sympathetic nervous system; occurs in females between the ages of 15 and 40 years.

Ocular

Spasm of retinal arteries; papillitis; retrobulbar neuritis; amaurosis fugax; cotton-wool spots; retinal hemorrhages; transient corneal opacification.

Clinical

Intermittent attacks of pallor or cyanosis in fingers, precipitated by cold or occasionally by emotional upsets; atrophy of terminal fat pads and digital skin; gangrenous ulcers.

Laboratory

Complete blood cell count, thyroid-stimulating hormone.

Treatment

Education and stopping any vasoconstricting agents, such as nicotine, are helpful. The use of calcium channel blockers, such as nifedipine, is more common. Angiotensin-converting inhibitors and intravenous prostaglandins have shown some benefits.

Additional Resource

1. Hansen-Dispenza H (2011). Raynaud Phenomenon. [online] Available from http://www.emedicine.com/med/TOPIC1993.HTM [Accessed April, 2012].

1274. REBEITZ-KOLODNY-RICHARDSON SYNDROME (EXOTROPIA)

General

Etiology unknown; possibly metabolic failure at cellular level; occurs in late middle age; neural achromasia with corticodentatonigral degeneration.

Ocular

Paralysis of ocular muscles.

Clinical

Clumsiness, slowness of movement of left limbs; severe impairment in control of muscular movements; postural abnormalities; tremor; severe contractures; dysphagia; speech impairment; Babinski sign.

Laboratory

Workup is focused in eliminating other diagnosis.

Treatment

Nonsurgical treatment involves correction of refractive error occlusion therapy for amblyopia, orthoptics, and botulinum toxin injections. Treatment of neurologic defect is also important. Surgery is only considered when the patient has poor control of the deviation, diplopia and severe asthenopia.

Bibliography

1. Magalini SI, Scrascia E. Dictionary of Medical Syndromes, 2nd edition. Philadelphia: JB Lippincott; 1981.
2. Rebeiz JJ, Kolodny EH, Richardson EP. Corticodentatonigral degeneration with neuronal achromasia. Arch Neurol. 1968;18:20-33.

1275. RECURRENT HYPHEMA

General

Trauma although bleeding may occur spontaneously in conditions, such as rubeosis iridis, leukemia, hemophilia, anticoagulation therapy, retinoblastoma or juvenile xanthogranuloma of iris. Recurrent hyphemas may be the result of iris nevus, rubbing of the iris on loops of older styles of intraocular lens or when the initial therapy for the traumatic hyphema is not adequate.

Clinical

None

Ocular

Tear and bleeding from the iris, ciliary body or elevated intraocular pressure may occur.

Laboratory

Diagnosis is made by clinical findings.

Treatment

Cycloplegia decreased the inflammation and discomfort associated with traumatic iritis. Topical beta-adrenergic antagonists are the therapy of choice for elevated intraocular pressures. Recurrent hyphemas following an initial trauma may require bedrest and sometimes sedation (especially in active children). If the recurrent hyphema is due to an intraocular lens loop rubbing on an iris vessel, laser may be necessary to cauterize the vessel.

Additional Resource

1. Sheppard JD (2011). Hyphema. [online] Available from http://www.emedicine.com/oph/TOPIC765.HTM [Accessed April, 2012].

1276. REFSUM SYNDROME (HEREDOPATHIA ATACTICA POLYNEURITIFORMIS SYNDROME; PHYTANIC ACID OXIDASE DEFICIENCY; PHYTANIC ACID STORAGE DISEASE; REFSUM-THIEBAUT SYNDROME)

General

Autosomal recessive; disorder of lipid metabolism; interstitial hypertrophic polyneuropathy; delamination of myelin sheaths; onset usually between the ages of 4 and 7 years; caused by deficiency of phytanic acid hydroxylase.

Ocular

Progressive external ophthalmoplegia; night blindness; visual field constriction; pupillary abnormalities; corneal opacities; retinal degeneration beginning in macula; atypical retinitis pigmentosa; cataracts.

Clinical

Spinocerebellar ataxia; deafness (progressive); polyneuritis-like effect on limbs; central nervous system degeneration; ichthyosis; sensory changes; wasting of extremities; complete heart block; relapses and remissions in adolescence; normal intelligence.

Laboratory

Check phytanic acid in serum.

Treatment

Dietary restriction of phytanic acid, plasma exchange; vitamin A 15,000 IU/day is thought to slow the decline of retinal function, dark sunglasses for outdoor use, surgery for cataract, genetic counseling.

Additional Resource

1. Zalewska A (2011). Refsum Disease. [online] Available from http://www.emedicine.com/derm/TOPIC705.HTM [Accessed April, 2012].

1277. REIMANN SYNDROME (HYPERVISCOSITY SYNDROME) NYSTAGMUS

General

Frequently found in association with Waldenström syndrome, other hyperglobulinemias, and occasionally with myeloma, reticulum sarcoma and other tumors; increase in y-globulin or other dysproteinemias that affect blood viscosity (see Bing-Neel Syndrome; Waldenström Syndrome); leukemia.

Ocular

Nystagmus; tortuosity of conjunctival vessels; sludging phenomenon with aggregation of intra-vascular erythrocytes; retinal vascular tortuosity and sludging; retinal hemorrhages and exudates; microaneurysms of various degrees and sizes; central retinal vein occlusion.

Clinical

Mucous membrane; hemorrhages; headaches; paraesthesia; ataxia; heart failure and low pulse pressure; partial loss of hearing; anorexia; vertigo; dyspnea; syncope; convulsions; peripheral edema; sausage-shaped veins.

Laboratory

Determine blood viscosity.

Treatment

Plasmapheresis is the treatment of choice, consult a hematologist for further evaluation.

Additional Resource

1. Hemingway TJ (2012). Hyperviscosity Syndrome. [online] Available from http://www.emedicine.com/emerg/TOPIC756.HTM [Accessed April, 2012].

1278. REIS-BUCKLERS CORNEAL DYSTROPHY (CORNEAL DYSTROPHY OF BOWMAN'S LAYER, GRANULAR CORNEAL DYSTROPHY TYPE III, SUPERFICIAL VARIANT OF GRANULAR DYSTROPHY)

General

Bilateral, progressive, autosomal dominant corneal dystrophy, manifests in early childhood.

Clinical

None

Ocular

Recurrent corneal epithelial erosions, corneal scarring, opacification at level of Bowman's layer and superficial stroma.

Laboratory

Mutation in *TGFBI* gene on chromosome 5q31 in many cases.

Treatment

Ocular lubricants, topical antibiotics, cycloplegic agents and hyperosmotic agents are useful. Debridement of loose epithelium, therapeutic contact lens, anterior stromal micropuncture, phototherapeutic keratectomy (PTK), lamellar keratoplasty or penetrating keratoplasty may be necessary.

Additional Resource

1. Afshari N (2010). Granular Dystrophy. [online] Available from http://www.emedicine.com/oph/TOPIC92.HTM [Accessed April, 2012].

1279. REITER SYNDROME (CONJUNCTIVO-URETHRO-SYNOVIAL SYNDROME; FIESSINGER-LEROY SYNDROME; IDIOPATHIC BLENNORRHEAL ARTHRITIS SYNDROME; POLYARTHRITIS ENTERICA)

General

Etiology unknown; more common in males; onset age 16–42 years; probably a combined infectious/autoimmune pathogenetic mechanism; reactive arthritis probably associated with infection with many different species of microorganisms; HLA-B27 confers disease susceptibility to infection.

Ocular

Sterile mucopurulent conjunctivitis, usually bilateral; photophobia; epiphora; iritis; keratitis;

uveitis; paralysis of extraocular muscles; optic neuritis; secondary glaucoma; hypopyon; hyphema.

Clinical

Skin erythema; genital ulcerations; urethritis with discharge; cystitis with dysuria, abacterial pyuria and hematuria; arthritis with pain, swelling, heat and effusion; fever; weight loss; fatigue; malaise; diarrhea; oral mucosal lesions; arthralgia.

Laboratory

Giemsa stain may reveal Gram-negative intracellular diplococci associated with gonorrhea. Stool cultures may also be helpful for enteric pathogens. Hla-b27 antigen testing will not provide a diagnosis but may be useful.

Treatment

Systemic antibiotics are useful. Topical corticosteroids and mydriatics should be administered early to minimize tissue damage. Nonsteroidal anti-inflammatory drugs (NSAIDs) may help reduce ocular inflammation.

Additional Resource

1. Bashour M (2012). Ophthalmologic Manifestations of Reactive Arthritis. [online] Available from http://www.emedicine.com/oph/TOPIC524. HTM [Accessed April, 2012].

1280. RELAPSING FEVER (RECURRENT FEVER)

General

Acute infectious disease caused by *Borrelia* transmitted by lice; characterized by recurrent bouts of fever separated by relatively asymptomatic periods; there is an endemic form of rheumatic fever transmitted by tick vectors and spirochetes of the genus *Borrelia*.

Ocular

Extraocular muscle paralysis; uveitis; interstitial keratitis; hypopyon; conjunctivitis; optic nerve atrophy; subconjunctival and retinal hemorrhages; ptosis; mydriasis; retinal venous occlusion.

Clinical

Toxemia and febrile paroxysms separated by afebrile periods.

Laboratory

Diagnosis is confirmed by bone marrow aspirates, cerebrospinal fluids or spirochetes in peripheral smears.

Treatment

The drugs of choice include doxycycline, penicillin G, chloramphenicol or erythromycin.

Additional Resource

1. Akhter K (2012). Relapsing Fever. [online] Available from http://www.emedicine.com/med/TOPIC1999. HTM [Accessed April, 2012].

1281. RELAPSING POLYCHONDRITIS (JAKSCH-WARTENHOST SYNDROME; MEYENBURG-ALTHERZ-VEHLINGER SYNDROME; VON MEYENBERG II SYNDROME)

General

Episodic, yet generally progressive; onset usually in middle life; possibly caused by lysosomal labilizing factor of endogenous or exogenous toxic nature or immunologic reactions; possible association with Reiter syndrome.

Ocular

Conjunctivitis; corneal ulcer; exophthalmos; panophthalmitis; phthisis bulbi; proptosis; optic neuritis; papilledema; retinal detachment; blue sclera; episcleritis; scleromalacia; vitreous opacity; cataracts; nystagmus; retinal artery thrombosis; keratoconjunctivitis sicca; secondary glaucoma; scotoma; uveitis; paresis of third or sixth nerve; conjunctival mass (salmon patch); chorioretinitis.

Clinical

Destruction of cartilage and eventual replacement with connective tissue; polyarthritis; chondritis; tracheal collapse; bronchial collapse; anemia; liver dysfunction; death; malaise; fever; dyspnea; changes in pitch of voice; hearing impairment; vertigo; deformed ears; aortic valve insufficiency.

Laboratory

No specific serologic markers.

Treatment

No therapy.

Additional Resource

1. http://www.emedicine.com/oph/TOPIC375.HTM [Accessed April, 2012].

1282. RENAL FAILURE

General

Absence of renal function.

Ocular

Cotton-wool spots; retinal edema; optic disk edema; conjunctival calcium deposits; band keratopathy; cortical blindness; severe retinopathy is more likely to be found in patients with renal insufficiency; patients undergoing hemodialysis are at increased risk of elevated intraocular pressure, particularly in eyes that have undergone vitrectomy.

Clinical

Hypertension; azotemia; hypervolemia; metabolic disturbances; hyponatremia; hypercalcemia.

Laboratory

Hyperkalemia electrolyte abnormalities, serum potassium is usually measured.

Treatment

Intravenous (IV) fluids should be used in cases of frank shock.

Additional Resource

1. Krause RS (2011). Dialysis Complications of Chronic Renal Failure. [online] Available from http://www.emedicine.com/emerg/TOPIC501.HTM [Accessed April, 2012].

1283. RENDU-OSLER SYNDROME [BABINGTON DISEASE; HEREDITARY HEMORRHAGIC TELANGIECTASIS; OSLER SYNDROME (2); RENDU-OSLER-WEBER SYNDROME]

General

Etiology unknown; autosomal dominant in Jews; repeated epistaxis begins in childhood; gastrointestinal hemorrhages with melena and hematemesis manifest in middle and later life.

Ocular

Star-shaped angiomas of the palpebral conjunctiva; intermittent filamentary keratitis; small retinal angiomas and occasionally retinal hemorrhages; subconjunctival hemorrhages; small retinal arteriovenous malformations; bloody tears; conjunctival telangiectasias.

Clinical

Epistaxis; hematuria; melena; angiomata of the pharynx and oral and nasal mucosa; angiomas on lips, face and upper extremities; cyanosis; polycythemia.

Laboratory

Anemia usually present, hematuria and stool evaluation. CT and/or MRI to evaluate internal arteriovenous malformations.

Treatment

In mild cases of hereditary hemorrhagic telangentacia (HHT), no treatment is necessary. In severe cases estrogen therapy may be useful.

Additional Resource

1. Soriano PA (2008). Osler-Weber-Rendu Disease. [online] Available from http://www.emedicine.com/derm/TOPIC782.HTM [Accessed April, 2012].

1284. RETICULAR DEGENERATION OF PIGMENT EPITHELIUM (RDPE)

General

Etiology unknown; associated with age-related macular degeneration (AMD).

Ocular

Hypopigmentation of retinal pigment epithelium interspersed with hyperpigmented lines forming a coarse netlike pattern of irregular polygons; multiple drusen of peripheral fundus; choroidal nevus; central retinal vein occlusion.

Clinical

Reduced vision with disturbance of pigment epithelium

Laboratory

Diagnosis is made by clinical findings.

Treatment

Macular degeneration: No treatment is available for non-neovascular AMD. Preventative therapy includes no smoking, control of hypertension, cholesterol, and blood sugar, exercise and vitamins. Neovascular AMD treatment consists of laser, Avastin and Lucentis.

Bibliography

1. el Baba F, Green WR, Fleischmann J, et al. Clinicopathologic correlation of lipidization and detachment of the retinal pigment epithelium. Am J Ophthalmol. 1986;101:576-83.
2. Gass JD. Drusen and disciform macular detachment and degeneration. Arch Ophthalmol. 1973; 90:206-17.
3. Lewis H, Straatsma BR, Foos RY, et al. Reticular degeneration of the pigment epithelium. Ophthalmology. 1985;92:1485-95.

1285. RETICULAR PIGMENTARY RETINAL DYSTROPHY OF POSTERIOR POLE (SJÖGREN DISEASE)

General

Autosomal recessive; characterized by peculiar network of black-pigmented lines in posterior pole of retina.

Ocular

Fishnet-like knots on posterior pole of retina; drusen.

Clinical

None

Laboratory

Diagnosis is made by clinical findings.

Treatment

None

Bibliography

1. Deutman AF, Rümke AM. Reticular dystrophy of the retinal pigment epithelium. Dystrophia reticularis laminae pigmentosa retinae of H. Sjögren. Arch Ophthalmol. 1969;82:4-9.
2. Deutman AF. Macular dystrophies. In: Ryan SJ (Ed). Retina, 2nd edition. St. Louis: CV Mosby; 1994. pp. 1216-7.
3. McKusick VA. Mendelian Inheritance in Man: A Catalog of Human Genes and Genetic Disorders, 12th edition. Baltimore: The Johns Hopkins University Press; 1998.
4. McKusick-Nathans Institute for Genetic Medicine, Johns Hopkins University and National Center for Biotechnology Information, National Library of Medicine. (2007). Online Mendelian Inheritance in Man (OMIM). [online] Available from http://www.ncbi.nlm.nih.gov/omim [Accessed April, 2012].
5. Wocheslünder E, Bartl G, Fellinger C, et al. Die retikulare pigmentdystrophie nach Sjögren. Klin Monatsbl Augenheilkd. 1980;177:684-8.

1286. RETICULUM CELL SARCOMA (NON-HODGKIN LYMPHOMA)

General

Autosomal recessive; large-cell lymphoma with chronic inflammation with a predominance of cells in vitreous cavity; average age at the time of diagnosis is 60 years; female to male ratio is approximately 2:1; 80% bilateral (frequently asymmetrical).

Ocular

Chronic uveitis; chorioretinal lesions; mycosis fungoides; necrosis of orbital tissues; phthisis bulbi; endophthalmos; exophthalmos; exudative retinal detachment; iris neovascularization; glaucoma; branch retinal vein occlusion; macular edema; optic neuropathy; vitreous hemorrhage; partial cranial nerve III palsy; multiple retinal pigment epithelium masses.

Clinical

Lymphocytic hyperplasia; fever; anemia; thrombocytopenia; liver and spleen enlargement; associated with immune dysfunction states, such as acquired immunodeficiency syndrome, or following transplantation.

Laboratory

Computed tomography (CT) or MRI scan, HIV evaluation, CBC, lumbar puncture.

Treatment

Radiation and chemotherapy.

Additional Resource

1. http://www.emedicine.medscape.com/article/203399-overview.

1287. RETINAL ARTERIES, TORTUOSITY (RETINAL HEMORRHAGE)

General

Autosomal dominant; retinal vascular tortuosity is the isolated physical finding but may be associated with a variety of ocular and systemic anomalies; tortuosity predominantly found in the arteriolar tree.

Ocular

Retinal vascular tortuosity; foveal hemorrhage; macular and paramacular hemorrhages; retinal hemorrhages; peripapillary retinal hemorrhage; juxtapapillary retinal hemorrhage; conjunctival hemorrhage; retinal telangiectasia; asteroid hyalitis; amblyopia; myopia; hyperopia; glaucoma; Coats disease; von Hippel-Lindau syndrome; racemose aneurysms of the retina; arteriolar ectasia.

Clinical

Polycythemia; splenomegaly; recurrent nosebleeds; nasal telangiectasia; pulmonary emphysema; systemic hypertension; aortic coarctation; hereditary hemorrhagic telangiectasia; leukemia; macroglobulinemia; cryoglobulinemia; sickle cell disease; familial dysautonomia; Maroteaux-Lamy syndrome; Fabry disease; hypogammaglobulinemia; intracranial or facial aneurysmal abnormalities; migraine headaches; psoriasis; colitis; diabetes mellitus; hypertension.

Laboratory

Retinal angiogram demonstrates retinal vascularity tortuosity, retinal hemorrhage

Treatment

Retinal tortuosity: It may be treated with laser.

Glaucoma: Its medication should be the first plan of action. If medication is unsuccessful, a filtering surgical procedure with or without antimetabolites may be beneficial.

Bibliography

1. Goldberg MF, Pollack IP, Green WR. Familial retinal arteriolar tortuosity with retinal hemorrhage. Am J Ophthalmol. 1972;73:183-91.
2. McKusick VA. Mendelian Inheritance in Man: A Catalog of Human Genes and Genetic Disorders, 12th edition. Baltimore: The Johns Hopkins University Press; 1998.
3. McKusick-Nathans Institute for Genetic Medicine, Johns Hopkins University and National Center for Biotechnology Information, National Library of Medicine. (2007). Online Mendelian Inheritance in Man (OMIM). [online] Available from http://www.ncbi.nlm.nih.gov/omim [Accessed April, 2012].

1288. RETINAL ARTERY OCCLUSION

General

This condition involves a sudden, painless visual loss.

Clinical

Temporal arteritis, jaw claudication, scalp tenderness.

Ocular

Ophthalmoscopic examination, a diffuse retinal pallor and a cherry-red spot in macula are noted.

Laboratory

To determan etiology; CBC to evaluate blood disorders, erythrocyte sedimentation rate (ESR), blood cultures, carotis ultrasound imaging, fluorescein angiogram.

Treatment

Intraocular pressure lowering medications, carbogen therapy, hyperbaric oxygen. Vitrectomy may be necessary.

Additional Resource

1. Graham RH (2012). Central Retinal Artery Occlusion. [online] Available from http://www.emedicine.com/oph/TOPIC387.HTM [Accessed April, 2012].

1289. RETINAL CAPILLARITIS

General

Rare; frequently associated with uveitis.

Clinical

Turbulointerstitial nephritis; inflammatory bowel disease.

Ocular

Decreased visual acuity; dilation and leakage of capillary.

Laboratory

Fluorescein angiography; OCT/SLO; ICGA; FAF.

Treatment

Traditional treatment for uveitis with topical steroids.

Bibliography

1. Ozmert E, Batioglu F. An unusual case of acute unilateral uveitis with retinal capillaritis. Ann Ophthalmol (Skokie). 2009;41:184-8.

1290. RETINAL CONE DEGENERATION

General

Autosomal dominant; diffuse cone degeneration; progressive loss of visual acuity; macular lesion has a bull's-eye appearance produced by a central area of uninvolved epithelium.

Ocular

Photophobia; defective color vision; loss of side vision; night blindness; macular lesion; poor central acuity and visual field scotomata closer to fixation compared to patients with retinal rod degeneration.

Clinical

None

Laboratory

Diagnosis is made by clinical findings.

Treatment

Low vision aids.

Bibliography

1. Heckenlively JR, Martin DA, Rosales TO. Telangiectasia and optic atrophy in cone-rod degenerations. Arch Ophthalmol. 1981;99:1983-91.
2. Krill AE, Deutman AF, Fishman M. The cone degenerations. Doc Ophthalmol. 1973;35:1-80.
3. McKusick VA. Mendelian Inheritance in Man: A Catalog of Human Genes and Genetic Disorders, 12th edition. Baltimore: The Johns Hopkins University Press; 1998.
4. McKusick-Nathans Institute for Genetic Medicine, Johns Hopkins University and National Center for Biotechnology Information, National Library of Medicine. (2007). Online Mendelian Inheritance in Man (OMIM). [online] Available from http://www.ncbi.nlm.nih.gov/omim [Accessed April, 2012].
5. Miller NR (Ed). Walsh and Hoyt's Clinical Neuro-Ophthalmology, 6th edition. Baltimore: Williams & Wilkins; 2004.
6. Rabb MF, Tso MO, Fishman GA. Cone-rod dystrophy. A clinical and histopathologic report. Ophthalmology. 1986;93:1443-51.
7. Weleber RG. Retinitis pigmentosa and allied disorders. In: Ryan SJ (Ed). Retina, 2nd edition. St. Louis: CV Mosby; 1994. pp. 359-60.

1291. RETINAL DETACHMENT

General

Separation of the neurosensory retina from the adjacent retinal pigment epithelium.

Clinical

Diabetes, Marfan syndrome, Stickler syndrome, Coats disease, Eales disease, Morning glory syndrome.

Ocular

Visual field defect, photopsia, vitreous floaters.

Laboratory

Diagnosis is made by clinical findings.

Treatment

Pneumatic retinopexy, sclera buckling, cryotherapy, pars plana vitrectomy.

Additional Resources

1. Wu L (2010). Retinal Detachment, Exudative. [online] Available from http://www.emedicine.com/oph/TOPIC407.HTM [Accessed April, 2012].
2. Wu L. (2011). Rhegmatogenous Retinal Detachment. [online] Available from http://www.emedicine.com/oph/TOPIC410.HTM [Accessed April, 2012].
3. Wu L. (2010). Retinal Detachment, Tractional. [online] Available from http://www.emedicine.com/oph/TOPIC411.HTM [Accessed April, 2012].
4. Wu L. (2010). Retinal Detachment, Postoperative. [online] Available from http://www.emedicine.com/oph/TOPIC408.HTM [Accessed April, 2012].

1292. RETINAL DETACHMENT, POSTOPERATIVE

General

Subretinal fluid accumulates in the space between the neurosensory retina and the underlying retinal pigment epithelium. Intraocular surgery is a major risk for the development of the detachment. Retinal tears can occur and liquefied vitreous can seep under the tear leading to the detachment.

Clinical

None

Ocular

Vitreous traction, cut in visual field; vitreous floaters; decreased visual acuity; scleritis.

Laboratory

Diagnosis is generally made by clinical observation. Ultrasound may be necessary if the media is hazy.

Treatment

Scleral buckle and vitrectomy are the treatments of choice for this type of detachment.

Additional Resource

1. Wu L (2010). Retinal Detachment, Postoperative. [online] Available from http://www.emedicine.medscape.com/article/1224609-overview [Accessed April, 2012].

1293. RETINAL DETACHMENT, PROLIFERATIVE

General

Subretinal fluid accumulates in the space between the neurosensory retina and the underlying retinal pigment epithelium. Proliferative vitreoretinopathy is the most common cause of failure in retinal detachment surgery.

Clinical

Diabetes; injury; following pneumatic retinopexy, cryotherapy, laser retinopexy, scleral buckling or vitrectomy.

Ocular

Vitreous traction, cut in visual field; vitreous floaters; decreased visual acuity; scleritis; retinal breaks.

Laboratory

Diagnosis is generally made by clinical observation. Ultrasound may be necessary if the media is hazy.

Treatment

Corticosteroids (topical, subconjunctival or retrobulbar) are beneficial at the time of surgery. Scleral buckle and vitrectomy are the treatments of choice for this type of detachment.

Additional Resource

1. Charles S (2012). Proliferative Retinal Detachment. [online] Available from http://www.emedicine.medscape.com/article/1226426-overview [Accessed April, 2012].

1294. RETINAL DETACHMENT, TRACTIONAL

General

Subretinal fluid accumulates in the space between the neurosensory retina and the underlying retinal pigment epithelium. Caused by traction on the retina secondary to injury, subretinal membranes, retinopathy of prematurity and proliferative vitreoretinopathy.

Clinical

Diabetes; injury.

Ocular

Vitreous traction, cut in visual field; vitreous floaters; decreased visual acuity; scleritis; retinal breaks.

Laboratory

Diagnosis is generally made by clinical observation. Ultrasound may be necessary if the media is hazy.

Treatment

Scleral buckle and vitrectomy are used to relieve vitreoretinal traction.

Additional Resource

1. Wu L (2010). Retinal Detachment, Tractional. [online] Available from http://www.emedicine. medscape.com/article/1224891-overview [Accessed April, 2012].

1295. RETINAL DETACHMENT, EXUDATIVE

General

Subretinal fluid accumulates in the space between the neurosensory retina and the underlying retinal pigment epithelium.

Clinical

Rheumatoid arthritis; preeclampsia; Coats disease; Vogt-Koyanagi-Harada; sarcoidosis; syphilis; toxoplasmosis; cytomegalovirus; Lyme disease; lupus; renal disease.

Ocular

Bullous retinal detachment, cut in visual field; vitreous floaters; decreased visual acuity; scleritis.

Laboratory

Diagnosis is generally made by clinical observation. Ultrasound may be necessary if the media is hazy.

Treatment

Medical and surgical treatments of exudative retinal detachment are tailored to the underlying condition and may include laser, cryotherapy and vitrectomy.

Additional Resource

1. Wu L (2010). Retinal Detachment, Exudative. [online] Available from http://www.emedicine. medscape.com/article/1224509-overview [Accessed April, 2012].

1296. RETINAL DISINSERTION SYNDROME (KERATOCONUS)

General

None

Ocular

Subluxation of the lens; microphthalmos; bilateral keratoconus; retinal detachment.

Clinical

None

Laboratory

Diagnosis is made by clinical findings.

Treatment

Keratoconus: Spectacle correction, hard contacts and avoid eye rubbing may be useful. If hydrops occurs discontinue contact lens, use NaCl drops and ointment, patching and short course of steroids. As the disease advances penetrating keratoplasty, deep anterior lamellar keratoplasty, intacs with laser grooves or collagen stabilization of cornea.

Subluxation of the lens: Careful phacoemulsification, topical steroids to control ocular inflammation.

Bibliography

1. Ryan SJ (Ed). Retina, 2nd edition. St. Louis: CV Mosby; 1994.
2. Hovland KR, Schepens CL, Freeman HM. Developmental giant retinal tears associated with lens coloboma. Arch Ophthalmol. 1968;80:325-31.
3. Shammas HJ, McGaughey AS. Retinal disinsertion syndrome: report of a case. J Pediatr Ophthalmol Strabismus. 1979;16:284-6.

1297. RETINAL ISCHEMIC SYNDROME (OULAR ISCHEMIC SYNDROME)

Ocular

Bilateral conjunctival injection; iris rubeosis; posterior synechia; retinal vascular tortuosity; retinal detachment; Axenfeld's syndrome; central retinal artery occlusion; glaucoma; corneal anesthesia; uveitis; ischemic retinopathy.

Clinical

Associated with partial occlusion of carotid artery; diabetes, hypercholesterolemia; tetralogy of Fallot.

Laboratory

Evaluation of the erythrocyte sedimentation rate (ESR) and C-reactive protein is recommended.

Treatment

Antiplatelet therapy.

Additional Resource

1. Leibovitch I (2011). Ocular Ischemic Syndrome. [online] Available from http://www.emedicine.com/oph/TOPIC487.HTM [Accessed April, 2012].

1298. RETINAL VASCULAR HYPOPLASIA WITH PERSISTENCE OF PRIMARY VITREOUS

General

Bilateral congenital retinopathy characterized by retinal vascular hypoplasia and persistence of primary vitreous; etiology unknown.

Ocular

Buphthalmos; microphthalmia; fixed and dilated pupils; neovascularization of iris; glaucoma; cataract; white opaque fibrovascular retrolental membrane; retinal detachment; vitreous hemorrhage; retinal vascular hypoplasia.

Clinical

None

Laboratory

Diagnosis is made by clinical findings.

Treatment

Cataract: Change in glasses can sometimes improve a patient's visual function temporarily; however, the most common treatment is cataract surgery.

Retinal detachment: Scleral buckle, pneumatic retinopexy and vitrectomy may be used to close all the breaks.

Bibliography

1. Ryan SJ (Ed). Retina, 2nd edition. St. Louis: CV Mosby; 1994.
2. Pollard ZF. Treatment of persistent hyperplastic primary vitreous. J Pediatr Ophthalmol Strabismus. 1985;22:180-3.
3. Pruett RC. The pleomorphism and complications of posterior hyperplastic primary vitreous. Am J Ophthalmol. 1975;80:625-9.
4. Sneed PJ, Augsburger JJ, Shields JA, et al. Bilateral retinal vascular hypoplasia associated with persistence of the primary vitreous: a new clinical entity? J Pediatr Ophthalmol Strabismus. 1988;25:77-85.

1299. RETINAL VENOUS OBSTRUCTION

General

Occlusion at the level of either the branch or central retinal venous system, causing a reduction in venous return.

Clinical

None

Ocular

Painless visual loss, ischemic central retinal vein occlusion, branch retinal vein occlusion.

Laboratory

Fluorescein angiography, OCT for assessment of macular edema.

Treatment

Anticoagulation, surgical adventitial sheathotomy, radial optic neurotomy, intravitreal injection of triamcinolone acetonide for macular edema. Vitrectomy may be necessary.

Bibliography

1. Campochiaro PA, Hafiz G, Channa R, et al. Antagonism of vascular endothelial growth factor for macular edema caused by retinal vein occlusions: two-year outcomes. Ophthalmology. 2010;117: 2387-94.

2. Scott IU, VanVeldhuisen PC, Oden NL, et al. Baseline predictors of visual acuity and retinal thickness outcomes in patients with retinal vein occlusion: standard care versus corticosteroid for retinal vein occlusion study report 10. Ophthalmology. 2011;118:345-52.

Additional Resource

1. Kooragayala LM (2011). Central Retinal Vein Occlusion. [online] Available from http://www.emedicine.com/oph/TOPIC388.HTM [Accessed April, 2012].

1300. RETINITIS PIGMENTOSA

General

Inherited progressive retinal disorder may have changes in ear or kidney.

Clinical

Hearing defect and kidney defect can be associated with the disease.

Ocular

Waxy-pole optic nerve, bonespickle pigmentation, posterior subcapsular cataract, visual field defect.

Laboratory

Diagnosis is made by clinical findings. A diagnostic genetic test is available and differentiates between Simplex retinitis pigmentosa (RP) and autosomal recessive RP.

Treatment

Retinitis pigmentosa: Vitamin A 15,000 IU/day is thought to slow the decline of retinal function, dark sunglasses for outdoor use, surgery for cataract, genetic counseling.

Bibliography

1. Clark GR, Crowe P, Muszynska D, et al. Development of a diagnostic genetic test for simplex and autosomal recessive retinitis pigmentosa. Ophthalmology. 2010;117:2169-77.

Additional Resource

1. Telander DG (2012). Retinitis Pigmentosa. [online] Available from http://www.emedicine.com/oph/TOPIC704.HTM [Accessed April, 2012].

1301. RETINITIS PIGMENTOSA, DEAFNESS, MENTAL RETARDATION, AND HYPOGONADISM

General

Autosomal recessive; similar to Laurence-Moon-Biedl-Bardet, Alstrom, and Usher syndromes, with the difference being the absence of polydactyly.

Ocular

Nystagmus; hyperplasia and thickening of prickle cell layer to lids or comer of eyes; myopia; retinitis pigmentosa; keratoconus.

Clinical

Acanthosis nigricans; multiple keloids; gyneco-mastia, small testes in males; oligomenorrhea; mental retardation; deafness; hypogonadism; glucose intolerance; hyperinsulinism.

Laboratory

Diagnosis is made by clinical findings.

Treatment

Keratoconus: It may be treated with spectacle correction, hard contacts and avoid eye rubbing. If hydrops occurs discontinue contact lens, use NaCl drops and ointment, patching and short course of steroids. As the disease advances penetrating keratoplasty, deep anterior lamellar keratoplasty, intacs with laser grooves or collagen stabilization of cornea.

Retinitis pigmentosa: Vitamin A 15,000 IU/day is thought to slow the decline of retinal function, dark sunglasses for outdoor use, surgery for cataract, genetic counseling.

Bibliography

1. Edwards JA, Sethi PK, Scoma AJ, et al. A new familial syndrome characterized by pigmentary retinopathy, hypogonadism, mental retardation, nerve deafness and glucose intolerance. Am J Med. 1976;60:23-32.
2. McKusick VA. Mendelian Inheritance in Man: A Catalog of Human Genes and Genetic Disorders, 12th edition. Baltimore: The Johns Hopkins University Press; 1998.
3. McKusick-Nathans Institute for Genetic Medicine, Johns Hopkins University and National Center for Biotechnology Information, National Library of Medicine. (2007). Online Mendelian Inheritance in Man (OMIM). [online] Available from http://www.ncbi.nlm.nih.gov/omim [Accessed April, 2012].

1302. RETINOBLASTOMA

General

Malignant tumor arising in one or both retinas of young children, usually under the age of 2 years; usually unilateral; autosomal dominant; most common intraocular malignancy of childhood; incidence is one in 20,000 live births; origin is questionably neuroectodermal cells capable of multipotentiality; one-third of patients have heritable (bilateral or have a positive family history) autosomal dominant and two-thirds are sporadic; genetic transmission obeys two-mutation hypothesis of Knudson; trilateral retinoblastoma is bilateral retinoblastoma plus midline central nervous system tumor (most commonly pinealoma); most common second tumor is an osteogenic sarcoma (begins in the second decade).

Ocular

Hyphema; hypopyon; corneal tumor; lid edema; endophthalmitis; exophthalmos; intraocular cal-cification of globe; heterochromia; neovascularization of iris or retina; papilledema; panophthalmitis; retinoblastoma extension into orbit and choroid; cat's-eye reflex; leukocoria; mydriasis; vitreous hemorrhage tumor seeding; esotropia; exotropia; glaucoma; visual loss.

Clinical

Metastasis into the lymph system, bone marrow and subarachnoid space; basal meningitis; death.

Laboratory

Computed tomography (CT)—calcification of lesion hallmark of disease; ultrasound demonstrates calcification and MRI demonstrates presence and extent of extraocular disease.

Treatment

External beam radiation therapy is recommended on patients with significant vitreous seeding.

Radioactive isotope plaques and chemotherapy are also an option. Removal of the tumor is the standard management for retinoblastoma.

Bibliography

1. Abramson DH, Dunkel IJ, Brodie SE, et al. Superselective ophthalmic artery chemotherapy as primary treatment for retinoblastoma (chemosurgery). Ophthalmology. 2010;117:1623-9.

Additional Resource

1. Isidro MA (2011). Retinoblastoma. [online] Available from http://www.emedicine.com/oph/TOPIC346.HTM [Accessed April, 2012].

1303. RETINOHYPOPHYSARY SYNDROME (BENIGN RETINOHYPOPHYSARY SYNDROME; LIJO PAVIA-LIS SYNDROME) OPTIC NEURITIS

General

Alterations of the bony structure of the sella turcica with decalcifications and osteolysis of the posterior clinoid process; all ages; more frequent in women.

Ocular

Superior nasal field contraction; narrowing of retinal vessels; macular edema; optic neuritis; optic atrophy; visual field defects.

Clinical

Glycosuria; headache; vertigo; psychic disturbances.

Laboratory

Diagnosis is made by clinical findings.

Treatment

Symptomatic

Bibliography

1. Geeraets WJ. Ocular Syndromes, 3rd edition. Philadelphia: Lea & Febiger; 1976.
2. Lijo Pavia J Retino-hypophysary syndrome: treatment with gonadotropin. Four new cases. Rev Otoneurooftal. 1947;22:5, Am J Ophthalmol. 1948; 31:382(abst).

1304. RETINOPATHY, PIGMENTARY, AND MENTAL RETARDATION (MIRHOSSEINI-HOLMES-WALTON SYNDROME)

General

Autosomal recessive; this disorder may be the same as (or alleli) to Cohen syndrome.

Ocular

Pigmentary retinal degeneration; cataract; keratoconus.

Clinical

Microcephaly; severe mental retardation; hyperextensible joints; scoliosis; arachnodactyly; hypogonadism.

Laboratory

Diagnosis is made by clinical findings.

Treatment

Retinitis pigmentosa: Vitamin A 15,000 IU/day is thought to slow the decline of retinal function, dark sunglasses for outdoor use, surgery for cataract, genetic counseling.

Bibliography

1. McKusick VA. Mendelian Inheritance in Man: A Catalog of Human Genes and Genetic Disorders, 12th edition. Baltimore: The Johns Hopkins University Press; 1998.
2. McKusick-Nathans Institute for Genetic Medicine, Johns Hopkins University and National Center for Biotechnology Information, National Library of Medicine. (2007). Online Mendelian Inheritance in Man (OMIM). [online] Available from http://www.ncbi.nlm.nih.gov/omim [Accessed April, 2012].
3. Mendez HM, Paskulin GA, Vallandro C. The syndrome of retinal pigmentary degeneration, microcephaly, and severe mental retardation (Mirhosseini-Holmes-Walton syndrome): report of two patients. Am J Med Genet. 1985;22:223-8.
4. Steinlein O, Tariverdian G, Boll HU, et al. Tapetoretinal degeneration in brothers with apparent Cohen syndrome: nosology with Mirhosseini-Holmes-Walton syndrome. Am J Med Genet. 1991;41:196-200.

1305. RETINOSCHISIS (RS)

General

Sex-linked; may not manifest until middle life.

Ocular

Intraretinal splitting due to degeneration or detachment of retina; retinal atrophy with sclerosis of the choroid; cystic maculopathy.

Clinical

None

Laboratory

Optical coherence tomography (OCT) provides high resolution of the macula region. Fluorescein angiography, indocyanine green and electroretinogram, are helpful tools in finding a diagnosis.

Treatment

No treatment is available.

Additional Resource

1. Song MK (2010). Retinoschisis, Juvenile. [online] Available from http://www.emedicine.com/oph/TOPIC639.HTM [Accessed April, 2012].

1306. RETINOSCHISIS, ACQUIRED [ACQUIRED RETINOSCHISIS (RS)]

General

Present in 4–22% of normal population over age 40 years; splitting in the outer plexiform layer; occasionally in the inner nuclear layer; generally asymptomatic.

Ocular

Slowly progressive; may cause retinal detachment when there are breaks in both outer and inner layers of retinoschisis.

Clinical

None

Laboratory

Visual field-absolute scotoma vs relative scotoma in retinal detachment; ultrasonography including B-scan ultrasonography and ultrasonic biomicroscopy; OCT to differentiate between schisis and detachment.

Treatment

Photocoagulation and/or cryotherapy can be used if retinoschisis is extending into the posterior pole.

Additional Resource

1. Phillpotts BA (2010). Retinoschisis, Senile. [online] Available from http://www.emedicine.com/oph/TOPIC640.HTM [Accessed April, 2012].

1307. RETINOSCHISIS, AUTOSOMAL DOMINANT

General

Autosomal dominant; degenerative abnormal splitting of retinal sensory layers.

Ocular

Loss of retinal function; retinal degeneration; macular degeneration.

Clinical

None

Laboratory

Diagnosis is made by clinical findings.

Treatment

Photocoagulation and/or cryotherapy.

Additional Resource

1. http://www.emedicine.medscape.com/article/1225958-overview.

1308. RETINOSCHISIS, CONGENITAL

General

X-linked recessive; nearly always found in males.

Ocular

Retinal splitting usually occurs in the nerve fiber layer; slow progression; frequently affects the macula; associated with vitreous hemorrhage; strabismus; nystagmus; retinal folds radiating from the fovea; macular pigmentary mottling; retinal detachment (rare complication).

Clinical

None

Laboratory

Diagnosis is made by clinical findings.

Treatment

Photocoagulation and/or cryotherapy.

Bibliography

1. Condon GP, Brownstein S, Wang NS, et al. Congenital hereditary (juvenile X-linked) retinoschisis. Histopathologic and ultrastructural findings in three eyes. Arch Ophthalmol. 1986;104:576-83.

2. Hirose T. Retinoschisis. In: Albert DM, Jakobiec FA (Eds). Principles and Practice of Ophthalmology. Philadelphia: WB Saunders; 1994. pp. 1071-84.

3. Regillo CD, Tasman WS, Brown GC. Surgical management of complications associated with X-linked retinoschisis. Arch Ophthalmol. 1993;111:1080-6.

1309. RETINOSCHISIS OF FOVEA

General

Autosomal recessive.

Ocular

Foveal dystrophy; rod-cone dystrophy; nyctalopia; hyperopia; paramacular tapetal sheen reflex.

Clinical

None

Laboratory

Diagnosis is made by clinical findings.

Treatment

Photocoagulation and/or cryotherapy.

Bibliography

1. McKusick VA. Mendelian Inheritance in Man: A Catalog of Human Genes and Genetic Disorders, 12th edition. Baltimore: The Johns Hopkins University Press; 1998.

2. McKusick-Nathans Institute for Genetic Medicine, Johns Hopkins University and National Center for Biotechnology Information, National Library of Medicine. (2007). Online Mendelian Inheritance in Man (OMIM). [online] Available from http://www.ncbi.nlm.nih.gov/omim [Accessed April, 2012].

3. Noble KG, Carr RE, Siegel IM. Familial foveal retinoschisis associated with a rod-cone dystrophy. Am J Ophthalmol. 1978;85:551-7.

1310. RETROLENTAL FIBROPLASIA (RLF; RETINOPATHY OF PREMATURITY)

General

Bilateral disease seen primarily in premature infants with immature retinal vessels; excessive use of oxygen responsible for the majority of cases, but disease is seen despite oxygen restrictions or even when no oxygen supplementation is used; known factors that correlate with degrees of retinopathy of prematurity are low birth weight, short gestational age, length of time with supplemental oxygen, length of time on a mechanical ventilator; role of excessive light in newborn nurseries also has been proposed.

Ocular

Anterior or posterior synechiae; neovascularization of iris; pallor of optic disk; dragged disk; attenuated vessels; retinal detachment; dilation of veins; retinal folds; retinal hemorrhage; retrolental mass; vascular tortuosity; vasoconstriction of retina; retinal pigmentary changes; vitreous haze; vitreous traction; vitreous hemorrhages; cataract; glaucoma; leukocoria; myopia; shallow anterior chamber; opaque retrolental membrane; ciliary body drawn anteriorly; ciliary process around dilated pupil; absent pupillary reflexes; keratoconus; associated strabismus; amblyopia.

Clinical

Low-birth-weight; prematurity.

Laboratory

Diagnosis is made by clinical findings.

Treatment

Cryotherapy and laser surgery can be effective. Vitrectomy may be necessary.

Bibliography

1. Wu WC, Yeh PT, Chen SN, et al. Effects and complications of bevacizumab use in patients with retinopathy of prematurity: a multicenter study in Taiwan. Ophthalmology. 2011;118:176-83.

Additional Resource

1. Bashour M (2012). Retinopathy of Prematurity. [online] Available from http://www.emedicine.com/oph/TOPIC413.HTM [Accessed April, 2012].

1311. RETROPAROTID SPACE SYNDROME (POSTERIOR RETROPAROTID SPACE SYNDROME; VILLARET SYNDROME) ENOPHTHALMOS

General

Lesions (traumatic, inflammatory, tumors) involving cranial nerves IX to XII and the cervical sympathetic [see Jugular Foramen Syndrome (Vernet Syndrome)].

Ocular

Enophthalmos; ptosis; lagophthalmos; epiphora; miosis; may produce sympathetic overactivity resulting in increased sympathetic outflow (i.e. pupillary dilation, widened palpebral fissure and facial sweating).

Clinical

Homolateral paralysis cranial nerves IX to XII, with dysphagia and loss of taste in posterior third of the tongue; dysphonia; paralysis of sternocleidomastoid and trapezium muscles; paralysis cranial nerve VII occasionally.

Laboratory

Clinical

Treatment

Ptosis: If visual acuity is affected most cases require surgical correction, and there are several procedures that may be used including levator resection, repair or advancement and Fasanella-Servat.

Bibliography

1. Garrett D, Ansell LV, Story JL. Villaret's syndrome: a report of two cases. Surg Neurol. 1993;39:282-5.
2. Geeraets WJ. Ocular Syndromes, 3rd edition. Philadelphia: Lea & Febiger; 1976.
3. Magalini SI, Scrascia E. Dictionary of Medical Syndromes, 2nd edition. Philadelphia: JB Lippincott; 1981.
4. Villaret M. Le Syndrome Nerveux de l'Espace Retroparotidien Posterieur. Rev Neurol. 1916;23:188.

1312. REYE SYNDROME (ACUTE ENCEPHALOPATHY SYNDROME)

General

Etiology unknown, although some relation to ingestion of aspirin with febrile illnesses, especially varicella and influenza, have been reported; both sexes; onset between the ages of 6 months and 10 years; acute metabolic encephalopathy largely affecting children and adolescents; pathogenesis is controversial, although there is new evidence for a generalized defect in intramitochondrial enzyme processing resulting in lowered ratio of adenosine triphosphate to adenosine diphosphate.

Ocular

Cortical blindness; dilated pupils with absent or sluggish reaction to light; papilledema.

Clinical

Respiratory infections with recovery between 3 and 21 days; vomiting after recovery from infection; dyspnea; hypotonia; coma; convulsions; fever; flexion of elbows and hands.

Laboratory

Liver function testing, anion gap test, lactic dehydrogenase and glucose level may be abnormal. Head CT scan.

Treatment

Maintain patient's breathing and circulation; dextrose may be introduce to manage hypoglycemia; but no specific treatment exists at this point.

Additional Resource

1. Weiner DL (2011). Reye Syndrome. [online] Available from http://www.emedicine.com/emerg/TOPIC399.HTM [Accessed April, 2012].

1313. RHABDOMYOSARCOMA (CORNEAL EDEMA)

General

Most common malignant orbital neoplasm of childhood; usually occurs before age 10 years; more commonly seen in males; rarely may develop in adults; shows evidence of striated muscle differentiation; has been divided into three histopathologic types: (1) embryonal, (2) alveolar and (3) pleomorphic.

Ocular

Choroidal folds; corneal edema; exposure keratitis; rhabdomyosarcoma (RMS) of orbit or extraocular muscles; decreased motility; proptosis; papilledema; orbital edema; enlarged optic foramen; erosion of bony walls of orbit; pupil irregularity; epiphora; glaucoma; visual loss; nasolacrimal duct obstruction; conjunctival mass.

Clinical

Metastasis to the lymph system, bone marrow and lungs; headaches.

Laboratory

Live, renal and cytogenetic testing. CT and bone scanning. MRI, ultrasonography and echocardiography.

Treatment

Chemotherapy radiation and surgically removing the tumor are used to treat patients with RMS.

Additional Resource

1. Cripe TP (2011). Pediatric Rhabdomyosarcoma. [online] Available from http://www.emedicine.com/ped/TOPIC2005.HTM [Accessed April, 2012].

1314. RHE SYNDROME (RETINO-HEPATO-ENDOCRINOLOGIC SYNDROME) COLOR BLINDNESS

General

More common in females.

Ocular

Total color blindness; thinning of retinal vessels with atrophy; optic disk pallor; poor photopic vision; progressive cone dystrophy.

Clinical

Degenerative liver disease; endocrine dysfunction; hypothyroidism; diabetes mellitus; repeated abortions or infertility; elevated blood creatine phosphokinase.

Laboratory

Diagnosis is made by clinical findings.

Treatment

Treat systemic disease.

Bibliography

1. Berg K, Larsen IF, Hansen E. Familial syndrome of progressive cone dystrophy, degenerative liver disease and endocrine dysfunction. III. Genetic studies. Clin Genet. 1978;13:190-200.
2. Larsen IF, Hansen E, Berg K. Familial syndrome of progressive cone dystrophy, degenerative liver disease and endocrine dysfunction. II. Clinical and metabolic studies. Clin Genet. 1978;13:176-89.
3. McKusick VA. Mendelian Inheritance in Man: A Catalog of Human Genes and Genetic Disorders, 12th edition. Baltimore: The Johns Hopkins University Press; 1998.
4. McKusick-Nathans Institute for Genetic Medicine, Johns Hopkins University and National Center for Biotechnology Information, National Library of Medicine. (2007). Online Mendelian Inheritance in Man (OMIM). [online] Available from http://www.ncbi.nlm.nih.gov/omim [Accessed April, 2012].

1315. RHEGMATOGENOUS RETINAL DETACHMENT

General

Subretinal fluid accumulates in the space between the neurosensory retina and the underlying retinal pigment epithelium. Most common type of retinal detachment and occurs with a retinal tear that allows liquefied vitreous to seep under the tear leading to the detachment.

Clinical

None

Ocular

Vitreous traction, cut in visual field; vitreous floaters; decreased visual acuity; scleritis.

Laboratory

Diagnosis is generally made by clinical observation. Ultrasound may be necessary if the media is hazy.

Treatment

Retinal detachment: Scleral buckle, pneumatic retinopexy and vitrectomy are used for this type of detachment and the goal is to close all the breaks.

Additional Resource

1. Wu L (2011). Rhegmatogenous Retinal Detachment Treatment & Management. [online] Available from http://www.emedicine.medscape.com/article/1224737-treatment [Accessed April, 2012].

1316. RHEUMATIC FEVER

General

Streptococcal infection; mechanisms may involve immune cross-reactivity between bacterial heat shock proteins and similar proteins in normal human tissues.

Ocular

Lid edema; characteristic arborizations of conjunctiva; subconjunctival hemorrhages; episcleritis; scleritis; tenonitis; uveitis; retinal detachment; central retinal artery occlusion; optic neuritis.

Clinical

Hematuria; proteinuria; proliferative glomerulonephritis; microembolization; calcific emboli; sore throat; fever; chorea; erythema marginatum; disseminated encephalomyelitis.

Laboratory

Throat culture, antigen detection and antibody titer test can confirm the diagnosis.

Treatment

Antistreptococcal prophylaxis to prevent attacks.

Additional Resource

1. Wallace MR (2009). Rheumatic Fever. [online] Available from http://www.emedicine.com/med/TOPIC3435.HTM [Accessed April, 2012].

1317. RHEUMATOID ARTHRITIS (ADULT)

General

Systemic disease of unknown cause; more common in women (3:1); thought to have a strong autoimmune pathogenesis with positive immunoglobulins M, G, and A directed against the Fc portion of immunoglobulin G.

Ocular

Sjögren syndrome; episcleritis; scleritis; keratitis; corneal ulcers; corneal perforation; uveitis; motility disorders; dry eyes; posterior scleritis (rare).

Clinical

Synovitis; stiffness; swelling; cartilaginous hypertrophy; joint pain; fibrous ankylosis; malaise; weight loss; vasomotor disturbance.

Laboratory

About 80% are positive for rheumatoid factor but is also found in systemic lupus erythematosus, Sjögren syndrome, sarcoidosis, hepatitis B and tuberculosis.

Treatment

Nonsteroidal anti-inflammatory drugs (NSAIDs), disease-modifying antirheumatologic drugs (DMARDs), corticosteroids and immunosuppressant can be use.

Additional Resource

1. Temprano K (2011). Rheumatoid Arthritis. [online] Available from http://www.emedicine.com/emerg/TOPIC48.HTM [Accessed April, 2012].

1318. RHINOSCLEROMA (KLEBSIELLA RHINOSCLEROMATIS)

General

Chronic granulomatous disease; Gram-negative bacillus; cicatricial deformities; chronic progressive granulomatous infection of the upper airways caused by the bacterium *Klebsiella rhinoscleromatis*.

Ocular

Conjunctivitis; chronic dacryocystitis; lid inflammation.

Clinical

Granulomas affecting nose and upper respiratory tract causing sclerosis and deformities; airway obstruction; leprosy; paracoccidioidomycosis; sarcoidosis; basal cell carcinoma; Wegener granulomatosis; also may occur in immunocompromised human immunodeficiency virus patients.

Laboratory

Culturing in MacConkey agar are positive in only 50–60% of patients. CT scan and MRI are useful.

Treatment

Bronchoscopy can be used as the initial treatment. Long-term antimicrobial and in cases were obstruction in suspected, surgical intervention may be necessary.

Additional Resource

1. Schwartz RA (2011). Rhinoscleroma. [online] Available from http://www.emedicine.com/derm/TOPIC831.HTM [Accessed April, 2012].

1319. RHINOSPORIDIOSIS

General

Rare fungal infection, primarily affecting the mucous membranes of the nose and eye. Causative agent is *Rhinosporidium seeberi*.

Clinical

Respiratory mucosa, vaginal mucosa, skin and metastatic-like involvement of the internal organs

Ocular

Conjunctival lesions, photophobia and conjunctival infection

Treatment

Complete surgical excision remains the most effective treatment. Cautery or cryopexy to the base of the excised lesion may be beneficial to prevent recurrence.

Bibliography

1. Roy FH, Fraunfelder FW, Fraunfelder FT. Roy and Fraunfelder's Current Ocular Therapy, 6th edition. Philadelphia: WB Saunders; 2008.

1320. RIEGER SYNDROME (AXENFELD POSTERIOR EMBRYOTOXON-JUVENILE GLAUCOMA; AXENFELD-RIEGER SYNDROME; DYSGENESIS MESODERMALIS CORNEAE ET IRIDES; DYSGENESIS MESOSTROMALIS)

General

Autosomal dominant; neural crest abnormality; 50% of patients develop glaucoma.

Ocular

Microphthalmia; congenital glaucoma; iris hypoplasia; deformed and acentric pupil; anterior synechiae; aniridia; microcornea; corneal opacities in Descemet's membrane parallel to the limbus; dislocated lens; optic atrophy; cataract; strabismus; ptosis; hypertelorism; keratoconus; posterior embryotoxon; broad iris processes to embryotoxon; iris stromal hypoplasia; corectopia; polycoria; secondary glaucoma.

Clinical

Face wide; hypodontia; underdeveloped maxilla; teeth deformities; myotonic dystrophy; facial anomalies: maxillary hypoplasia, protrusion of the lower lip, broad, flat nose; dental anomalies include absent teeth, piglike incisors, and decreased crown size; hypospadias.

Laboratory

Diagnosis is made by clinical findings.

Treatment/Ocular

Congenital glaucoma can be treated with beta-blockers, prostaglandin analogs and carbonic anhydrase inhibitors. Surgery such as goniotomy or trabeculectomy can be use if IOP is not controlled.

Bibliography

1. Eagle RC. Congenital, developmental and degenerative disorders of the iris and ciliary body. In: Albert DM, Jakobiec FA (Eds). Principles and Practice of Ophthalmology. Philadelphia: WB Saunders; 1994. pp. 367-87.
2. Montes JG, Montes JCG. Syndrome de Rieger, Anomalie de Axenfeld con Glaucoma Juvenil Familiar. Arch Soc Ophth Hisp Am. 1967;27:93.
3. Rieger H. Beitrage zur Kenntnis seltener Missbildungen der Iris. Graefes Arch Clin Esp Ophthalmol. 1935;133:602.
4. Wesley RK, Baker JD, Golnick AL. Rieger's syndrome: (oligodontia and primary mesodermal dysgenesis of the iris) clinical features and report of an isolated case. J Pediatr Ophthalmol Strabismus. 1978;15:67-70.

1321. RIFT VALLEY FEVER

General

Acute viral infection transmitted by mosquito that occurs in regions of Africa.

Ocular

Central serous retinitis; central scotoma; macular scarring; retinal vascular occlusion; uveitis; retinitis; choroiditis.

Clinical

Fever; chills; severe headache; muscle and joint pain; leukopenia; bradycardia.

Laboratory

Skin tests for C immitis, chest X-ray to rule out pulmonary involvement.

Treatment

Patients with uveitis often have other systemic conditions such as pulmonary or disseminated diseases are usually hospitalized and are given intravenous antifungal therapy. Intracameral amphotericin B is considered in patients if vision is threatened by uveitis.

Bibliography

1. Weiss KE. Rift Valley fever: a review. Bull Epizoot Dis Afr. 1957;5:431-58.
2. Wilson ML. Rift Valley fever virus ecology and the epidemiology of disease emergence. Ann N Y Acad Sci. 1994;740:169-80.

1322. RILEY-DAY SYNDROME (CONGENITAL FAMILIAL DYSAUTONOMIA)

General

Autosomal recessive; occurs in Ashkenazi Jewish population; impaired catechol metabolism; manifested in the first few days of life; characterized by developmental loss of neurons from the sensory and autonomic nervous systems.

Ocular

Congenital failure of tear production; corneal anesthesia; neuroparalytic keratitis; keratitis sicca; corneal ulcers; optic atrophy.

Clinical

Excessive salivation; failure to thrive; recurrent respiratory infections; diarrhea; insensitivity to pain; spontaneous fractures; pandysautonomia; orthostatic hypotension; gastrointestinal paresis; decreased fungiform papillae on the tongue.

Laboratory

DNA test is use to confirm the diagnosis.

Treatment

Artificial drops and/or gels are useful in any dry eye condition. Tarsorrhaphy is an effective treatment of the decompensated neurotrophic cornea.

Additional Resource

1. D'Amico RA (2011). Familial Dysautonomia. [online] Available from http://www.emedicine. com/oph/TOPIC678.HTM [Accessed April, 2012].

1323. RILEY-SMITH SYNDROME (BANNAYAN-RILEY-RUVALCABA SYNDROME) PSEUDOPAPILLEDEMA

General

Etiology unknown; possibly heterozygous condition (single autosomal gene); macrocephaly-pseudopapilledema-multiple hemangiomas; noted at birth; has been proposed that there is overlap with the Bannayan-Zonana syndrome and the Ruvalcaba-Myhre syndrome; autosomal dominant inherited condition.

Ocular

Pseudopapilledema; prominent Schwalbe line; visible corneal nerves; ocular hypertelorism; strabismus; amblyopia.

Clinical

Macrocephaly; subcutaneous hemangiomas; pulmonary infections; mild-to-severe mental retardation; skin hemangiomas; hypotonus; gastrointestinal polyps; pigmented maculae on the skin.

Laboratory

Complete blood count, stools for occult blood, genetic testing, serum albumin levels, liver function and alpha-fetoprotein level test.

Treatment

Medical care and management of cutaneous cysts, osteomas, fibromas, polyposis and neoplasia.

Additional Resource

1. Hsu EK (2011). Intestinal Polyposis Syndromes. [online] Available from http://www.emedicine. com/ped/TOPIC828.HTM [Accessed April, 2012].

1324. RING CHROMOSOME 6 (ANIRIDIA, CONGENITAL GLAUCOMA, AND HYDROCEPHALUS)

General

Rare disorder associated with various congenital anomalies; autosomal dominant with recessive sporadically reported.

Ocular

Microphthalmia; aniridia; congenital uveal ectropion; Rieger anomaly; congenital glaucoma; corneal clouding; prominent Schwalbe line with attached iris strands; hypopigmented fundi; hypoplasia of iris stroma; strabismus; ptosis; nystagmus; megalocornea; iris coloboma; optic atrophy; hypertelorism; antimongoloid slant of palpebral fissures; ectopic pupils; angle anomalies; posterior embryotoxon; microcornea; colobomatous.

Clinical

Hydrocephalus; agenesis of corpus callosum; congenital heart defects; mental retardation; low-set malformed ears; broad nasal bridge; micrognathia; short neck; hand anomalies; high-arched palate; widely spaced nipples; deformity of feet; respiratory distress syndrome; hyperbilirubinemia; hypocalcemia; anemia; seizure; bulging anterior fontanelle.

Laboratory

Diagnosis is made by clinical findings.

Treatment

Ptosis: If visual acuity is affected most cases require surgical correction, and there are several procedures that may be used including levator resection, repair or advancement and Fasanella-Servat.

Bibliography

1. Bateman JB. Chromosomal anomalies and the eye. In: Wright KW (Ed). Pediatric Ophthalmology and Strabismus. St. Louis: CV Mosby; 1995. p. 595.
2. Chitayat D, Hahm SY, Iqbal MA, et al. Ring chromosome 6: report of a patient and literature review. Am J Med Genet. 1987;26:145-51.
3. deLuise UP, Anderson DR. Primary infantile glaucoma (congenital glaucoma). Surv Ophthalmol. 1983;28:1-19.
4. Levin H, Ritch R, Barathur R, et al. Aniridia, congenital glaucoma, and hydrocephalus in a male infant with ring chromosome 6. Am J Med Genet. 1986;25:281-7.

1325. RING D CHROMOSOME (HYPERTELORISM)

General

Variant of the chromosome 13 deletion syndrome; ring chromosomes.

Ocular

Hypertelorism; epicanthal folds; ptosis; microphthalmos; uveal colobomas; abnormal palpebral fissure; strabismus; retinoblastoma.

Clinical

Aplasia of thumbs; mental and physical retardation; trigonocephaly; malrotation of ear; micrognathia; hypoplastic nipple; widely spaced first and second toes.

Laboratory

Diagnosis is made by clinical findings.

Treatment

Strabismus: Equalized vision with correct refractive error; surgery may be helpful in patient with diplopia.

Retinoblastoma: External beam radiation therapy is recommended on patients with significant vitreous seeding. Radioactive isotope plaques and chemotherapy are also an option. Removal of the tumor is the standard management for retinoblastoma.

Bibliography

1. Collins JF. Handbook of Clinical Ophthalmology. New York: Masson; 1982.
2. Magalini SI, Scrascia E. Dictionary of Medical Syndromes, 2nd edition. Philadelphia: JB Lippincott; 1981. p. 711.

1326. RING DERMOID SYNDROME (AMBLYOPIA)

General

Autosomal dominant; usually bilateral.

Ocular

Dermoid choristoma; conjunctival plaques of keratinization; corneal lipid deposition; irregular corneal astigmatism; amblyopia; concomitant strabismus.

Laboratory

Diagnosis is made by clinical findings.

Treatment

Strabismus: Equalized vision with correct refractive error; surgery may be helpful in patient with diplopia.

Bibliography

1. Henkind P, Marinoff G, Manas A, et al. Bilateral corneal dermoids. Am J Ophthalmol. 1973;76: 972-7.
2. Mattos J, Contreras F, O'Donnell FE. Ring dermoid syndrome. A new syndrome of autosomal dominantly inherited, bilateral, annular limbal dermoids with corneal and conjunctival extension. Arch Ophthalmol. 1980;98:1059-61.
3. McKusick VA. Mendelian Inheritance in Man: A Catalog of Human Genes and Genetic Disorders, 12th edition. Baltimore: The Johns Hopkins University Press; 1998.
4. McKusick-Nathans Institute for Genetic Medicine, Johns Hopkins University and National Center for Biotechnology Information, National Library of Medicine. (2007). Online Mendelian Inheritance in Man (OMIM). [online] Available from http://www.ncbi.nlm.nih.gov/omim [Accessed April, 2012].
5. Oakman JH, Lambert SR, Grossniklaus HE. Corneal dermoid: case report and review of classification. J Pediatr Ophthalmol Strabismus. 1993; 30:388-91.

1327. RINX DISEASE (VSX1 MUTATION)

General

Mutation of the homeobox transcription factor gene VSX1 (RINX) Wide interpupillary distance; hypertelorism; anomalies of corneal endothelium; abnormal cone bipolar cells.

Clinical

Empty sella turcica; posterior fossa cyst; anterior encephalocele; hydrocephalus.

Ocular

Hypertelorism, anomalies of corneal endothelium, wide interpupillary distance.

Laboratory

None

Treatment

None

Bibliography

1. Mintz-Hittner HA, Semina EV, Frishman LJ, et al. VSX1 (RINX) mutation with craniofacial anomalies, empty sella, corneal endothelial changes, and abnormal retinal and auditory bipolar cells. Ophthalmology. 2004;111:828-36.

1328. ROBERTS PSEUDOTHALIDOMIDE SYNDROME (GLAUCOMA)

General

Rare, autosomal recessive disorder characterized by prenatal and postnatal growth retardation, limb defects and craniofacial anomalies.

Ocular

Cataracts; glaucoma; microcornea; corneal clouding.

Clinical

Patients usually do not survive past 1 month; patients often are mentally retarded.

Laboratory

Diagnosis is made by clinical findings.

Treatment

Cataract: Change in glasses can sometimes improve a patient's visual function temporarily; however, the most common treatment is cataract surgery.

Glaucoma: Its medication should be the first plan of action. If medication is unsuccessful, a filtering surgical procedure with or without antimetabolites may be beneficial.

Bibliography

1. Holden KR, Jabs EW, Sponseller PD. Roberts/pseudothalidomide syndrome and normal intelligence: approaches to diagnosis and management. Dev Med Child Neurol. 1992;34:534-9.
2. Otano L, Matayoshi T, Gadow EC. Roberts syndrome: first-trimester prenatal diagnosis. Prenat Diagn. 1996;16:770-1.

1329. ROBINOW-SILVERMAN-SMITH SYNDROME (ACHONDROPLASTIC DWARFISM; MESOMELIC DWARFISM; ROBINOW DWARFISM)

General

Autosomal dominant; both sexes affected; present from birth.

Ocular

Hypertelorism; epicanthal folds.

Clinical

Dwarfism; shortened forearms; bulging forehead; depressed nasal bridge; hypoplastic mandible; small, upturned nose; micrognathia; crowded teeth; penile hypoplasia.

Laboratory

Radiography, CT scan, MRI and ultrasound.

Treatment

No specific treatment exists.

Additional Resource

1. Khan AN (2011). Achondroplasia Imaging. [online] Available from http://www.emedicine.com/radio/TOPIC809.HTM [Accessed April, 2012].

1330. ROCHON-DUVIGNEAUD SYNDROME (SUPERIOR ORBITAL FISSURE SYNDROME) OPTIC ATROPHY

General

Inflammatory, traumatic, tumor, or vascular lesions such as meningioma of the sphenoid, carotid aneurysm, and arachnoiditis; infections originating in the maxillary sinus.

Ocular

Mild exophthalmos; lid edema; partial or complete ophthalmoplegia (III, IV, and VI); decreased corneal sensitivity; papilledema; optic atrophy.

Clinical

Decreased sensitivity in area of nasociliary, lacrimal, frontal, and ophthalmic nerve distribution; may result from a metastatic tumor.

Laboratory

Complete blood count, erythrocyte sedimentation rate (ESR), thyroid function test, fluorescent treponemal antibody (FTA), antinuclear antibody (ANA), lupus erythematosus (LE) preparation, antineutrophil cytoplasmic antibody (ANCA), serum protein electrophoresis, Lyme titer, angiotensin-converting enzyme (ACE) level, and HIV titer are helpful. Cerebrospinal fluid, anti-GQ1b antibodies, and MRI of the brain and the orbits.

Treatment

Corticosteroids are the treatment of choice.

Bibliography

1. Falcone F, Lazow SK, Berger JR, et al. Superior orbital fissure syndrome. Secondary to infected dentigerous cyst of the maxillary sinus. N Y State Dent J. 1994;60:62-4.
2. Hedstrom J, Parsons J, Maloney PL, et al. Superior orbital fissure syndrome: report of a case. J Oral Surg. 1974;32:198-201.
3. Phanthumchinda K, Hemachuda T. Superior orbital fissure syndrome as a presenting symptom in hepatocellular carcinoma. J Med Assoc Thai. 1992;75:62-5.
4. Rochon-Duvigneaud A. Quelques Cas de Paralysie de Tous les Nerfs Orbitaires (Ophtalmoplegie Totale avec Amaurose et Anesthesie dans le Domaine de l'Ophtalmique d'Origine Syphilitique). Arch Ophthalmol. 1896;16:746.

1331. ROCKY MOUNTAIN SPOTTED FEVER

General

Acute systemic disease caused by *Rickettsia rickettsii* transmitted by a wood tick or dog tick.

Ocular

Conjunctivitis; optic atrophy; cotton-wool spots; scotoma; uveitis; optic neuritis; paralysis of accommodation; paralysis of extraocular muscles; retinal vascular occlusion; vitreal opacity; hypopyon; anterior uveitis with fibrin clots.

Clinical

Fever; chills; headache; muscle aches; rash.

Laboratory

Early diagnosis depends on clinical and epidemiologic grounds. Polymerase chain reaction has high sensitivity and specifity.

Treatment

Intravenous tetracycline and chloramphenicol should be started as soon as possible. Oral doxycycline, tetracycline and chloramphenicol may be considered but only if patient is not acutely ill.

Additional Resource

1. Cunha BA (2011). Rocky Mountain Spotted Fever. [online] Available from http://www.emedicine.com/oph/TOPIC503.HTM [Accessed April, 2012].

1332. ROLLET SYNDROME (ORBITAL APEX-SPHENOIDAL SYNDROME) OPTIC NEURITIS

General

Lesion in the apex of the orbit (neoplastic, hemorrhagic or inflammatory) involving the III, IV and VI cranial nerves, the ophthalmic branch of the fifth sympathetic fibers when they pass through the sphenoidal fissure, and the optic nerve; manifestations vary greatly with extent of lesion; pain is frequent early sign; orbital fissure syndrome and sphenocavernous syndrome are similar; sudden onset.

Ocular

Exophthalmos; ptosis; hyperesthesia or anesthesia of the upper lid; ophthalmoplegia (partial or complete); wide pupil with loss of reaction on accommodation; neuralgic pain in the region of the ophthalmic branch of cranial nerve V; anesthesia of the cornea; papilledema; optic neuritis; optic atrophy; diplopia; herpes zoster ophthalmicus.

Clinical

Hyperesthesia or anesthesia of the forehead; inflammation of cavernous sinuses; meningoencephalitis.

Laboratory

Diagnosis is made by clinical findings.

Treatment

Exophthalmos: Reversing the problem, which is causing the exophthalmos, is the treatment of choice and will minimize the ocular complications. Ocular lubricants are beneficial for control of the corneal exposure.

Bibliography

1. Bourke RD, Pyle J. Herpes zoster ophthalmicus and the orbital apex syndrome. Aust N Z J Ophthalmol. 1994;22:77-80.

2. Goldberg RA, Hannani K, Toga AW. Microanatomy of the orbital apex. Computed tomography and microcryoplaning of soft and hard tissue. Ophthalmology. 1992;99:1447-52.

1333. ROMBERG SYNDROME (FACIAL HEMIATROPHY; PARRY-ROMBERG SYNDROME; PROGRESSIVE FACIAL HEMIATROPHY; PROGRESSIVE HEMIFACIAL ATROPHY) ENOPHTHALMUS

General

Autosomal dominant; irritation in the peripheral trophic sympathetic system; onset in the second decade of life; both sexes affected.

Ocular

Enophthalmos; outer canthus lowered; absence of nasal portion of eyebrow; ptosis; paresis of ocular muscles; miosis; iritis; iridocyclitis; heterochromia iridis; keratitis; neuroparalytic keratitis; cataracts; choroiditis; Fuchs heterochromic cyclitis; retinal vascular abnormalities; association with Coats syndrome and exudative stellate neuroretinopathy; scleral melting.

Clinical

Atrophy of soft tissue on one side of the face, including tongue; trigeminal neuralgia and/or paresthesia; alopecia and poliosis not uncommon.

Laboratory/Ocular

Neuroimaging, CT scan of the orbits, MRI and bone scans.

Treatment/Ocular

Chemotherapy, ionizing radiation or immunosuppressive treatments.

Bibliography

1. Aracena T, Roca FP, Barragan M. Progressive hemifacial atrophy (Parry-Romberg syndrome): report of two cases. Ann Ophthalmol. 1979;11:953-8.
2. Gass JD, Harbin TS, Del Piero EJ. Exudative stellate neuroretinopathy and Coats' syndrome in patients with progressive hemifacial atrophy. Eur J Ophthalmol. 1991;1:2-10.
3. Hoang-Xuan T, Foster CS, Jakobiec FA, et al. Romberg's progressive hemifacial atrophy: an association with scleral melting. Cornea. 1991;10: 361-6.
4. La Hey E, Baarsma GS. Fuchs' heterochromic cyclitis and retinal vascular abnormalities in progressive hemifacial atrophy. Eye (Lond). 1993;7:426-8.
5. Parry CH. Collections from Unpublished Papers. London: Underwood; 1825.
6. Romberg MH. Trophoneurosen Kliniske Ergenbrisse. Berlin: A. Forster; 1846.

1334. ROSENBERG-CHUTORIAN SYNDROME (OPTIC ATROPHY)

General

Recessive inheritance; inheritance is considered X-linked semidominant.

Ocular

Optic atrophy.

Clinical

Polyneuropathy; neural hearing loss.

Laboratory

Diagnosis is made by clinical findings.

Treatment

Intravenous steroids may be used with optic neuritis or ischemic optic neuritis.

Bibliography

1. Geeraets WJ. Ocular Syndromes, 3rd edition. Philadelphia: Lea & Febiger; 1976.

2. Konigsmark BW, Knox DL, Hussels IE, et al. Dominant congenital deafness and progressive optic nerve atrophy. Occurrence in four generations of a family. Arch Ophthalmol. 1974;91:99-103.

3. McKusick VA. Mendelian Inheritance in Man: A Catalog of Human Genes and Genetic Disorders, 12th edition. Baltimore: The Johns Hopkins University Press; 1998.

4. McKusick-Nathans Institute for Genetic Medicine, Johns Hopkins University and National Center for Biotechnology Information, National Library of Medicine. (2007). Online Mendelian Inheritance in Man (OMIM). [online] Available from http://www.ncbi.nlm.nih.gov/omim [Accessed April, 2012].

5. Rosenberg RN, Chutorian A. Familial opticoacoustic nerve degeneration and polyneuropathy. Neurology. 1967;17:827-32.

1335. ROSENTHAL-KLOEPFER SYNDROME (CORNEAL OPACITY)

General

Autosomal dominant; unilateral or bilateral; onset in early childhood; hyperplasia and furrowing of skin, especially of face and scalp, beginning about the fourth decade of life; etiology unknown; affects both sexes.

Ocular

Prominent lateral aspect of the supraorbital arch of the frontal bone; corneal leukomas (initially superficial stromal infiltrations that develop to thick and dense corneal opacities).

Clinical

Acromegaly; thickening of the bony skull; prominent lower jaw; skin changes (with verticis gyrata); abnormal ridges and creases of the palms.

Laboratory

Diagnosis is made by clinical findings.

Treatment

Consult dermatologist.

Bibliography

1. McKusick VA. Mendelian Inheritance in Man: A Catalog of Human Genes and Genetic Disorders, 12th edition. Baltimore: The Johns Hopkins University Press; 1998.

2. McKusick-Nathans Institute for Genetic Medicine, Johns Hopkins University and National Center for Biotechnology Information, National Library of Medicine. (2007). Online Mendelian Inheritance in Man (OMIM). [online] Available from http://www.ncbi.nlm.nih.gov/omim [Accessed April, 2012].

3. Rosenthal JW, Kloepfer HW. An acromegaloid, cutis verticis gyrata, corneal leukoma syndrome. A new medical entity. Arch Ophthalmol. 1962;68:722-6.

1336. ROTHMUND SYNDROME (CONGENITAL POIKILODERMA WITH JUVENILE CATARACT; ECTODERMAL SYNDROME; ROTHMUND-THOMSON SYNDROME; TELANGIECTASIA-PIGMENTATION-CATARACT SYNDROME) KERATOCONUS

General

Autosomal recessive; more common in females (2:1); Werner syndrome in adults has certain similarities to this syndrome; inflammatory phase progresses to atrophy and telangiectasia; onset age 3–6 months.

Ocular

Eyebrows may be sparse or absent; hypertelorism; cilia sometimes are diminished or absent; trichiasis; epiphora; cataracts (anterior subcapsular, posterior stellate or perinuclear type); corneal lesions; retinal hyperpigmentation; keratoconus; strabismus; epibulbar dermoids.

Clinical

Poikiloderma; hypogonadism; hypomenorrhea; head deformity (enlarged with depressed nasal bridge as well as microcephaly); small stature, with short or malformed distal phalanges; aplasia cutis congenita (congenital absence of skin in one or more areas); alopecia.

Laboratory

Skeletal radiograph by age 5.

Treatment

Sun blocker with UVA and UVB should be used often. Keratolytics and retinoids are used to treat hyperkeratotic lesions.

Additional Resource

1. Hsu S (2011). Rothmund-Thomson Syndrome. [online] Available from http://www.emedicine.com/derm/TOPIC379.HTM [Accessed April, 2012].

1337. ROUSSY-CORNIL SYNDROME

General

Etiology unknown; sporadic hypertrophic neuropathy; onset in the second to third decade of life or later; progressive; occasionally, remissions and exacerbations.

Ocular

Sluggish pupils; disturbed vision.

Clinical

Nerves palpable and tender; peripheral atrophy; tendon reflexes diminished or abolished; scoliosis; muscle fasciculations; ataxia; lancinating pains.

Laboratory

Diagnosis is made by clinical findings.

Treatment

None

Bibliography

1. Magalini SI, Scrascia E. Dictionary of Medical Syndromes, 2nd edition. Philadelphia: JB Lippincott; 1981.
2. Roussy G, Cornil L. Nevrite Hypertrophique Progressive Non-Familiale de l'Adulte. Ann Med. 1919;6:296-305.
3. Suarez GA, Giannini C, Smith BE, et al. Localized hypertrophic neuropathy. Mayo Clin Proc. 1994;69:747-8.

1338. ROY SYNDROME (CATARACT, POSTERIOR)

General

Long history of smoking tobacco.

Ocular

Cataract, usually unilateral, posterior subcapsular, and cortical.

Clinical

Emphysema; cardiac disorder; cancer.

Laboratory

Diagnosis is made by clinical findings.

Treatment

Cataract: Change in glasses can sometimes improve a patient's visual function temporarily; however, the most common treatment is cataract surgery.

Bibliography

1. Roy H. Cigarette smoking and risk of cataracts. JAMA. 1993;269:748.

1339. ROY SYNDROME II (CATARACT, NUCLEAR)

General

Long history of smoking tobacco.

Ocular

Cataract; nuclear cataract may be cortical or posterior subcapsular cataract.

Clinical

Emphysema; cardiac disorder; cancer.

Laboratory

Diagnosis is made by clinical findings.

Treatment

Cataract: Change in glasses can sometimes improve a patient's visual function temporarily; however, the most common treatment is cataract surgery.

Bibliography

1. Klein BE, Klein R, Linton KL, et al. Cigarette smoking and lens opacities: the Beaver Dam Eye Study. Am J Prev Med. 1993;9:27-30.
2. Roy H. Cigarette smoking and risk of cataracts. JAMA. 1993;269:748.

1340. RUBELLA SYNDROME (CONGENITAL RUBELLA SYNDROME; GERMAN MEASLES; GREGG SYNDROME)

General

Rubella infection of the mother during first trimester of pregnancy; ocular disease is the most commonly found abnormality in patients with congenital rubella syndrome (75%), multiorgan disease is common (greater than 75%); no significant association has been found between gestational age and time of maternal infection and incidence of individual ocular conditions.

Ocular

Nystagmus; glaucoma; corneal haziness; cataracts; retinal pigmentary changes; appearance and central distribution of lesions are quite distinguishable from retinitis pigmentosa; retinopathy is not progressive and has little, if any, effect on vision; waxy atrophy of optic disk; conjunctivitis; megalocornea or microcornea; buphthalmos; microphthalmos; uveitis; iris atrophy; spherophakia; strabismus.

Clinical

Low-birth-weight; diarrhea; pneumonia; urinary infection; hearing loss; heart disease; hepatosplenomegaly; mental retardation; inguinal hernias; ataxia; cardiac abnormalities.

Laboratory

Diagnosis is made by clinical findings, if in doubt, a rising titer of immunoglobulin M will indicate a recent infection.

Treatment

Treatment for rubella of the eye centers on glaucoma and cataract.

Additional Resource

1. Lombardo PC (2011). Dermatologic Manifestations of Rubella. [online] Available from http://www.emedicine.com/derm/TOPIC380.HTM [Accessed April, 2012].

1341. RUBEOSIS IRIDIS

General

Neovasc015riztion of the iris.

Clinical

None

Ocular

Intractable type of secondary glaucoma, rubeosis iridis, diabetic retinopathy, retinal vein occlusion, carotid occlusive disease, iritis.

Laboratory

Diagnosis is made by clinical findings. Check for diabetes.

Treatment

Trabeculectomy with the antifibrotic agents mitomycin-C and 5-fluorouracil (5-FU) is one modality. Trabeculectomy in NVG has a significant failure rate. Using standard trabeculectomy (without antifibrosis), an IOP of less than 25 mm Hg on one medication or less has been reported to occur in 67–100% of patients in three studies.

Using injections of 5-FU subconjunctivally in the postoperative period, the surgical success has been reported to be 68% over 3 years. Inject 0.1 mL of 5 mg/mL 5-FU subconjunctivally either superiorly above the bleb or inferiorly (just above the lower fornix). Mitomycin-C used intraoperatively has been shown to be more effective than 5-FU in routine trabeculectomies. No significant follow-up studies exist on the use of mitomycin-C with trabeculectomy in NVG.

Valve implant surgery is another modality and is indicated when trabeculectomy fails or extensive conjunctival scarring exists, thereby preventing a standard filtering procedure. Molteno, Krupin and Ahmed valve implants commonly are used. One large series using the Krupin valve reported 79% of eyes with NVG had a 67% success rate in controlling IOP (< 24 mm Hg) with mean follow-up of 23 months. Long-term results are mixed. Using the Molteno implant, 60 eyes with NVG achieved a satisfactory IOP (< 21 mm Hg) and maintenance of visual acuity over 5 years of only 10.3%. If combined with the need for vitrectomy, consideration of pars plana tube-shunt insertion may reduce anterior segment complications.

Avastin injections have shown some promise for the control of iris neovascularization.

Complications include postoperative hypotony with associated complications, blockage of internal fistula, blockage of external filtration site (fibrosis of the filtering bleb), and corneal endothelial loss.

Additional Resource

1. Freudenthal J (2011). Neovascular Glaucoma. [online] Available from http://www.emedicine.com/oph/TOPIC135 [Accessed April, 2012].

1342. RUBINSTEIN-TAYBI SYNDROME (OPTIC ATROPHY)

General

Inheritance polygenic or multifactorial; rare.

Ocular

Antimongoloid slant of lid fissure; epicanthus; long eyelashes and highly arched brows; strabismus; myopia; hyperopia; iris coloboma; cataract; optic atrophy; ptosis; retinal detachment.

Clinical

Motor and mental retardation; broad thumbs and toes; highly arched palate; allergies; heart murmurs; anomalies of size, shape, and position of ears; dwarfism; cryptorchidism.

Laboratory

Computed tomography (CT) scan, MRI, chromosomal karyotype analysis, fluorescence in situ hybridization and CBP gene analysis.

Treatment

Physical therapy, speech and feeding therapy. Cardiothoracic intervention may be needed in patients with congenital heart defect.

Additional Resource

1. Mijuskovic ZP (2011). Dermatologic Manifestations of Rubinstein-Taybi Syndrome. [online] Available from http://www.emedicine.com/derm/TOPIC711.HTM [Accessed April, 2012].

1343. RUD SYNDROME

General

Etiology unknown; immature nerve cells and decreased number of cells; Betz cells in the motor cortex show chronic chromatolysis; excess of oligodendroglia in the frontal cortex; relationship to tuberous sclerosis and neurofibromatosis; X-linked inheritance has been reported.

Ocular

Retinal pigmentary degeneration.

Clinical

Epilepsy; infantilism; idiocy; congenital ichthyosis; muscular atrophy; male hypogonadism.

Laboratory

Diagnosis is made by clinical findings.

Treatment

Retinitis pigmentosa: It may be treated with vitamin A 15,000 IU/day and is thought to slow the decline of retinal function, dark sunglasses for outdoor use, surgery for cataract, genetic counseling.

Bibliography

1. Duke-Elder S (Ed). System of Ophthalmology. St. Louis: CV Mosby; 1976. p. 1130.

2. McKusick VA. Mendelian Inheritance in Man: A Catalog of Human Genes and Genetic Disorders, 12th edition. Baltimore: The Johns Hopkins University Press; 1998.

3. McKusick-Nathans Institute for Genetic Medicine, Johns Hopkins University and National Center for Biotechnology Information, National Library of Medicine. (2007). Online Mendelian Inheritance in Man (OMIM). [online] Available from http://www.ncbi.nlm.nih.gov/omim [Accessed April, 2012].

4. Rud E. Et Tilfaelde af Infantilsms med Tetani, Epilepsy, Polyneuritis, Ichthiosis og Anaemi of Pernicios Type. Hospitalstidende. 1927;70:525.

5. Wisniewski K, Levis AR, Shanske AL. X-linked inheritance of the Rud syndrome. Am J Hum Genet. 1985;37:A83.

1344. RUSSELL SYNDROME (NYSTAGMUS)

General

Onset between the ages of 3 months and 2 years; caused by tumors of the anterior portion of the thalamus (usually astrocytoma), optic chiasm, midcerebellar region, and midline ependymoma; erosion under the anterior clinoid processes that causes a characteristic J-shaped sella in lateral skull films.

Ocular

Lid retraction; nystagmus (horizontal, vertical or rotatory); homonymous hemianopsia; optic nerve atrophy.

Clinical

Extreme emaciation; euphoria; pale skin.

Laboratory

Diagnosis is made by clinical findings.

Treatment

Lid retraction: Identify systemic abnormalities such as thyroid. Treatment must be given for 6 months for stabilizing before performing eyelid surgery. Local-ocular lubrication (drops or ointment). Botulism type A may also be useful.

Bibliography

1. Ciccarelli EC, Huttenlocher PR. Diencephalic tumor. A cause of infantile nystagmus and cachexia. Arch Ophthalmol. 1967;78:350-3.

2. Geeraets WJ. Ocular Syndromes, 3rd edition. Philadelphia: Lea & Febiger; 1976.

3. Russell A. A diencephalic syndrome: emaciation in infancy and childhood. Arch Dis Child. 1951; 26: 274.

1345. SABIN-FELDMAN SYNDROME (CHORIORETINITIS)

General

Etiology unknown; similar to toxoplasmosis; results of toxoplasma dye and complement fixation tests are negative; onset in early infancy.

Ocular

Microphthalmia; strabismus; fixed pupils; posterior lenticonus; microcornea; chorioretinitis or atrophic degenerative chorioretinal changes; optic atrophy.

Clinical

Cerebral calcifications (infrequent); convulsions (frequent); microcephaly; hydrocephalus.

Laboratory

Diagnosis is made by clinical findings.

Treatment

Lens extraction with irrigation-aspiration.

Bibliography

1. Geeraets WJ. Ocular Syndromes, 3rd edition. Philadelphia: Lea & Febiger; 1976.
2. Sabin AB, Feldman HA. Chorioretinopathy associated with other evidence of cerebral damage in childhood: a syndrome of unknown etiology separable from congenital toxoplasmosis. J Pediatr. 1949;35:296-309.

1346. SAETHRE-CHOTZEN SYNDROME (ACROCEPHALOSYNDACTYLY III)

General

Genetic condition characterized by craniosynostosis, facial asymmetry and characteristic appearance of the ear.

Ocular

Ptosis, antimongoloid palpberal fissure, hypertelorism.

Clinical

Small pinna with a prominat crus of the ear, syndactyly of digits, developmental delays, short stature, parietal foramina, vertebral fusions, hearing loss and heart defects.

Laboratory

Diagnosis is made by clinical findings.

Treatment

Cranioplasty to prevent progressive facial asymmetry.

Bibliography

1. Bianchi E, Arico M, Podesta AF, et al. A family with the Saethre-Chotzen syndrome. Am J Med Genet. 1985;22:649-58.
2. Chun K, Teebi AS, Jung JH, et al. Genetic analysis of patients with the Saethre-Chotzen phenotype. Am J Med Genet. 2002;110:136-43.

1347. SAINT ANTHONY FIRE (ERYSIPELAS)

General

Acute localized inflammation of the skin and subcutaneous tissue; erysipelas is a febrile infection of the skin and subcutaneous tissue, most commonly caused by *Streptococcus*, characterized by the acute onset of a red, indurated expanding plaque that nearly disappears with the use of antibiotics; sometimes caused by *Staphylococcus*.

Ocular

Conjunctivitis; blepharitis; elephantiasis and gangrene of lid; ptosis; dacryocystitis; cellulitis of orbit; keratitis; panophthalmitis; uveitis; eyelid involvement.

Clinical

Edema; fever; rigor; vesicles; tenderness; headache; vomiting; localized pain.

Laboratory

Blood cultures, needle aspirates or biopsy yields less than 10% positive cultures; direct immunofluorescence is useful to detct streptococcus in skin specimens.

Treatment

Systemic treatment is penicillin G. Ocular treatment is to clean and debridement of wound and use of a broad spectrum antibiotic ointment.

Bibliography

1. Binford RT, Lindo SD. Dermatologlc conditions affecting the eye. In: Dunlap EA (Ed). Gordon's Medical Management of Ocular Disease, 2nd edition. New York: Harper & Row; 1976. pp. 91-110.
2. Bratton RL, Nesse RE. St. Anthony's fire: diagnosis and management of erysipelas. Am Fam Physician. 1995;51:401-4.
3. Duane TD. Clinical Ophthalmology. Philadelphia: JB Lippincott; 1987.
4. Roy FH, Fraunfelder FW, Fraunfelder FT. Roy and Fraunfelder's Current Ocular Therapy, 6th edition. Philadelphia: WB Saunders; 2008.
5. McHugh D, Fison PN. Ocular erysipelas. Arch Ophthalmol. 1992;110:1315.

1348. SALDINO-MAINZER SYNDROME (RETINITIS PIGMENTOSA)

General

Autosomal recessive; Leber congenital amaurosis associated with familial juvenile nephronophthisis and cone-shaped epiphysis of the hands; similar to Senior-Loken syndrome, with the difference being cone-shaped epiphysis.

Ocular

Tapetoretinal degeneration; retinal atrophy; Leber congenital amaurosis; retinitis pigmentosa.

Clinical

Nephronophthisis; cone-shaped epiphyses of hands and feet; flared ribs; hypoplastic pelvis; brachydactyly; hyperparathyroidism; osteomalacia; osteopetrosis; renal failure.

Laboratory

Diagnosis is made by clinical findings.

Treatment

None

Bibliography

1. Ellis DS, Heckenlively JR, Martin CL, et al. Leber's congenital amaurosis associated with familial juvenile nephronophthisis and cone-shaped epiphyses of the hands (the Saldino-Mainzer syndrome). Am J Ophthalmol. 1984;97:233-9.
2. Foxman SG, Heckenlively JR, Bateman JB, et al. Classification of congenital and early onset retinitis pigmentosa. Arch Ophthalmol. 1985;103:1502-6.

1349. SANDHOFF DISEASE [GANGLIOSIDOSIS TYPE 2 (GM2)] VISUAL LOSS

General

Hereditary cerebromacular degeneration-sphingolipidoses; onset by age 6 months; autosomal recessive inheritance; enzyme defect; caused by deficiency of hexosaminidases A and B; defect localized to chromosome 5 (5q13).

Ocular

Cherry-red spot of macula; visual loss; clinically identical to Tay-Sachs disease.

Clinical

Motor retardation; doll-like facies; dementia; hyperacusis; frequent respiratory infections; variable hepatosplenomegaly.

Laboratory

Enzyme assay and DNA diagnostic evaluation.

Treatment

No treatment is available.

Additional Resource

1. Tegay DH (2012). GM2 Gangliosidoses. [online] Available from http://www.emedicine.com/ped/TOPIC3016.HTM [Accessed April, 2012].

1350. SANDIFER SYNDROME (HIATAL HERNIA-TORTICOLLIS SYNDROME) EXOTROPIA

General

Inheritance not known; males affected; hiatal hernia.

Ocular

Strabismus (not related to existing torticollis).

Clinical

Rotation of the head to one shoulder with stretching of the neck (more pronounced during eating and reading); epigastric pain associated with vomiting, primarily in infancy; malnutrition; hiatal hernia; asthenia.

Laboratory

pH monitoring, cranial MRI, video-EEG and endoscopy.

Treatment

No treatment is required.

Additional Resource

1. Eslami P (2009). Sandifer Syndrome. [online] Available from http://www.emedicine.com/ped/TOPIC2039.HTM [Accessed April, 2012].

1351. SANDS OF THE SAHARA SYNDROME (DIFFUSE LAMELLAR KERATITIS)

General

Interface inflammation after laser in situ keratomileusis (LASIK).

Ocular

Interface inflammation after LASIK is a rare, but potential sight-threatening complication; syndrome presents 1–5 days after LASIK; affected patients often complain of decreased or cloudy vision, foreign body sensation, and photophobia; symptoms may be mild or severe; cause of the interface debris is unknown, but microkeratome material is implicated.

Laboratory

Diagnosis is made by clinical findings.

Treatment

Increments in strength and frequency of topical steroids and discontinuing nonsteroidal anti-inflammatory drugs.

Bibliography

1. Kaufman SC, Maitchouk DY, Chiou AG, et al. Interface inflammation after laser in situ keratomileusis. Sands of the Sahara syndrome. J Cataract Refract Surg. 1998;24:1589-93.

2. Smith RJ, Maloney RK. Diffuse lamellar keratitis. A new syndrome in lamellar refractive surgery. Ophthalmology. 1998;105:1721-6.

1352. SANDWICH INFECTIOUS KERATITIS SYNDROME (SIK SYNDROME)

General

Bacterial and fungal organisms infiltration of the interface between donor and host corneas following DLEK, DALK, DSAEK and ALK.

Clinical

None

Ocular

Infectious infiltrates in the interface of the corneal which are white small irregular or circular.

Laboratory

Careful slit lamp examination is essential and any interface infiltrate should be monitored closely.

Cultures are difficult to get because the infection is intracorneal.

Treatment

Intensive antibiotic treatment regimen is necessary, if fungal infection is identified the use of antifungal agents are recommended. If medical treatment fail a TKP may be necessary.

Bibliography

1. John T, Park T. New techniques, new corneal complication. Review of Ophthalmology. 2009;16:3.
2. John T. Selective tissue corneal transplantation: a great step forward in global visual restoration. Expert Rev Ophthalmol. 2006;1:5-7.

1353. SANFILIPPO-GOOD SYNDROME (HEPARITINURIA; MUCOPOLYSACCHARIDOSIS III; MPS III)

General

Autosomal recessive; excess urinary excretion of heparitin sulfate (see Hunter Syndrome; Hurler Syndrome; Maroteaux-Lamy Syndrome; Morquio Syndrome; Scheie Syndrome). Lack of a beta-galactosaminidase-like enzyme causing accumulation of glycolipids, acid mucopolysaccharides, and their precursors; both sexes affected; death occurs by second decade in the majority of cases; autosomal recessive; divided into type A (with decreased levels of heparan sulfatase) and type B (with decreased levels of N-acetyl-a-D-glucosaminidase).

Ocular

Night blindness; slight narrowing of retinal vessels; pigment deposits in the fundi; bushy eyebrows; coarse eyelashes; acid mucopolysaccharide deposits in cornea, iris, lens and sclera; retinal degeneration; optic nerve atrophy.

Clinical

Mental deficiency progressing to severe degrees within a few years; seizures; gargoyle features very mild; dwarfism; stiff joints; hepatosplenomegaly; hirsutism; mitral valve insufficiency.

Laboratory

Urine-excessive heparin sulfate MPS urine spot test is positive.

Treatment

Bone marrow transplant improves systemic health, but there is no therapy to prevent long-term function.

Additional Resource

1. Bittar T (2010). Mucopolysaccharidosis. [online] Available from http://www.emedicine.com/orthoped/TOPIC203.HTM [Accessed April, 2012].

1354. SAVIN SYNDROME

General

Congenital ichthyosis combined with urticarial manifestations.

Ocular

Nodular thickening in parenchyma of cornea.

Clinical

Dry, scaly skin; atopic dermatitis; pruritus.

Laboratory

Diagnosis is made by clinical findings.

Treatment

Topical steroids and muro 128 ointment may be useful.

Bibliography

1. Korting GW. The Skin and the Eye: A Dermatologic Correlation of Diseases of the Periorbital Region. Philadelphia: WB Saunders; 1973. p. 72.
2. Savin LH. Corneal dystrophy associated with congenital ichthyosis and allergic manifestations in male members of a family. Br J Ophthalmol. 1956;40:82-9.

1355. SCALDED SKIN SYNDROME (EPIDERMOLYSIS ACUTA TOXICA; LYELL SYNDROME; NECROLYSIS; RITTER DISEASE; STAPHYLOCOCCAL SCALDED SKIN SYNDROME; TOXIC EPIDERMAL; TOXIC EPIDERMAL NECROLYSIS OF LYELL; TOXIC EPIDERMAL NECROLYSIS) SYMBLEPHARON

General

Generalized exfoliative dermatitis frequently affecting neonates and resulting from an initial focal staphylococcal infection (i.e. staphylococcal ophthalmia neonatorum); toxic epidermal necrolysis usually refers to manifestation in the adult secondary to a drug reaction but affects all ages; immunopathogenetic mechanisms probably initiated with drug-skin binding with aberrant immune responses, including complement and immunoglobulin G deposition with the epidermis and mucosa; recent reports suggest that patients with the acquired immunodeficiency syndrome (AIDS) are at higher risk for developing mucocutaneous reactions, such as toxic epidermal necrolysis; mortality rate approximately 30%.

Ocular

Necrotic areas of lids, conjunctiva, and cornea; symblepharon; loss of corneal epithelium; corneal ulcer; leukoma; perforation of globe; abolition of lacrimal secretion; conjunctival chemosis; blepharitis; entropion; periorbital swelling; trichiasis; distichiasis; fornix shortening.

Clinical

Widespread reddening and tenderness of the skin followed by the exfoliation of large areas of skin; in children, erythema starts usually around the mouth and spreads over the entire body within hours, followed by blisters and large exudative lesions; fever; shock.

Laboratory

Culture and biopsy of the lesion.

Treatment

Intravenous penicillinase-resistant and antistaphylococcal antibiotics. Cloxacillin is the treatment of choice.

Bibliography

1. Lopez-Garcia JS, Rivas Jara LR, Garcia-Lozano CI, et al. Ocular features and histopathologic changes during follow-up of toxic epidermal necrolysis. Ophthalmology. 2011;118:265-71.

Additional Resource

1. Kim JH (2012). Dermatologic Manifestations of Staphylococcal Scalded Skin Syndrome. [online] Available from http://www.emedicine.com/derm/TOPIC402.HTM [Accessed April, 2012].

1356. SCAPHOCEPHALY SYNDROME (PAPILLEDEMA)

General

Craniofacial dysostoses with failure in the development of the primitive mesoderm; facial features result from premature fusion of the sagittal cranial suture; males more commonly affected (4:1).

Ocular

Shallow orbits; proptosis; nystagmus; exotropia; aniridia; cataract; papilledema; optic atrophy; aniridia; dislocated lens.

Clinical

Long anteroposterior head diameter; short transverse diameter of the head; increased intracranial pressure; flat forehead with absent superciliary arches; prominent nose; mental retardation.

Laboratory

Plain skull radiograph, ultrasound, CT scan and MRI.

Treatment

Molding therapy (helmets) during the first year and surgical intervention.

Additional Resource

1. Podda S (2011). Craniosynostosis Management. [online] Available from http://www.emedicine.com/plastic/TOPIC534.HTM [Accessed April, 2012].

1357. SCHAFER SYNDROME (KERATOSIS PALMOPLANTARIS SYNDROME; RICHER-HANHART SYNDROME; TYROSINE TRANSAMINASE DEFICIENCY) CORNEAL ULCER

General

Etiology unknown; dominant form manifested as an ectodermal dysplasia with disseminated follicular keratosis and leukokeratosis of the oral mucosa; recessive form also involves cornea; oculocutaneous syndrome; autosomal recessive phenotype associated with tyrosine transaminase deficiency.

Ocular

Dustlike, randomly distributed corneal lesions in the lower portion of the cornea; herpetoid corneal lesions; cataract; herpetiform corneal ulcers.

Clinical

Keratosis of palms and soles; pachyonychia; alopecia; microcephaly; dwarfism; oligophrenia; painful punctate keratoses of digits, palms and soles.

Laboratory

Diagnosis is made by clinical findings.

Treatment

Cataract: Change in glasses can sometimes improve a patient's visual function temporarily; however, the most common treatment is cataract surgery.

Corneal ulcer: Corneal cultures may be taken and treatment initiated. Treatment includes a broad spectrum of antibiotics and cycloplegic drops.

Bibliography

1. Beinfang DC, Kuwabara T, Pueschel SM. The Richer-Hanhart syndrome: report of a case with associated tyrosinemia. Arch Ophthalmol. 1976;94:1133-7.
2. Grayson M. Corneal manifestations of keratosis plantaris and palmaris. Am J Ophthalmol. 1965;59: 483-6.
3. McKusick VA. Mendelian Inheritance in Man: A Catalog of Human Genes and Genetic Disorders, 12th edition. Baltimore: The Johns Hopkins University Press; 1998.
4. McKusick-Nathans Institute for Genetic Medicine, Johns Hopkins University and National Center for Biotechnology Information, National Library of Medicine. (2007). Online Mendelian Inheritance in Man (OMIM). [online] Available from http://www.ncbi.nlm.nih.gov/omim [Accessed April, 2012].
5. Schafer E. Zur Lehre von den Congenitalen Dyskeratosen. Arch Dermatol Syphil (Germ). 1925;148:425.

1358. SCHAUMANN SYNDROME (BESNIER-BOECK-SCHAUMANN SYNDROME; BOECK SARCOID; SARCOIDOSIS)

General

Etiology unknown; theories include tuberculosis, hypersensitivity to pine pollen, virus infection; affects blacks most often; chronic course with spontaneous re-missions (see Heerfordt Syndrome); hilar or paratracheal nodes with erythema nodosum; onset most often in middle and old age; ocular involvement in 20–25% of all cases.

Ocular

Orbital granulomatous mass; bony defects; cutaneous and subcutaneous nodules; myogenic palsy; lacrimal gland adenopathy; decreased tear formation; secondary glaucoma; granulomatous uveitis with iris nodules, cells, and flare; mutton fat keratitic precipitates; keratitis sicca; vitreous floaters; band-shaped keratitis; complicated cataract; inflammatory retinal exudates; "candle wax drippings"; optic nerve atrophy; neuritis; eyelid nodules; ocular nerve enlargement (granuloma).

Clinical

Lymphadenopathy; hilar nodes; fatigue; cystic, punched-out or reticulated changes in small bones (mainly hands and feet); muscle wasting; contractures; weakness in legs and arms.

Laboratory

Chest X-ray, CT scan and MRI of the brain.

Treatment

Glucocorticoids are the treatment of choice.

Additional Resource

1. Sharma GD (2011). Pediatric Sarcoidosis. [online] Available from http://www.emedicine.com/ped/TOPIC2043.HTM [Accessed April, 2012].

1359. SCHEIE SYNDROME (MPS IS; MPS V; MUCOPOLYSACCHARIDOSIS IS; MUCOPOLYSACCHARIDOSIS V)

General

Autosomal recessive; chondroitin sulfate B excreted in excess in the urine; formerly MPS V (see Hurler Syndrome; Hunter Syndrome; Sanfilippo-Good Syndrome; Morquio Syndrome; Maroteaux-Lamy Syndrome). Both sexes affected; deficiency of a-L-iduronidase; increased urinary dermatan and heparan sulfate; fibrous long-spacing collagen on histopathologic examination; least severe form of mucopolysaccharidosis.

Ocular

Night blindness; fields may show general constriction; ring scotomata; diffuse corneal haze to marked corneal clouding (progressive); bushy eyebrows; coarse eyelashes; optic atrophy; anisocoria; cataracts; proptosis; acid mucopolysaccharide deposits in the iris and sclera; tapetoretinal degeneration; glaucoma.

Clinical

Normal intelligence; broad facies; thickened joints; aortic valvular disease; psychosis; claw hand; carpal tunnel syndrome; excessive body hair; progressive juxta-articular cystic lesions.

Laboratory

Thin layer chromatography and radiography.

Treatment

Enzyme replacement therapy. Patients with joint contractures may need surgery. Corneal transplant may be necessary if vision problems are severe.

Additional Resource

1. Banikazemi M (2012). Genetics of Mucopolysaccharidosis Type I. [online] Available from http://www.emedicine.com/ped/TOPIC2052.HTM [Accessed April, 2012].

1360. SCHILDER DISEASE (ENCEPHALITIS PERIAXIALIS DIFFUSA)

General

Lesions situated in the subcortical white matter (area 17); occurs in males; any age; etiology unknown; possibly toxic, infectious, or abiotrophic neural defects.

Ocular

Nystagmus; extraocular muscle palsy, either nuclear or supranuclear; hemianopsia (in occipital lobe involvement); optic nerve, chiasm, and tract involvement can lead to blindness; papilledema; optic neuritis; optic atrophy; central scotomata.

Clinical

Progressive spastic paralysis; progressive mental deterioration; irritability and peevishness; deafness if the temporal lobe becomes involved; tremor; dullness; characteristically bilateral lesions in the brain.

Laboratory

Electroencephalography (EEG)and CSF analysis. MRI and lumbar puncture should be performed.

Treatment

No available treatment at this point.

Additional Resource

1. Rust RS (2012). Diffuse Sclerosis. [online] Available from http://www.emedicine.com/neuro/TOPIC92. HTM [Accessed April, 2012].

1361. SCHISTOSOMIASIS (BILHARZIASIS)

General

Parasitic infection caused by *Schistosoma mansoni*.

Ocular

Hyphema; parasite in anterior chamber; granuloma of conjunctiva, lid, lacrimal gland, and orbit; uveitis; keratitis; iritis; retinitis; dacryoadenitis; cataract; posterior uveitis; choroiditis; blepharitis; optic atrophy.

Clinical

Dermatitis; fever; allergic reaction; short-lasting hepatosplenomegaly, inflammation, granuloma formation, and fibrosis; meningitis; cor pulmonale.

Laboratory

Stool or Urine analysis, egg viability test and liver function test.

Treatment

Praziquantel (Biltricide) drug is the treatment of choice.

Additional Resource

1. Ahmed SH (2011). Schistosomiasis. [online] Available from http://www.emedicine.com/med/ TOPIC2071.HTM [Accessed April, 2012].

1362. SCHIZOPHRENIA

General

Organic brain syndrome due to degeneration or toxic, infectious, or metabolic conditions; acute or insidious onset; disturbances of thinking, mood, and behavior; etiology unknown.

Ocular

Miosis; ocular hallucinations; associated with retinitis pigmentosa in one pedigree; abnormal smooth-pursuit eye movement; visual perceptual dysfunction: low amplitude of accommodation, esophoria or exophoria, and vergence duction suppression.

Clinical

Paranoia; depression; fear; anxiety; catatonia; delusions; hallucinations; misinterpretation of reality; lack of will or enthusiasm; hypochondriasis; preoccupation with own thoughts; meaningless repetitive speech; meaningless repetitive motions; sensorineural deafness; mental retardation associated in one pedigree.

Laboratory

No laboratory results are found.

Treatment

Neuroleptic medication or tranquilizers are used to treat schizophrenia.

Additional Resource

1. Frankenburg FR (2012). Schizophrenia. [online] Available from http://www.emedicine.com/med/TOPIC2072.HTM [Accessed April, 2012].

1363. SCHNYDER'S CRYSTALLINE CORNEAL DYSTROPHY

General

Rare, autosomal dominant disorder with abnormal bilateral deposition of cholesterol and lipid in the cornea.

Clinical

Hypercholesterolemia and genu valgam.

Ocular

Central corneal haze, subepithelial cholesterol crystal deposition, midperipheral, panstromal haze and arcus lipoides.

Laboratory

Serum lipid analysis because hyperlipidemia.

Treatment

Phototherapeutic keratectomy (PTK) can be used to treat subepithelial crystals and penetrating keratoplasty may be necessary.

Additional Resource

1. Weiss JS (2011). Crystalline Dystrophy. [online] Available from http://www.emedicine.com/oph/TOPIC548.HTM [Accessed April, 2012].

1364. SCHOMBERG DISEASE (SUBCONJUNCTIVAL HEMORRHAGE)

General

Blood dyscrasias; associated with thrombocytopenia.

Ocular

Subconjunctival hemorrhage.

Clinical

Petechiae may occur in any tissue; bleeding from any orifice.

Laboratory

Diagnosis is made by clinical findings.

Treatment

None

Bibliography

1. Duke-Elder S (Ed). System of Ophthalmology. St. Louis: CV Mosby; 1976. pp. 33-9.
2. Givner I. Noninfectious conjunctival congestion. In: Infectious Diseases of the Conjunctiva and Cornea. Symposium of the New Orleans Academy of Ophthalmology. St. Louis: CV Mosby; 1963. p. 48.

1365. SCHONENBERG SYNDROME (DWARF-CARDIOPATHY SYNDROME) BLEPHAROPHYMOSIS

General

Consanguinity and familial occurrence; etiology obscure.

Ocular

Blepharophimosis; epicanthal folds; pseudoptosis.

Clinical

Dwarfism (proportionate); congenital heart disease.

Laboratory

Diagnosis is made by clinical findings.

Treatment

None

Bibliography

1. Geeraets WJ. Ocular Syndromes, 3rd edition. Philadelphia: Lea & Febiger; 1976.
2. Schonenberg H. Uber ein Neues Kombinationsbild Multipler Abartungen. (Minderwuchs, Vitium Cordis, Beiderseitige Congenitale Ptose). Ann Pediatr. 1954;182:229.

1366. SCHWARTZ SYNDROME (RETINAL DETACHMENT)

General

Glaucoma associated with retinal detachment; caused by inflammation of trabecula or pigment granules obstructing outflow; photoreceptor outer segments identified in the aqueous humor of patients with this syndrome are thought to playa role in the elevation of intraocular pressure.

Ocular

Secondary open-angle glaucoma; retinal detachment; uveitis; myopia; blepharophimosis; long eyelashes; microcornea.

Clinical

Small stature; myotonia; expressionless facies; joint limitation in hips; dystrophy of epiphyseal cartilage, vertical shortness of vertebrae, short neck; low hairline.

Laboratory

Blood test, muscle biopsy, EMG and nerve conduction studies.

Treatment

Botulinum toxin type A is used to treat problems such as blepharospasm, blepharophimosis and ptosis; surgery may also be necessary.

Additional Resource

1. Ault J (2012). Schwartz-Jampel Syndrome. [online] Available from http://www.emedicine.com/neuro/TOPIC337.HTM [Accessed April, 2012].

1367. SCLERAL RUPTURES AND LACERATIONS

General

Ruptures caused by large, blunt objects that exert pressure on the eye. Lacerations are caused by sharp objects that enter the eye a the point of contact.

Clinical

None

Ocular

Iris prolapse, endophthalmitis, cataract vitreous hemorrhage, hemorrhagic chemosis and decreased visual acuity.

Laboratory

Diagnosis is made on clinical findings.

Treatment

Complete vitrectomy, repair of laceration, systemic and local antibiotic therapy.

Bibliography

1. Roy FH, Fraunfelder FW, Fraunfelder FT. Roy and Fraunfelder's Current Ocular Therapy, 6th edition. Philadelphia: WB Saunders; 2008.

1368. SCLERAL STAPHYLOMAS AND DEHISCENCES

General

Staphylomas may be congenital or acquired. They are anterior or posterior.

Clinical

None

Ocular

Posterior staphylomas are associated with myopia greater than 8 diopters as well as Ehler-Danlos and Marfan syndromes, elevated intraocular pressure.

Laboratory

Diagnosis is made by clinical findings.

Treatment

Lower IOP with topical agents if elevated, consider pars plana vitrectomy internal drainage with endophotocoagulation and air-gas exchange.

Bibliography

1. Roy FH, Fraunfelder FW, Fraunfelder FT. Roy and Fraunfelder's Current Ocular Therapy, 6th edition. Philadelphia: WB Saunders; 2008.

1369. SCLEROCORNEA

General

Autosomal dominant; feature of cornea plana.

Ocular

Malformation of cornea; indistinct limits of cornea and sclera.

Clinical

Found in a patient with monosomy 21; may be found in association with hypertelorism, syndactyly, ambiguous genitalia and epidermolysis bullosa dystrophica.

Laboratory

Diagnosis is made by clinical findings.

Treatment

Check for elevated intraocular pressure. Medical treatment includes the use of hyperosmotic drops, nonsteroidal and steroid eye drops. Corneal transplant may be necessary.

Bibliography

1. Bloch N. Les Differents Types de Sclerocornea, Lewis Modes d'Heredite et les Malformations Congenitales Concornitantes. J Genet Hum. 1965;14:133-72.
2. Doane JF, Sajjadi H, Richardson WP. Bilateral penetrating keratoplasty for sclerocornea in an infant with monosomy 21. Case report and review of the literature. Cornea. 1994;13:454-8.
3. Martinez-Frias ML, Bermejo E, Sánchez Otero T, et al. Sclerocornea, hypertelorism, syndactyly, and ambiguous genitalia. Am J Med Genet. 1994;49:195-7.
4. McKusick VA. Mendelian Inheritance in Man: A Catalog of Human Genes and Genetic Disorders, 12th edition. Baltimore: The Johns Hopkins University Press; 1998.
5. McKusick-Nathans Institute for Genetic Medicine, Johns Hopkins University and National Center for Biotechnology Information, National Library of Medicine. (2007). Online Mendelian Inheritance in Man (OMIM). [online] Available from http://www.ncbi.nlm.nih.gov/omim [Accessed April, 2012].
6. Sharkey JA, Kervick GN, Jackson AJ, et al. Cornea plana and sclerocornea in association with recessive epidermolysis bullosa dystrophica. Case report. Cornea. 1992;11:83-5.

1370. SCLEROMALACIA PERFORNS

General

Scleritis mainly in postmenopausal women with long-standing rheumatoid arthritis.

Clinical

Multiple areas of deep scleral ulceration that coalesce to release uveal tissue.

Ocular

Corneal apeptic, necrosis, pannus and ulceration; limitation of motion, tendonitis, episcleritis, scleritis, anterior staphyloma, cataract retinal vasculitis, secondary glaucoma, uveitis.

Laboratory

Test for rheumatoid arthritis and AIDS.

Treatment

Topical steroid, systemic prednisone, cyclosporine A, reinforce areas of thinned sclera with scleral autograft or preserved sclera.

Bibliography

1. Roy FH, Fraunfelder FW, Fraunfelder FT. Roy and Fraunfelder's Current Ocular Therapy, 6th edition. Philadelphia: WB Saunders; 2008.

1371. SEBACEOUS GLAND CARCINOMA

General

Ocular adnexa contains various sebaceous glands from which carcinomas may arise; predilection for the upper lids but may involve both lids; usually in older age groups; slight female preponderance.

Ocular

Blepharitis; madarosis; meibomianitis; sebaceous carcinoma of lids or orbit; orbital edema; proptosis; conjunctivitis; superficial keratitis; lacrimal gland tumor.

Clinical

Metastasis to preauricular or cervical lymph nodes, or submandibular area.

Laboratory

Biopsy diagnostic in chronic non-healing chalazia or suspicious unresolved chronic blepharitis.

Treatment

Moh's technique appears to have the hightest success rate.

Additional Resource

1. Glassman ML (2012). Sebaceous Gland Carcinoma. [online] Available from http://www.emedicine. com/oph/TOPIC716.HTM [Accessed April, 2012].

1372. SECKEL SYNDROME (ATELIOSIS; BIRD-HEADED DWARF SYNDROME; INTRAUTERINE GROWTH RETARDATION; LOW-BIRTH-WEIGHT DWARFISM; NANOCEPHALIC DWARFISM; PRIMORDIAL DWARFISM; VIRCHOW-SECKEL DWARFISM) EXOTROPIA

General

Autosomal recessive; syndrome shows variations in phenotypic appearance; both sexes affected; present at birth.

Ocular

Widely spaced eyes; incomplete eyebrow; strabismus; horizontal nystagmus; bilateral macular coloboma with pigmentation and umbilicated appearance; disk hypoplasia.

Clinical

Dwarfism; cranial deformity (bird head); developmental anomalies with short arms and clawlike hands; skeletal anomalies with narrow chest and beading of ribs; facial deformities with hypoplasia of maxilla and mandible; beaklike protrusion of central face; sparse hair; absent thumb; malformation of genitourinary tract and rectum; birdlike malformation of the face and further abnormalities; cardiac anomalies; hypophyseal hypoplasia; association with Legg-Calve Perthes disease.

Laboratory

Diagnosis is made by clinical findings.

Treatment

Strabismus: Equalized vision with correct refractive error; surgery may be helpful in patient with diplopia.

Bibliography

1. Di Blasi S, Belvedere M, Pintacuda S, et al. Seckel's syndrome: a case report. J Med. 1993;24:75-96.
2. Geeraets WJ. Ocular Syndromes, 3rd edition. Philadelphia: Lea & Febiger; 1976. p. 389.
3. Rappen U, von Brenndorff AL. Kardiale Symptomatik kei 2 Patienten mit Seckel-Syndrom. Monatschr Kinderheilkd. 1993;141:584-6.
4. Seckel HPC. Bird-Headed Dwarfs. Springfield, IL: Charles C. Thomas; 1960.

1373. SECOND EYE SYNDROME

General

Associated with the second cataract surgery within 1 month of the first.

Ocular

Increased pain during the second surgery.

Laboratory

Diagnosis is made by clinical findings.

Treatment

Iritis: Oral steroids if not responsive to topical steroids, immunosuppressants if bilateral disease that does not respond to oral steroids, periocular steroids for unilateral or posterior uveitis. Vitrectomy can be used for severe vitreous opacification. Cryotherapy and laser photocoagulation may be used for localized pars plana exudates.

Bibliography

1. Mathew MR, Webb LA, Hill R. Surgeon experience and patient comfort during clear corneal phacoemulsificiation under topical local anesthesia. J Cataract Refract Surg. 2002;28:1977-81.
2. O'Brian PD, Fulcher T, Wallace D, et al. Patient pain during different stages of phacoemulsification using topical anesthesia. J Cataract Refract Surg. 2001;27:880-3.

1374. SENTER SYNDROME [CORNEAL INVOLVEMENT, AND DEAFNESS (KERATITIS); KERATITIS-ICHTHYOSIS-DEAFNESS SYNDROME; KID SYNDROME; ICHTHYOSIFORM ERYTHRODERMA]

General

Autosomal recessive.

Ocular

Corneal involvement.

Clinical

Ichthyosiform erythroderma; deafness; hepatomegaly; hepatic cirrhosis; glycogen storage; short stature; mental retardation; hepatitis.

Laboratory

Diagnosis is made by clinical findings.

Treatment

Steroids or Antibiotics may be useful.

Bibliography

1. McKusick VA. Mendelian Inheritance in Man: A Catalog of Human Genes and Genetic Disorders, 12th edition. Baltimore: The Johns Hopkins University Press; 1998.
2. McKusick-Nathans Institute for Genetic Medicine, Johns Hopkins University and National Center for Biotechnology Information, National Library of Medicine. (2007). Online Mendelian Inheritance in Man (OMIM). [online] Available from http://www.ncbi.nlm.nih.gov/omim [Accessed April, 2012].
3. Senter TP, Jones KL, Sakati N, et al. Atypical ichthyosiform erythroderma and congenital neurosensory deafness—a distinct syndrome. J Pediatr. 1978;92:68-72.
4. Wilson GN, Squires RH, Weinberg AG. Keratitis, hepatitis, ichthyosis, and deafness: report and review of KID syndrome. Am J Med Genet. 1991;40:255-9.

1375. SHAKEN BABY SYNDROME (BATTERED-BABY SYNDROME; BATTERED-CHILD SYNDROME; CHILDABUSE SYNDROME; SILVERMAN SYNDROME)

General

Associated with parental abuse or accidents.

Ocular

Exophthalmos with orbital hemorrhages; lid hematoma; lid edema; secondary glaucoma; hyphema; vitreous hemorrhages; retinal exudates and hemorrhages (Berlin edema); choroidal atrophy; retinal detachment; papilledema; optic nerve sheath hemorrhage; preretinal, intraretinal, and subretinal hemorrhages; optic disk edema; choroidal hemorrhage.

Clinical

Soft tissue bruises; multiple fractures of long bones, ribs, and skull; pharyngeal bruising; subdural hematoma; seizures; failure to thrive; vomiting associated with lethargy or drowsiness; respiratory irregularities; coma or death; intracranial hemorrhage.

Laboratory

Computed tomography (CT) of head to quantify degree of head trauma. MRI to define intraparenchymal brain lesions and subdural hematoma skeletal survey detects fractures of bones.

Treatment

Vitreous hemorrage: If possible the source of the bleeding needs to be isolated and treated with laser. Vitrectomy may be necessary.

Retinal detachment: Scleral buckle, pneumatic retinopexy and vitrectomy may be used to close all the breaks.

Orbital hemorrhage: Topical medication to lower intraocular pressure, lateral canthotomy and inferior cantholysis.

Bibliography

1. Budenz DL, Farber MG, Mirchandani HG, et al. Ocular and optic nerve hemorrhages in abused

infants with intracranial injuries. Ophthalmology. 1994;101:559-65.

2. Coody D, Brown M, Montgomery D, et al. Shaken baby syndrome: identification and prevention for nurse practitioners. J Pediatr Health Care. 1994;8:50-6.

3. Lambert SR, Johnson TE, Hoyt CS, et al. Optic nerve sheath and retinal hemorrhages associated with the shaken baby syndrome. Arch Ophthalmol. 1986;104:1509-12.

4. Munger CE, Peiffer RL, Bouldin TW, et al. Ocular and associated neuropathologic observations in suspected whiplash shaken infant syndrome. A retrospective study of 12 cases. Am J Forensic Med Pathol. 1993;14:193-200.

1376. SHAMBERG DISEASE

General

Common benign skin disorder; self-limiting cutaneous vasculitis.

Ocular

Discrete foci of retinal periphlebitis associated with localized intraretinal hemorrhages and exudates; retinal and cutaneous vasculitides wax and wane concurrently; retinal vasculitis is self-limiting cause of visual disturbance and requires no therapy.

Clinical

Purpuric, erythematous patches appear on trunk and extremities; mononuclear perivascular infiltrate of involved skin.

Laboratory

Diagnosis is made by clinical findings.

Treatment

None

Bibliography

1. Bedrick JJ et al. Retinal vasculitis in Shamberg's disease. Ophthalmology. 1982;89:188.

1377. SHIGELLOSIS (BACILLARY DYSENTERY)

General

Caused by Shigellae; frequently passed through food and via food handlers; more commonly seen in countries with poor sanitation; evidence suggests that the ability of Shigellae to invade and multiply within the corneal epithelium is similar to the invasion in the intestinal epithelium.

Ocular

Scleroconjunctivitis; severe uveitis; conjunctival xerosis.

Clinical

Fever; abdominal pain; diarrhea; intestinal perforation; toxic megacolon; dehydration; there has been one case reported of an association with the Klüver-Bucy syndrome.

Laboratory

Stool culture and blood cultures.

Treatment

Oral rehydration and antibiotic treatment.

Additional Resource

1. Kroser JA (2011). Shigellosis. [online] Available from http://www.emedicine.com/med/TOPIC2112.HTM [Accessed April, 2012].

1378. SHORT SYNDROME

General

Autosomal recessive; short stature; hyperextensibility; hernia; ocular depression; Rieger anomaly; teething delay.

Ocular

Sunken eyes; ocular depression; Rieger syndrome; glaucoma.

Clinical

Short stature; hyperextensibility of joints; hernia; low-birth-weight; teething delay; delayed speech development; deafness; diabetes mellitus.

Laboratory

Serum levels, pituitary function, CBC test, wintrobre sedimentation rate, sweat chloride testing, renal and cardiac ultrasonography.

Treatment

Human growth hormone.

Additional Resource

1. Ferry RJ (2010). Short Stature. [online] Available from http://www.emedicine.com/ped/TOPIC2087.HTM [Accessed April, 2012].

1379. SHY-DRAGER SYNDROME (ORTHOSTATIC HYPOTENSION SYNDROME; SHY-MCGEE-DRAGER SYNDROME)

General

Etiology unknown; gradual onset; adults; progressive degeneration of the nervous system.

Ocular

External ophthalmoplegia; iris atrophy; ocular sympathetic and parasympathetic insufficiency (alternating Horner syndrome, cholinergic supersensitivity, decreased lacrimation, and corneal hypesthesia).

Clinical

Orthostatic hypotension; rigidity; tremor; adiadochokinesia; wasting of muscles; mental retardation; impotence; dysphagia; bilateral vocal cord paralysis; neurogenic bladder; anhydrosis; extremity weakness and paresthesia; dizziness; abnormal postural balance.

Laboratory

No laboratory studies are indicated.

Treatment

No effective systemic therapy is known.

Additional Resource

1. Dalvi AI (2012). Striatonigral Degeneration. [online] Available from http://www.emedicine.com/neuro/TOPIC354.HTM [Accessed April, 2012].

1380. SHY-GONATAS SYNDROME

General

Unknown etiology; similar to Hunter and Refsum syndromes; accumulation of lipids in muscles simulates gargoylism; present from birth.

Ocular

Mild proptosis; hypertelorism; ptosis; external ophthalmoplegia (progressive); concentric visual field constriction; keratopathy with possible corneal ulcer; lattice-like white opacities in the area of Bowman's membrane; retinal pigmentary degeneration (atypical retinitis pigmentosa) with difficulties with night vision.

Clinical

Weakness of extremities (proximal); myopathy and neuropathy; cerebellar ataxia.

Laboratory

Diagnosis is made by clinical findings.

Treatment

Ptosis: If visual acuity is affected most cases require surgical correction, and there are several procedures that may be used including levator resection, repair or advancement and Fasanella-Servat.

Corneal ulcer: Corneal cultures may be taken and treatment initiated. Treatment includes a broad spectrum of antibiotics and cycloplegic drops.

Bibliography

1. Geeraets WJ. Ocular Syndromes, 3rd edition. Philadelphia: Lea & Febiger; 1976.
2. Gonatas NK. A generalized disorder of nervous system, skeletal muscle and heart resembling Refsum's disease and Hurler's syndrome. II. Ultrastructure. Am J Med. 1967;42:169-78.
3. Shy GM, Silberberg DH, Appel SH, et al. A generalized disorder of nervous system, skeletal muscle and heart resembling Refsum's disease and Hurler's syndrome. I. Clinical, pathologic and biochemical characteristics. Am J Med. 1967;42:163-8.

1381. SIEGRIST SYNDROME (PIGMENTED CHOROIDAL VESSELS)

General

Rare; more common in females (2:1); malignant hypertension; onset in advanced age.

Ocular

Exophthalmos; granular pigmented spots in the choroid, fairly uniform, following the course of larger choroidal vessels with extension radially toward the periphery; changes related to arteriosclerotic choroidal changes and seen following chorioretinitis of pregnancy and albuminuric choroiditis; Elschnig spots.

Clinical

Hypertension; albuminuria.

Laboratory

Diagnosis is made by clinical findings.

Treatment

None

Bibliography

1. Archer D, Krill AE, Newell FW. Fluorescein studies of choroidal sclerosis. Am J Ophthalmol. 1971;71: 266-85.
2. Deutman AF, Oosterhuis JA, Boen-Tan TN, et al. Acute posterior multifocal placoid pigment epi-theliopathy. Pigment epitheliopathy of choriocap-illaritis? Br J Ophthalmol. 1972;56:863-74.
3. Duke-Elder S (Ed). Textbook of Ophthalmology. St. Louis: CV Mosby; 1941.
4. Schmidt D, Loffer KU. Elschnig's spots as a sign of severe hypertension. Ophthalmologica. 1993;206: 24-8.
5. Siegrist A. Report at the 9th International Congress. Utrecht; 1899. p. 36.

1382. SILENT SINUS SYNDROME

General

Spontaneous enophthalmos and hypoglobus associated with a small, ipsilateral maxillary sinus.

Ocular

Enophthalmos; hypoglobus.

Clinical

Patients usually undergo painless progressive sinking of the eye.

Laboratory

Imaging of maxillary sinus.

Treatment

Sinus surgery.

Bibliography

1. Davidson JK, Soparkar CN, Williams JB, et al. Negative sinus pressure and normal predisease imaging in silent sinus syndrome. Arch Ophthalmol. 1999;117:1653-4.
2. Eto RT, House JM. Enophthalmos, a sequela of maxillary sinusitis. AJNR Am J Neuroradiol. 1995;16:939-41.
3. Kass ES, Salman S, Montgomery WW. Manometric study of complete ostial occlusion in chronic maxillary atelectasis. Laryngoscope. 1996;106:1255-8.
4. Rose, GE, Sandy C, Hallberg L, et al. Clinical and radiologic characteristics of the imploding antrum or silent sinus syndrome. Ophthalmology. 2003;110:811-8.
5. Scharf KE, Lawson W, Shapiro JM, et al. Pressure measurements in the normal and occluded rabbit maxillary sinus. Laryngoscope. 1995;105:570-4.
6. Soparker CN, Patrinely JR, Cuaycong MJ, et al. The silent sinus syndrome. A cause of spontaneous enophthalmos. Ophthalmology. 1994;101:772-8.

1383. SILVER SYNDROME (CONGENITAL HEMIHYPERTROPHY)

General

Muscular hypertrophy of one side of face; etiology unknown; reported association of this condition with a small deletion in chromosome 13.

Ocular

Café-au-lait spots of the lid.

Clinical

Broad forehead; small triangular face; inverted V-shaped mouth; genitourinary abnormalities; precocious puberty; medullary sponge kidney; Wilms tumor.

Laboratory

Patient and parental blood test to evaluate for uniparental disomy of chromosome 7.

Treatment

Growth hormone therapy and physical therapy.

Additional Resource

1. Ferry RJ (2011). Silver-Russell Syndrome. [online] Available from http://www.emedicine.com/ped/TOPIC2099.HTM [Accessed April, 2012].

1384. SIMMONDS SYNDROME (HYPOPITUITARISM SYNDROME)

General

Anterior pituitary gland destroyed by various causes, such as hemorrhage, infarction, injuries or postparturition infections; females; late form of Simmonds syndrome is Snapper-Witts with achlorhydria and subacute combined degeneration, and hypochromic or hyperchromic anemia; onset during postpubertal period.

Ocular

Loss of eyebrow; loss of eyelashes; central scotomata; diabetic retinopathy tends to improve after development of this syndrome; optic nerve atrophy (descending type).

Clinical

Weight loss and generalized weakness (progressive); anorexia; amenorrhea; dry skin and brittle nails; hypotension with bradycardia; anemia; psychosis; loss of libido.

Laboratory

Hormonal studies should be performed such as: ACTH and Cortrosyn stimulation test, TSH and thyroxine, FSH and LH, prolactin and GH provocative test. MRI or computed axial tomography of the pituitary may be helpful.

Treatment

Hormone replacement therapy.

Additional Resource

1. Corenblum B (2011). Hypopituitarism (Panhypopituitarism). [online] Available from http://www.emedicine.com/med/TOPIC1137.HTM [Accessed April, 2012].

1385. SIPPLE SYNDROME (FAMILIAL CHROMAFFINOMATOSIS; MULTIPLE ENDOCRINE NEOPLASIA 2 OR 2A; MULTIPLE ENDOCRINE ADENOMATOSIS 2 OR 2A; MULTIPLE NEUROMA; MEN2 OR MEN2A; MEA2 OR MEA2A; PHEOCHROMOCYTOMA-THYROID MEDULLARY CARCINOMA; PCT)

General

Autosomal dominant; sporadic types have been described; both sexes affected; genetic mapping has assigned the genes responsible for these tumors to the pericentromeric region of chromosome 10.

Ocular

Prominent corneal nerves (rare).

Clinical

Association of medullary thyroid carcinoma and pheochromocytoma; parathyroid tumors; neurofibromas; diabetes mellitus; diarrhea.

Laboratory

Investigation of tumor expansion patterns.

Treatment

Surgery is the treatment of choice, for patients that are unable to undergo surgery, bisphosphonates may be useful.

Additional Resource

1. Lendel I (2010). Wermer Syndrome (MEN Type 1). [online] Available from http://www.emedicine.com/med/TOPIC2404.HTM [Accessed April, 2012].

1386. SJÖGREN-LARSSON SYNDROME (OLIGOPHRENIA ICHTHYOSIS SPASTIC DIPLEGIA SYNDROME)

General

Rare; autosomal recessive; consanguinity; loss of neurons and gliosis throughout gray matter; autosomal recessively inherited disorder characterized by the triad of congenital ichthyosis, spastic diplegia or tetraplegia, and mental retardation.

Ocular

Hypertelorism; ichthyosis of lid; chorioretinitis with macular and perimacular pigment degeneration or bright, glistening intraretinal dots; atypical retinitis pigmentosa; blepharitis; conjunctivitis; keratitis; tan/white areas of retinal pigment epithelium loss; maculopathy.

Clinical

Oligophrenia idiocy; ichthyosis (congenital); spastic disorders; epilepsy; speech defect.

Laboratory

Measurement of FALDH or fatty alcohol: NAD oxidoreductase on cultured skin fibroblast.

Treatment

Moisturizing creams and keratolyct agent, such as alpha-hydroxyacid, salicylic acid, and urea. Standard anticonvulsant are use to treat recurrent seizures. Surgery procedures, such as tendon lengthening, adduction release, dorsal root rhizotomy may help some patients with SLS.

Bibliography

1. van der Veen RL, Fuijkschot J, Willemsen MA, et al. Patients with Sjögren-Larsson syndrome lack macular pigment. Ophthalmology. 2010;117:966-71.

Additional Resource

1. Rizzo WB (2010). Genetics of Sjögren-Larsson Syndrome. [online] Available from http://www.emedicine.com/ped/TOPIC2111.HTM [Accessed April, 2012].

1387. SJÖGREN SYNDROME (GOUGEROT-SJÖGREN SYNDROME; SECRETOINHIBITOR SYNDROME; SICCA SYNDROME)

General

Etiology unknown; autosomal recessive; occurs in women over age 40 years; failure of the lacrimal and conjunctival glands to maintain adequate secretion; similarities exist with Mikulicz syndrome (Mikulicz-Radecki Syndrome); insidious onset; associated with collagen disorders; Epstein-Barr virus infection.

Ocular

Blepharoconjunctivitis; tears show no lysozyme; keratoconjunctivitis sicca; superficial corneal ulcers; thready, tenacious, yellow-white discharge of the conjunctiva; hypertrophy of lacrimal gland; decreased tear secretion with cellular and mucous debris in tear film; cicatrization of cornea and conjunctiva.

Clinical

Dryness of mouth and other mucous membranes; enlarged salivary glands; dysphagia; painless swelling of joints; polyarthritis; dental cavities; vaginitis; laryngitis; rhinitis sicca; hepatomegaly; focal myositis; alopecia; splenomegaly.

Laboratory

Tear osmolarity, fluorecein clearance test and tear function index. Parotid flow rate may determine xerostomia.

Treatment

Artificial tears and lubricating ointments are the treatment of choice. Topical autologous serum eye drops also provide therapeutic benefit.

Additional Resource

1. Aquavella JV (2011). Ophthalmologic Manifestations of Sjögren Syndrome. [online] Available from http://www.emedicine.com/oph/TOPIC477.HTM [Accessed April, 2012].

1388. SKEW DEVIATION SYNDROME (HERTWIG-MAGENDIE SYNDROME)

General

Vascular deficiency involving the brainstem and middle cerebral peduncle; observed after encephalitis, tumors of the cerebellum, and lesions of the labyrinth; this is a vertical strabismus due to a supranuclear lesion; bilateral and alternating skew deviation suggests midbrain or caudal medullar lesion.

Ocular

Alternating paresis of elevators of one eye combined with depressor paresis of the other eye or alternating hyperphorias; in skew deviation the eyes point in diagonally opposite directions; this effect is more pronounced in the eye contralateral to the lesion.

Clinical

Cerebellar ataxia.

Laboratory

Imaging studies of brainstem.

Treatment

Treat the findings.

Bibliography

1. Halmagyi GM. Central eye movement disorders. In: Albert DM, Jakobiec FA (Eds). Principles and Practice of Ophthalmology. Philadelphia: WB Saunders; 1994. p. 2411.
2. Keane JR. Alternating skew deviation: 47 patients. Neurology. 1985;35:725-8.
3. Miller NR. Walsh and Hoyt's Clinical Neuro-Ophthalmology, 6th edition. Baltimore: Williams & Wilkins; 2004.
4. Moster ML, Schatz NJ, Savino PJ, et al. Alternating skew deviation on lateral gaze (bilateral abducting hypertropic). Ann Neurol. 1988;23:190-2.
5. Silfverskiold BP. Skew deviation in Wallersberg's syndrome. Acta Neurol Scand. 1966;41:381-6.

1389. SLEEP APNEA (OBSTRUCTIVE SLEEP APNEA)

General

Interruption of normal breathing during sleep secondary to airway obstruction; life-threatening.

Ocular

Papilledema; optic disk edema; floppy eyelid syndrome, retinal microaneursym, macular edema.

Clinical

Obesity; hypertrophic tonsils and adenoids; excessive daytime sleepiness; snoring with periods of silence; memory loss; headache; increased intracranial pressure; personality changes; oscillopsia; pickwickian syndrome; chronic disequilibrium; increased intracranial pressure.

Laboratory

Thyrotropin hormone level, arterial blood gas should be obtained, if obesity hypoventilation syndrome is suspected. Lateral cephalometry, endoscopy, fluoroscopy, CT scanning, MRI, and radiography are used to identify the site of obstruction.

Treatment

Continuous positive airway pressure (CPAP) and positive pressure therapy is the most prescribed treatment. Weight loss and avoiding the use of sedatives, alcohol, and being in the spine position are useful methods to avoid surgery. Repositioning or advancement of the mandible.

Additional Resource

1. Downey R (2012). Obstructive Sleep Apnea. [online] Available from http://www.emedicine.com/med/TOPIC163.HTM [Accessed April, 2012].

1390. SLIT VENTRICLE SYNDROME

General

Self-limited episodes of shunt malfunction associated with a small or unchanged ventricular system; rare.

Ocular

Esotropia; nystagmus; optic atrophy.

Clinical

Hydroencephalus; headache; nausea and vomiting; altered levels of consciousness.

Laboratory

Check intracranial pressure.

Treatment

Neurological treatment.

Bibliography

1. Nguyen TN, Polomeno RC, Farmer JP, et al. Ophthalmic complications of slit-ventricle syndrome in children. Ophthalmology. 2002;109: 520-4.

1391. SLUDER SYNDROME (LOWER FACIAL NEURALGIA SYNDROME; SPHENOPALATINE GANGLION NEURALGIA SYNDROME)

General

Irritation of the sphenopalatine ganglion; attacks of pain last from minutes to days (see Charlin Syndrome).

Ocular

Severe orbital pain; increased lacrimation during episodes of pain.

Clinical

Unilateral facial pain, mainly root of nose, orbit, and mastoid area; episodes of headaches; nasal congestion.

Laboratory

Diagnosis is made by clinical findings.

Treatment

Identify pain and treat.

Bibliography

1. Geeraets WJ. Ocular Syndromes, 3rd edition. Philadelphia: Lea & Febiger; 1976.
2. Seltzer AP. Facial pain. J Natl Med Assoc. 1971;63:354-6.
3. Sluder G. The role of the sphenopalatine (or Meckel's) ganglion in nasal headaches. N Y Med J. 1908;87:989-90.

1392. SMALLPOX (VARIOLA)

General

Highly contagious cutaneous disease caused by viral infection.

Ocular

Conjunctivitis; keratitis; corneal ulcer; hypopyon; endophthalmitis; congenital corneal clouding; albinotic spots on iris; choroiditis; vitreous opacities; papillitis; extraocular muscle palsies; entropion; dacryocystitis; chorioretinitis; optic neuritis; and vesicles of the eyelid; preauricular adenopathy; eyelid ulcerating pustules; several conditions predispose to the spread of vaccinia, including eczema, hypogammaglobulinemia, steroid therapy and AIDS.

Clinical

Fever, headache and vomiting prior to appearance of the rash on the face, upper trunk and down to the extremities.

Laboratory

Brick-shaped virions viewed with electron microscopy examination, virus culture from live cells, or DNA analysis using polymerase chain reaction and smallpox skin specimen should be collected.

Treatment

No known treatment is effective.

Additional Resource

1. Hussain AN (2011). Smallpox. [online] Available from http://www.emedicine.com/med/TOPIC3545. HTM [Accessed April, 2012].

1393. SMITH-LEMLI-OPITZ SYNDROME (CEREBROHEPATORENAL SYNDROME)

General

Autosomal recessive; similarities with trisomy 18 syndrome; prognosis poor, with death in early infancy (Zellweger Syndrome); onset in fetal life; prevalent in males; reduced myelination in the cerebral hemispheres, cranial nerves, and peripheral nerves secondary to a defective cholesterol biosynthesis.

Ocular

Joining of the eyebrows (synophrys); ptosis (bilateral); pronounced epicanthal folds; strabismus; nystagmus; cataract; optic nerve demyelinization.

Clinical

Mental retardation; microcephaly; hypertonia; low-set ears; high-arched palate; failure to thrive; vomiting; hypospadias; cryptorchidism; metatarsus adductus.

Laboratory

Examination via slit-lamp may reveal strabismus, cataracts, ptosis and/or optic nerve abnormalities. Fetal ultrasonography, sterol analysis, MRI or CT scanning may reveal brain malformations. Renal ultrasonography is used to identify renal anomalies. Abdominal ultrasonography and barium swallow may help rule out pyloric stenosis.

Treatment

No treatment has proven effective for patients with Smith-Lemli-Opitz syndrome.

Additional Resource

1. Steiner RD (2011). Smith-Lemli-Opitz Syndrome. [online] Available from http://www.emedicine. com/ped/TOPIC2117.HTM [Accessed April, 2012].

1394. SMITH-MAGENIS SYNDROME (SMS)

General

Mental retardation, physical dysmorphia and behavior abnormalities due to a deletion at chromosome l7pl1.2.

Ocular

High myopia; retinal detachment; iris anomalies (absent collarette, nasal corectopia, stromal dysplasia); microcornea; strabismus; iris nodules called Wolfflin-Kruckmann spots.

Clinical

Wolfflin-Kruckmann spots may be confused with Brushfield spots, which are seen only in Down's syndrome patients.

Laboratory

DNA analysis of the *FraX* promoter region should be ordered. Karyotype at the 500 band level and FISH probes should also be ordered. Brain MRI, head CT scan and skeletal film.

Treatment

No treatment is available for SMS.

Bibliography

1. Finucane BM, Jaeger ER, Kurtz MB, et al. Eye abnormalities in the Smith-Magenis contiguous gene deletion syndrome. Am J Med Genet. 1993;45:443-6.
2. Barnicoat AJ, Moller HU, Palmer RW, et al. An unusual presentation of Smith-Magenis syndrome with iris dysgenesis. Clin Dysmorphol. 1996;5:153-8.

1395. SMITH SYNDROME (FACIO-SKELETO-GENITAL DYSPLASIA)

General

Autosomal recessive; more common in males.

Ocular

Ptosis; antimongoloid slant; epicanthus.

Clinical

Microcephaly; high-arched palate; large, low-set ears; mental retardation; broad nose; hypoplastic mandible; pedal syndactyly.

Laboratory

Diagnosis is made by clinical findings.

Treatment

Ptosis: If visual acuity is affected most cases require surgical correction, and there are several procedures that may be used including levator resection, repair or advancement and Fasanella-Servat.

Bibliography

1. Aita JA. Congenital Facial Anomalies with Neurologic Defects. Springfield, IL: Charles C. Thomas; 1969. p. 246.
2. Magalini SI, Scrascia E. Dictionary of Medical Syndromes, 2nd edition. Philadelphia: JB Lippincott; 1981.

1396. SNEDDON DISEASE

General

Livedo reticularis; neurologic abnormalities; labile hypertension; apparently autosomal dominant inheritance characterized by a rare potentially severe, arteriooclusive disorder; probably an immunologically mediated disorder leading to the migration and proliferation of smooth cells of small arteries, resulting in partial or complete narrowing of the vessel lumen.

Ocular

Central retinal artery occlusion; visual loss; optic atrophy; visual field defect; cherry-red spot of macula.

Clinical

Diffuse headaches; hemihypesthesia; transient aphasic attack; hemianopsia; reticular blue discoloration of skin; hypertension; transient global amnesia; livedo reticularis; progressive neurologic deterioration; multiple ischemic cerebrovascular episodes; renal cell carcinoma.

Laboratory

Diagnosis is made by clinical findings.

Treatment

Central retinal artery occlusion: Intraocular pressure lowering medications, carbogen therapy, hyperbaric oxygen. Vitrectomy may be necessary.

Bibliography

1. Carella F, Fetoni V, Pollo B, et al. Sneddon's syndrome and renal carcinoma. Case report. Funct Neurol. 1992;7:395-400.

2. Green KM, Lynfield YL, Davis DE. Livedo reticularis with ulcers and circulating immune complexes. Cutis. 1983;31:312-5.

3. Jonas J, Kölble K, Völcker HE, et al. Central retinal artery occlusion in Sneddon's disease associated with antiphospholipid antibodies. Am J Ophthalmol. 1986;102:37-40.

4. Lossos A, Ben-Hur T, Ben-Nariah Z, et al. Familial Sneddon's syndrome. J Neurol. 1995;242: 164-8.

5. Sepp N, Zelger B, Schuler G, et al. Sneddon's syndrome—an inflammatory disorder of small arteries followed by smooth muscle proliferation. Immunohistochemical and ultrastructural evidence. Am J Surg Pathol. 1995;19:448-53.

6. Sneddon IB. Cerebrovascular lesions and livedo reticularis. Br J Dermatol. 1965;77:180-5.

1397. SNOWFLAKE VITREORETINAL DEGENERATION

General

Autosomal dominant; very small yellow-white dots on the retina.

Ocular

Fibrillar vitreous degeneration; thickening of cortical vitreous; optically empty vitreous cavity; vitreous hemorrhage; posterior vitreous detachment with collapse; retinal detachment; retinal hemorrhage; retinal holes; marked retinal pigmentation; obliterated retinal vessels; sheathed retinal vessels; preretinal retraction; chorioretinal atrophy; corneal opacities; myopia; hyperopia; astigmatism; amblyopia; cataract; glaucoma.

Clinical

None

Laboratory

Diagnosis is made by clinical findings.

Treatment

Retinal detachment: Scleral buckle, pneumatic retinopexy and vitrectomy may be used to close all the breaks.

Bibliography

1. Gheiler M, Pollack A, Uchenik D, et al. Hereditary snowflake vitreoretinal degeneration. Birth Defects Orig Artic Ser. 1982;18:577-80.

2. McKusick VA. Mendelian Inheritance in Man: A Catalog of Human Genes and Genetic Disorders, 12th edition. Baltimore: The Johns Hopkins University Press; 1998.

3. McKusick-Nathans Institute for Genetic Medicine, Johns Hopkins University and National Center for Biotechnology Information, National Library of Medicine. (2007). Online Mendelian Inheritance in Man (OMIM). [online] Available from http://www.ncbi.nlm.nih.gov/omim [Accessed April, 2012].

1398. SNUFF-OUT SYNDROME (SNUFF SYNDROME)

General

Rare; sudden vision loss following ocular or laser surgery in patients with advanced glaucoma; etiology unknown, but probably involves several factors, including unrecognized increased intra-ocular pressure, sudden hypotony, nerve injury, or retrobulbar anesthesia.

Ocular

Loss of central fixation; reduction in visual acuity; reduction in visual field; cataract; glaucoma.

Clinical

None

Laboratory

Diagnosis is made by clinical findings.

Treatment

Glaucoma: Its medication should be the first plan of action. If medication is unsuccessful, a filtering surgical procedure with or without antimetabolites may be beneficial. Careful moni-toring in individuals with large cupping and visual field loss is important.

Bibliography

1. Harrington DO (Ed). The Visual Fields: A Textbook and Atlas of Clinical Perimetry, 5th edition. St. Louis: CV Mosby; 1981.
2. Kolker AE. Visual prognosis in advanced glau-coma: a comparison of medical and surgical therapy for retention of vision in 101 eyes with advanced glaucoma. Trans Am Ophthalmol Soc. 1977;75:539-55.
3. Lichter PR, Ravin JG. Risks of sudden visual loss after glaucoma surgery. Am J Ophthalmol. 1974;78:1009-13.
4. Sharma N, Ooi JL, Francis IC, et al. Sudden visual loss after uneventful cataract surgery: Snuff syndrome. J Cataract Refract Surg. 2004;30:2435-7.

1399. SOLAR RETINOPATHY

General

Photochemical injury to the retina.

Clinical

None

Ocular

Central scotoma, micron lamellar defect.

Laboratory

Optical coherence tomography (OCT) can be normal or tiny hyper-reflective spots.

Treatment

No effective treatment is available.

Bibliography

1. Roy FH, Fraunfelder FW, Fraunfelder FT. Roy and Fraunfelder's Current Ocular Therapy, 6th edition. Philadelphia: WB Saunders; 2008.

1400. SORSBY I SYNDROME (HEREDITARY MACULAR COLOBOMA SYNDROME)

General

Autosomal dominant; related to Laurence-Moon-Bardet-Biedl and Biemond syndromes; apical dystrophy of the extremities and bilateral macular colobomata; both sexes affected; onset from birth.

Ocular

Hypermetropia; nystagmus; bilateral macular colobomata with various degrees of pigmentation but sharply lined borders.

Clinical

Distal dystrophy of the hands and feet; rudimentary or absent index fingernails; absence of big toe; cleft palate.

Laboratory

Diagnosis is made by clinical findings.

Treatment

None

Bibliography

1. Francois J. Heredity in Ophthalmology. St. Louis: CV Mosby; 1961. p. 694.
2. Magalini SI, Scrascia E. Dictionary of Medical Syndromes, 2nd edition. Philadelphia: JB Lippincott; 1981.
3. Sorsby A. Congenital coloboma of the macula: together with an account of the familial occurrence of bilateral macular coloboma in association with apical dystrophy of hands and feet. Br J Ophthalmol. 1935;19:65-90.

1401. SORSBY II SYNDROME (SORSBY MACULAR DYSTROPHY)

General

Both sexes affected; onset in the third and fourth decades of life.

Ocular

Retinal hemorrhages; retinal exudates; chorioretinitis; macular dystrophy.

Clinical

None

Laboratory

Diagnosis is made by clinical findings.

Treatment

Retinal hemorrhage: If possible the source of the bleeding needs to be isolated and treated with laser. Vitrectomy may be necessary.

Chorioretinitis: Topical, systemic and regional steroids may be useful. Cyclosporine, ketoconazole and other immunomodulatory therapies may also be necessary.

Bibliography

1. Magalini SI, Scrascia E. Dictionary of Medical Syndromes, 2nd edition. Philadelphia: JB Lippincott; 1981.
2. Sorsby A. The dystrophies of the macula. Br J Ophthalmol. 1940;24:469-484.25.

1402. SORSBY III SYNDROME (SORSBY FUNDUS DYSTROPHY)

General

Both sexes are affected; onset in the fifth decade of life; autosomal dominant; mutations in the tissue inhibitor of metalloproteinases-3 have been associated with this condition; condition has been genetically linked to chromosome 22q 13-qter.

Ocular

Retinal hemorrhages; retinal exudates; retinal pigmentary deposits; choroid atrophy; choroidal neovascularization; abnormal color vision; generalized fine granularity of the retinal pigment epithelium and peripheral iris transillumination.

Clinical

None

Laboratory

Diagnosis is made by clinical findings.

Treatment

Retinal hemorrhage: If possible the source of the bleeding needs to be isolated and treated with laser. Vitrectomy may be necessary.

Bibliography

1. Magalini SI, Scrascia E. Dictionary of Medical Syndromes, 2nd edition. Philadelphia: JB Lippincott; 1981.
2. Sorsby A et al. A fundus dystrophy with unusual features (late onset and dominant inheritance of central retinal lesion showing edema, hemorrhage and exudates developing into generalized choroidal atrophy with massive pigment proliferation). Br J Ophthalmol. 1949;33:67-100.
3. Weber BH, Vogt G, Pruett RC, et al. Mutations in the tissue inhibitor of metalloproteinases-3 (TIMP3) in patients with Sorsby's fundus dystrophy. Nat Genet. 1994;8:352-6.
4. Wu G, Pruett RC, Baldinger J, et al. Hereditary hemorrhagic macular dystrophy. Am J Ophthalmol. 1991;111:294-301.

1403. SOTOS SYNDROME (CEREBRAL GIGANTISM)

General

Idiopathic disturbance of the diencephalon; etiology unknown; cerebral gigantism in childhood, Russell syndrome, and total lipodystrophy are related forms of the same entity.

Ocular

Hypertelorism; antimongoloid lid aperture; high refractive error (hyperopia); nystagmus; strabismus.

Clinical

Acromegaly; large skull with frontal bossing; mental retardation; incoordination; abnormal excessive growth, mainly during the first 2 years of life.

Laboratory

Diagnosis is made by clinical findings.

Treatment

Strabismus: Equalized vision with correct refractive error; surgery may be helpful in patient with diplopia.

Bibliography

1. Maino DM, Kofman J, Flynn MF, et al. Ocular manifestations of Sotos syndrome. J Am Optom Assoc. 1994;65:339-46.

2. Milunsky A, Cowie VA, Donoghue EC. Cerebral gigantism in childhood. A report of two cases and a review of the literature. Pediatrics. 1967;40:395-402.
3. Sotos JF, Dodge PR, Muirhead D, et al. Cerebral gigantism in childhood. A syndrome of excessively rapid growth with acromegalic features and a nonprogressive neurologic disorder. N Engl J Med. 1964;271:109-16.
4. Yeh H, Price RL, Lonsdale D. Cerebral gigantism (Sotos' syndrome) and cataracts. J Pediatr Ophthalmol Strabismus. 1978;15:231-2.

1404. SPANLANG-TAPPEINER SYNDROME (KERATOSIS PALMOPLANTARIS AND CORNEAL DYSTROPHY SYNDROME)

General

Autosomal dominant; etiology unknown; occurs in both sexes; onset age is 5–20 years; linear palmar and diffuse plantar keratosis with dystrophy of the cornea.

Ocular

Corneal opacities (yellowish, tongue-shaped, and not always involving the center of the cornea).

Clinical

Hyperkeratosis of palms and soles; nail dystrophy; hyperhidrosis.

Laboratory

Diagnosis is made by clinical findings.

Treatment

Bandage soft contact lenses, corneal graft (rare), and sodium chloride hypertonic ophthalmic solutions.

Additional Resource

1. Coupal DJ (2010). Posterior Polymorphous Corneal Dystrophy. [online] Available from http://www.emedicine.com/oph/TOPIC768.HTM [Accessed April, 2012].

1405. SPASMUS NUTANS SYNDROME

General

Etiology unknown; both sexes affected; onset between ages 6 and 18 months; disappears during sleep; aggravated by cold weather; spontaneous disappearance by age of 3 or 4 years; it is not clear whether head nodding is a compensatory mechanism to control the nystagmus or an involuntary movement of pathologic origin.

Ocular

Bilateral nystagmus; attempt at gaze fixation intensifies manifestations.

Clinical

Rhythmic movements of head in upright position.

Laboratory

Diagnosis is made by clinical findings.

Treatment

Baclofen for adults only. Retrobulbar or intramuscular injection of botulinum toxin provides temporarily relief. Strabismus surgery may be necessary in certain forms of nystagmus.

Additional Resource

1. Curtis T (2010). Nystagmus, Congenital. [online] Available from http://www.emedicine.com/oph/TOPIC688.HTM [Accessed April, 2012].

1406. SPASTIC PARAPLEGIA, OPTIC ATROPHY, DEMENTIA

General

Autosomal dominant.

Ocular

Pallor of optic disk; constricted visual fields; optic atrophy; visible deficit in retinal fiber layer; deficit in color vision; slight decrease in visual acuity; pupillary reflex sluggishness to light.

Clinical

Dementia; spastic paraparesis; stiff gait; increased deep tendon reflexes; bilateral extensor plantar responses; euphoria; pseudobulbar speech; incontinence.

Laboratory

Erythrocyte sedimentation rate (ESR), C-reactive protein (CRP).

Treatment

Control of blood pressure and diabetes. In giant cell arteritis, systemic steroids are used.

Additional Resource

1. Younge BR (2012). Anterior Ischemic Optic Neuropathy. [online] Available from http://www.emedicine.com/oph/TOPIC161.HTM [Accessed April, 2012].

1407. SPASTIC PARAPLEGIA, X-LINKED (SPPX)

General

X-linked; early onset; slow progression and long survival with eventual involvement of the cerebellum, cerebral cortex and optic nerves.

Ocular

Nystagmus; optic atrophy; poor vision; cataracts; convergent strabismus; red-green color vision defects.

Clinical

Spastic paraplegia; athetosis; mental retardation; dysarthria, ankle clonus; clubfeet; slow speech; spasticity of the legs; hyperactive reflexes; bilateral Babinski signs; toe walking; bilateral pes cavus; knee clonus; upward plantar reflexes; urinary incontinence; recurrent urinary infection; hematuria; progressive spastic gait disorder; hyperreflexia.

Laboratory

Genetic loci, preliminary genotype-phenotype, MRI and electrophysiologic studies are useful.

Treatment

Regular physical therapy is important.

Additional Resource

1. Paik NJ (2012). Hereditary Spastic Paraplegia. [online] Available from http://www.emedicine.com/pmr/TOPIC45.HTM [Accessed April, 2012].

1408. SPASTIC QUADRIPLEGIA, RETINITIS PIGMENTOSA, MENTAL RETARDATION

General

Autosomal recessive; consanguineous parents.

Ocular

Granular pigmented retina; pale optic disk; retinal degeneration; exotropia; miotic pupils; ptosis; nystagmus; small optic disk; retinitis pigmentosa.

Clinical

Expressionless face; drooling; spastic contractures; scissoring; spastic gait; mental retardation; brachydactyly; hypoplasia; tremors; hearing impairment.

Laboratory

Fluorescent treponemal antibody absorption test, inherited/syndromic disease lab test, neoplasm related lab test and optical coherence tomography (OCT) can be helpful.

Treatment/Ocular

Antioxidants may be useful, very high daily doses of vitamin A palmitate slow the progress of RP, beta-carotene have been recommended.

Additional Resource

1. Telander DG (2012). Retinitis Pigmentosa. [online] Available from http://www.emedicine.com/oph/TOPIC704.HTM [Accessed April, 2012].

1409. SPATIAL VISUALIZATION APTITUDE

General

Sex-linked; more prevalent in males.

Ocular

Aptitude for visualizing space.

Clinical

None

Laboratory

Diagnosis is made by clinical findings.

Treatment

None

Bibliography

1. McKusick VA. Mendelian Inheritance in Man: A Catalog of Human Genes and Genetic Disorders, 12th edition. Baltimore: The Johns Hopkins University Press; 1998.
2. McKusick-Nathans Institute for Genetic Medicine, Johns Hopkins University and National Center for Biotechnology Information, National Library of Medicine. (2007). Online Mendelian Inheritance in Man (OMIM). [online] Available from http://www.ncbi.nlm.nih.gov/omim [Accessed April, 2012].
3. Stafford RE. Sex differences in spatial visualization as evidence of sex-linked inheritance. Percept Mot Skills. 1961;13:428.

1410. SPHENOCAVERNOUS SYNDROME

General

Lesion in the cavernous sinus; similar to the superior orbital fissure syndrome (Rochon-Duvigneaud) and orbital apex syndrome (Rochon-Duvigneaud Syndrome).

Ocular

Proptosis; edema; paresis of cranial nerves III, IV and VI (paralysis of the abducens nerve precedes paralysis of the oculomotor nerve, because the abducens is situated between the internal carotid artery and the cavernous sinus wall); conjunctival edema.

Clinical

Paresis of the first (sometimes second and third) division of cranial nerve V; sinusitis.

Treatment

Proptosis: Ocular lubricants are beneficial for control of the corneal exposure.

Paresis of cranial nerves III: Prism therapy, surgical—muscle surgery on the affected muscle, occlusion of the involved eye to relieve diplopia.

Bibliography

1. Geeraets WJ. Ocular Syndromes, 3rd edition. Philadelphia: Lea & Febiger; 1976. p. 404.
2. Jefferson G. Concerning injuries, aneurysms and tumors involving the cavernous sinus. Trans Ophthalmol Soc UK. 1953;73:117-52.
3. Sekhar LN, Linskey ME, Sen CN, et al. Surgical management of lesions within the cavernous sinus. Clin Neurosurg. 1991;37:440-89.
4. Watson NJ, Dick AD, Hutchinson CH. A case of sinusitis presenting with spheno-cavernous syndrome: discussion of the differential diagnosis. Scott Med J. 1991;36:179-80.

1411. SPHENOMAXILLARY FOSSA SYNDROME (PTERYGOPALATINE FOSSA SYNDROME)

General

Malignant tumor, second division of which involves the sphenopalatine fossa, causing paralysis of cranial nerve V; similar to Trotter syndrome with unilateral deafness, mandibular pain, facial pain, defective mobility of the palate and trismus.

Ocular

Infraorbital anesthesia; optic nerve atrophy.

Clinical

Maxillary neuralgia with pain in the upper teeth; mandibular pain; displaced jaw toward involved side because of pterygoid muscle paralysis; deafness (middle ear, ipsilateral).

Laboratory

Blood test, CT scan and MRI are helpful in the diagnosis.

Treatment/Ocular

Optic nerve atrophy: Corticosteroids are useful in the this treatment.

Bibliography

1. Ford FR, Walsh FB. Raeder's paratrigeminal syndrome: a benign disorder, possibly a complication of migraine. Bull Johns Hopkins Hosp. 1958;103:296-8.
2. Klossek JM, Ferrie JC, Goujon JM, et al. Endoscopic approach of the pterygopalatine fossa: report of one case. Rhinology. 1994;32:208-10.
3. Magalini SI, Scrascia E. Dictionary of Medical Syndromes, 2nd edition. Philadelphia: JB Lippincott; 1981.

1412. SPIDER BITES

General

Venom of several different spiders can cause systemic poisoning in humans.

Ocular

Conjunctivitis; subconjunctival hemorrhages; conjunctival chemosis; lid edema; lid gangrene; necrosis of lid; ptosis; pupil constriction; retinal cyanosis; visual loss.

Clinical

Localized itching; vesicle and necrosis of tissue; secondary infection; abdominal rigidity; headache; sweating; nausea; facial congestion.

Laboratory

No laboratory tests are specific.

Treatment

For mild lesions, antibiotics and antihistamines are used.

Additional Resource

1. Bush SP (2010). Widow Spider Envenomation. [online] Available from http://www.emedicine. com/oph/TOPIC652.HTM [Accessed April, 2012].

1413. SPINA BIFIDA (RACHISCHISIS)

General

Defect of the bony spinal canal without defect of cord or meninges; myelocele sac containing meninges may protrude; failure of neural tube of embryo to close and separate from surface ectoderm.

Ocular

Anophthalmos; microphthalmos; choroidal coloboma; aplasia of retinal ganglion cells and optic nerve; macular aplasia; Horner syndrome; strabismus; lateral rectus palsy; papilledema; optic nerve atrophy.

Clinical

Progressive motor, sensory, vasomotor, and trophic disturbances; hydrocephalus.

Laboratory

Computer tomography, radiographs and MRI are important in the evaluation.

Treatment

Prolonged physical therapy.

Additional Resource

1. Foster MR (2011). Spina Bifida. [online] Available from http://www.emedicine.com/orthoped/ TOPIC557.HTM [Accessed April, 2012].

1414. SPINOCEREBELLAR ATROPHY WITH PUPILLARY PARALYSIS

General

Autosomal dominant; rare.

Ocular

Absence of pupillary reaction to light or convergence.

Clinical

Spinocerebellar atrophy.

Laboratory

Diagnosis is made by clinical findings.

Treatment

None

Bibliography

1. McKusick VA. Mendelian Inheritance in Man: A Catalog of Human Genes and Genetic Disorders, 12th edition. Baltimore: The Johns Hopkins University Press; 1998.
2. McKusick-Nathans Institute for Genetic Medicine, Johns Hopkins University and National Center for Biotechnology Information, National Library of Medicine. (2007). Online Mendelian Inheritance in Man (OMIM). [online] Available from http://www.ncbi.nlm.nih.gov/omim [Accessed April, 2012].
3. Sutherland JM et al. Atrophic Spino-Cerebelleuse (HDSC) Familiale avec Mydriase Fixe. Rev Neurol. 1963;108:439-42.

1415. SPINOCEREBELLAR DEGENERATION AND CORNEAL DYSTROPHY (CORNEAL CEREBELLAR SYNDROME; CORNEAL DYSTROPHY WITH SPINOCEREBELLAR DEGENERATION)

General

Autosomal recessive; consanguineous parents.

Ocular

Corneal opacification; thickened Descemet's membrane; degeneration of pannus; congenital cataracts; myopia; tilted optic disks.

Clinical

Mental retardation; progressive cerebellar abnormalities with variable dorsal column lesions; upper motor neuron involvement; histologic muscle abnormalities.

Laboratory

Diagnosis is made via slit-lamp examination.

Treatment

Treatment is based on the severity of the corneal decomposition. Hyperosmotic drops and ointments are used when corneal edema with corneal failure is present. Bandage contact lenses are used only as a temporary measure.

Bibliography

1. Der Kaloustian VM, Jarudi NI, Khoury MJ, et al. Familial spinocerebellar degeneration with corneal dystrophy. Am J Med Genet. 1985;20:325-39.
2. McKusick VA. Mendelian Inheritance in Man: A Catalog of Human Genes and Genetic Disorders, 12th edition. Baltimore: The Johns Hopkins University Press; 1998.
3. McKusick-Nathans Institute for Genetic Medicine, Johns Hopkins University and National Center for Biotechnology Information, National Library of

Medicine. (2007). Online Mendelian Inheritance in Man (OMIM). [online] Available from http://www.ncbi.nlm.nih.gov/omim/ [Accessed April, 2012].

4. Mousa AR, Al-Din AS, Al-Nassar KE, et al. Autosomally inherited recessive spastic ataxia, macular corneal dystrophy, congenital cataracts, myopia and vertically oval temporally tilted discs. Report of a Bedouin family—a new syndrome. J Neurol Sci. 1986;76:105-21.

1416. SPONGY DEGENERATION OF THE WHITE MATTER (CANAVAN DISEASE; VAN BOGAERT-BERTRAND SYNDROME)

General

Neurologic disorder of childhood; Jews; familial; autosomal recessive; this is a severe leukodystrophy caused by the deficiency of aspartoacylase (ASPA) and accumulation of N-acetylaspartic acid; a missense mutation recently was identified in the human ASPA coding sequence from patients with this disorder.

Ocular

Optic atrophy; nystagmus; strabismus; roving eye movements.

Clinical

Progressive megalocephaly; psychomotor deterioration; death.

Laboratory

Blood test, CT scans and MRI are essential in the evaluation and diagnosis.

Treatment

Corticosteroids are useful. Excision or decompression is needed when orbital tumors compress the optic nerve.

Bibliography

1. Cogan DG. Ocular manifestations of spongy degeneration. Birth Defects Orig Artic Ser. 1976;12:527-34.
2. Evans OB. Inborn errors of metabolism of the nervous system: Canavan's disease. In: Bradley WG (Ed). Neurology in Clinical Practice, 2nd edition. Boston: Butterworth-Heinemann; 1995. p. 1506.
3. Fenichel GM. Spongy degeneration of infancy (Canavan). In: Fenichel GM (Ed). Clinical Pediatric Neurology, 2nd edition. Philadelphia: WB Saunders; 1993. p. 136.
4. Harley RD (Ed). Pediatric Ophthalmology, 4th edition. Philadelphia: WB Saunders; 1998.

1417. SPORADIC CRETINISM (CONGENITAL HYPOTHYROIDISM)

General

Variable, from complete lack of thyroid function to reduced function because of enzyme defects; endemic in particular areas (Crete, Beotia, Alpine Valley); affects both sexes; occurs at birth; normal physical and mental development possible with correct treatment.

Ocular

Nystagmus;

Clinical

Excessive weight; lethargy; facies with heavy expression; large tongue; open mouth; drooling; yellowish tint on cheeks; hypothermia; altered tone of voice; persistent neonatal jaundice; protuberant stomach; umbilical hernia; dry skin; coarse hair; failure to thrive; poor appetite; constipation; cardiomegaly; slow pulse; delayed sexual development; dwarfism; imbecility; reported coexistence with the CHARGE association (bilateral papillary coloboma, congenital heart disease, dysmorphic ears, sensorineural deafness, psychomotor retardation, cryptorchidism, facial palsy and vesicoureteral reflux).

Laboratory

Confirm levels of serum thyroid hormone. Thyroid scanning and ultrasonography may be useful.

Treatment

Early diagnose and thyroid hormone replacement is the primary treatment for congenital hypothyroidism.

Additional Resource

1. Postellon DC (2011). Congenital Hypothyroidism. [online] Available from http://www.emedicine.com/ped/TOPIC501.HTM [Accessed April, 2012].

1418. SPOROTRICHOSIS

General

Chronic fungal infection caused by *Sporothrix schenckii*; lesion usually occurs on exposed skin and is characterized by nodules or pustules that may develop into small ulcers; infectious agent usually gains entrance into the skin by traumatic implantation of soil or plant materials; disseminated sporotrichosis is uncommon, usually occurring in alcoholics or immunosuppressed patients.

Ocular

Conjunctivitis; keratitis; corneal ulcer; blepharitis; endophthalmitis; iris atrophy; dacryocystitis; osteitis; periosteitis; scleritis; erosion of bony walls of the orbit.

Clinical

Enlargement of regional lymph nodes; pulmonary lesions; granulomas in the joints and genitourinary system.

Laboratory

Cultured on Sebouraud dextrose agar, cream-colored to black, folded and leathery.

Treatment

Potassium iodide drops as a saturated solution is the treatment of choice. Amphotericin B may be necessary in more severe forms with visceral and intraocular or orbital involvement.

Additional Resource

1. Greenfield RA (2012). Sporotrichosis. [online] Available from http://www.emedicine.com/med/TOPIC2161.HTM [Accessed April, 2012].

1419. SPRENGEL SYNDROME (HIGH SCAPULA CONGENITA)

General

Etiology unknown; nonprogressive.

Ocular

Hypertelorism

Clinical

One scapula short in vertical axis and wider in transverse and closer to the midline than the other scapula; scoliosis; torticollis; vertebral malformations.

Laboratory/Ocular

Diagnosis is made by clinical findings.

Treatment

None

Bibliography

1. Beals RK, Robbins JR, Rolfe B. Anomalies associated with vertebral malformations. Spine. 1993;18:1329-32.
2. Magalini SI, Scrascia E. Dictionary of Medical Syndromes, 2nd edition. Philadelphia: JB Lippincott; 1981.
3. Sprengel AE. Die Angeborene Verschiebung des Schulterblattes Nach Oben. Arch Klin Chir (Berlin). 1891;42:545-9.

1420. SQUAMOUS CELL CARCINOMA OF EYELID

General

Relatively rare periocular malignancy which usually occurs in the lower eyelid.

Clinical

None

Ocular

Tumor of the eyelid.

Laboratory

Careful biopsy and histologic examination.

Treatment

Systemic or intralesional chemotherapy, or both has been effective when used in conjunction with surgery or radiation.

Additional Resource

1. Monroe M (2011). Head and Neck Cutaneous Squamous Cell Carcinoma. [online] Available from http://www.emedicine.medscape.com/article/1212601-overview [Accessed April, 2012].

1421. SQUAMOUS CELL CARCINOMA, CONJUNCTIVAL

General

Malignant epithelial neoplasm characterized by basement membrane invation or distant metastasis. Believed to arise from limbal stem cells and present as a mass in the interpalpebral fissure. Seen more frequently in caucasians and individuals with exposure to sunlight but multiple infectious agents may play a role in the development. Human papilloma virus, HIV, actinic exposure, the use of petroleum products, cigarette smoking may also be factors.

Clinical

Human papilloma virus, HIV, actinic exposure, the use of petroleum products, cigarette smokers.

Ocular

Gelatinous and velvety papilliform or leukoplakic mass on the nasal or temporal limbal area; irritation, chronic conjunctivitis.

Laboratory

Excisional biopsy is used to make positive diagnosis.

Treatment

Excisional biopsy is the treatment of choice. Careful monitoring is necessary to look for orbital invasion. Oncologist should be consulted if metastatic disease is suspected.

Additional Resource

1. Monroe M (2011). Head and Neck Cutaneous Squamous Cell Carcinoma. [online] Available from http://www.emedicine.medscape.com/article/1192041-overview [Accessed April, 2012].

1422. STANESCO SYNDROME (OSTEOCHONDROSIS-OSTEOPETROSIS; STANESCO DYSOSTOSIS SYNDROME)

General

Autosomal dominant; present from birth; both sexes are affected.

Ocular

Exophthalmos

Clinical

Small stature; brachycephaly; depression at frontoparietal sutures; narrow maxilla; small mandible; crowded teeth; exostoses; fractures.

Laboratory/Ocular

Thyroid function test is recommended. Complete blood counts, blood and nasal cultures in patients with orbital cellulitis is advised. CT scan, X-rays, MRI and ocular ultrasonography are recommended.

Treatment/Ocular

Ocular lubricants are recommended to prevent dryness.

Bibliography

1. McKusick VA. Mendelian Inheritance in Man: A Catalog of Human Genes and Genetic Disorders, 12th edition. Baltimore: The Johns Hopkins University Press; 1998.
2. McKusick-Nathans Institute for Genetic Medicine, Johns Hopkins University and National Center for Biotechnology Information, National Library of Medicine. (2007). Online Mendelian Inheritance in Man (OMIM). [online] Available from http://www.ncbi.nlm.nih.gov/omim/ [Accessed April, 2012].
3. Stanesco V et al. Syndrome Hereditaire Dominant Reussissant une Dyostose Cranio-Faciale de Type Particulier, Une Insuffisance de Croissance d' Aspect Chondrodystrophlque et un Epaississement Massif de la Corticale des Os Longs. Rev Fr Endocrinol Clin. 1963;4:219-31.

1423. STANNUS CEREBELLAR SYNDROME

General

Vitamin B (riboflavin) deficiency.

Ocular

Nystagmus; increased lacrimation; asthenopia; blepharitis; angular conjunctivitis; iris nodules; perilimbal vasodilation and pigmentation; corneal vascularization; superficial, diffuse keratitis; epithelial edema and corneal opacities; cataracts; brownish retinal patches.

Clinical

Muscular asthenia; hypotonia; ataxia; dysdiadochokinesia; mucocutaneous lesions resembling monilial intertrigo and glossitis.

Treatment

Nystagmus: See-saw nystagmus—visual field to consider neoplastic or vascular etiologies. Upbeat nystagmus—may indicate multiple sclerosis, cerebellar degeneration, tumors or infarcts. Treatment is directed toward identification and resolution of underlying cause. Downbeat nystagmus—affects the cerebellum or craniocervical junction including Arnold-Chiari malformation, multiple sclerosis, trauma, tumor, infarction and many toxic metabolic entities. MRI may indicate a surgically correctable lesion. Periodic alternating nystagmus is continuous horizontal nystagmus from stroke, tumor, multiple sclerosis, trauma, infection and drug intoxication. Can occur from cataract, vitreous hemorrhage or optic atrophy.

Corneal vascularization: Check for elevated intraocular pressure. Medical treatment includes the use of hyperosmotic drops, nonsteroidal and steroid eye drops. Corneal transplant may be necessary.

Cataract: Change in glasses can sometimes improve a patient's visual function temporarily; however, the most common treatment is cataract surgery.

Bibliography

1. Osuntokun BO, Langman MJ, Wilson J, et al. Controlled trial of combinations of hydroxocobalamin-cystine and riboflavin-cystine, in Nigerian ataxic neuropathy. J Neurol Neurosurg Psychiatry. 1974;37:102-4.
2. Roe DA. Riboflavin deficiency: mucocutaneous signs of acute and chronic deficiency. Semin Dermatol. 1991;10:293-5.
3. Stannus HS. Problems in riboflavin and allied deficiencies-I. Br Med J. 1944;2:103-5.
4. Stannus HS. Problems in riboflavin and allied deficiencies-II. Br Med J. 1944;2:140-4.

1424. STAPHYLOCOCCUS

General

Gram-positive coccus *Staphylococcus aureus*; most common cause of suppurative infection in humans; more common in patients with a previous disorder, such as diabetes, thyroid disease, renal failure, or malnutrition; although most *S. aureus* isolates from other sources are encapsulated, capsules have not been noted in ocular isolates.

Ocular

Uveitis; hypopyon; conjunctivitis; keratitis; cellulitis of lid; meibomianitis; ptosis; blepharitis; endophthalmitis; dacryocystitis; increased intraocular pressure; orbital periosteitis.

Clinical

Tissues hypertonic, edematous and painful; lesion liquefies, forming creamy-yellow pus; fever; nausea; vomiting; cough; dyspnea; abdominal pain; diarrhea; bloody stools; dehydration; shock.

Laboratory

Aerobic Gram-positive cocci bacteria grow in grape-like clusters. Coagulase positive indicates pathogenicity.

Treatment

Specific antimicrobial therapy is chosen based on the site and severity of the infection and the antimicrobial sensitivities of the organism involved.

Additional Resource

1. Tolan RW (2012). Staphylococcus Aureus Infection. [online] Available from http://www.emedicine.com/ped/TOPIC2704.HTM [Accessed April, 2012].

1425. STARGARDT DISEASE (JUVENILE MACULAR DEGENERATION)

General

Onset between the ages of 8 and 14 years; variable appearance in different families.

Ocular

Heredomacular dystrophy; bilateral lesions showing some degree of symmetry; chorioretinal heredodegeneration; abnormal color vision.

Clinical

Possible association with neurologic deficits, including spastic tetraparesis and cerebellar involvement.

Laboratory

Diagnosis is made by clinical findings.

Treatment

No effective treatment. Ultraviolet sunglasses may be beneficial.

Bibliography

1. Cibis GW, Morey M, Harris DJ. Dominantly inherited macular dystrophy with flecks (Stargardt). Arch Ophthalmol. 1980;98:1785-9.
2. Hadden OB, Gass JD. Fundus flavimaculatus and Stargardt's disease. Am J Ophthalmol. 1976;82: 527-39.
3. Kalfakis N, Grivas I, Panayiotidou E, et al. Stargardt's disease with neurological involvement: case report. Funct Neurol. 1994;9:97-100.
4. Mantyjarvi M, Tuppurainen K. Color vision in Stargardt's disease. Int Ophthalmol. 1992;16:423-8.
5. Moloney JB, Mooney DJ, O'Connor MA. Retinal function in Stargardt's disease and fundus flavimaculatus. Am J Ophthalmol. 1983;96:57-65.
6. Noble KG, Carr RE. Stargardt's disease and fundus flavimaculatus. Arch Ophthalmol. 1979;97:1281-5.

1426. STEELE-RICHARDSON-OLSZEWSKI SYNDROME (PROGRESSIVE SUPRANUCLEAR PALSY)

General

Nerve cell degeneration centered in the brainstem; resemblance to Lhermitte pyramidopallidal syndrome and to Jakob disease with dementia and rigidity; onset in the sixth decade of life; prominent in males.

Ocular

Supranuclear ophthalmoplegia affecting chiefly vertical gaze, especially downward.

Clinical

Pseudobulbar palsy; dysarthria; dystonic rigidity of neck and upper trunk; axial rigidity; bradykinesia; pyramidal signs; parkinsonism; frontal lobe-type dementia.

Laboratory

No specific laboratory or imaging findings.

Treatment

No medication is effective and only few patients respond to dopaminergic or anticholinergic drugs.

Additional Resource

1. Eggenberger ER (2012). Progressive Supranuclear Palsy. [online] Available from http://www.emedicine.com/neuro/TOPIC328.HTM [Accessed April, 2012].

1427. STEVENS-JOHNSON SYNDROME [BAADER DERMATOSTOMATITIS SYNDROME; DERMATOSTOMATITIS; ERYTHEMA MULTIFORME EXUDATIVUM; FUCHS (2) SYNDROME; MUCOSAL-RESPIRATORY SYNDROME; MUCOCUTANEOUS OCULAR SYNDROME; SYNDROMA MUCOCUTANEO-OCULARE]

General

Etiology unknown; affects all ages; most frequently seen in the first and third decades of life; prevalent in males; drugs are the most commonly identified etiologic factor in this condition.

Ocular

Hypopyon; iritis; keratitis; corneal ulcers; keratoconjunctivitis sicca; chemosis; conjunctivitis; widespread fibrinoid necrosis of conjunctival vessels; blepharitis; endophthalmitis; phthisis bulbi; uveitis; cataracts; pannus; optic neuritis; keratoconus; adenoviral conjunctivitis has been reported to have precipitated Stevens-Johnson syndrome; orbital cyst may be a complication.

Clinical

General malaise, headaches, chills and fever; severe skin and mucous membrane eruptions (erythema multiforme); dorsa of hands and feet are most frequently affected; rhinitis; balanitis; vulvovaginitis; urethritis (nonspecific); cystitis; patients with AIDS are at higher risk of developing Stevens-Johnson syndrome.

Laboratory

No laboratory tests are specific to Stevens-Johnson syndrome. Diagnosis is made from clinical findings.

Treatment

Systemic treatment with steroids is controversial. Antibiotics are used based on clinical course. Eyelid hygiene should be performed as needed.

Additional Resource

1. Plaza JA (2011). Erythema Multiforme. [online] Available from http://www.emedicine.com/med/TOPIC727.HTM [Accessed April, 2012].

1428. STICKLER SYNDROME (HEREDITARY PROGRESSIVE ARTHROOPHTHALMOPATHY)

General

Autosomal dominant; onset in childhood; severe and debilitating connective tissue disorder inherited as an autosomal dominant syndrome with a variable phenotype; linkage analysis has provided statistical evidence for linkage of collagen type II (COL2A1) gene with this syndrome in some but not all families.

Ocular

Phthisis bulbi; glaucoma; chronic uveitis; keratopathy; complicated cataracts; chorioretinal degeneration; total retinal detachment during the first decade of life; myopia; giant retinal tears.

Clinical

Bony enlargement of joints with abnormal development of the articular surfaces and premature degenerative changes; hypermobility of joints with abnormality in connective tissues supporting the joints; possible skeletal deformities.

Laboratory

Bone radiographs, and a full genetic evaluation is appropriate.

Treatment

The primary concern is airway obstruction. Tracheotomy tube is effective in bypassing the obstruction. If feeding difficulties, special cleft nursing bottles are available. If this is not enough, gavage or feeding tubes can provide temporary nutrition.

Additional Resource

1. Tolarova MM (2012). Pierre Robin Malformation. [online] Available from http://www.emedicine.com/ped/TOPIC2680.HTM [Accessed April, 2012].

1429. STRACHAN SYNDROME (TROPICAL NUTRITIONAL NEUROPATHY)

General

Possibly nutritional vitamin A deficiency, chronic cyanide poisoning, and/or infectious agents.

Ocular

Optic atrophy; blurred vision, usually bilateral and symmetric; retrobulbar neuritis; scotoma; decreased vision; bilateral and symmetrical central or cecocentral scotomata; loss of color vision due to selective lesion of the maculopapillary bundles.

Clinical

Ataxic neuropathy; sensorineural deafness; high prevalence of goiter.

Laboratory

Diagnosis is made by clinical findings.

Treatment

Optic atrophy: Intravenous steroids may be used with optic neuritis or ischemic neuropathy. Stem cell treatment may be the future treatment of choice.

Bibliography

1. Dreyfus PM. Nutritional disorder of obscure etiology. Med Sci. 1966;17:44-8.
2. Strachan H. On a form of multiple neuritis prevalent in the West Indies. Practitioner. 1897;59:477-84.

1430. STRAW PETER SYNDROME (SLOVENLY PETER SYNDROME; STRUWWELPETER SYNDROME)

General

Etiology unknown; combination of organic and environmental factors; affects 5–20% of the general school population; in preschool-aged children, manifested as clumsiness, abnormal activity level, and disorganized thought process; in school-aged children, manifested as distractibility and learning disability.

Ocular

Strabismus; impaired visual perception.

Clinical

Hyperkinesia; restlessness; fidgetiness; disorganized thought process; hypokinesia; impulsivity; poor coordination of fingers; motor awkwardness; impaired auditory perception.

Laboratory

Diagnosis is made by clinical findings.

Treatment

None

Bibliography

1. Clements SD, Peters JE. Minimal brain dysfunctions in the school-age child. Diagnosis and treatment. Arch Gen Psychiatry. 1962;6:185-97.
2. Hoffmann H. "Struwwelpeter." JAMA. 1967;202:28-9.
3. Magalini SI, Scrascia E. Dictionary of Medical Syndromes, 2nd edition. Philadelphia: JB Lippincott; 1981.

1431. STREPTOCOCCUS (SCARLET FEVER)

General

Gram-positive bacteria that can invade any tissue.

Ocular

Conjunctivitis; corneal ulcer; blepharitis; scarlatinal rash of lid; erysipelas dermatitis of lid; gangrene of lid; endophthalmitis; proptosis; dacryocystitis; optic neuritis; orbital cellulitis; uveitis; hypopyon; secondary glaucoma; paralysis of extraocular muscles; infectious crystalline keratopathy; scleritis.

Clinical

Pharyngitis; impetigo; scarlet fever; pneumonia; bacteremia; rheumatic fever; glomerulonephritis.

Laboratory

Gram-positive cocci growing in pairs or chains. Throat culture and sensitivity useful.

Treatment

Penicillin is the drug of choice.

Additional Resource

1. Balentine J (2010). Scarlet Fever in Emergency Medicine. [online] Available from http://www.emedicine.com/emerg/TOPIC518.HTM [Accessed April, 2012].

1432. STRING SYNDROME

General

Following encircling operations or circular diathermy, chemosis, and excess protein exudation into the anterior chamber; onset between postoperative days 4 and 19; suture causing vascular obstruction; configuration of eye is a predisposing factor.

Ocular

Necrosis of iris; necrosis of ciliary body; corneal ring abscess; iritis; deep anterior chamber; proptosis; lid edema; chemosis of conjunctiva; ocular hypertension; iris assumes a green color; retinal detachment.

Clinical

None

Laboratory

Diagnosis is made by clinical findings.

Treatment

Iritis: Oral steroids if not responsive to topical steroids, immunosuppressants if bilateral disease that does not respond to oral steroids, periocular steroids for unilateral or posterior uveitis. Vitrectomy can be used for severe vitreous opacification. Cryotherapy and laser photocoagulation may be used for localized pars plana exudates.

Retinal detachment: Scleral buckle, pneumatic retinopexy and vitrectomy may be used to close all the breaks.

Corneal ulcer: Corneal cultures may be taken and treatment initiated. Treatment includes a broad spectrum of antibiotics and cycloplegic drops.

Bibliography

1. Magalini SI, Scrascia E. Dictionary of Medical Syndromes, 2nd edition. Philadelphia: JB Lippincott; 1981.
2. Manson N. The string syndrome: seen as a complication of Arruga's cerclage suture. Br J Ophthalmol. 1964;48:70-4.
3. Pau H. Differential Diagnosis of Eye Diseases. New York: Thieme; 1987.

1433. STRUMPELL-LEICHTENSTERN SYNDROME (ACUTE HEMORRHAGIC ENCEPHALITIS)

General

Etiology viral, postvaccinal, drug-induced or allergic; both sexes affected; onset at all ages but prevalent in children.

Ocular

Optic atrophy; acute retinal necrosis syndrome.

Clinical

Fever; convulsions; mental dullness; delirium; coma; ataxia; neck rigidity; tachypnea; myoclonus; aphasia; acute disseminated encephalomyelitis.

Laboratory

Diagnosis is made by clinical findings.

Treatment

Optic atrophy: Intravenous steroids may be used with optic neuritis or ischemic neuropathy. Stem cell treatment may be the future treatment of choice.

Bibliography

1. Ahmadieh H, Sajjadi SH, Azarmina M, et al. Association of herpetic encephalitis with acute retinal necrosis syndrome. Ann Ophthalmol. 1991;23:215-9.
2. Dangond F, Lacomis D, Schwartz RB, et al. Acute disseminated encephalomyelitis progressing to hemorrhagic encephalitis. Neurology. 1991;41: 1697-8.
3. Magalini SI, Scrascia E. Dictionary of Medical Syndromes, 2nd edition. Philadelphia: JB Lippincott; 1981.
4. von Strumpell A. Ueber Primaere Acute Encephlitis. Dtsch Arch Klin Med. 1890;47:53-74.

1434. STURGE-WEBER SYNDROME (ENCEPHALOFACIAL ANGIOMATOSIS; ENCEPHALOTRIGEMINAL SYNDROME; MENINGOCUTANEOUS SYNDROME; NEURO-OCULOCUTANEOUS ANGIOMATOSIS; VASCULAR ENCEPHALOTRIGEMINAL SYNDROME)

General

Trisomy 22 or Partial trisomy inheritance. Variations include Jahnke syndrome (neuro-oculocutaneous angiomatosis without glaucoma), Schirmer syndrome (oculocutaneous angiomatosis with early glaucoma), Lawford syndrome (oculocutaneous angiomatosis with late glaucoma and no increase in volume of globe) and Mille syndrome (oculocutaneous syndrome with choroidal angioma but no glaucoma).

Ocular

Unilateral hydrophthalmos; secondary glaucoma (late) conjunctival angiomata (telangiectases); iris decoloration; nevoid marks or vascular dilation of the episclera; glioma; serous retinal detachment; choroidal angiomata; deep anterior chamber angle; port-wine stain of eyelid; buphthalmos; optic nerve cupping; anisometropia; hemianopsia; increased corneal diameter; enophthalmos; exophthalmos; optic atrophy; choroidal hemangioma; anterior chamber angle vascularization.

Clinical

Vascular port-wine nevus (face, scalp, limbs, trunk, leptomeninges); acromegaly; facial hemihypertrophy; intracranial angiomas; convulsion; mental retardation; obesity; limb atrophy.

Laboratory

Neuroimaging studies and the clinical examination have been the procedures of choice to establish the diagnosis.

Treatment

Anticonvulsants for seizure control, symptomatic and prophylactic therapy for headache and glaucoma treatment to reduce the IOP.

Additional Resources

1. Takeoka M (2010). Pediatric Sturge-Weber Syndrome. [online] Available from http://www.emedicine.com/neuro/TOPIC356.HTM [Accessed April, 2012].

2. Del Monte MA (2012). Sturge-Weber Syndrome. [online] Available from http://www.emedicine.com/oph/TOPIC348.HTM [Accessed April, 2012].

1435. SUBACUTE BACTERIAL ENDOCARDITIS

General

Inflammation of the lining of the heart typically caused by *Staphylococcus epidermidis*.

Ocular

Optic neuritis; papillitis; choroiditis; conjunctival and retinal petechiae; retinal hemorrhages; Roth spots; floaters in aqueous and vitreous; rare embolic occlusion of the central retinal artery; ophthalmoplegia; papilledema.

Clinical

Fever; anemia; splenomegaly; heart murmur.

Laboratory

Multiple blood cultures, CBC, erythrocyte sedimentation rate (ESR), echocardiography and MRI.

Treatment

Prolonged parenteral therapy is needed to kill all the bacteria. Penicillin G is used to treat streptococcal endocarditis on native cardiac valves.

Additional Resource

1. Gewitz MH (2011). Pediatric Bacterial Endocarditis. [online] Available from http://www.emedicine.com/ped/TOPIC2511.HTM [Accessed April, 2012].

1436. SUBCLAVIAN STEAL SYNDROME

General

Reversal of blood flow through the vertebral artery caused by stenosis of one subclavian artery proximal to the origin of the vertebral artery; arteriosclerosis; atresia of the proximal subclavian artery; aortic coarctation; subclavian artery may siphon (steal) blood from the vertebral artery; causes fluctuating symptoms of basilar artery insufficiency.

Ocular

Ptosis; nystagmus; temporary visual loss during activity of one arm; visual disturbances.

Clinical

Brachial vascular insufficiency; claudication; tingling of the arm; syncope; decrease of blood pressure in affected arm by at least 20 mm Hg;

numbness; coldness; pain; facial paresthesia; headache; syncopal attacks; vertigo; intermittent claudication of the involved upper extremity.

Laboratory

Lipid profile, blood glucose, duplex ultrasonography, CT angiography, chest X-ray, and MRI.

Treatment

No medical therapy is known.

Additional Resource

1. McIntyre KE (2012). Subclavian Steal Syndrome. [online] Available from http://www.emedicine.com/med/TOPIC2771.HTM [Accessed April, 2012].

1437. SUBMANDIBULAR, OCULAR, AND RECTAL PAIN WITH FLUSHING

General

Autosomal dominant; brief, severe pain of submandibular, ocular and rectal areas with flushing of surrounding skin.

Ocular

Ocular pain.

Clinical

Jaw aches; severe rectal pain.

Laboratory

Diagnosis is made by clinical findings.

Treatment

Treat pain.

Bibliography

1. Hayden R, Grossman M. Rectal, ocular, and submaxillary pain; a familial autonomic disorder related to proctalgia fugax: report of a family. AMA J Dis Child. 1959;97:479-82.
2. McKusick VA. Mendelian Inheritance in Man: A Catalog of Human Genes and Genetic Disorders, 12th edition. Baltimore: The Johns Hopkins University Press; 1998.
3. McKusick-Nathans Institute for Genetic Medicine, Johns Hopkins University and National Center for Biotechnology Information, National Library of Medicine. (2007). Online Mendelian Inheritance in Man (OMIM). [online] Available from http://www.ncbi.nlm.nih.gov/omim [Accessed April, 2012].

1438. SUDDEN VISUAL LOSS

General

Usually lasts a few minutes, but can persist for hours. The frequency varies from a single episode to many episodes during a day; it may continue for years, but more often lasts from seconds to hours. Most common cause is ischemia, often by mechanical obstruction, can affect any aspect of the visual system.

Clinical

Athersclerotic disease; smokers; hypercholesterolemia; hypertension; cancer; drug abuse.

Ocular

Transient visual obstruction; amaurosis fugax; transient monocular or bilateral visual loss; ocular infarction.

Laboratory

Fluorescein angiography is helpful for detection of retinal vascular occlusion. Since common causes are ischemic, comanagment with an internist is recommended to help determine and treat the cause.

Treatment

Aspirin is used in patients with no hemo-dynamically significant disease of the carotid artery; modification of risk factors, such as hypertension, cholesterol level, etc. is important.

Additional Resource

1. Farina GA (2011). Sudden Visual Loss. [online] Available from http://www.emedicine.medscape.com/article/1216594-overview [Accessed April, 2012].

1439. SULFITE OXIDASE DEFICIENCY

General

Rare abnormality of sulfur metabolism in which there is an accumulation of S-sulfocysteine, thiosulfate, and sulfate and a deficiency of sulfite; present at birth; death occurs before age 3 years.

Ocular

Dislocated lens; nystagmus; ectopia lentis.

Clinical

Muscular rigidity; eccentric behavior; coarse face; broad nasal bridge; long philtrum (in association with Leigh syndrome).

Laboratory

Plasma and urine aminoacid levels; urinary urothion, urinary thiosulfate and cranial CT or MRI.

Treatment

No known treatment that will improve neurological outcome is available.

Additional Resource

1. Arnold GL (2012). Sulfite Oxidase Deficiency. [online] Available from http://www.emedicine.com/ped/TOPIC2172.HTM [Accessed April, 2012].

1440. SUNRISE SYNDROME

General

Occurs when the intraocular lens (IOL) optic is displaced superiorly out of the visual axis.

Ocular

Edge of IOL in pupil; decreased visual acuity; glare.

Clinical

None

Laboratory

Diagnosis is made by clinical findings.

Treatment

Constrict pupil with either alphagan or pilocarpine. May have to remove IOL and replace with AC IOL.

Bibliography

1. Akkin C, Ozler SA, Mentes J. Tilt and decentration of bag-fixated intraocular lenses: a comparative study between capsulorhexis and envelope techniques. Doc Ophthalmol. 1994;87:199-209.
2. Davison JA. Capsule contraction syndrome. J Cataract Refract Surg. 1993;19:582-9.
3. Smiddy WE, Ibanez GV, Alfonso E, et al. Surgical management of dislocated intraocular lenses. J Cataract Refract Surg. 1995;21:64-9.
4. Smith SG, Lindstrom RL. Malpositioned posterior chamber lenses: etiology, prevention, and management. J Am Intraocul Implant Soc. 1985;11:584-91.
5. Smith SG, Lindstrom RL. Report and management of the sunrise syndrome. J Am Intraocul Implant Soc. 1984;10:218-20.
6. Wilson DJ, Jaeger MJ, Green WR. Effects of extracapsular cataract extraction on the lens zonules. Ophthalmology. 1987;94:467-70.

1441. SUNSET SYNDROME

General

Occurs when the capsule or zonules have been sufficiently damaged to allow the posterior chamber IOL to slip gradually into the inferior vitreous in the postoperative period.

Ocular

Superior edge of IOL in pupil; IOL in vitreous body; retinal detachment; decreased visual acuity; glare; zonular disinsertions.

Clinical

None

Laboratory

Diagnosis is made by clinical findings.

Treatment

Constrict pupil with either alphagan or pilocarpine. May have to remove IOL and replace with AC IOL.

Bibliography

1. Akkin C, Ozler SA, Mentes J. Tilt and decentration of bag-fixated intraocular lenses: a comparative study between capsulorhexis and envelope techniques. Doc Ophthalmol. 1994;87:199-209.
2. Allara RD, Weinstein GW. A new surgical technique for managing sunset syndrome. Ophthalmic Surg. 1987;18:811-4.
3. Davison JA. Capsule contraction syndrome. J Cataract Refract Surg. 1993;19:582-9.
4. Smiddy WE, Ibanez GV, Alfonso E, et al. Surgical management of dislocated intraocular lenses. J Cataract Refract Surg. 1995;21:64-9.
5. Smith SG, Lindstrom RL. Malpositioned posterior chamber lenses: etiology, prevention, and management. J Am Intraocul Implant Soc. 1985;11: 584-91.

1442. SUPERIOR LIMBIC KERATOCONJUNCTIVITIS (SLK; THEODORES SUPERIOR LIMBIC KERATOCONJUNCTIVITIS)

General

Corneal disease affecting the superior limbus.

Clinical

None

Ocular

Hyperemia, thickened upper bulbar conjunctiva in a "corridor-like" distribution, fine papillary inflammation of superior palpebral conjunctival, punctate erosion over the superior and perilimbal cornea and superior filamentary keratopathy.

Laboratory

Giemsa stained scraping of upper conjunctiva demonstrate keratinized cells.

Treatment

Topical lubricants and mast cell stabilizers, punctal plugs, silver nitrate treatment on upper tarsal and bulbar conjunctiva, bandage contact lens, brief focal applications of thermal cautery and recession of involved superior bulbar conjunctiva.

Additional Resource

1. Oakman JH (2011). Superior Limbic Kerato-conjunctivitis. [online] Available from http://www.emedicine.com/oph/TOPIC103.HTM [Accessed April, 2012].

1443. SUPERIOR OBLIQUE (IV NERVE) PALSY

General

Unilateral or Bilateral, can be caused by head trauma, tumor, vascular abnormality, diabetes and following sinus or orbital surgery.

Clinical

None

Ocular

Children—head tilt and V-pattern esotropia. Adult—chin depression, intermittent diplopia, torsional diplopia a head tilt and turn to the side opposite the affected eye in unilateral cases.

Laboratory

Diagnosis is made by clinical findings.

Treatment

Class I—greatest vertical deviation in field of action of inferior oblique, weaken inferior oblique; Class II—greatest vertical deviation in field of action of the underacting superior oblique-superior oblique strengthening; Class III—equal vertical deviation of inferior oblique and superior oblique either inferior oblique or superior oblique surgery.

Bibliography

1. Jiang L, Demer JL. Magnetic resonance imaging of the functional anatomy of the inferior rectus muscle in superior oblique muscle palsy. Ophthalmology. 2008;115:2079-86.

2. Petermann SH, Newman NJ. Pituitary macroadenoma manifesting as an isolated fourth nerve palsy. Am J Ophthalmol. 1999;127:235-6.

1444. SUPERIOR OBLIQUE MYOKYMIA

General

Twitching of superior oblique, rare, occurs in adults, frequently chronic.

Clinical

None

Ocular

Oscillopsia (microtremor, twitching and vertical and/or torsional diplopia).

Laboratory

Magnetic resonance imaging (MRI) to identify vascular compression.

Treatment

Systemic—regretol, topical—betoxalol, surgical—weaken the affected superior oblique and ipsilateral inferior oblique.

Bibliography

1. Roy FH, Fraunfelder FW, Fraunfelder FT. Roy and Fraunfelder's Current Ocular Therapy, 6th edition. Philadelphia: WB Saunders; 2008.

1445. SUPERIOR VENA CAVA SYNDROME (VENA CAVA SUPERIOR SYNDROME)

General

Compression or Obstruction of the superior vena cava by aortic aneurysms, mediastinal neoplasms, thyroid adenoma, or carcinoma of the lung; found in males in their 50s.

Ocular

Glaucoma; conjunctival vasodilation; retinal hemorrhages (Valsalva retinopathy); eyelid edema; optic disk edema; engorgement of the conjunctival and episcleral vessels; periorbital edema.

Clinical

Cyanosis and edema of face, neck, and upper trunk with a rather sharp demarcation line (short cape edema); dysphagia; epistaxis; hoarseness; vertigo; tinnitus; may be caused by Graves' disease and as a presentation of Behçet disease.

Laboratory

Thoracic CT scan, radiographs and venography.

Treatment

Attention to breathing, airway, and circulation is important; steroids as needed.

Additional Resource

1. Beeson MS (2010). Superior Vena Cava Syndrome in Emergency Medicine. [online] Available from http://www.emedicine.com/emerg/TOPIC561.HTM [Accessed April, 2012].

1446. SUPRARENAL SYMPATHETIC SYNDROME (ADRENAL MEDULLA TUMOR SYNDROME; ADRENAL SYMPATHETIC SYNDROME; PHEOCHROMOCYTOMA SYNDROME)

General

Tumors producing increased secretion of nor-epinephrine and epinephrine deriving from chromaffin cells of the adrenal medulla; more common in males (3:2); symptoms occur in paroxysms or attacks; precipitated by emotional upsets; predilection for the right adrenal.

Ocular

Spasm of retinal arteries with associated cotton-wool exudates; flame-shaped hemorrhages; papilledema; pupillary dilation; neovasculariza-tion of retina; following removal of the tumor there may be macular scarring and optic atrophy.

Clinical

Hypertension; tachycardia; severe anxiety; head-ache; nervous tension; sweating; pallor; nausea; polyuria; polydipsia; association with neuro-fibromatosis and von Hippel disease.

Laboratory

Plasma metanephrine testing, 24-hour collection for catecholamines and metanephrines. MRI and CT scan may be beneficial.

Treatment

Surgically removing the tumor is the treatment of choice.

Additional Resource

1. Blake MA (2011). Pheochromocytoma. [online] Available from http://www.emedicine.com/med/TOPIC1816.HTM [Accessed April, 2012].

1447. SUSAC SYNDROME

General

Rare; unknown origin; characterized by the triad of encephalopathy, fluctuation hearing loss and visual loss resulting from microangiopathy of the brain, cochlea and retina.

Ocular

Cotton-wool spot; central retinal vein occlusion.

Clinical

Hearing loss; encephalopathy.

Laboratory

Diagnosis is made by clinical findings.

Treatment

Central vein occlusion: Intraocular pressure lowering medications, carbogen therapy, hyper-baric oxygen. Vitrectomy may be necessary.

Bibliography

1. Gross M, Banin E, Eliashar R, et al. Susac syndrome. Otol Neurotol. 2004;25:470-3.
2. McLeod DS, Ying HS, McLeod CA, et al. Retinal and optic nerve head pathology in Susac's syndrome. Ophtalmology. 2011;118:548-52.
3. Xu MS, Tan CB, Umapathi T, et al. Susac syndrome: serial diffusion-weighted MR imaging. Magn Reson Imaging. 2004;22:1295-8.

1448. SWEET SYNDROME (ACUTE FEBRILE NEUTROPHILIC DERMATOSIS) GLAUCOMA

General

Cause unknown; common in middle-aged women; associated with acute leukemia; acute febrile neutrophilic dermatosis; neurologic symptoms.

Ocular

Conjunctivitis; episcleritis; glaucoma; limbal nodules.

Clinical

Cutaneous eruption with fever; nondeforming, asymmetrical, large-joint arthritis; albuminuria; anemia; oral aphthae; genital ulcers; association with Behçet disease has been reported.

Laboratory

Complete blood count, ESR and CRP levels, urinalysis and chest radiographs.

Treatment

Prednisone is effective; topical steroids are used in localized lesions.

Additional Resource

1. Yoon-Soo Cindy Bae-Harboe (2012). Acute Febrile Neutrophilic Dermatosis. [online] Available from http://www.emedicine.com/derm/TOPIC11. HTM [Accessed April, 2012].

1449. SYLVESTER DISEASE

General

Dominant inheritance.

Ocular

Optic atrophy.

Clinical

Ataxia; moderate and slowly progressive hearing loss.

Laboratory/Ocular

Diagnosis is made by clinical findings.

Treatment/Ocular

Optic atrophy: Intravenous steroids may be used with optic neuritis or ischemic neuropathy. Stem cell treatment may be the future treatment of choice.

Bibliography

1. Konigsmark BW, Knox DL, Hussels IE, et al. Dominant congenital deafness and progressive optic nerve atrophy. Occurrence in four generations of a family. Arch Ophthalmol. 1974;91: 99-103.

1450. SYMONDS SYNDROME (BENIGN INTRACRANIAL HYPERTENSION; OTITIC HYDROCEPHALUS SYNDROME; PSEUDOTUMOR CEREBRI; SEROUS MENINGITIS SYNDROME)

General

Children and adolescents; protracted course; increased cerebrospinal fluid, but without increase in protein or cells.

Ocular

Sixth nerve palsy, ipsilateral side with otitis media; retinal hemorrhages and exudates; moderate-to-marked papilledema followed by secondary optic atrophy; unilateral or bilateral swelling of the optic nerve head have been reported; cranial nerve III and IV involvement; bilateral retinal vein occlusion.

Clinical

Greatly increased pressure of spinal fluid, often greater than 300 mm, without increased cells or protein; intermittent headaches; otitis media; chronic renal failure; chronic myeloid leukemia.

Laboratory

Imaging studies such as MRI to rule out tumors of brain and spinal cord and lumbar puncture.

Treatment

Carbonic anhydrase inhibitors such as acetazolamide and furosemide are useful.

Bibliography

1. Chang D, Nagamoto G, Smith WE. Benign intracranial hypertension and chronic renal failure. Cleve Clin J Med. 1992;59:419-22.
2. Chari C, Rao NS. Benign intracranial hypertension—its unusual manifestations. Headache. 1991;31:599-600.
3. Chern S, Magargal LE, Brav SS. Bilateral central retinal vein occlusion as an initial manifestation of pseudotumor cerebri. Ann Ophthalmol. 1991; 23:54-7.
4. Roy FH, Fraunfelder FW, Fraunfelder FT. Roy and Fraunfelder's Current Ocular Therapy, 6th edition. Philadelphia: WB Saunders; 2008.
5. Venable HP. Pseudo-tumor cerebri. J Natl Med Assoc. 1970;62:435-40.
6. Venable HP. Pseudo-tumor cerebri: further studies. J Natl Med Assoc. 1973;65:194-7.

1451. SYMPATHETIC OPHTHALMIA

General

Trauma or Injury to one eye and later onset of inflammation in the other eye.

Ocular

Iridocyclitis (acute inflammation of iris, ciliary body and anterior chamber); choroiditis; chronic persistent keratitic precipitates; posterior synechiae; phthisis bulbi; has been reported following laser cyclocoagulation.

Clinical

None

Laboratory

Diagnosis is made by clinical findings.

Treatment

Aggressive treatment with steroids and nonsteroids.

Bibliography

1. Bechrakis NE, Müller-Stolzenburg NW, Helbig H, et al. Sympathetic ophthalmia following laser cyclocoagulation. Arch Ophthalmol. 1994;112:80-4.

2. Boniuk V, Boniuk M. The incidence of phthisis bulbi as a complication of cataract surgery in the congenital rubella syndrome. Trans Am Acad Ophthalmol Otolaryngol. 1970;74:360-8.

3. Duane TD. Clinical Ophthalmology. Philadelphia: JB Lippincott; 1987.

1452. SYNECHIAE, PERIPHERAL ANTERIOR

General

Consequence of altered anterior chamber anatomy and anterior chamber inflammation. Apposition of the iris against the trabecular meshwork as a result of pupil block without any inflammation can result in periphral anterior synechiae. With inflammation or cellular proliferation, a membrane is form between the iris and the trabecular meshwork, creating peripheral anterior synechiae.

Clinical

Inflammatory syndromes such as: juvenile rheumatoid arthritis, intestinal keratitis, sarcoidosis, Posner-Schlossman syndrome, herpes simplex, herpes zoster, toxoplasmosis and syphilis.

Ocular

Primary angle-closure glaucoma, iris bombe, pupil block, posterior uveitis, CRVO, nanophthalmos, suprachoroidal hemorrhage, ciliary block, posterior segment tumors, retinoblastoma, choroidal melanoma, retinopathy of prematurity.

Laboratory

Ultrasound biomicroscopy is helpful in evaluating the angle. Provocative testing is used to measure IOP while dilating and constricting of the pupil.

Treatment

No specific medical treatment exists. The following medications may be considered depending on the diagnosis: topical beta-blockers, alpha-agonists, carbonic anhydrase inhibitors, oral carbonic anhydrase inhibitors, topical prostaglandin analogs, miotics, cycloplegics and topical corticosteroids. Surgical: YAG/laser iridotomy, surgical iridotomy, argon laser peripheral iridoplasty, argon laser pupilloplasty, and glaucoma filtering procedures such as: trabeculectomy, primary tube shunt.

Additional Resource

1. Khan BU (2012). Peripheral Anterior Synechia. [online] Available from http://www.emedicine.medscape.com/article/1189962-diagnosis [Accessed April, 2012].

1453. TAKAYASU SYNDROME (AORTIC ARCH SYNDROME; MARTORELL SYNDROME; PULSELESS DISEASE; REVERSED COARCTATION SYNDROME)

General

Two types are: (1) occlusive inflammatory lesion (seen in young Japanese women) and (2) occlusive vascular disease without inflammation, associated with atherosclerosis and syphilis; onset in the fifth and sixth decades of life; both sexes affected; can involve the aorta and its major branches as well as the coronary, hepatic, mesenteric, pulmonary and renal arteries.

Ocular

Iris atrophy; cataracts; retinal microaneurysms; sausage-shaped venous dilations; reduced central retinal artery pressure; optic atrophy; cotton-wool spots; anterior segment ischemia; retinal arteriovenous shunts.

Clinical

Diminished or Absent pulsation of arteries (head, neck, upper limbs); orthostatic syncope; facial atrophy; epileptiform seizures; intermittent claudication.

Laboratory

Arteriography, magnetic resonance angiography (MRA), MRI, CT scan, Gallium-67 radionuclide scan, or chest radiography.

Treatment

Corticosteroids, methotrexate or intravenous cyclophosphamide can be used in patients with glucocorticoid-resistant TA.

Additional Resource

1. Hom C (2011). Pediatric Takayasu Arteritis. [online] Available from http://www.emedicine. com/ped/TOPIC1956.HTM [Accessed April, 2012].

1454. TANGIER SYNDROME (ALPHA-LIPOPROTEIN DEFICIENCY; FAMILIAL HIGH-DENSITY LIPOPROTEIN DEFICIENCY; FISH EYE DISEASE; LIPOPROTEIN DEFICIENCY)

General

First seen on Chesapeake Bay Island; rare; autosomal recessive; inability to synthesize polypeptide required in the elaboration of high-density lipoprotein; cholesterol esters are stored; occurs in both sexes; onset from childhood to fifth decade of life; disorder appears to be a variant of familial lecithin-cholesterol acyltransferase (LCAT) deficiency in which the enzyme remains partly active.

Ocular

Corneal infiltrates; fine, dotted stromal opacities, most marked in posterior central third of corneal stroma; wasting of orbicularis oculi muscle.

Clinical

Maculopapular rash; orange-yellow striped tonsils; hepatosplenomegaly; lymphadenopathy; intermittent diarrhea; bilateral motor weakness.

Laboratory

Diagnosis is made by clinical findings.

Treatment

None

Bibliography

1. Chu FC, Kuwabara T, Cogan DG, et al. Ocular manifestations of familial high-density lipoprotein deficiency (Tangier disease). Arch Ophthalmol. 1979;97:1926-8.
2. Hoffman HN, Fredrickson DS. Tangier disease (familial high density lipoprotein deficiency). Clinical and genetic features in two adults. Am J Med. 1965;39:582-93.
3. Kastelein JJ, Pritchard PH, Erkelens DW, et al. Familial high density-lipoprotein deficiency causing corneal opacities (fish eye disease) in a family of Dutch descent. J Intern Med. 1992;231: 413-9.

1455. TAPETAL-LIKE REFLEX SYNDROME

General

Rare

Ocular

Ring scotoma; discrete bright yellow spots in posterior polar region deep to the retinal vessels; tapetal-like reflex and retinitis pigmentosa may be present in members of the same family.

Clinical

None

Laboratory/Ocular

Infectious lab test, fluorescent treponemal antibody absorption test, veneral disease research laboratory test, inherited/syndromic disease lab test and neoplasm related lab test are used to detect conditions associated with retinitis pigmentosa.

Treatment/Ocular

Refraction and low-vision evaluation, annual evaluations including visual field testing. Vitamin A/beta-carotene and systemic acetazolamide.

Bibliography

1. Ciccarelli EC. A new syndrome of tapetal-like fundic reflexes with ring scotomata. Report of two cases. Arch Ophthalmol. 1962;67:316-20.

1456. TAR SYNDROME (THROMBOCYTOPENIA ABSENT RADIUS SYNDROME)

General

Bilateral absence of the radius and hypomegakaryocytic thrombocytopenia.

Ocular

May have cataracts, glaucoma, megalocornea and blue sclera.

Clinical

Patients have foreshortened forearms and radially deviated hands; infrequently associated with mental retardation (7%); also may have lower extremity deformity.

Laboratory

Complete blood count, genetic testing, ultrasonography and bone marrow biopsy.

Treatment

Platelet transfusion is the most important treatment.

Additional Resource

1. Wu JK (2009). Thrombocytopenia-Absent Radius Syndrome. [online] Available from http://www.emedicine.com/ped/TOPIC2237.HTM [Accessed April, 2012].

1457. TAY-SACHS SYNDROME (FAMILIAL AMAUROTIC IDIOCY; GANGLIOSIDOSIS GM2 TYPE 1; HEXOSAMINIDASE DEFICIENCY; NORMAN-WOOD SYNDROME)

General

Similar to ceroid lipofuscinosis; autosomal recessive; occasional dominant inheritance; onset birth to 10 months; affects Jewish females; death during the first 2 years; stored ganglioside (see Ceroid Lipofuscinosis); decreased hexosaminidase A localized to chromosome 15 (15q22–15q25.1).

Ocular

Nystagmus; strabismus; whitish-gray macular area with cherry-red spot in the center; retinal pigmentary changes with involvement of the macula occasionally may be seen instead of the typical red spot; grayish coloration of the macula is due to the swollen ganglion cells in the perifoveal macular region; retinal vessels become narrowed; progressive ascending optic atrophy; cortical blindness by age of 12–18 months with reactive pupils; deterioration of ocular motor function.

Clinical

Hyperacusis; mental retardation; convulsions; muscles, initially flaccid, becoming spastic with progression; infants normal at birth but fail to thrive after 4–8 months; hypotonia; death; occurs primarily in Jewish children; biochemical heterogeneity; absence of hexosaminidase A most common (type 1); absence of hexosaminidase A and B in Sandhoff variant (type 2); feeding difficulties; doll-like facies; fine hair; macrocephaly; abnormal acoustic-motor reaction.

Laboratory/Ocular

Diagnosis is made by clinical findings.

Treatment/Ocular

Nystagmus: See-saw nystagmus—visual field to consider neoplastic or vascular etiologies. Upbeat nystagmus—may indicate multiple sclerosis, cerebellar degeneration, tumors or infarcts. Treatment is directed toward identification and resolution of underlying cause. Downbeat nystagmus—affects the cerebellum or craniocervical junction including Arnold-Chiari malformation, multiple sclerosis, trauma, tumor, infarction and many toxic metabolic entities. MRI may indicate a surgically correctable lesion. Periodic alternating nystagmus is continuous horizontal nystagmus from stroke, tumor, multiple sclerosis, trauma, infection and drug intoxication. Can occur from cataract, vitreous hemorrhage or optic atrophy.

Bibliography

1. Gravel RA, Triggs-Raine BL, Mahuran DJ. Biochemistry and genetics of Tay-Sachs disease. Can J Neurol Sci. 1991;18(3 Suppl):419-23.
2. Honda Y, Sudo M. Electroretinogram and visually evoked cortical potential in Tay-Sachs disease: a report of two cases. J Pediatr Ophthalmol. 1976;13:226-9.
3. Nagashima K, Kikuchi F, Suzuki Y, et al. Retinal amacrine cell involvement in Tay-Sachs disease. Acta Neuropathol. 1981;53:333-6.
4. Sachs B. An arrested cerebral development with special reference to its cortical pathology. J Nerv Ment Dis. 1887;14:541.
5. Schmitt HP, Berlet H, Volk B. Peripheral intra-axonal storage in Tay-Sachs' disease (GM2-gangliosidosis type 1). J Neurol Sci. 1979;44:115-24.
6. Smith LH. Inherited metabolic disease with pediatric ocular manifestations. In: Albert DM, Jakobiec FA (Eds). Principles and Practice of Ophthalmology. Philadelphia: WB Saunders; 1994. pp. 2777-90.
7. Tay W. Symmetrical changes in the region of the yellow spot in each eye of an infant. Trans Ophthalmol Soc U K. 1881;1:55-7.

1458. TEMPORAL ARTERITIS SYNDROME (CRANIAL ARTERITIS SYNDROME; GIANT CELL ARTERITIS; HUTCHINSON-HORTON-MAGATH-BROWN SYNDROME)

General

Etiology unknown; mainly females; mainly whites; between the ages of 55 and 80 years; temporal artery shows inflammatory thickening; arteritis of the vessels supplying the optic nerve.

Ocular

Transient ptosis; partial or complete loss of vision on the affected side; retinal detachment; exudates and hemorrhages; narrowing of retinal vessels; obstruction of the central retinal artery; optic atrophy; ischemic optic neuropathy; acute decreased intraocular pressure; corneal hypesthesia; palsies of extraocular muscles; hemorrhagic glaucoma; diplopia; hemorrhages on or around the disk.

Clinical

Throbbing headache; hyperalgesia of the scalp; malaise; anorexia; weakness; weight loss; fever; nodular pulmonary nodules; cough; otitis with deafness.

Laboratory

Elevated erythrocyte sedimentation rate (ESR) greater than 50 mm/h, positive temporal artery biopsy.

Treatment

Systemic corticosteroids are the therapy of choice.

Additional Resource

1. Allen AW (2011). Temporal Arteritis Imaging. [online] Available from http://www.emedicine.com/radio/TOPIC675.HTM [Accessed April, 2012].

1459. TERRIEN DISEASE (GUTTER DYSTROPHY; PERIPHERAL FURROW KERATITIS; SENILE MARGINAL ATROPHY; TERRIEN MARGINAL DEGENERATION)

General

Rare; no known cause; 75% of patients are males from age 10 to 70 years.

Ocular

Usually bilateral; may be asymmetrical; peripheral, fine, yellow-white, punctate stromal opacities associated with mild, superficial corneal vascularization; progressive thinning leads to peripheral gutter formation; decrease in visual acuity; loss of Bowman's membrane and anterior stromal lamella with partial replacement of these tissues by a vascularized connective tissue; fatty deposits; thin stroma; thickness changes in

Descemet's membrane; regular recurring attacks of pain and inflammation; keratoconus; reported association with Terrien marginal degeneration.

Clinical

None

Laboratory/Ocular

Diagnosis is made by clinical findings.

Treatment

Mild cases can be observed and soft contact lenses are helpful, penetrating keratoplasty may be necessary, graft recurrences treated by superficial keratectomy, phototherapeutic keratectomy or repeat penetrating keratoplasty.

Bibliography

1. Ashenhurst M, Slomovic A. Corneal hydrops in Terrien's marginal degeneration: an unusual complication. Can J Ophthalmol. 1987;22:328-30.
2. Austin P, Brown SI. Inflammatory Terrien's marginal corneal disease. Am J Ophthalmol. 1981;92:189-92.
3. Friedlaender MH. Allergy and Immunology of the Eye. Hagerstown, Maryland: Harper & Row; 1979. p. 190.
4. Kremer I. Terrien's marginal degeneration associated with vernal conjunctivitis. Am J Ophthalmol. 1991;111:517-8.
5. Lopez JS, Price FW, Whitcup SM, et al. Immunohistochemistry of Terrien's and Mooren's corneal degeneration. Arch Ophthalmol. 1991;109: 988-92.

1460. TERSON SYNDROME (SUBARACHNOID HEMORRHAGE SYNDROME)

General

Spontaneous rupture of aneurysm or traumatic intracerebral hemorrhage; onset at all ages.

Ocular

Weakness of extraocular muscles; disarranged and uncoordinated gaze; severe intraocular hemorrhage; preretinal hemorrhages; peripapillary hemorrhages; papilledema secondary to optic nerve sheath hemorrhages; pigmentary changes in macula and retina; preretinal membrane formation; vitreous detachment; amblyopia; anisocoria; bilateral retinal detachments have been associated with this disorder; epiretinal membranes (sequelae).

Clinical

Sudden unconsciousness; elevated cerebrospinal fluid pressure.

Laboratory

Sickle cell preparation, CT scan, MRI and angiography.

Treatment

Vitrectomy is required if vitreous hemorrhage does not clear by itself.

Bibliography

1. Ko F, Knox DL. The ocular pathology of Terson's syndrome. Ophthalmology. 2010;117:1423-9.

Additional Resource

1. Ou RJ (2012). Terson Syndrome. [online] Available from http://www.emedicine.com/oph/TOPIC753. HTM [Accessed April, 2012].

1461. THALASSELIS SYNDROME

General

Keratoconus-tetany-menopause.

Ocular

Spontaneous keratoconus.

Clinical

Syndrome describes an association between hormone deficiency, magnesium deficiency, allergy, keratoconus and type B behavior.

Laboratory/Ocular

Diagnosis is made by clinical findings.

Treatment/Ocular

Keratoconus: It may be treated with spectacle correction, hard contacts and avoid eye rubbing.

If hydrops occurs discontinue contact lens, use NaCl drops and ointment, patching and short course of steroids. As the disease advances penetrating keratoplasty, deep anterior lamellar keratoplasty, intacs with laser grooves or collagen stabilization of cornea.

Bibliography

1. Rabinowitz YS. Keratoconus. Surv Ophthalmol. 1998;42:297-319.
2. Thalasselis A, Selim AA. Keratoconus-tetany-menopause: the new association. Optom Vis Sci. 1991;68:357-63.

1462. THANATOPHORIC DWARFISM

General

Etiology unknown, but autosomal recessive inheritance is suspected; seen most frequently in males; onset in fetal life; death usually within first 3 days of life; possible association with drug administration has been reported.

Ocular

Exophthalmos

Clinical

Head enlarged; small face; enlarged fontanelles; high forehead; frontal bossing; saddle nose; abdomen protuberant; thorax narrow; short rib; hypotonia; respiratory distress; cardiac failure; marked shortening of the extremities; macrocephaly.

Laboratory/Ocular

Imaging studies should direct laboratory studies. Patients should undergo thyroid function testing. Complete blood counts, blood and nasal cultures in patients with orbital cellulitis are advised. CT scan, X-rays, MRI and ocular ultrasonography are recommended.

Treatment/Ocular

Ocular lubricants are recommended to prevent dryness.

Additional Resource

1. Mercandetti M (2010). Exophthalmos. [online] Available from http://www.emedicine.com/oph/TOPIC616.HTM [Accessed April, 2012].

1463. THELAZIASIS (UVEITIS)

General

Ocular infection caused mainly by the nematode *Thelazia callipardon*; natural habitat is the lacrimal gland of the dog.

Ocular

Uveitis; parasites in the conjunctiva, cornea, lacrimal system, and anterior chamber; corneal opacity; corneal abrasion; increased tear secretion.

Clinical

None

Laboratory/Ocular

Serum ACE level, chest X-ray, Veneral Disease Reaserch Laboratory test, fluorescent treponemal antibody absorption test and CBC.

Treatment/Ocular

Topical prednisolone acetate 1% only treats the anterior segment inflammation. Periocular injections of corticosteroids are also useful. Oral prednisolone may be the treatment of choice.

Additional Resource

1. Janigian RH (2011). Intermediate Uveitis. [online] Available from http://www.emedicine.com/oph/TOPIC445.HTM [Accessed April, 2012].

1464. THERMAL BURNS

General

May occur to any body tissue.

Ocular

Conjunctival necrosis; corneal ulcer; exposure keratitis; ectropion; contracture deformity of lids; lid edema; entropion; endophthalmitis; proptosis; dacryocystitis; chronic epiphora; cellulitis; corneal perforation; symblepharon.

Clinical

Bums of any body tissue; edema; contractures; secondary infections.

Laboratory

Diagnosis is made by clinical findings.

Treatment

Pain management and topical medication are two therapeutic interventions.

Additional Resource

1. Jenkins JA (2011). Emergent Management of Thermal Burns. [online] Available from http://www.emedicine.com/emerg/TOPIC72.HTM [Accessed April, 2012].

1465. THOMPSON SYNDROME

General

Autosomal dominant inheritance.

Ocular

Congenital optic atrophy; nystagmus; blindness.

Clinical

None

Laboratory/Ocular

Diagnosis is made by clinical findings.

Treatment/Ocular

Optic atrophy: Intravenous steroids may be used with optic neuritis or ischemic neuropathy. Stem cell treatment may be the future treatment of choice.

Bibliography

1. Magalini SI, Scrascia E. Dictionary of Medical Syndromes, 2nd edition. Philadelphia: JB Lippincott; 1981.

2. Thompson AH, Cashell GT. A pedigree of congenital optic atrophy embracing sixteen affected cases in six generations. Proc R Soc Med. 1935;28:1415-25.

1466. THOMSEN SYNDROME (CONGENITAL MYOTONIA SYNDROME; MYOTONIA CONGENITA)

General

Dominant; inheritance manifestations before age of 5 years; prevalent in males; possibly caused by excessive production of acetylcholine neuromuscular junction; emotions and cold enhance symptoms; warmth decreases symptoms; there are two types of this disorder: (1) an autosomal dominant and (2) an autosomal recessive, both with the same clinical features; has been linked to chromosome 7q35 in the region of the human skeletal muscle chloride channel gene (HUMCLC).

Ocular

Inability to open eyelids for a few seconds after closure; spasm of the orbicularis oculi muscle; extraocular muscle paresis.

Clinical

Myotonia with muscles of upper and lower extremities primarily affected; muscle hypertrophy; pronounced delay in relaxation of contracted voluntary muscles.

Laboratory/Ocular

Diagnosis is made by clinical findings.

Treatment

None

Bibliography

1. Adams RD, Victor M. Congenital myotonia. In: Adams RD, Victor M (Eds). Principles of Neurology, 5th edition. New York: McGraw-Hill; 1993. pp. 1275-8.

2. Ashworth B. Ocular myotonia. Bristol Med Chir J. 1975;90:31-5.

3. Brooke NM, Cwik VE. Disorders of skeletal muscle: myotonia congenita. In: Bradley WG (Ed). Neurology in Clinical Practice, 2nd edition. Boston: Butterworth-Heinemann; 1995. pp. 2026-7.

4. George AL, Crackower MA, Abdalla JA, et al. Molecular basis of Thomsen's disease (autosomal dominant myotonia congenita). Nat Genet. 1993;3:305-10.

5. Miller NR (Ed). Walsh and Hoyt's Clinical Ophthalmology, 6th edition. Baltimore: Williams & Wilkins; 2004.

6. Thomsen AJT. Myotonia Congenita: Tonische Krampfe in Willkurlich Beweglichen Muskeln in Folge von Ererbter Physischer Disposition (Ataxia Muscularis?). Arch Psych. 1876;6:702.

1467. THROMBOCYTOPENIA

General

Decrease in platelets.

Ocular

Retinal hemorrhages; papilledema; visual field defects; oculomotor nerve palsy; optic nerve atrophy.

Clinical

Anemia; cranial nerve palsies; thrombotic thrombocytopenic purpura; intracranial hemorrhage; neuro-ophthalmologic signs and symptoms.

Laboratory/Ocular

Diagnosis is made by clinical findings.

Treatment/Ocular

Papilledema: Underlying cause should be determined and treated. Systemic acetazolamide is the medical therapy of choice.

Bibliography

1. Collins JF. Handbook of Clinical Ophthalmology. New York: Masson; 1982. p. 235.
2. Elewaut C, Meire F, Van Coster R, et al. Optic atrophy as a complication of neonatal alloimmune thrombocytopenia. Bull Soc Belg Ophthalmol. 1991:241:85-8.
3. Miyao S, Takano A, Teramoto J, et al. Oculomotor nerve palsy due to intraneural hemorrhage in idiopathic thrombocytopenic purpura: a case report. Eur Neurol. 1993;33:20-2.

1468. THYGESON SYNDROME (KERATITIS SUPERFICIALIS PUNCTATA)

General

Etiology probably of viral origin; recurrence every 3–4 years.

Ocular

Punctate lesions of cornea; keratitis.

Clinical

None

Laboratory/Ocular

Diagnosis is made by clinical findings.

Treatment/Ocular

Keratitis: Local treatment is used for prevention and reduction of corneal damage. Systemic therapy is used for controlling the underlying disease. Tissue adhesives may be necessary for impending perforation. Keratectomy, conjunctival resection, amniotic membrane transplantation and keratoplasty may necessary.

Bibliography

1. Magalini SI, Scrascia E. Dictionary of Medical Syndromes, 2nd edition. Philadelphia: JB Lippincott; 1981.
2. Thygeson P. Superficial punctate keratitis. J Am Med Assoc. 1950;144:1544-9.

1469. THYROCEREBRORETINAL SYNDROME (FAMILIAL THYROCEREBRAL RETINAL SYNDROME)

General

Autosomal recessive; renal, neurologic, and thyroid disease.

Ocular

Retinal hemorrhages; central vision defect; retinal edema; optic atrophy.

Clinical

Thrombocytopenia; chronic renal disease; colloid goiter.

Laboratory

Blood test, CT scans and MRI are essential in the evaluation and diagnosis.

Treatment/Ocular

Corticosteroids are useful. Excision or decompression is needed when orbital tumors compress the optic nerve.

Bibliography

1. McKusick VA. Mendelian Inheritance in Man: A Catalog of Human Genes and Genetic Disorders, 12th edition. Baltimore: The Johns Hopkins University Press; 1998.

1470. TIC DOULOUREUX (TRIGEMINAL NEURALGIA)

General

Brief, sharp, unilateral facial pain that usually occurs in the middle or lower face; occurs more often in females; occurs most frequently in persons over age 40 years; right side affected more than left side.

Ocular

Ipsilateral hyperemia with the pain of conjunctiva; periorbital pain; ipsilateral lacrimation during the pain; decreased corneal sensitivity; photophobia.

Clinical

Pain triggered by chewing, swallowing, laughing, brushing teeth, shaving, or combing hair; may be present with multiple sclerosis.

Laboratory

Magnetic resonance imaging (MRI) and magnetic resonance angiography will demonstrate structural compression of the trigeminal rootlet.

Treatment

Systemic medications, such as carbamazepine and phenytoin, are particularly useful.

Additional Resource

1. Huff JS (2010). Trigeminal Neuralgia in Emergency Medicine. [online] Available from http://www.emedicine.com/emerg/TOPIC617.HTM [Accessed April, 2012].

1471. TILTED DISK SYNDROME

General

Relatively common congenital anomaly (1–2% of the population) consisting of inferonasal "tilting" of the disk, with the upper and temporal portion of the disk laying anterior to the inferonasal portion.

Ocular

"Tilting" of the disk with associated findings of an obliquely directed long axis of the disk, inferonasal crescent, posterior staphyloma of the affected inferonasal region of the fundus, and upper and temporal emergence of the retinal vessels rather than the nasal (situs inversus); lenticular astigmatism.

Clinical

Patients tend to have myopic astigmatism and superotemporal or bitemporal visual field depression; patients are at increased risk for retinal serous detachment.

Laboratory/Ocular

Diagnosis is made by clinical findings.

Treatment

None

Bibliography

1. Apple DJ, Rabb MF, Walsh PM. Congenital anomalies of the optic disc. Surv Ophthalmol. 1982;27:3-41.
2. Brazitikos PD, Safran AB, Simona F, et al. Threshold perimetry in tilted disc syndrome. Arch Ophthalmol. 1990;108:1698-1700.
3. Cohen SY, Quentel G, Guiberteau B, et al. Macular serous retinal detachment caused by subretinal leakage in tilted disc syndrome. Ophthalmology. 1998;105:1831-4.
4. Dorrell D. The tilted disc. Br J Ophthalmol. 1978;62:16-20.
5. Gass JDM. Stereoscopic Atlas of Macular Diseases: Diagnosis and Treatment, 4th edition. St. Louis: CV Mosby; 1997. pp. 986-7.
6. Gunduz A, Evereklioglu C, Er H, et al. Lenticular astigmatism in tilted disc syndrome. J Cataract Refract Srug. 2002;28:1836-40.
7. Young SE, Walsh FB. Knox DL. The tilted disk syndrome. Am J Ophthalmol. 1976;82:16-23.

1472. TOLOSA-HUNT SYNDROME (PAINFUL OPHTHALMOPLEGIA)

General

Symptoms last from days to weeks; attacks recur at intervals of months or years; inflammatory lesion of cavernous sinus; onset most frequent in the fifth decade of life; recurrent Tolosa-Hunt syndrome has been observed in some patients.

Ocular

Steadily "growing" retro-orbital pain; ptosis; involvement of cranial nerves III, IV, VI, and first division of V; scintillating scotomata; sluggish pupil reaction to light; corneal sensitivity diminished; optic neuritis.

Clinical

Inflammatory lesions of cavernous sinus.

Laboratory

Magnetic resonance imaging (MRI) with axial and coronal views of brain, typically showing thickening and enhancement of involved cavernous sinus. Cerebral angiography to rule out aneurysm. Blood count, erythrocyte sedimentation rate, antinuclear antibody, antineutrophil cytoplasmic antibody and angiotension-converting enzyme levels may be abnormal.

Treatment

Corticosteroids are often used to treat the chronic granulomatous inflammation of the cavernous sinus.

Additional Resource

1. Taylor DC (2010). Tolosa-Hunt Syndrome. [online] Available from http://www.emedicine.com/neuro/TOPIC373.HTM [Accessed April, 2012].

1473. TOLUENE ABUSE

General

Caused by inhalation of toluene and other toluene-containing substances, such as glue.

Ocular

Jerking movements of the eyes; bilateral optic neuropathy.

Clinical

Progressive tremor of the limbs, trunk, and head; dizziness; slurred speech; bilateral hearing loss; mild impairment of memory and concentration; reduced magnetic resonance signal intensity in the brain; distal renal tubular acidosis.

Laboratory

Serum electrocyte and glucose levels. Blood urea nitrogen and creatinine are use to monitor kidney function. Level of serum hippuric acid and toluene. Toxicological screens to measure levels of alcohol, cocaine, and salicylates.

Treatment

Provide oxygen as soon as possible; avoid mouth-to-mouth breathing; move patient to a safer area so that rescue workers can avoid contamination. Irrigation of the skin and eyes should be immediate specially if burns are present.

Additional Resource

1. McKeown NJ (2011). Toluene Toxicity. [online] Available from http://www.emedicine.com/emerg/TOPIC594.HTM [Accessed April, 2012].

1474. TOPLESS OPTIC DISK SYNDROME

General

Superior segmental optic hypoplasia.

Ocular

Relative superior entrance of the central retinal artery; thinning of the superior peripapillary nerve fiber layer; superior peripapillary scleral halo; pallor of the superior disk.

Clinical

Patients usually have good visual acuity and an inferior altitudinal or sector-like field defect; all reported patients either are children of mothers with type I diabetes mellitus or are Japanese.

Laboratory

Diagnosis is made by clinical findings.

Treatment

None

Bibliography

1. Hashimoto M, Ohtsuka K, Nakagawa T, et al. Topless optic disk syndrome without maternal diabetes mellitus. Am J Ophthalmol. 1999;128:111-2.
2. Kim RY, Hoyt WF, Lessell S, et al. Superior segmental optic hypoplasia. A sign of maternal diabetes. Arch Ophthalmol. 1989;107:1312-5.
3. Landau K, Bajka JD, Kirchschlager BM. Topless optic disks in children of mothers with type I diabetes mellitus. Am J Ophthalmol. 1998;125:605-11.
4. Petersen RA, Walton DS. Optic nerve hypoplasia with good visual acuity and visual field defects: a study of children of diabetic mothers. Arch Ophthalmol. 1977;95:254-8.

1475. TORIELLO-CAREY SYNDROME

General

Rare, genetic condition first described in 1988. Manin manifestations include agenesis of the corpus callosum, telecanthus, short palpebral fissures, small nose with anteverted nares, retrognathia, abnormal ears, laryngeal and cardiac anomalies.

Clinical

Corpus callosum agenesis, small nose, anteverted nostrils, Robin sequence, malformed ears, redundant neck skin, laryngeal abnormalities, heart defect, short hands, hypotonia, developmental delay.

Ocular

Telecanthus; short palpebral fissures.

Laboratory

Diagnosis is made by clinical findings.

Treatment

None

Bibliography

1. Chinen Y, Tohma T, Izumikawa Y, et al. Two sisters with Toriello-Carey syndrome. Am J Med Genet. 1999;87:262-4.
2. Lacombe D, Creusot G, Battin J. New case of Toriello-Carey syndrome. Am J Med Genet. 1992;42:374-6.

1476. TORRE-MUIR SYNDROME

General

Multiple sebaceous gland tumors of nonglabrous skin and visceral malignancy (primarily colonic) and keratoacanthomas; like Torre syndrome but associated with keratoacanthomas; benign skin tumors accompany and sometimes precede development of internal visceral malignancy; autosomal dominant inheritance.

Ocular

Sebaceous cell carcinoma of lid; carcinoma of caruncle; keratoacanthomas; tumor of the meibomian gland.

Clinical

Visceral carcinoma of gastrointestinal tract, breast and prostate.

Laboratory

Genetic studies, stool guaiac is useful in finding colonic carcinomas. The presence of MSI can be established with immunostaining of a biopsy specimen.

Treatment

Oral isotretinoin may prevent some neoplasms in patients with MTS. Benign sebaceous tumors and keratoacanthomas can be treated with excision or cryotherapy. Sebaceous carcinoma need to be completely excised and followed-up frequently for possible metastases.

Additional Resource

1. Prieto VG (2010). Muir-Torre Syndrome. [online] Available from http://www.emedicine.com/derm/TOPIC275.HTM [Accessed April, 2012].

1477. TORRE SYNDROME

General

Multiple sebaceous gland tumors of nonglabrous skin and visceral malignancy (primarily colonic).

Ocular

Sebaceous cell carcinoma of lid; carcinoma of caruncle; tumor of the meibomian gland.

Clinical

Visceral carcinoma of gastrointestinal tract, breast and prostate.

Laboratory

Diagnosis is made by clinical findings.

Treatment

Sebaceous cell carcinoma: Moh's technique appears to have the highest success rate.

Bibliography

1. Descalzi ME, Rosenthal S. Sebaceous adenomas and keratoacanthomas in a patient with malignant lymphoma. A new form of Torre's syndrome. Cutis. 1981;28:169-70.
2. Jakobiec FA. Sebaceous adenoma of the eyelid and visceral malignancy. Am J Ophthalmol. 1974;78:952-60.
3. Tillawi I, Katz R, Pellettiere EV. Solitary tumors of meibomian gland origin and Torre's syndrome. Am J Ophthalmol. 1987;104:179-82.
4. Torre D. Multiple sebaceous tumors. Arch Dermatol. 1968;98:549-51.

1478. TOURAINE-SOLENTE-GOLE SYNDROME (ACROPACHYDERMA; AUDRY II SYNDROME; BRUGSCH SYNDROME; FRIEDRICH-ERB-ARNOLD SYNDROME; HEHLINGER SYNDROME; PACHYDERMOPERIOSTOSIS)

General

Rare; hereditary; predominant in males; onset in puberty to third decade of life.

Ocular

Elephantiasis of the lids caused by meibomian gland cysts and connective tissue hypertrophy; ptosis.

Clinical

Thick and furrowed skin of forehead, face, scalp, hands, and feet; hyperhidrosis of hands and feet; increased subcutaneous secretion; enormous hands and feet; watch crystal-like nails; cylindrical arms and legs; effusions of ankles, knees, and other joints; finger clubbing; facial enlargement; periostitis; cutaneous mucinosis.

Laboratory

Levels of thyrotropin and growth hormone should be tested. Radionucleotide bone imaging may be helpful.

Treatment

Nonsteroidal anti-inflammatory drugs (NSAIDs) or corticosteroids may provide comfort from the polyarthritis. Vagotomy may alleviate the swelling and articular pain.

Additional Resource

1. Goyal S (2011). Pachydermoperiostosis. [online] Available from http://www.emedicine.com/derm/TOPIC815.HTM [Accessed April, 2012].

1479. TOURETTE SYNDROME (BRISSAUD II SYNDROME; CAPROLALIA GENERALIZED TIC; GILLES DE LA TOURETTE SYNDROME; GUINON MYOSPASIA IMPULSIVA)

General

Etiology unknown; occurs at age 7–8 years; emotional trauma is frequent precipitating factor; disturbed parent-child relationship frequently encountered.

Ocular

Blepharospasm; oculogyric deviations; dystonic neck movements.

Clinical

Chorea; caprolalia; echolalia tic; blinking and facial twitching.

Laboratory

No laboratory is available.

Treatment

Alpha2-adrenergic agonists and D2 dopamine medications are used to suppress tics.

Additional Resource

1. Hawley JS (2012). Pediatric Tourette Syndrome. [online] Available from http://www.emedicine. com/med/TOPIC3107.HTM [Accessed April, 2012].

1480. TOXIC LENS SYNDROME (TASS; TOXIC ANTERIOR SEGMENT SYNDROME)

General

Syndrome occurs within a few days to several weeks of implantation of an intraocular lens; with therapy, vision is restored in the majority of cases; increased incidence of disease caused by use of ethylene oxide sterilization (dry pack intraocular lenses); toxic lens syndrome may be prevented by treating the lens with sodium hydroxide and by using modem lathe-cut or compression-molded lenses with polypropylene loops; risk factors include uveitis in history, pseudo-exfoliation syndrome, inadequate mydriasis at the start of surgery, problems with intraocular lens implantation, and pigment effusion during surgery.

Ocular

Pigment precipitation on the surface of an intraocular lens; hypopyon; vitreous opacification; chronic uveitis; secondary glaucoma.

Clinical

None

Laboratory

Anterior chamber aspiration, vitreous tap, and/or vitreous biopsy for Gram stain and microbiologic cultures.

Treatment

Topical steroids and NSAIDs; patients should be evaluated the same or the next day to rule out infectious endophthalmitis, in which case, steroids would worsen the condition.

Additional Resource

1. Al-Ghoul AR (2010). Toxic Anterior Segment Syndrome. [online] Available from http://www. emedicine.com/oph/TOPIC779.HTM [Accessed April, 2012].

1481. TOXIC SHOCK SYNDROME

General

Multisystem illness caused by toxin-producing *Staphylococcus aureus* infection; occurs in all sexes and ages but most frequently in women; seen in association with tampon use; onset may be sudden.

Ocular

Eyelid necrosis; periorbital abscess; neonatal conjunctivitis; conjunctival hyperemia; preseptal cellulitis.

Clinical

Fever; rash; desquamation; hypotension; syncope; dizziness; shock; cardiovascular collapse; coma; death.

Laboratory

Electrolyte levels, CBC, liver function test, urinalysis, creatine kinase levels, chest radiograph, echocardiogram, and CT scan.

Treatment

Aggressive fluid resuscitation and oxygen should be administered. Intravenous immunoglobulin has been effective.

Additional Resource

1. Venkataraman R (2010). Toxic Shock Syndrome. [online] Available from http://www.emedicine. com/emerg/TOPIC600.HTM [Accessed April, 2012].

1482. TOXIC/NUTRITIONAL OPTIC NEUROPATHY

General

Caused by deficit nutrition or abuse of ethanol and tobacco; seen more frequently in underdeveloped countries, but is seen in US undernourished tobacco and alcohol abusers. Can also be associated with ingestion of toxic substances, workplace exposure or systemic medications.

Clinical

Alcoholism; drug and tobacco abuse.

Ocular

Papillomacular bundle damage; central scotoma; decreased color vision; bilateral vision loss; hyperemic disk; optic atrophy; temporal disk pallor; flame-shaped hemorrhages.

Laboratory

Clinical observation is used to make the diagnosis. Blood work for serum B-12 and red cell folate levels should be obtained. Urinalysis and other blood work may be needed to identify the possible toxin.

Treatment

Correction of the underlying etiology includes improving nutrition and eliminating the toxin is critical.

Additional Resource

1. Zafar A (2011). Toxic/Nutritional Optic Neuropathy. [online] Available from http://www.emedicine.medscape.com/article/1217661-overview [Accessed April, 2012].

1483. TRACHOMA

General

Most common in rural communities of the Middle East, Africa, Asia, and South and Central America; caused by *Chlamydia trachomatis*; associated with poor sanitation and medical care.

Ocular

Chronic keratoconjunctivitis; papillae follicles; keratitis; opacities of cornea; scars of palpebral conjunctiva; ptosis; tearing; entropion.

Clinical

Rhinitis; otitis media; upper respiratory tract infection.

Laboratory

Most endemic areas, lab tests are unavailable. Commercial polymerase chain reaction (PCR) based assay has high sensitivity and specifity.

Treatment

Tetracycline eye ointment for 6 weeks or a single dose azithromycin systemically.

Bibliography

1. Biebesheimer JB, House J, Hong KC, et al. Complete local elimination of infectious trachoma from severely affected communities after six biannual mass azithromycin distributions. Ophthalmology. 2009;116:2047-50.

Additional Resource

1. Solomon AW (2011). Trachoma. [online] Available from http://www.emedicine.com/oph/TOPIC118.HTM [Accessed April, 2012].

1484. TRANSIENT LIGHT SENSITIVITY SYNDROME (UVEITIS)

General

Associated with femtosecond laser keratome; may be related to the pulse energy used in flap creation.

Ocular

Transient postoperative photosensitivity.

Clinical

None

Laboratory

Diagnosis is made by clinical findings.

Treatment

Uveitis: Topical steroids and cycloplegic medication should be the initial treatment of choice. Oral steroids if not responsive to topical steroids, immunosuppressants if bilateral disease that does not respond to oral steroids, periocular steroids for unilateral or posterior uveitis. Vitrectomy can be used for severe vitreous opacification. Cryotherapy and laser photocoagulation may be used for localized pars plana exudates.

Bibliography

1. Kurtz RM, Liu X, Elner VM, et al. Photodisruption in the human cornea as a function of laser pulse width. J Cataract Refract Surg. 1997;13:653-8.
2. Stonecipher KG, Dishler JG, Ignacio TS, et al. Transient light sensitivity after femtosecond laser flap creation: clinical findings and management. J Cataract Refract Surg. 2006;32:91-4.

1485. TRANSIENT LOSS OF VISION

General

Monocular or Bilateral and last from seconds to hours. Episodes are usually ischemic in origin. Causes of ischemic transient visual loss include cerebrovascular ischemia, retinal arteriolar emboli, and amaurosis fugax syndrome. In children causes may include migraine and epileptic seizure.

Clinical

Hypotension, cardiac arrhythmias, anemia; epilepsy, heart failure, atherosclerotic disease, angiospasm, migraine.

Ocular

Amaurosis fugax; ocular migraine; transient visual disturbance mononcular or bilateral; afferent pupillary defect; decreased visual acuity.

Laboratory

Lab work and neuroimaging studies may be necessary if a cause can not be determined.

Treatment

If possible cause should be determined and patient referred to the appropriate specialist.

Additional Resource

1. Tatham AJ (2011). Transient Loss of Vision. [online] Available from http://www.emedicine.medscape.com/article/1435495-overview [Accessed April, 2012].

1486. TRAUMATIC CATARACT

General

Injury resulting in lens opacification which can be diagnosed at the time of the trauma or years later.

Clinical

None

Ocular

Visual loss, amblyopia, trauma to cornea, loose iris zonules.

Laboratory

Diagnosis is made by clinical findings.

Treatment

Extracapsular cataract extraction or phacoemulsification is the procedure of choice.

Additional Resource

1. Graham RH (2012). Traumatic Cataract. [online] Available from http://www.emedicine.com/oph/TOPIC52.HTM [Accessed April, 2012].

1487. TRAUMATIC ENCEPHALOPATHY SYNDROME (POSTCONCUSSION SYNDROME; POST-TRAUMATIC GENERAL CEREBRAL SYNDROME; PUNCH-DRUNK SYNDROME) NYSTAGMUS

General

Small focal hemorrhages within the cerebrum and/or cerebellum causing functional brain damage; minor traumatic brain injury is the most common type of traumatic encephalopathy.

Ocular

Nystagmus or Nystagmoid ocular movements.

Clinical

Personality change; rigid face without expression; staggering gait; dysphonia.

Laboratory

Computed tomography (CT) and MRI can detect intracranial abnormalities.

Treatment

No specific treatment has been proven effective.

Additional Resource

1. Legome EL (2011). Postconcussive Syndrome in Emergency Medicine. [online] Available from http://www.emedicine.com/emerg/TOPIC865. HTM [Accessed April, 2012].

1488. TRAUMATIC OPTIC NEUROPATHY

General

Related to head or ocular trauma in the absence of another etiology. Motor vehicle and bicycle accidents are the most frequent causes.

Clinical

Head trauma, blood in the sphenoid sinus.

Ocular

Optic neuropathy, decreased visual acuity, decreased color vision, afferent pupillary defect and optic canal fracture.

Laboratory

Computed tomography (CT) scanning is the most important evaluation and is superior to MRI.

Treatment

No treatment is advised for anterior or direct optic nerve injuries. Posterior, indirect injuries may benefit from intravenous corticosteroids. If improvement occurs oral prednisone should be given. If no improvement surgical decompression should be considered.

Additional Resources

1. O'Brien EK (2011). Optic Nerve Decompression for Traumatic Optic Neuropathy. [online] Available from http://www.emedicine.com/ent/TOPIC168. HTM [Accessed April, 2012].
2. Zoumalan CI (2012). Traumatic Optic Neuropathy. [online] Available from http://www. emedicine.com/ent/TOPIC167.HTM [Accessed April, 2012].

1489. TREFT SYNDROME (OPTIC ATROPHY)

General

Autosomal dominant; usually appears by age of 11 years.

Ocular

Optic atrophy; visual loss; ptosis; ophthalmoplegia.

Clinical

Hearing loss by age of 14 years; myopathic changes; balance difficulty.

Laboratory

Diagnosis is made by clinical findings.

Treatment

Optic atrophy: Intravenous steroids may be used with optic neuritis or ischemic neuropathy. Stem cell treatment may be the future treatment of choice.

Bibliography

1. McKusick VA. Mendelian Inheritance in Man: A Catalog of Human Genes and Genetic Disorders, 12th edition. Baltimore: The Johns Hopkins University Press; 1998.
2. McKusick-Nathans Institute for Genetic Medicine, Johns Hopkins University and National Center for Biotechnology Information, National Library of Medicine. (2007). Online Mendelian Inheritance in Man (OMIM). [online] Available from http://www.ncbi.nlm.nih.gov/omim/ [Accessed April, 2012].
3. Treft RL, Sanborn GE, Carey J, et al. Dominant optic atrophy, deafness, ptosis, ophthalmoplegia, dystaxia, and myopathy. A new syndrome. Ophthalmology. 1984;91:908-15.

1490. TRIANGULAR SYNDROME (RETINAL TEAR)

General

Rare; follows trauma of excessive compression during surgery, such as Faden operation.

Ocular

Choroidal ischemia; retinal tear; sectorial infarction of choroid; occlusion of posterior ciliary vessel with triangular chorioretinal scar.

Clinical

None

Laboratory

Diagnosis is made by clinical findings.

Treatment

Retinal tear: Perfluoron can be used to unravel the retina and then laser is applied to reattach the retina.

Bibliography

1. Alio JL, Faci A. Fundus changes following faden operation. Arch Ophthalmol. 1984;102:211-3.
2. Brini A, Risse JF, Flament J. Post-contusional triangular syndrome of the posterior pole. Bull Soc Ophthalmol. 1973;73:985-8.

1491. TRICHIASIS

General

Acquired condition in which previous normal eyelashes are misdirected toward the globe.

Clinical

Stevens-Johnson syndrome, toxic epidermal necrolysis and ocular cicatrical pemphigoid.

Ocular

Ocular irritation, chronic eyelid inflammation or infection, foreign body sensation.

Laboratory

Diagnosis is made by clinical findings.

Treatment

Epilation, argon laser ablation, cryosurgery, radio surgery and full-thickness wedge resection or eyelid margin rotation procedures are all possible therapies.

Additional Resource

1. Graham RH (2012). Trichiasis. [online] Available from http://www.emedicine.com/oph/TOPIC609.HTM [Accessed April, 2012].

1492. TRICHINELLOSIS (TRICHINOSIS)

General

Parasite *Trichinella* enters the body by ingestion of infected meat (usually poorly cooked pork).

Ocular

Conjunctivitis; splinter hemorrhages of conjunctiva; paralysis of sixth nerve; exophthalmos; proptosis; uveitis; optic neuritis; papilledema; retinal hemorrhages; dyschromatopsia; scotoma; secondary glaucoma; encysted parasites in the extraocular muscles.

Clinical

Fever; urticaria; respiratory symptoms; muscle pain; myalgias and severe proximal muscle weakness; impaired coordination.

Laboratory

Leukocytosis and eosinophilia elevated serum levels of lactic dehydrogenase, aldolase and creatine phosphokinese (50% cases).

Treatment

Mebendazole orally is the treatment of choice. In severe cases, prednisone may be used in conjunction with antihelminthic agent.

Additional Resource

1. Arnold LK (2010). Trichinellosis/Trichinosis. [online] Available from http://www.emedicine.com/emerg/TOPIC612.HTM [Accessed April, 2012].

1493. TRICHOMEGALY WITH MENTAL RETARDATION, DWARFISM, AND PIGMENTARY DEGENERATION OF THE RETINA (OLIVER MCFARLANE SYNDROME) NYSTAGMUS

General

Autosomal recessive.

Ocular

Excessive growth of eyelashes and eyebrow hair; pigmentary degeneration of retina; horizontal nystagmus; bilateral choroidoretinal pigmentary degeneration; ring heterochromia of the iris.

Clinical

Bulging of occipital and frontal bones; low-birth-weight; dwarfism; cryptorchidism; underdevelopment of penis; frontal alopecia.

Laboratory

Diagnosis is made by clinical findings.

Treatment

None

Bibliography

1. Delleman JW, Van Walbeek K. The syndrome of trichomegaly, tapetoretinal degeneration and growth disturbances. Ophthalmologica. 1975;171:313-5.
2. McKusick VA. Mendelian Inheritance in Man: A Catalog of Human Genes and Genetic Disorders, 12th edition. Baltimore: The Johns Hopkins University Press; 1998.
3. McKusick-Nathans Institute for Genetic Medicine, Johns Hopkins University and National Center for Biotechnology Information, National Library of Medicine. (2007). Online Mendelian Inheritance in Man (OMIM). [online] Available from http://www.ncbi.nlm.nih.gov/omim [Accessed April, 2012].

1494. TRIPLOIDY SYNDROME (IRIS COLOBOMA)

General

Extra set of chromosomes due to diandry or digyny; stillbirth or early neonatal death.

Ocular

Iris coloboma; microphthalmia; hypertelorism.

Clinical

Large placenta; prenatal growth deficits; large fontanelles; syndactyly; heart defects; cleft lip; genital, brain, ear, and kidney malformations; meningomyelocele; micrognathia.

Laboratory/Ocular

Diagnosis is made by clinical findings.

Treatment

None

Bibliography

1. Arvidsson CG, Hamberg H, Johnsson H, et al. A boy with complete triploidy and unusually long survival. Acta Paediatr Scand. 1986;75:507-10.
2. Crane JP, Beaver HA, Cheung SW. Antenatal ultrasound findings in fetal triploidy syndrome. J Ultrasound Med. 1985;4:519-24.

3. Kaufman MH. New insights into triploidy and tetraploidy, from an analysis of model systems for these conditions. Hum Reprod. 1991;6:8-16.

4. Magalini SI, Scrascia E. Dictionary of Medical Syndromes, 2nd edition. Philadelphia: JB Lippincott; 1981.

5. O'Brien WF, Knuppel RA, Kousseff B, et al. Elevated maternal serum alpha-fetoprotein in triploidy. Obstet Gynecol. 1988;71(6 Pt 2):994-5.

6. Rubenstein JB, Swayne LC, Dise CA, et al. Placental changes in fetal triploidy syndrome. J Ultrasound Med. 1986;5:545-50.

7. Strobel SL, Brandt JT. Abnormal hematologic features in a live-born female infant with triploidy. Arch Pathol Lab Med. 1985;109:775-7.

8. Walker S, Andrews J, Gregson NM, et al. Three further cases of triploidy in man surviving to birth. J Med Genet. 1973;10:135-41.

1495. TRISOMY 10q SYNDROME (10q+ SYNDROME) OPTIC DISK

General

Chromosome 10q trisomy (duplication) syndrome.

Ocular

Microphthalmia; deep-set eyes; epicanthus; bilateral, enlarged, gray optic disks; distended retinal vessels; bilateral punctate yellow deposits near the macula and optic disk.

Clinical

Mental retardation; microcephaly; prominent forehead; upturned nose; bow-shaped mouth; micrognathia; thick and flat helices of the ears; long slender limbs.

Laboratory

Diagnosis is made by clinical findings.

Treatment

None/Ocular.

Bibliography

1. Neely K, Mets MB, Wong P, et al. Ocular findings in partial trisomy 10q syndrome. Am J Ophthalmol. l988;106:82-7.

1496. TRISOMY 13 SYNDROME (PATAU SYNDROME, REESE SYNDROME, TRISOMY D1 SYNDROME) IRIS COLOBOMA

General

Extra chromosome in the D group; fatal in the first few months of life; trisomy 13–15 resembles trisomy D1.

Ocular

Anophthalmos; microphthalmos; iris coloboma; cataracts; retinal dysplasia; optic nerve coloboma; optic atrophy; iris dysplasia; calcified lens; retinal detachment; optic nerve hypoplasia; orbital cysts.

Clinical

Apneic spells; developmental deficiency of the nervous system; seizures (minor motor); deafness; cleft lip and palate; hemangiomata; horizontal palmar creases; hyperconvex fingernails; interventricular septal defects; renal abnormalities; cardiovascular changes; respiratory involvement; gastrointestinal disease; urogenital involvement; cerebral hypoplasia with hydrocephalus; mental retardation.

Laboratory

Immediate conventional cytogenetic test. Ultrasonography for any anomalies. Trisomy 13 is best identified through cytogenetic study of amniotic fluid.

Treatment

Surgical care is usually withheld for the first few months of life.

Additional Resource

1. Best RG (2012). Patau Syndrome. [online] Available from http://www.emedicine.com/ped/TOPIC1745.HTM [Accessed April, 2012].

1497. TRISOMY 17p SYNDROME (HYPERTELORISM)

General

Trisomy 17p duplication syndrome.

Ocular

Hypertelorism, antimongoloid (up-slanting) palpebral fissures.

Clinical

Growth retardation; microcephaly; long philtrum with a thin upper lip; micrognathia; high-arched palate.

Laboratory

Diagnosis is made by clinical findings.

Treatment

None/Ocular.

Bibliography

1. Schrander-Stumpel C, Schrander J, Fryns JP, et al. Trisomy 17p due to a t(8;17) (p23;p11.2) pat translocation. Case report and review of the literature. Clin Genet. 1990;37:148-52.

1498. TRISOMY 18 SYNDROME (E SYNDROME; EDWARDS SYNDROME) CONGENITAL GLAUCOMA

General

Chromosome 18 present in triplicate; more common in females (3:1); age of mother over 40 years; onset from fetal life.

Ocular

Unilateral ptosis; epicanthal folds; congenital glaucoma; corneal opacities; lens opacities; optic atrophy.

Clinical

Low-set ears; micrognathia; high-arched palate; prominent occiput; cryptorchidism; failure to thrive; ventricular septal defect; hypertonicity with rigidity in flexion of limbs; mental retardation; umbilical and inguinal hernias.

Laboratory

Cytogenetic test, echocardiography, Ultrasono-graphy, and skeletal radiography are use to detect any abnormalities.

Treatment

Treat infections as appropriate. For feeding difficulties nasogastric and gastrostomy supplementation is recommended.

Additional Resource

1. Chen H (2011). Trisomy 18. [online] Available from http://www.emedicine.com/ped/TOPIC652.HTM [Accessed April, 2012].

1499. TRISOMY 20 SYNDROME (EXOTROPIA)

General

Trisomy 20q (duplication) syndrome.

Ocular

Oblique palpebral fissures, strabismus.

Clinical

Round face; cardiac and vertebral abnormalities; mild psychomotor retardation with poor coordination and speech impediment; anencephaly.

Laboratory

Diagnosis is made by clinical findings.

Treatment

Strabismus: Equalized vision with correct refractive error; surgery may be helpful in patient with diplopia.

Bibliography

1. Archidiacono N, Tecilazich D, Tonini G, et al. Trisomy 20p from maternal t(3;20) translocation. J Med Genet. 1979;16:229-32.
2. Zumel RM, Darnaude MT, Delicado A, et al. Trisomy 20p from maternal translocation and anencephaly. Case report and genetic review. Ann Genet. 1989;32:247-9.

1500. TRISOMY 21q- SYNDROME (21q DELETION SYNDROME)

General

Chromosome 21q deletion syndrome.

Ocular

Blepharochalasis; microphthalmia with persistent hypoplastic primary vitreous.

Clinical

Mental and physical retardation; generalized hypertonia; high nasal bridge; micrognathia; malformed ears with preauricular pits, and overlying fingers.

Laboratory

Amniocentesis, fetal chromosome analysis and prenatal echography.

Treatment

Knowing the systemic and ocular findings is important in the treatment of patients with trisomy 21.

Additional Resource

1. Izquierdo NJ (2011). Ophthalmologic Manifestations of Down Syndrome. [online] Available from http://www.emedicine.com/oph/TOPIC522.HTM [Accessed April, 2012].

1501. TRISOMY 22 SYNDROME

General

Trisomy for chromosome 21/22; trisomy 22 may be very mild form of Down's syndrome (trisomy 21).

Ocular

High myopia.

Clinical

Schizophrenia; micrognathia; large nostrils; flat occiput; hyperextension of elbows; macrocephaly; hydrocephalus; holoprosencephaly; facioauriculovertebral (Goldenhar) sequence.

Laboratory

Diagnosis is made by clinical findings.

Treatment

Myopia: Generally treated with glasses, contact lens and refractive surgery.

Bibliography

1. Collins JF. Handbook of Clinical Ophthalmology. New York: Masson; 1982.
2. Fahmi F, Schmerler S, Hutcheon RG. Hydrocephalus in an infant with trisomy 22. J Med Genet. 1994;31:141-4.
3. Hayward MD, Bower BD. Chromosomal trisomy associated with the Sturge-Weber syndrome. Lancet. 1960;2:844-6.
4. Kobrynski L, Chitayat D, Zahed L, et al. Trisomy 22 and facioauriculovertebral (Goldenhar) sequence. Am J Med Genet. 1993;46:68-71.
5. Kucerova M, Polivkova Z. A case of a girl with a 21 ring chromosome. Hum Hered. 1974;24:100-4.

1502. TRISOMY 2q SYNDROME (q33-qTER) CONGENITAL GLAUCOMA

General

Associated with monosomy 9p (p24-pter); autosomal recessive or X-linked inheritance.

Ocular

Congenital glaucoma; hypertelorism; epicanthus.

Clinical

Low-set and malformed ears; short saddle nose with anteverted nostrils; long, hypoplastic philtrum; thin upper lip; hypospadias; short fingers; muscular hypotonia; psychomotor retardation; clinodactyly; scoliosis; broad, flat nasal bridge; short neck; short esophagus; tubular stomach.

Laboratory

Diagnosis is made by clinical findings.

Treatment

Congenital glaucoma: Primary congenital glaucoma almost always is managed surgically, both goniotomy and trabeculectomy may be useful. When multiple goniotomies and/or trabeculectomies fail, the surgeon usually resorts to a filtering procedure.

Bibliography

1. De Grouchy J, Turleau C. Clinical Atlas of Human Chromosomes, 2nd edition. New York: John Wiley and Sons; 1984.
2. Katsushima H, Kii T, Soma K, et al. Primary congenital glaucoma in a patient with trisomy 2q (q33-qter) and monosomy 9p(p24-pter). Case report. Arch Ophthalmol. 1987;105:323.
3. Porter J, Klein VR, Wilson GN, et al. Gastrointestinal malformation in genetic disorders: a case of partial trisomy 2q with short esophagus and tubular stomach. Clin Pediatr (Phila). 1991;30:559-62.
4. Romain DR, Mackenzie NG, Moss D, et al. Partial trisomy for 2q in a patient with dir dup(2) (q33.1q35). J Med Genet. 1994;31:652-3.

1503. TRISOMY 6q SYNDROME (DUPLICATION 6q+6q SYNDROME) HYPERTELORISM

General

Chromosome 6q trisomy syndrome.

Ocular

Hypertelorism; mongoloid (down-slanting) palpebral fissures.

Clinical

Cleft soft palate; bow-shaped mouth; micrognathia; short, laterally webbed neck; microcephaly; clubbing of hands and feet; syndactyly; growth retardation; mental retardation; "carp" mouth.

Laboratory/Ocular

Diagnosis is made by clinical findings.

Treatment

None/Ocular.

Bibliography

1. Chen H, Tyrkus M, Cohen F, et al. Familial partial trisomy 6q syndromes resulting from inherited ins (5;6) (q33; q15q27). Clin Genet. 1976;9:631-7.
2. Franchino CJ, Beneck D, Greco MA, et al. Partial trisomy 6q: case report with necropsy findings. J Med Genet. 1987;24:300-3.
3. Zneimer SM, Ziel B, Bachman R. Partial trisomy of chromosome 6q: an interstitial duplication of the long arm. Am J Med Genet. 1998;80:133-5.

1504. TRISOMY 8 MOSAICISM SYNDROME (EXOTROPIA)

General

Chromosomally abnormal cell line with each cell containing an extra chromosome 8; other cell lines normal; both sexes affected; present from birth.

Ocular

Strabismus; hypertelorism; deep-set eyes.

Clinical

Mild-to-moderate mental retardation; low-set or malformed ears; broad, bulbous nose; palatal deformity; congenital cardiovascular disorders; hydronephrosis; cryptorchidism; poor coordination; prominent forehead; enlarged nares; full lips; cupped ears; camptodactyly of fingers and toes; reported as a nonrandom secondary change in myxoid liposarcoma.

Laboratory/Ocular

Diagnosis is made by clinical findings.

Treatment

Strabismus: Equalized vision with correct refractive error; surgery may be helpful in patient with diplopia.

Bibliography

1. Fineman RM, Ablow RC, Howard RO, et al. Trisomy 8 mosaicism syndrome. Pediatrics. 1975;56:762-7.
2. Geeraets WJ. Ocular Syndromes, 3rd edition. Philadelphia: Lea & Febiger; 1976.

1505. TRISOMY 9q SYNDROME (HYPERTELORISM)

General

Congenital mental retardation syndrome due to 9p trisomy.

Ocular

Hypertelorism; deep-set eyes; antimongoloid (up-slanting) eyes.

Clinical

Mental retardation; short stature; down-turned corners of the mouth; slightly or moderately bulbous nose; moderately large ears; nail dysplasia and hypoplasias; clinodactyly; abnormal dermatoglyphs.

Laboratory

Diagnosis is made by clinical findings.

Treatment

None

Bibliography

1. Centerwall WR, Miller KS, Reeves LM. Familial 'partial 9p' trisomy: six cases and four carriers in three generations. J Med Genet. 1976;13:57-61.
2. Wahlstrom J, Gustavasson KH. Trisomy 9p syndrome and syndrome in siblings. Clin Genet. 1978;13:511.
3. Young RS, Reed T, Hodes ME, et al. The dermatoglyphic and clinical features of the 9p trisomy and partial 9p monosomy syndromes. Hum Genet. 1982;62:31-9.

1506. TRISOMY D1 SYNDROME (PATAU SYNDROME; REESE SYNDROME; TRISOMY 13) IRIS COLOBOMA

General

Extra chromosome in the D group; fatal in the first few months of life; trisomy 13-15 resembles trisomy D1.

Ocular

Anophthalmos; microphthalmos; iris coloboma; cataracts; retinal dysplasia; optic nerve coloboma; optic atrophy; iris dysplasia; calcified lens; retinal detachment; optic nerve hypoplasia; orbital cysts.

Clinical

Apneic spells; developmental deficiency of nervous system; seizures (minor motor); deafness; cleft lip and palate; hemangiomata (capillary type); horizontal palmar creases; hyperconvex fingernails; interventricular septal defects; renal abnormalities; cardiovascular changes; respiratory involvement; gastrointestinal disease; urogenital involvement; cerebral hypoplasia with hydrocephalus; mental retardation.

Laboratory/Ocular

Diagnosis is made by clinical findings.

Treatment

Anophthalmos: Orbital expansion with serial implants in the growing orbit, increase horizontal length of palpebral fissure, dermis fat graft, inflatable silicone expander.

Bibliography

1. Apple DJ, Holden JD, Stallworth B. Ocular pathology of Patau's syndrome with an unbalanced D-D translocation. Am J Ophthalmol. 1970;70:383-91.
2. Cogan DG, Kuwabara T. Ocular pathology of the 13–15 trisomy syndrome. Arch Ophthalmol. 1964;72:246-53.
3. Ginsberg J, Bove KE. Ocular pathology of trisomy 13. Ann Ophthalmol. 1974;6:113.
4. Kukharenko V, Sheleg S, Freudine M, et al. Down's syndrome, Edward's syndrome, Patau's syndrome—synthesis of glycosaminoglycans. Hum Genet. 1994;94:80-2.

1507. TRISTICHIASIS

General

Autosomal dominant.

Ocular

Three rows of eyelashes.

Clinical

None

Laboratory

Diagnosis is made by clinical findings.

Treatment

Trichiasis: Epilation, argon laser ablation, cryosurgery, radio surgery and full-thickness wedge resection or eyelid margin rotation procedures are all possible therapies.

Bibliography

1. Loeffler L. Erbbiologie des Menschlichen Hautorgans. In: Hanbuch der Erbbiologie des Menschen. Berlin: Springer Verlag; 1940.
2. McKusick VA. Mendelian Inheritance in Man: A Catalog of Human Genes and Genetic Disorders, 12th edition. Baltimore: The Johns Hopkins University Press; 1998.
3. McKusick-Nathans Institute for Genetic Medicine, Johns Hopkins University and National Center for Biotechnology Information, National Library of Medicine. (2007). Online Mendelian Inheritance in Man (OMIM). [online] Available from http://www.ncbi.nlm.nih.gov/omim [Accessed April, 2012].

1508. TRITANOPIA (BLUE COLOR BLINDNESS; COLOR BLINDNESS)

General

Autosomal dominant; more common in males; defective blue color vision is characteristic; two amino acid substitutions in the gene encoding the blue-sensitive opsin have been detected.

Ocular

Lacking blue and yellow sensory mechanisms while retaining those for red and green; optic atrophy.

Clinical

None

Laboratory

Diagnosis is made by clinical findings.

Treatment

Optic atrophy: Intravenous steroids may be used with optic neuritis or ischemic neuropathy. Stem cell treatment may be the future treatment of choice.

Bibliography

1. Boger WP, Petersen RA. Pediatric ophthalmology. Protan and deutan color blindness. In: Pavan-Langston D (Ed). Manual of Ocular Diagnosis and Therapy, 4th edition. Boston: Little, Brown and Company; 1995. pp. 285-6.
2. McKusick VA. Mendelian Inheritance in Man: A Catalog of Human Genes and Genetic Disorders, 12th edition. Baltimore: The Johns Hopkins University Press; 1998.
3. McKusick-Nathans Institute for Genetic Medicine, Johns Hopkins University and National Center for Biotechnology Information, National Library of Medicine. (2007). Online Mendelian Inheritance in Man (OMIM). [online] Available from http://www.ncbi.nlm.nih.gov/omim [Accessed April, 2012].
4. Merin S. The cone dystrophies and color vision disorders. In: Merin S (Ed). Inherited Eye Diseases. New York: Marcel Dekker; 1991. pp. 176-96.
5. Miyake Y, Yagasaki K, Ichikawa H. Differential diagnosis of congenital tritanopia and dominantly inherited juvenile optic atrophy. Arch Ophthalmol. 1985;103:1496-501.
6. Weitz CJ, Miyake Y, Shinzato K, et al. Human tritanopia associated with two amino acid substitutions in the blue-sensitive opsin. Am J Hum Genet. 1992;50:498-507.

1509. TROPICAL PANCREATIC DIABETES (TPD) (BACKGROUND RETINOPATHY)

General

Secondary diabetes as a result of chronic calcific pancreatitis; limited geographically to a few tropical countries; highest prevalence in Southern India; male predominance; onset at young age; associated with protein calorie malnutrition; possible cause is cassava ingestion; malnutrition has been postulated as a possible etiology.

Ocular

Background retinopathy; proliferative retinopathy; fibrous retinitis proliferans; microaneurysms; macular edema; hemorrhages; exudates; decreased visual acuity.

Clinical

Chronic pancreatitis; recurrent abdominal pain; steatorrhea.

Laboratory/Ocular

Fasting glucose and hemoglobin A1C.

Treatment/Ocular

Laser photocoagulation.

Additional Resource

1. Bhavsar AR (2011). Diabetic Retinopathy. [online] Available from http://www.emedicine.com/oph/TOPIC414.HTM [Accessed April, 2012].

1510. TUBERCULOSIS

General

Communicable disease caused by the acid-fast bacillus *Mycobacterium tuberculosis*.

Ocular

Conjunctivitis; subconjunctival nodules (tuberculomas); keratitis; pannus; corneal ulcer; blepharitis; cellulitis; meibomianitis; uveitis; dacryocystitis; chronic orbital cellulitis; retinitis; scleritis; scleral perforation; hypopyon; vitreous hemorrhages; optic neuritis; optic atrophy; tuberculous panophthalmitis; choroidal tubercles; intraorbital extraocular lesions.

Clinical

Pulmonary infection; pyuria; hematuria; epididymitis; dysuria; flank pain; distorted calyces; productive cough.

Laboratory

Acid-fast bacillus culture of body fluids including vitreous and aqueous. Polymerase chain reaction 89% positive for pulmonary infection.

Treatment

A course of chemothrerapy (isoniazid, vifampin, pyrazinamide and ethambutol or streptomycin) for a period of 6 months is the recommended therapy.

Bibliography

1. Collins JF. Handbook of Clinical Ophthalmology. New York: Masson; 1982.
2. D'Souza P, Garg R, Dhaliwal RS, et al. Orbital tuberculosis. Int Ophthalmol. 1994;18:149-52.
3. Devoe AG, Locatcher-Khorazo D. The external manifestations of ocular tuberculosis. Trans Am Ophthalmol Soc. 1964;62:203-12.
4. Roy FH, Fraunfelder FW, Fraunfelder FT. Roy and Fraunfelder's Current Ocular Therapy, 6th edition. Philadelphia: WB Saunders; 2008.
5. Gupta V, Gupta A, Arora S, et al. Presumed tubercular serpiginouslike choroiditis: clinical presentations and management. Ophthalmology. 2003;110:1744-9.
6. Patkar S, Singhania BK, Agrawal A. Intraorbital extraocular tuberculosis: a report of three cases. Surg Neurol. 1994;42:320-1.
7. Tejada P, Mendez MJ, Negreira S. Choroidal tubercles with tuberculous meningitis. Int Ophthalmol. 1994;18:115-8.

1511. TUNBRIDGE-PALEY DISEASE (OPTIC ATROPHY)

General

Onset in childhood; familial; optic atrophy and deafness seen in conjunction with juvenile diabetes mellitus.

Ocular

Optic atrophy; ptosis; retinal pigmentation.

Clinical

Hearing loss; perceptive deafness; juvenile diabetes mellitus; neurogenic bladder; Friedreich ataxia; Refsum syndrome; amentia; epilepsy; Laurence-Moon-Biedl-Bardet syndrome.

Laboratory

Diagnosis is made by clinical findings.

Treatment

Ptosis: If visual acuity is affected most cases require surgical correction, and there are several procedures that may be used including levator resection, repair or advancement and Fasanella-Servat.

Bibliography

1. Ikkos DG, Fraser GR, Matsouki-Gavra E, et al. Association of juvenile diabetes mellitus, primary optic atrophy and perceptive hearing loss in three sibs, with additional idiopathic diabetes mellitus insipidus in one case. Acta Endocrinol. 1970;65:95-102.

2. Konigsmark BW, Knox DL, Hussels IE, et al. Dominant congenital deafness and progressive optic nerve atrophy. Occurrence in four generations of a family. Arch Ophthalmol. 1974;91:99-103.

3. Paley RG, Tunbridge RE. Primary optic atrophy in diabetes mellitus. Diabetes. 1956;5:295-6.

1512. TUOMAALA-HAAPANEN SYNDROME (NUCLEAR CATARACT)

General

Unknown etiology; features similar to pseudo-hypoparathyroidism.

Ocular

Antimongoloid lid fissures; hypoplastic tarsus; distichiasis; nystagmus; strabismus; myopia; cataract; hypoplasia of the fovea.

Clinical

Dwarfism; short fingers and toes; wide nose bridge; small maxilla; oxycephaly; cutaneous depigmentation; alopecia; micrognathia; anodontia.

Laboratory

Diagnosis is made by clinical findings.

Treatment

Cataract: Change in glasses can sometimes improve a patient's visual function temporarily; however, the most common treatment is cataract surgery.

Bibliography

1. Albright R, Burnett CH, Smith PH, et al. Pseudo-hypoparathyroidism—example of "Seabright-Bantam syndrome", report of three cases. Endocrinology. 1942;30:922-32.

2. Tuomaala P, Haapanen E. Three siblings with similar anomalies in the eyes, bones and skin. Acta Ophthalmol. 1968;46:365-71.

1513. TURNER SYNDROME (BONNEVIE-ULLRICH SYNDROME; GENITAL DWARFISM SYNDROME; GONADAL DYSGENESIS; PTERYGOLYMPHANGIECTASIA SYNDROME; TURNER-ALBRIGHT SYNDROME; ULLRICH-BONNEVIE SYNDROME; ULLRICH-TURNER SYNDROME) CATARACT, POSTERIOR

General

Ovarian or gonadal agenesis; 45 chromosomes with an XO sex chromosome constitution; females; rare in males; onset in childhood.

Ocular

Exophthalmos; hypertelorism; ptosis; epicanthal folds; blue sclera; corneal nebulae; cataracts; conjunctival lymphoedema; keratoconus.

Clinical

Webbed neck (pterygium colli); diminished growth; mandibulofacial disproportion; cubitus valgus; masculine chest and trunk; late appearance of pubic and axillary hair; congenital deafness; mental retardation; coarctation of aorta.

Laboratory

Karyotyping is needed for diagnosis. Y chromosomal test. LH and FSH levels, thyroid function test, fasting glucose levels, echocardiography and MRI.

Treatment

Growth hormone therapy is used to prevent short stature. Estrogen replacement therapy is usually started by the age of 12–15 years old.

Additional Resource

1. Postellon DC (2011). Turner Syndrome. [online] Available from http://www.emedicine.com/ped/TOPIC2330.HTM [Accessed April, 2012].

1514. UGH SYNDROME (UVEITIS-GLAUCOMA-HYPHEMA SYNDROME) GLAUCOMA

General

Caused by a defective anterior chamber lens; can be caused by toxic substance incorporated into the plastic of lens during manufacture or warped intraocular lens; syndrome may rarely occur after extracapsular cataract extraction (ECCE) with implantation of a posterior chamber intraocular lens.

Ocular

Uveitis, glaucoma, hyphema (UGH).

Clinical

None

Laboratory

Diagnosis is made by clinical findings.

Treatment

Uveitis: Topical steroids and cycloplegic medication should be the initial treatment of choice. Oral steroids if not responsive to topical steroids, immunosuppressants if bilateral disease that does not respond to oral steroids, periocular steroids for unilateral or posterior uveitis. Vitrectomy can be used for severe vitreous opacification. Cryotherapy and laser photocoagulation may be used for localized pars plana exudates.

Glaucoma: Its medication should be the first plan of action. If medication is unsuccessful, a filtering surgical procedure with or without antimetabolites may be beneficial.

Hyphema: Cycloplegia decreased the inflammation and discomfort associated with traumatic iritis. Topical beta-adrenergic antagonists are the therapy of choice for elevated intraocular pressures; laser may be used to cauterize the bleeding vessel.

Bibliography

1. Percival SP, Das SK. UGH syndrome after posterior chamber lens implantation. J Am Intraocul Implant Soc. 1983;9:200-1.
2. Masket S. Pseudophakic posterior iris chafing syndrome. J Cataract Refract Surg. 1986;12:252-6.
3. Van Liefferinge T, Van Oye R, Kestelyn P. Uveitis-glaucoma-hyphema syndrome: a late complication of posterior chamber lenses. Bull Soc Belg Ophthalmol. 1994;252:61-5.

1515. ULCERATIVE COLITIS (INFLAMMATORY BOWEL DISEASE; REGIONAL ENTERITIS)

General

Chronic inflammatory disease of unknown etiology; both sexes affected; onset at all ages, most frequently between the ages of 20 and 40 years; usually abrupt onset; psychosomatic pathogenesis possible.

Ocular

Iritis; uveitis; episcleritis; papillomatous changes of palpebral conjunctiva; scleritis; serous retinal detachment; choroidal infiltrates; retrobulbar neuritis; papillitis; retinal pigment epithelium disturbance; choroidal folds.

Clinical

Abdominal pain; cramps; diarrhea; arthritis; weight loss; erythema nodosum; aphthous stomatitis; pallor; tenderness over colon; nutritional deficiency; carcinoma; associations with Sjögren syndrome and Takayasu disease have been reported.

Laboratory

Elevated white blood count and erythrocyte sedimentation rate. Radiography demonstrates the "sting sign" of narrowed lumen in the terminal ileum.

Treatment

Systemic corticosteroids, metronidazole, pain medication and antispasmodic drugs give relief.

Additional Resource

1. Khan AN (2011). Ulcerative Colitis Imaging. [online] Available from http://www.emedicine.com/radio/TOPIC785.HTM [Accessed April, 2012].

1516. ULLRICH SYNDROME (DYSCRANIOPYLOPHALANGY; ULLRICH-FEICHTIGER SYNDROME) CORNEAL ULCER

General

Belongs to trisomy 13–15; unknown etiology; sporadic occurrence.

Ocular

Microphthalmia to anophthalmia; hypertelorism; narrow lid fissures; strabismus; glaucoma;

aniridia; cloudy cornea; corneal ulcers; chorio-retinal coloboma.

Clinical

Hypoplastic mandible; broad nose; polydactyly; spina bifida; bicornuate uterus or septa vagina; congenital heart disease.

Laboratory/Ocular

Antinuclear antibody (ANA) test, serum muscle enzyme levels.

Treatment

Topical cycloplegic agents, topical cyclosporine and topical antibiotics.

Bibliography

1. Geeraets WJ. Ocular Syndromes, 3rd edition. Philadelphia: Lea & Febiger; 1976.

1517. ULTRAVIOLET KERATITIS

General

Radiation injury, UV absorbed by cornea, most commonly from welder's equipment but suntan beds, flood lamps, lightning, and electric sparks can also be the cause.

Ocular

Foreign-body sensation; irritation; pain; photophobia; reduced visual acuity; tearing and blepharospasm.

Laboratory

Slit-lamp examination with fluorescein uptake and straining along with history.

Treatment

Topical cycloplegic drops, and antibiotic ointment; pressure patch is the traditional therapy. Some physicians feel that a pressure patch delays re-epithelialization and opt for cycloplegics and antibiotics only.

Additional Resource

1. Brozen R (2011). Ultraviolet Keratitis. [online] Available from http://www.emedicine.medscape.com/article/799025-overview [Accessed April, 2012].

1518. ULTRAVIOLET RADIATION

General

Eye and skin are the only organs of the body particularly sensitive to the nonionizing wavelengths of radiation normally present in the environment.

Ocular

Photokeratitis; pterygia; band keratopathy; herpes simplex keratitis; recurrent corneal erosions; discoloring of lens; retinal degeneration; cataract formation; questionable alterations to the corneal endothelium.

Clinical

Actinic keratosis; edema; erythema of skin, blisters of skin; depigmentation of skin; skin carcinoma.

Laboratory

Patients with sever sunburn and diagnosis is unclear, laboratory studies are needed; and monitor for electrolyte and fluid imbalance.

Treatment

For severe sunburn admission to a sunburn unit for parenteral fluid replacement, pain control, and prophylaxis against infection.

Additional Resource

1. Brozen R (2011). Ultraviolet Keratitis. [online] Available from http://www.emedicine.com/emerg/ TOPIC759.HTM [Accessed April, 2012].

1519. UNNA II SYNDROME (MARIE-UNNA SYNDROME)

General

Both sexes are affected; rare; autosomal dominant; onset in children.

Ocular

Eyebrows and eyelashes missing.

Clinical

Loss of hair; scant growth of axillary and pubic hair, teeth, and nails; loss of hair in the eyebrows, eyelashes, and body.

Laboratory

Diagnosis is made by clinical findings.

Treatment

None/Ocular.

Bibliography

1. Magalini SI, Scrascia E. Dictionary of Medical Syndromes, 2nd edition. Philadelphia: JB Lippincott; 1981.
2. McKusick VA. Mendelian Inheritance in Man: A Catalog of Human Genes and Genetic Disorders, 12th edition. Baltimore: The Johns Hopkins University Press; 1998.
3. McKusick-Nathans Institute for Genetic Medicine, Johns Hopkins University and National Center for Biotechnology Information, National Library of Medicine. (2007). Online Mendelian Inheritance in Man (OMIM). [online] Available from http://www.ncbi.nlm.nih.gov/omim [Accessed April, 2012].
4. Unna M. Ueber Hypotricosis congenita hereditaria. Dermatol Wochenschr. 1925;81:1167-78.

1520. UNVERRICHT SYNDROME (FAMILIAL MYOCLONIA SYNDROME; LAFORA DISEASE) AMAUROSIS FUGAX

General

Fatal hereditary form of diffuse neuronal disease; autosomal recessive; late childhood; death within 2–10 years from onset of symptoms.

Ocular

Amaurosis; laminated Lafora bodies in ganglion cell and inner nuclear layers of the retina, either intracellular or extracellular, in inner plexiform and nerve fiber layers, and in the optic nerve.

Clinical

Major epilepsy; widespread myoclonus; dementia; tetraplegia; pseudobulbar palsy; generalized tonic-clonic seizure; behavioral changes; brisk tendon reflexes; cerebellar signs.

Laboratory

Diagnosis is made by clinical findings.

Treatment

None

Bibliography

1. Acharya JN, Satishchandra P, Asha T, et al. Lafora's disease in south India: a clinical, electrophysiologic, and pathologic study. Epilepsia. 1993; 34:476-87.
2. Kaufman MA, Dwork AJ, Willson NJ, et al. Late-onset Lafora's disease with typical intraneuronal inclusions. Neurology. 1993;43:1246-8.
3. Riehl JL, Lee DK, Andrews JM, et al. Electrophysiological and neuropharmacological studies in a patient with Unverricht-Lafora's disease. Neurology. 1967;17:502-11.
4. Unverricht H. Die myokionie. Berlin: Franz Denticke; 1891.

1521. URBACH-WIETHE SYNDROME (HYALINOSIS CUTIS ET MUCOSAE; LIPOID PROTEINOSIS; LIPOPROTEINOSIS; PROTEINOSIS-LIPOIDOSIS; ROSSLE-URBACH-WIETHE SYNDROME) DRY EYES

General

Rare autosomal recessive disorder in which hyaline material is deposited in the skin, mucous membranes, and brain; both sexes affected; onset in infancy; relatively benign progressive course; association with diabetes mellitus.

Ocular

Margin of eyelids may show beadlike excrescences with loss of cilia; itching of eyes; dry eyes.

Clinical

Skin about face covered with small, yellowish-white, waxy nodules; alopecia; hoarseness of voice at birth or within first few years of life; tongue large, thick; hyper-keratotic lesions on knees, elbows, and fingers; inability to cry; dry mouth.

Laboratory

Erythrocyte sedimentation rate, polymerase chain amplification and direct neuclotide sequence of the *ECM1* gene.

Treatment

No cure is known.

Additional Resource

1. Cordoro KM (2011). Lipoid Proteinosis. [online] Available from http://www.emedicine.com/derm/ TOPIC241.HTM [Accessed April, 2012].

1522. URRETS-ZAVALIA SYNDROME

General

Etiology uncertain. Fixed dilated pupil following ocular procedures which include penetrating keratoplasty, phakic intraocular lens, trabeculectomy, argon laser and peripheral idioplasty.

Clinical

None

Ocular

Fixed dilated pupil, iris atrophy.

Laboratory

Diagnosis is made by clinical findings.

Treatment

None

Bibliography

1. Espana EM, Ioannidis A, Tello C, et.al. Urrets-Zavalia syndrome as a complication of argon laser peripheral iridoplasty. Br J Ophthalmol. 2007;91: 427-9.
2. Yuzbasioglu E, Helvacioglu F, Sencan S. Fixed, dilated pupil after phakic intraocular lens implantation. J Cataract Refract Surg. 2006;32:174-6.
3. Srinivasan M, Patnaik L. Fixed dilated pupil (Urrets-Zavalia syndrome) in corneal dystrophies. Cornea. 2004;23:81-3.

1523. USHER SYNDROME (HEREDITARY RETINITIS PIGMENTOSA-DEAFNESS SYNDROME) RETINITIS PIGMENTOSA

General

Retinitis pigmentosa associated with deaf-mutism; dominantly inherited; anatomic and metabolic condition; onset unknown (Hallgren Syndrome).

Ocular

Concentric contraction of visual fields; retinitis pigmentosa with dotted, fine pigmentation in midperiphery; bone-corpuscle configured pigment deposits mainly along the vessels toward the periphery; yellow-white dots in outer retina and choroid; poor night vision.

Clinical

Deaf-mutism; however, deafness is not always complete; multiple sclerosis.

Laboratory

Diagnosis is made by clinical findings.

Treatment

Retinitis pigmentosa: It may be treated with vitamin A 15,000 IU/day is thought to slow the decline of retinal function, dark sunglasses for outdoor use, surgery for cataract, genetic counseling.

Bibliography

1. Berson EL, Adamian M. Ultrastructural findings in an autopsy eye from a patient with Usher's syndrome type II. Am J Ophthalmol. 1992;114:748-57.
2. Holland MG, Cambie E, Kloepfer W. An evaluation of genetic carriers of Usher's syndrome. Am J Ophthalmol. 1972;74:940-7.
3. Lynch SG, Digre K, Rose JW. Usher's syndrome and multiple sclerosis. Review of an individual with Usher's syndrome with a multiple sclerosis-like illness. J Neuroophthalmol. 1994;14:34-7.
4. Muftuoglu AU, Akman N, Savaş I. Polycythemia vera associated with Usher's syndrome. Am J Ophthalmol. 1975;80:93-5.
5. Usher CH. On the inheritance of retinitis pigmentosa with notes of cases. R Lond Ophthalmol Hosp Rep. 1913/1914;19:130.

1524. UVEA TOUCH SYNDROME (CORNEAL DYSTROPHY)

General

Caused by intraocular lens coming in contact with uveal tissue; seen most frequently with intracapsular cataract extraction and anterior chamber intraocular lens implant.

Ocular

Corneal decompensation; endothelial dystrophy; retinal edema; pigment dispersion; painful eye; disorders of motility.

Clinical

None

Laboratory

Diagnosis is made by clinical findings.

Treatment

Cycloplegics, steroids, and possibly intraocular lens exchange.

Bibliography

1. Binkhorst CD. The uvea-touch syndrome and how to avoid it. Personal thoughts about lens implantation. Acta Ophthalmol. 1985;63:609-23.
2. Smith SG, Cameron JD, Lindstrom RL. An experimental model for uveal touch syndrome. J Cataract Refract Surg. 1988;14:182-6.

1525. UVEAL EFFUSION SYNDROME (EXUDATIVE RETINAL DETACHMENT)

General

Congenital anomaly of sclera and, in some cases, the vortex vein; inability to transport extravascular protein across abnormal sclera; condition typically affects middle-aged men and causes recurrent, spontaneous serous retinal and ciliochoroidal detachments, often resulting in significant visual impairment.

Ocular

Exudative retinal detachment; sclera abnormally thick; vortex vein obstruction; idiopathic central serous choroidopathy; vitreous cells; ciliochoroidal detachment; nanophthalmos.

Clinical

Viral infection; elevated blood pressure; allergic reaction; minor trauma.

Laboratory

Diagnosis is made by clinical findings.

Treatment

Retinal detachment: Scleral buckle, pneumatic retinopexy and vitrectomy may be used to close all the breaks.

Bibliography

1. Brubaker RF, Pederson JE. Ciliochoroidal detachment. Surv Ophthalmol. 1983;27:281-9.
2. Gass JD. Uveal effusion syndrome. A new hypothesis concerning pathogenesis and technique of surgical treatment. Retina. 1983;3:159-63.
3. Morita H, Funata M, Kusakari T, et al. Recurrence of nanophthalmic uveal effusion. Ophthalmologica. 1993;207:30-6.
4. Stelmach MZ, O'Day J, Ryan H. Uveal effusion syndrome. Aust N Z J Ophthalmol. 1994;22:139-43.

1526. UVEITIS (INTERMEDIATE AND POSTERIOR UVEITIS, IRIDOCYSTITIS, IRITIS, NONINFECTIOUS CHORIORETINITIS)

General

Most idiopathic or post-traumatic but other causes include infections, malignancies, autoimmune diseases and pharmaceutical.

Clinical

None

Ocular

Photophobia, ciliary flush, decreased vision.

Laboratory

Chest X-ray—sarcoid, purified protein derivative (PPD), fluorescent treponemal antibody absorption (FTA-ABS)—syphilis, Lyme C6 peptide—Lyme disease.

Treatment

Oral steroids if not responsive to topical steroids, immunosuppressants if bilateral disease that does not respond to oral steroids, periocular steroids for unilateral or posterior uveitis. Vitrectomy can be used for severe vitreous opacification. Cryotherapy and laser photocoagulation may be used for localized pars plana exudates.

Additional Resources

1. Walton RC (2010). Uveitis, Anterior, Childhood. [online] Available from http://www.emedicine.com/oph/TOPIC585.HTM [Accessed April, 2012].
2. Al-Fawaz A (2010). Uveitis, Anterior, Nongranulomatous. [online] Available from http://www.emedicine.com/oph/TOPIC587.HTM [Accessed April, 2012].

1527. UVEITIS MASQUERADE SYNDROME(S) (VMS) UVEITIS

General

Uveitis masquerade syndrome is a group of disorders that mimic uveitis; cells seen may be of noninflammatory origin or are inflammatory and secondary to another disorder.

Ocular

Uveitis; panuveitis; pars planitis; vitreitis; papillitis; anterior segment cells; hypopyon; vitreal infiltrates.

Clinical

Causes may be malignant, such as lymphoma, leukemia, retinoblastoma, melanoma, and lung cancer metastasis, or nonmalignant, such as ocular toxoplasmosis, diabetic retinopathy, hypertension, and radiation retinopathy.

Laboratory/Ocular

Diagnosis is made by clinical findings.

Treatment/Ocular

Uveitis: Topical steroids and cycloplegic medication should be the initial treatment of choice. Oral steroids if not responsive to topical steroids, immunosuppressants if bilateral disease that does not respond to oral steroids, periocular steroids for unilateral or posterior uveitis. Vitrectomy can be used for severe vitreous opacification. Cryotherapy and laser photocoagulation may be used for localized pars plana exudates.

Bibliography

1. Nussenblatt RB, Witcup SM, Palestine AG. Uveitis: Fundamentals and Clinical Practice, 2nd edition. St. Louis: CV Mosby; 1996. pp. 385-95.
2. Ranking GA, Jakobiec FA, Hidayat AA. Intraocular lymphoproliferations simulating uveitis. In: Albert DM, Jacobiec FA (Eds). Principles and Practice of Ophthalmology. Philadelphia: WB Saunders; 1994. pp. 524-48.

1528. UVEITIS, ANTERIOR, GRANULOMATOUS (IRITIS)

General

Ocular inflammation of the iris and ciliary body. Etiology is idiopathic but certain systemic diseases may be the underlying cause.

Clinical

Herpes zoster, sarcoidosis, syphilis, Lyme disease, tuberculosis, multiple sclerosis, leprosy, toxoplasmosis, coccidiodomycosis, Vogt-Koyanagi-Harada disease, brucellosis.

Ocular

Photophobia, red eye, dull aching eye pain, perilimbal injection, keratic precipitates, flare and cell of anterior chamber, posterior synechiae, lenticular precipitates.

Laboratory

Diagnosis is made by clinical findings. If granulomatous iritis is recurrent, studies are necessary to determine the cause. ELISA, serologic testing for syphilis, sarcoidosis and Lyme may be indicated.

Treatment

Topical corticosteroids are the mainstay of therapy. Subconjunctival corticosteroids may be necessary in non-responding cases. Cycloplegia is useful for control of pain and photophobia.

Additional Resource

1. Al-Fawaz A (2010). Uveitis, Anterior, Granulomatous. [online] Available from http://www.emedicine.com/oph/TOPIC586.HTM [Accessed April, 2012].

1529. UVEITIS, ANTERIOR, NONGRANULOMATOUS (CHRONIC, IRITIS)

General

Ocular inflammation. Etiology is idiopathic but certain systemic diseases may be the underlying cause.

Clinical

HLA-B27, Behçet disease, herpes zoster, sarcoidosis, syphilis, Lyme disease, juvenile idiopathic arthritis, Fuchs heterochromic iridocyclitis, tuberculosis.

Ocular

Photophobia, red eye, dull aching eye pain, perilimbal injection, keratic precipitates, flare and cell of anterior chamber, posterior synechiae, lenticular precipitates.

Laboratory

Diagnosis is made by clinical findings. If nongranulomatous iritis is recurrent studies are necessary to determine the cause. HLA-B27 typing, serologic testing for syphilis, sarcoidosis rheumatoid factor and Lyme may be indicated.

Treatment

Topical corticosteroids are the mainstay of therapy. Subconjunctival corticosteroids may be necessary in non-responding cases. Cycloplegia is useful for control of pain and photophobia.

Additional Resource

1. Al-Fawaz A (2010). Uveitis, Anterior, Nongranulomatous. [online] Available from http://www.emedicine.com/oph/TOPIC587.HTM [Accessed April, 2012].

1530. UVEITIS, JUVENILE IDIOPATHIC ARTHRITIS

General

Uveitis in children are approximately 6% of all cases. the most frequent cause of juvenile uveitis is juvenile idiopathic arthritis (JIA).

Ocular

The affected eye is often healthy in appearance, yet 30–40% of patients with JIA uveits have demonstrate severe loss of vision due to the condition.

Clinical

Past medical and ocular history. Chief complaint and history of illnesses. Other manifestations such as anemia, fever, rash, back pain, diarrhea, weight loss, fatigue.

Laboratory

Atinuclear antibody, rheumatoid factor, human leukocyte antigen B27. X-ray of joint. Additional serologic test may include; Syphilis serologies, Lyme titers, serum lysozyme, angiotensin-converting enzyme (ACE).

Treatment

Initial treatment should began with topical corticosteroids. If vitreous cells are present, the risk of CME increases, continuing corticosteroids and additional nonsteroidal anti-inflammatory drugs may be helpful.

Additional Resource

1. Roque MR (2010). Uveitis, Juvenile Idiopathic Arthritis. [online] Available from http://www.emedicine.medscape.com/article/1209891-overview [Accessed April, 2012].

1531. UYEMURA SYNDROME (FUNDUS ALBIPUNCTATUS WITH HEMERALOPIA AND XEROSIS) NIGHT BLINDNESS

General

Rare; resembles retinitis punctata albescens, fundus albipunctatus, and congenital idiopathic night blindness or Oguchi disease; avitaminosis A; affects both sexes.

Ocular

Night blindness; conjunctival xerosis; Bitot spots; white spots on the fundus.

Clinical

None

Laboratory

Diagnosis is made by clinical findings.

Treatment

None

Bibliography

1. Krill AE, Martin D. Photopic abnormalities in congenital stationary nightblindness. Invest Ophthalmol. 1971;10:625-36.
2. Uyemura M. Uber eine Merkwurdige Augenhintergrundsveranderung bei zwei Fallen von Idiopathischer Hemeralopie. Klin Monatsbl Augenheilkd. 1928;81:471.
3. Venkataswamy G. Ocular manifestations of vitamin A deficiency. Br J Ophthalmol. 1967;51:854-9.

1532. V-ESOTROPIA SYNDROME

General

Esotropia greater looking down by 15 prism diopters than looking up; may have underaction of superior oblique or overaction of inferior oblique; antimongoloid (downward) slant of lid fissures; may have accommodative, nonaccommodative or paralytic esotropia components.

Clinical

Fusion obtained by chin depression.

Laboratory

Diagnosis is made by clinical findings.

Treatment

Recess the medial rectus bilaterally with a half tendon downward. If unilateral surgery recess medial rectus with downshift and resect the lateral rectus (LR) with a half tendon upshift. With significant oblique overaction—recess the medial rectus bilaterally or recess the medial rectus and resect the LR unilaterally for esotropia in primary position weaken the superior oblique bilaterally if 25 diopters from up to down.

Additional Resource

1. Thacker N (2011). V-Pattern Esotropia and Exotropia. [online] Available from http://www.emedicine.com/oph/TOPIC561.HTM [Accessed April, 2012].

1533. V-EXOTROPIA SYNDROME

General

Exotropia greater looking up by 15 diopters than looking down; underaction of superior oblique or overaction of inferior oblique muscles; anti-mongoloid (downward) slant of lid fissures.

Clinical

Fusion obtained by chin elevation.

Laboratory

Diagnosis is made by clinical findings.

Treatment

Recess the lateral rectus with upshift. If unilateral surgery recess the lateral rectus with upshift and resect the medial rectus with downshift. With oblique dysfunction—recess the rectus bilateral and weaken the superior oblique bilaterally.

Additional Resource

1. Thacker N (2011). V-Pattern Esotropia and Exotropia. [online] Available from http://www.emedicine.com/oph/TOPIC561.HTM [Accessed April, 2012].

1534. V-PATTERN STRABISMUS

General

Divergence of about 15 prism diopters in the upward position than downward position.

Clinical

None

Ocular

V-exotropia, V-esotropia, amblyopia.

Laboratory

Diagnosis is made by clinical findings.

Treatment

V-pattern esotropia without oblique dysfunction—recess medial rectus bilateral with downshift or recess the medial rectus with downshift and resect lateral rectus with upshift in one eye. V-pattern esotropia with superior oblique overaction—recess the medial rectus bilaterally or recess medial rectus and resect lateral rectus unilaterally and weaken superior oblique by tenectomy. V-pattern exotropia without oblique dysfunction—recess the lateral rectus bilaterally with upshift or unilaterally recess the lateral rectus with a upshift and resect the medial rectus with a downshift. V-pattern exotropia with superior oblique overaction—recess the lateral rectus bilaterally or unilaterally recess the lateral rectus and resect the medial rectus and weaken the superior oblique bilaterally by tenectomy.

Additional Resource

1. Thacker N (2011). V-Pattern Esotropia and Exotropia. [online] Available from http://www.emedicine.com/oph/TOPIC561.HTM [Accessed April, 2012].

1535. VACCINIA (KERATITIS)

General

Laboratory virus used for vaccination against smallpox.

Ocular

Pustules of lids; edema of lids; conjunctivitis; orbital cellulitis; keratitis; pannus; corneal perforation; iridocyclitis; central serous retinopathy; perivasculitis; pseudoretinitis pigmentosa; ocular palsies papillitis; optic atrophy.

Clinical

Vesicles; pustules; erythema; fever; malaise; axillary lymphadenopathy; necrosis of skin; vaccinia gangrenosa; encephalomyelitis; drowsiness; vomiting; coma; death.

Laboratory

Immune deficiency workup should be considered as well as imaging studies.

Treatment

Vaccinia immunoglobulin (VIG) can be helpful in selected patients.

Additional Resource

1. Lee JJ (2012). Vaccinia. [online] Available from http://www.emedicine.com/med/TOPIC2356.HTM [Accessed April, 2012].

1536. VAN BOGAERT-HOZAY SYNDROME (ESOTROPIA)

General

Manifest after age 3 years; similar to Rubinstein-Taybi syndrome; etiology unknown; affects both sexes.

Ocular

Hypertelorism; hypoplastic cilia and eyebrows; ptosis; esotropia; astigmatism; myopia.

Clinical

Facial dysplasia; broad nasal bridge and zygomatic arch; flat, wide nose; arched palate; skeletal anomalies with short, thick phalangeal joints; finger and toes appear infantile; flat nasal bridge; thickened cheeks; deformed ears; micrognathia.

Laboratory/Ocular

Diagnosis is made by clinical findings.

Treatment

Hypertelorism: The primary correction involves orbital reconstruction and the nasal deformity correction that is universally associated with this deformity.

Bibliography

1. Hozay J. Sur une Dystrophic Familiale Particuliere. Inhibition Precoce de la Croissance et Osteolyse Non Mutilante Acrales avec Dysmorphie Faciale. Rev Neurol. 1953;89:245-58.
2. McKusick VA. Mendelian Inheritance in Man: A Catalog of Human Genes and Genetic Disorders, 12th edition. Baltimore: The Johns Hopkins University Press; 1998.
3. McKusick-Nathans Institute for Genetic Medicine, Johns Hopkins University and National Center for Biotechnology Information, National Library of Medicine. (2007). Online Mendelian Inheritance in Man (OMIM). [online] Available from http://www.ncbi.nlm.nih.gov/omim [Accessed April, 2012].
4. Roy FH, Summitt RL, Hiatt RL, et al. Ocular manifestations of the Rubinstein-Taybi syndrome. Case report and review of the literature. Arch Ophthalmol. 1968;79:272-8.
5. Van Bogaert L. Essai de Classement et d'Interpretation de Quelques Acro-osteolyses Mutilantes et Non Mutilantes Actuellement Connues. Acta Neural Psychiatr Belg. 1953;53:90-115.

1537. VAN BOGAERT-SCHERER-EPSTEIN SYNDROME (FAMILIAL HYPERCHOLESTEROLEMIA SYNDROME; PRIMARY HYPERLIPIDEMIA) CATARACT NUCLEAR

General

Autosomal dominant; high serum lipoprotein; both sexes are affected; onset at all ages.

Ocular

Xanthelasma; arcus juveniles of the cornea; lipid keratopathy; cataract; retinopathy with yellowish deposits and cholesterol crystals have been reported but are more rare manifestations.

Clinical

Xanthelasmatosis of skin and tendons; progressive atherosclerosis; coronary insufficiency; cardiac infarcts; dementia; progressive ataxia; cerebral infarction; polyneuropathy.

Laboratory

Diagnosis is made by clinical findings.

Treatment

Control blood lipids.

Bibliography

1. Blodi FC, Yarbrough JC. Ocular manifestations of familial hypercholesterolemia. Am J Ophthalmol. 1963;55:714-8.
2. Geeraets WJ. Ocular Syndromes, 3rd edition. Philadelphia: Lea & Febiger; 1976.
3. Hoeg JM. Familial hypercholesterolemia. What the zebra can teach us about the horse. JAMA. 1994;271:543-6.

4. Ihara Y, Nobukuni K, Namba R, et al. A family of familial hypercholesterolemia with cerebral infarction and without coronary heart disease. An unusual case with corneal opacity, polyneuropathy and carpal tunnel syndrome in the family: therapy with probucol and tocopherol nicotinate. J Neurol Sci. 1991;106:10-8.

5. Van Bogaert L, Scherer HJ, Epstein E. Une Forme Cerebrale de la Cholesterinose Generalisee. Paris: Masson; 1937.

1538. VAN DER HOEVE SYNDROME (BRITTLE BONE DISEASE; EDDOWES SYNDROME; EKMAN SYNDROME; LOBSTEIN SYNDROME; OSTEOGENESIS IMPERFECTA; OSTEOPSATHYROSIS; SPURWAY SYNDROME; VROLIK SYNDROME) GLAUCOMA

General

Autosomal dominant.

Ocular

Glaucoma; blue sclera; keratoconus; cataract; optic nerve atrophy; retinopathy; retinal detachment.

Clinical

Brittle bones; deafness; hyperflexibility of ligaments; dental defects; developmental delay.

Laboratory

DNA blood test, analysis of type I, III and V collagens synthesized by fibroblast, prenatal sonography.

Treatment

Synthetic analogs of pyrophosphate, cyclic intravenous pamidronate, growth hormone.

Additional Resource

1. Ramachandran M (2012). Osteogenesis Imperfecta. [online] Available from http://www.emedicine.com/orthoped/TOPIC530.HTM [Accessed April, 2012].

1539. VASCULOPATHIC OPTIC NEUROPATHIES

General

Caused by optic nerve damage through ischemia, leading to axonal stasis.

Clinical

Giant cell arteritis, temporal pain, headaches, jaw claudication, tongue pain, proximal muscle weakness.

Ocular

Sudden visual loss, optic disk hemorrhages, disk edema and pallor of optic nerve.

Laboratory

Diagnosis is made by clinical findings.

Treatment

Systemic and intravenous corticosteroids.

Additional Resource

1. Younge BR (2012). Anterior Ischemic Optic Neuropathy. [online] Available from http://www.emedicine.com/oph/TOPIC161.HTM [Accessed April, 2012].

1540. VELOCARDIOFACIAL SYNDROME (DIGEORGE SYNDROME)

General

Autosomal dominant; anomaly of neural crest derivatives; most common syndrome of clefting; possible association with microdeletion at 22q11.

Ocular

Retinal vascular tortuosity; posterior embryotoxon; narrow palpebral fissures; suborbital discoloration; small optic nerves; iris nodules; cataracts; prominent corneal nerves; strabismus; hyperopia; myopia; astigmatism; anisometropic astigmatism.

Clinical

Cleft palate; learning disability; ventricular septal defect with or without the tetralogy of Fallot; right-sided aortic arch; prominent nose; retrognathia; helical thickening; small auricles; auricular protrusion; microcephaly; small stature; inguinal or umbilical hernia; scoliosis; slender hands and digits; small vermis; small posterior fossa; developmental delay; heart malformations; late-onset psychosis.

Laboratory

Fluorescence in situ hybridization, perform immune studies, chest radiography may show heart defect, and MRI is use on severe cases.

Treatment

Medical therapy may be needed to treat heart failure, hypocalemia, immune deficiency, feeding problems and inadequate growth.

Additional Resource

1. Horenstein MS (2012). Velocardiofacial Syndrome. [online] Available from http://www.emedicine.com/ped/TOPIC2395.HTM [Accessed April, 2012].

1541. VERMIS SYNDROME (PAPILLEDEMA)

General

Medulloblastomas arising primarily in the posterior vermis but invading the fourth ventricle secondarily and compressing the bulb; frequent in children.

Ocular

Nystagmus; papilledema; abnormal saccades.

Clinical

Enlargement of the head; vomiting (early sign); stiffness and pain of the neck and shoulders; equilibratory disturbances; incoordination of the limbs.

Laboratory

Computed tomography (CT) scan of the head.

Treatment

Seek neurological assistance.

Bibliography

1. Baker GS. Physiologic abnormalities encountered after removal of brain tumors from the floor of the fourth ventricle. J Neurosurg. 1965;23:338-43.
2. Geeraets WJ. Ocular Syndromes, 3rd edition. Philadelphia: Lea & Febiger; 1976.
3. Halmagyi GM. Central eye movement disorders. In: Albert DM, Jakobiec FA (Eds). Principles and Practice of Ophthalmology. Philadelphia: WB Saunders; 1994. p. 2411.

4. Ranalli PJ, Sharpe JA. Contrapulsion of saccades and ipsilateral ataxia: a unilateral disorder of the rostral cerebellum. Ann Neurol. 1986;20:311-6.

5. Van Bogaert L, Martin P. Les Tumeurs du IV. Vent, et le Syndrome Cerebelleux de la Ligne Mediane. Rev Neurol. 1928;2:431.

1542. VERNAL KERATOCONJUNCTIVITIS (ALLERGIC CONJUNCTIVITIS, ATOPIC KERATOCONJUNCTIVITIS, GIANT PAPILLARY CONJUNCTIVITIS)

General

Bilateral, chronic, severe allergy, more frequent in young males and during the springtime.

Clinical

Atopy present in half of cases.

Ocular

Giant papillae conjunctivitis.

Laboratory

Diagnosis is made by clinical findings.

Treatment

Ocular lubricants, nonsteroidal anti-inflammatory and steroid drops, oral nonsteroidal anti-inflammatory or steroids. Supratarsal steroids. Surgical excision, cryotherapy and beta-irradiation of papillae.

Additional Resource

1. Ventocilla M (2012). Allergic Conjunctivitis. [online] Available from http://www.emedicine.com/oph/TOPIC85.HTM [Accessed April, 2012].

1543. VERTEBRAL BASILAR ARTERY SYNDROME (INTRANUCLEAR OPHTHALMOPLEGIA)

General

"Whiplash" injury with hyperextension of the neck followed by rapid forward movement of the head or osteoarthritis of the cervical spine, cervical ribs (see Cranio-cervical Syndrome).

Ocular

Nystagmus (postural); internuclear ophthalmoplegia; visual deterioration; visual hallucinations may be associated with a decrease in consciousness; homonymous hemianopsia (bilateral); contralateral hemianopic visual field defect.

Clinical

Severe, throbbing occipital headache associated with neck pain; vertigo from ischemia of the internal auditory artery, from the temporoparietal cortex or from ischemia in the lateral tegmentum of the pons; nausea and vomiting; ataxia; hemiparesis; quadriplegia; dysarthria; dysphagia; deafness; dyslexia; atonia; confusion; coma; tremor.

Laboratory/Ocular

Diagnosis is made by clinical findings.

Treatment

Nystagmus: See-saw nystagmus—visual field to consider neoplastic or vascular etiologies. Upbeat nystagmus—may indicate multiple sclerosis, cerebellar degeneration, tumors or infarcts. Treatment is directed toward identification and resolution of underlying cause. Downbeat nystagmus—affects the cerebellum or craniocervical junction including Arnold-Chiari malformation, multiple sclerosis, trauma, tumor, infarction and many toxic metabolic entities. MRI may indicate a surgically correctable lesion. Periodic alternating nystagmus is continuous horizontal nystagmus from stroke, tumor, multiple sclerosis, trauma, infection and drug intoxication. Can occur from cataract, vitreous hemorrhage or optic atrophy.

Bibliography

1. Caplan LR. Posterior cerebral artery syndrome. In: Vinken PJ, Bruyn GW, Klawans HL (Eds). Handbook of Clinical Neurology: Vascular Diseases. Amsterdam: Elsevier Science; 1988.
2. Caplan LR. "Top of the basilar" syndrome. Neurology. 1980;30:72-9.
3. Hoyt WF. Transient bilateral blurring of vision. Considerations of an episodic ischemic symptom of vertebral-basilar insufficiency. Arch Ophthalmol. 1963;70:746-51.
4. Millikan CH, Siekert RG. Studies in cerebrovascular disease. I. The syndrome of intermittent insufficiency of the basilar arterial system. Proc Staff Meet Mayo Clin. 1955;30:61-8.

1544. VESELL SYNDROME (DEAFNESS-STRABISMUS SYMPHALANGIA SYNDROME) EXOTROPIA

General

Etiology unknown; possibly autosomal dominant inheritance.

Ocular

Strabismus

Clinical

Symphalangism; hearing loss.

Laboratory/Ocular

Diagnosis is made by clinical findings.

Treatment

Strabismus: Equalized vision with correct refractive error; surgery may be helpful in patient with diplopia.

Bibliography

1. Magalini SI, Scrascia E. Dictionary of Medical Syndromes, 2nd edition. Philadelphia: JB Lippincott; 1981.
2. Vesell ES. Symphalangism, strabismus and hearing loss in mother and daughter. N Engl J Med. 1960;263:839-42.

1545. VESTIBULAR PARALYSIS, BILATERAL (NYSTAGMUS)

General

Infective process bilaterally affecting the vestibular system in any site between the semicircular canals and the vestibular nuclei in the brain; usually vasculitic-type lesion.

Ocular

Nystagmus; no depth perception with eyes closed, no difficulty with eyes open.

Clinical

Staggering; inability to swim; disorientation in water; loss of hearing; vertigo.

Laboratory/Ocular

Diagnosis is made by clinical findings.

Treatment

Nystagmus: See-saw nystagmus—visual field to consider neoplastic or vascular etiologies. Upbeat nystagmus—may indicate multiple sclerosis, cerebellar degeneration, tumors or infarcts. Treatment is directed toward identification and resolution of underlying cause. Downbeat nystagmus—affects the cerebellum or craniocervical junction including Arnold-Chiari malformation, multiple sclerosis, trauma, tumor, infarction and many toxic metabolic entities. MRI may indicate a surgically correctable lesion. Periodic alternating nystagmus is continuous horizontal nystagmus from stroke, tumor, multiple sclerosis, trauma, infection and drug intoxication. Can occur from cataract, vitreous hemorrhage or optic atrophy.

Bibliography

1. Chusid J et al. Syndrome of bilateral vestibular paralysis. J Nerv Ment Dis. 1946;103:172-80.
2. Magalini SI, Scrascia E. Dictionary of Medical Syndromes, 2nd edition. Philadelphia: JB Lippincott; 1981.
3. Ryu JH. Vestibular neuritis: an overview using a classical case. Acta Otolaryngol Suppl. 1993;503: 25-30.

1546. VINCENT INFECTION (GINGIVITIS; TRENCH MOUTH)

General

Onset usually sudden; remission, but may reoccur; young adults.

Ocular

Conjunctivitis; corneal ulcer; dacryocystitis; dacryoadenitis; orbititis; uveitis.

Clinical

Painful, bleeding gingiva characterized by necrosis and ulceration of gingival papillae and margins; lymphadenopathy; foul mouth odor; fever; leukocytosis.

Laboratory

Smear to identify agent.

Treatment

Proper oral hygiene, warm saline rinse.

Additional Resource

1. Stephen JM (2010). Gingivitis. [online] Available from http://www.emedicine.com/emerg/ TOPIC217.HTM [Accessed April, 2012].

1547. VISUAL DISORIENTATION SYNDROME (RIDDOCH SYNDROME) HOMONYMOUS QUADRANTANOPIA

General

Parietal lobe lesion.

Ocular

Visual agnosia; stereoscopic vision and central vision unimpaired; homonymous quadrantanopsia.

Clinical

Contralateral numbness and tingling; loss of static or postural sensation when postcentral convolution affected.

Laboratory

Computed tomography (CT) scan of the head.

Treatment

Seek neurological assistance.

Bibliography

1. Geeraets WJ. Ocular Syndromes, 3rd edition. Philadelphia: Lea & Febiger; 1976.
2. Riddoch G. Dissociation of visual perceptions due to occipital injuries, with special reference to appreciation of movement. Brain. 1917;40:15-57.
3. Riddoch G. Visual disorientation in homonymous half-fields. Brain. 1935;58:376-82.

1548. VISUAL PARANEOPLASTIC SYNDROME (VISUAL FIELD DEFECT)

General

Loss of visual acuity and loss of visual field due to malignant disease without metastasis to visual system; most often occurs with small cell carcinoma of lung; visual symptoms may be only symptom, before neoplastic disease is diagnosed; can occur associated with cutaneous melanoma.

Ocular

Visual field defects; impaired color vision; narrowing of arterioles; changes in retinal pigment epithelium; orbital myositis; optic neuropathy.

Clinical

Endometrial carcinoma, small cell lung carcinoma.

Laboratory

Computed tomography (CT) scan of the head.

Treatment

Seek neurological assistance.

Bibliography

1. Apple DJ, Rabb MF. Ocular Pathology: Clinical Applications and Self Assessment. St. Louis: CV Mosby; 1985.
2. Crofts JW, Bachynski BN, Odel JG. Visual paraneoplastic syndrome associated with undifferentiated endometrial carcinoma. Can J Ophthalmol. 1988;23:128-32.
3. Harris GJ, Murphy ML, Schmidt EW, et al. Orbital myositis as a paraneoplastic syndrome. Arch Ophthalmol. 1994;112:380-6.
4. Kim RY, Retsas S, Fitzke FW, et al. Cutaneous melanoma-associated retinopathy. Ophthalmology. 1994;101:1837-43.
5. Malik S, Furlan AJ, Sweeney PJ, et al. Optic neuropathy: a rare paraneoplastic syndrome. J Clin Neuroophthalmol. 1992;12:137-41.

1549. VITAMIN A DEFICIENCY

General

Worldwide cause of blindness; onset in childhood; dietary vitamin A insufficiency; interference of absorption from the intestinal tract and transport or storage in the liver, as with diarrhea or vomiting; most frequent in young children.

Ocular

Bitot spots; conjunctival xerosis; corneal xerosis; keratomalacia with perforation; photophobia; enlarged tarsal glands; corneal ulcer; nyctalopia; hemeralopia; obstruction of the tear ducts.

Clinical

Diarrhea; malabsorption syndrome; follicular hyperkeratosis; lesions on buttocks, legs, and arms; xerosis of skin; tracheitis; bronchitis; pneumonia; chronic obstruction of pancreatic or biliary ducts; increased infant mortality.

Laboratory

Serum retinol study, serum RBP study, zinc levels, CBC, electrolyte evaluation and liver function studies.

Treatment

Vitamin A rich foods such as beef, chicken, sweet potatoes, mangoes, carrots, eggs, fortified milk and leafy green vegetables.

Additional Resource

1. Ansstas G (2012). Vitamin A Deficiency. [online] Available from http://www.emedicine.com/med/TOPIC2381.HTM [Accessed April, 2012].

1550. VITILIGO

General

Patchy depigmentary disorder of the skin; progressive; etiology unknown; autosomal dominant; associated with Vogt-Koyanagi-Harada disease and uveitis.

Ocular

Posterior uveitis; depigmentation of lids, lashes, iris, and retina; retinal atrophy.

Clinical

Loss of pigment in hair; depigmentation of skin; halo nevi.

Laboratory

Diagnosis is made by clinical findings, occasionally skin biopsy is helpful.

Treatment

Narrowband UV-B phototherapy, systemic steroids, topical tacrolimus ointment.

Additional Resource

1. Groysman V (2011). Vitiligo. [online] Available from http://www.emedicine.com/derm/TOPIC453.HTM [Accessed April, 2012].

1551. VITREOCORNEAL TOUCH SYNDROME (DESCEMENT FOLDS)

General

After cataract extraction, vitreous bulges through the pupillary space, coming in contact with and finally attaching to the corneal endothelium; onset 2–3 weeks after cataract extraction.

Ocular

Area of decreased transparency of the central cornea; Descemet's folds; striate keratopathy where the intact vitreous face is touching the corneal endothelium; corneal edema; iris bombs; bullous keratopathy.

Clinical

None

Laboratory

Diagnosis is made by clinical findings.

Treatment

Anterior vitrectomy.

Bibliography

1. Gostin SB. Vitreocorneal touch syndrome: management by vitreous face discission via posterior approach. South Med J. 1972;65: 741-4.
2. Leahey BD. Bullous keratitis from vitreous contact. AMA Arch Ophthalmol. 1951;46: 22-32.

1552. VITREORETINAL SKELETAL SYNDROME [RETINAL BREAK(S)]

General

Associated with various systemic skeletal abnormalities; autosomal dominant.

Ocular

Optically empty posterior vitreous; fibrillar anterior vitreous preretinal membrane; retinal breaks.

Clinical

Cleft palate; hypermobility of joints; mild skeletal abnormalities; pelvic bone deformities; hearing loss.

Laboratory

Diagnosis is made by clinical findings.

Treatment

None/Ocular.

Bibliography

1. Jones KL, Smith DW, Harvey MA, et al. Older paternal age and fresh gene mutation: data on additional disorders. J Pediatr. 1975;86:84-8.
2. Regenbogen L, Godel V. Hereditary vitreoretinal degeneration, cleft lip and palate, deafness, and skeletal dysplasia. Am J Ophthalmol. 1980;89:414-8.

1553. VITREORETINOCHOROIDOPATHY (VRCP; AUTOSOMAL DOMINANT VITREORETINOCHOROIDOPATHY; ADVIRC) CHOROIDAL ATROPHY

General

Autosomal dominant.

Ocular

Chorioretinal hypopigmentation or hyperpigmentation; preretinal punctate opacities; retinal arteriolar narrowing and occlusion; choroidal atrophy; diffuse retinal vascular incompetence; cystoid macular edema; presenile cataracts; fibrillar condensation and moderate pleocytosis of vitreous; myopia; optically empty vitreous; lattice degeneration; retinal breaks; retinal detachment; glaucoma; spontaneous vitreous hemorrhage.

Clinical

None

Laboratory

Diagnosis is made by clinical findings.

Treatment

Cataract: Change in glasses can sometimes improve a patient's visual function temporarily; however, the most common treatment is cataract surgery.

Bibliography

1. Blair NP, Goldberg MF, Fishman GA, et al. Autosomal dominant vitreoretinochoroidopathy. Br J Ophthalmol. 1984;68:2-9.

2. McKusick VA. Mendelian Inheritance in Man: A Catalog of Human Genes and Genetic Disorders, 12th edition. Baltimore: The Johns Hopkins University Press; 1998.

3. McKusick-Nathans Institute for Genetic Medicine, Johns Hopkins University and National Center for Biotechnology Information, National Library of Medicine. (2007). Online Mendelian Inheritance in Man (OMIM). [online] Available from http://www.ncbi.nlm.nih.gov/omim [Accessed April, 2012].

4. Traboulsi EL, Payne JW. Autosomal dominant vitreoretinochoroidopathy. Report of the third family. Arch Ophthalmol. 1993;111:194-6.

1554. VITREOUS HEMORRHAGE

General

Hemorrhage into vitreous.

Clinical

Reduced vision secondary to bleeding in vitreous.

Ocular

Retinal vascular with proliferation or nonproliferation of retinal vessels, traction on retinal vessel, trauma, uveal tract.

Laboratory

Identify the cause with CBC, sickle cell prep, FBS, clotting time, B-scan ultrasonography.

Treatment

Prophylaxis—treat the underlying pathology, vitreous surgery—vitrectomy for nonclearing.

Additional Resource

1. Phillpotts BA (2011). Vitreous Hemorrhage. [online] Available from http://www.emedicine.com/oph/TOPIC421.HTM [Accessed April, 2012].

1555. VITREOUS TUG SYNDROME (VITREOUS WICK SYNDROME) RETINAL DETACHMENT

General

Vitreous strand passes through the pupillary space and becomes attached or incarcerated in a corneal wound either post-traumatic or after intraocular surgery (Irvine Syndrome); associated with endophthalmitis.

Ocular

Sensation of light flashes due to vitreous pull on the retina; irregular pupil; vitreous strands passing through pupil to attach to corneal wound or scar; loss of foveal reflex on ophthalmoscopic examination; circumscribed retinal edema; occasional posterior retinal detachment.

Clinical

None

Laboratory

Diagnosis is made by clinical findings.

Treatment

Consider anterior vitrectomy.

Additional Resource

1. Roque MR (2010). Vitreous Wick Syndrome. [online] Available from http://www.emedicine. com/oph/TOPIC649.HTM [Accessed April, 2012].

1556. VITREOUS WICK SYNDROME

General

Vitreous incarcerated in corneal or cornoscleral wound.

Clinical

None

Ocular

Anterior chamber cells and flare, hypoyon, strands of vitreous in anterior chamber, distorted pupil, cystoid macular edema, retinal tears, retinal detachment.

Laboratory

Fluoroscein angiography.

Treatment

Topical steroids for 2 weeks, followed by non-steroid drops, if no improvement sub-Tenon's injection of steroids. Surgical sponge vitrectomy at the time of initial surgery.

Additional Resource

1. Roque MR (2010). Vitreous Wick Syndrome. [online] Available from http://www.emedicine. com/oph/TOPIC649.HTM [Accessed April, 2012].

1557. VOGT-KOYANAGI-HARADA DISEASE (HARADA DISEASE; UVEITIS-VITILIGO-ALOPECIA-POLIOSIS SYNDROME)

General

Viral infection; occurs predominantly among Italian and Japanese individuals; young adults; chronic.

Ocular

White lashes; secondary glaucoma; bilateral uveitis; sympathetic ophthalmitis; exudative iridocyclitis; vitreous opacities; bilateral serous retinal detachment and edema with spontaneous reattachment after weeks; depigmentation and patches of scattered pigment later; bilateral acute diffuse exudative choroiditis; papilledema; macular hemorrhage; cataracts; phthisis bulbi; poliosis; scleromalacia; intraocular lymphoma.

Clinical

Poliosis; vitiligo; hearing defect; headache; vomiting; meningeal irritation; reported to occur rarely in children.

Laboratory

Immunohistochemistry specimens demonstrates inflitration of CD4+ T-cells, epitheloid cells and multinucleated giant cells.

Treatment

Systemic therapy involves the use of high-dose corticosteroids. Topical steroids may be needed in conjunction with the use of systemic steroids.

Additional Resource

1. Walton RC (2010). Vogt-Koyanagi-Harada Disease. [online] Available from http://www.emedicine.com/oph/TOPIC459.HTM [Accessed April, 2012].

1558. VON BEKHTEREV-STRUMPELL SYNDROME (ANKYLOSING SPONDYLITIS; BEKHTEREV DISEASE; MARIE-STRUMPELL SPONDYLITIS; PIERRE-MARIE SYNDROME; RHEUMATOID SPONDYLITIS) OPTIC ATROPHY

General

Variant of rheumatoid arthritis; etiology unknown; autosomal dominant; male preponderance; onset age is 20–40 years; although genetic background determines susceptibility to uveitis, the disease pattern suggests the possibility of random environmental triggers unrelated to the course of the underlying rheumatologic disorder.

Ocular

Nongranulomatous anterior uveitis; optic nerve atrophy (occasionally); hypopyon; band keratopathy; spontaneous hyphema.

Clinical

Spondylitis of vertebra and sacroiliac joints; ankylosis; general arthralgia; kyphosis; scoliosis; displaced head and total rigidity of spine.

Laboratory

Histocompatibility antigen HLA-B27 and a negative rheumatoid factor and antinuclear antibody; X-ray evidence of narrowing of sacroiliac joint space and sclerosis.

Treatment

Oral nonsteroidal anti-inflammatory drugs, urethritis in Reiters disease should be treated with tetracycline, topical steroids and cycloplegic agents.

Additional Resource

1. Vives MJ (2011). Rheumatoid Arthritis of the Cervical Spine Overview of Rheumatoid Spondylitis. [online] Available from http://www.emedicine.com/orthoped/TOPIC551.HTM [Accessed April, 2012].

1559. VON ECONOMO SYNDROME (ENCEPHALITIS LETHARGICA; ICELAND DISEASE; SLEEPING SICKNESS) NYSTAGMUS

General

Etiology not understood; may be caused by filterable virus; both sexes affected; onset at all ages; epidemic form.

Ocular

Nystagmus; strabismus; diplopia; muscle imbalance; lid retraction; homonymous hemianopsia; cortical blindness.

Clinical

Fever; headache; cramps; lethargy; insomnia; athetoid or choreiform movements; convulsions; depression; unsteady gait; fatigue; parkinsonism; oculogyric crisis; behavior disorder.

Laboratory

Diagnosis is made by clinical findings.

Treatment

Nystagmus: See-saw nystagmus—visual field to consider neoplastic or vascular etiologies. Upbeat nystagmus—may indicate multiple sclerosis, cerebellar degeneration, tumors or infarcts. Treatment is directed toward identification and resolution of underlying cause. Downbeat nystagmus—affects the cerebellum or craniocervical junction including Arnold-Chiari malformation, multiple sclerosis, trauma, tumor, infarction and many toxic metabolic entities. MRI may indicate a surgically correctable lesion. Periodic alternating nystagmus is continuous horizontal nystagmus from stroke, tumor, multiple sclerosis, trauma, infection and drug intoxication. Can occur from cataract, vitreous hemorrhage or optic atrophy.

Bibliography

1. Magalini SI, Scrascia E. Dictionary of Medical Syndromes, 2nd edition. Philadelphia: JB Lippincott; 1981.
2. Pruskauer-Apostol B, Popescu-Pretor R, Plăiaşu D, et al. The present status of encephalitis lethargica. Neurol Psychiatr (Bucur). 1977;15:125-8.
3. von Economo C. Encephalitis lethargica. Wien Klin Wochenschr. 1917;30:581.

1560. VON GIERKE DISEASE (GLYCOGEN STORAGE DISEASE TYPE I; GLYCOGENOSIS TYPE I; GLUCOSE-6-PHOSPHATASE DEFICIENCY)

General

Condition simulating congenital glaucoma; affects both sexes during the first year of life.

Ocular

Corneal clouding; discrete, nonelevated, yellow flecks in macular area.

Clinical

Convulsions; failure to thrive; epistaxis; bleeding tendency; steatorrhea; lumbar lordosis; adiposity; hepatomegaly; enlarged kidney; renal tubular acidosis type I and kidney stones.

Laboratory

Serum glucose and electrolyte levels, serum lactate levels, blood pH serum uric acid level, serum triglyceride and cholesterol levels, gamma glutamyltransferase level, CBC, urinalysis, serum alkaline phosphatase, calcium, phosphorus, urea, and creatinine levels.

Treatment

No specific treatment is available.

Additional Resource

1. Stojanov L (2012). Glycogen Storage Diseases Types I-VII. [online] Available from http://www.emedicine.com/derm/TOPIC723.HTM [Accessed April, 2012].

1561. VON HERRENSCHWAND SYNDROME (SYMPATHETIC HETEROCHROMIA) PTOSIS

General

Congenital anomaly; heterochromia with Horner syndrome; sympathetic palsy from cervical ribs, tumor of the thyroid gland, enlarged cervical lymph nodes, scars following tuberculosis, or syringomyelia in apex of the pleura.

Ocular

Enophthalmos; ptosis; heterochromia (ipsilateral iris); miosis; iris on the side of the sympathetic denervation usually shows subtle hypochromia.

Clinical

Decrease of sweating ipsilateral side of face as part of the sympathetic paralysis.

Laboratory

Computed tomography (CT) scan of neck.

Treatment

Seek specialist assistance.

Bibliography

1. Durham DG. Congenital hereditary in Horner's syndrome. AMA Arch Ophthalmol. 1958;60:939-40.
2. Eagle RC. Congenital, developmental and degenerative disorders of the iris and ciliary body. In: Albert DM, Jakobiec FA (Eds). Principles and Practice of Ophthalmology. Philadelphia: WB Saunders; 1994. p. 367.
3. Margo CE, Hamed LM. Horner's syndrome. In: Margo CE, Mames R, Hamed LM (Eds). Diagnostic Problems in Clinical Ophthalmology. Philadelphia: WB Saunders; 1994. p. 729.
4. Volpe JJ. Brachial plexus injury. In: Volpe JJ (Ed). Neurology of the Newborn, 3rd edition. Philadelphia: WB Saunders; 1995. pp. 781-4.
5. von Herrenschwand F. Zur Sympathikusheterochromie. Klin Wochenschr. 1923;2:1059.

1562. VON HIPPEL-LINDAU SYNDROME (ANGIOMATOSIS RETINAE; CEREBELLORETINAL HEMANGIOBLASTOMATOSIS; LINDAU SYNDROME; RETINAL CAPILLARY HAMARTOMA; RETINOCEREBRAL ANGIOMATOSIS) GLAUCOMA

General

Dominant inheritance; angiomata in the cerebellum and the walls of the fourth ventricle; young adults.

Ocular

Secondary glaucoma; angiomatosis of the iris; vitreous hemorrhages; tortuosity of dilated retinal artery and vein (feeder vessels); retinal exudates and hemorrhages; retinitis proliferans; angiomata of optic nerve and retina; papilledema; retinal detachment; lipid accumulation in macula; keratoconus; bilateral macular holes; choroid plexus papilloma; bilateral optic nerve hemangioblastomas.

Clinical

Cerebellar angiomatosis; epilepsy; psychic disturbances to dementia.

Laboratory

Diagnosis is made from clinical findings.

Treatment

Smaller tumors can be treated with argon laser photocoagulation. Cryotherapy is used to treat larger posterior angiomas. Vitreoretinal surgery is effective for the treatment of severe VHL retinal hemangiomas.

Bibliography

1. Gaudric A, Krivosic V, Duguid G, et.al. Vitreoretinal surgery for severe retinal capillary hemangiomas in Von Hippel-Lindau Disease. Ophthalmology. 2011;118:142-9.

Additional Resource

1. Khan AN (2011). Imaging in Von Hippel-Lindau Syndrome. [online] Available from http://www.emedicine.com/radio/TOPIC742.HTM [Accessed April, 2012].

1563. VON MONAKOW SYNDROME (MONAKOW ANTERIOR CHOROIDAL ARTERY SYNDROME) VISUAL FIELD DEFECT

General

Rupture or thrombosis of anterior choroidal artery; aneurysm; tumor.

Ocular

Visual field defect; hemianopia.

Clinical

Hemiplegia; hemianesthesia.

Laboratory

Visual field.

Treatment

Consult specialist for assistance.

Bibliography

1. Magalini SI, Scrascia E. Dictionary of Medical Syndromes, 2nd edition. Philadelphia: JB Lippincott; 1981.
2. Steegmann AT, Roberts DJ. The syndrome of the anterior choroidal artery. JAMA. 1935;104:1695-7.
3. Takahashi S, Fukasawa H, Ishii K, et al. The anterior choroidal artery syndrome. I. Microangiography of the anterior choroidal artery. Neuroradiology. 1994;36:337-9.

1564. VON RECKLINGHAUSEN SYNDROME (NEURINOMATOSIS; NEUROFIBROMATOSIS TYPE I)

General

Dominant inheritance activated at puberty, during pregnancy, and at menopause; strong evidence supports the existence of NFl as a tumor suppresser gene.

Ocular

Proptosis; displacement of the globe; pulsation of the globe; ptosis; elephantiasis of the lids; pigment spots on lids; hydrophthalmos; nodular swelling of corneal nerves; cataracts; optic atrophy; choroidal melanoma; neurofibroma of the choroid, iris, eyelid, and ciliary body; enlarged optic foramen; underdevelopment of orbital bones; cafe-au-lait spots on fundus; hamartoma of retina; congenital glaucoma; focal iris nodules; choroidal nevi; optic nerve gliomas; orbital neurofibroma; keratoconus.

Clinical

Cafe-au-lait skin pigmentations; fibroma molluscum; lipomas and sebaceous adenomas; schwannomas; growth abnormalities; spontaneous fractures; facial hemihypertrophy.

Laboratory

T2-weighted MRI images demonstrate multiple bright lesions in the basal ganglia, cerebellum, and brain in 80% optic nerve gliomas often develop perineural arachnoidal hyperplasia which appears as an expanded CSF space around the nerve.

Treatment

Oral ketotifen may reduce the pain, tenderness and itchiness associated with neurofibromas.

Additional Resource

1. Dahl AA (2011). Ophthalmologic Manifestations of Neurofibromatosis Type 1. [online] Available from http://www.emedicine.com/oph/TOPIC338. HTM [Accessed April, 2012].

1565. VON REUSS SYNDROME (GALACTOKINASE DEFICIENCY; GALACTOSEMIA; GALACTOSEMIC SYNDROME) NYSTAGMUS

General

Autosomal recessive; consanguinity; conversion of galactose into glucose is blocked, leading to galactosemia; onset after a few days or weeks of milk ingestion; deficiency of galactose-1-phosphate uridyltransferase.

Ocular

Searching-type nystagmus; bilateral nuclear or cortical cataracts appear clinically as oil droplets; bilateral zonular cataracts with fine punctate opacities in the lens periphery.

Clinical

Vomiting; refusal of food; diarrhea; weight loss; hepatomegaly with ascites; jaundice; galactosuria; aminoaciduria; dehydration; hypoglycemic crisis; failure to thrive; hypotonia; lethargy; severe mental and neurologic manifestations.

Laboratory

Test for galactosuria and aminoaciduria.

Treatment

Dietary and cataract treatment as needed.

Bibliography

1. Cordes FC. Galactosemia cataract: a review. Am J Ophthalmol. 1960;50:1151.
2. Roy FH, Fraunfelder FW, Fraunfelder FT. Roy and Fraunfelder's Current Ocular Therapy, 6th edition. Philadelphia: WB Saunders; 2008.
3. Lerman S. The lens in congenital galactosemia. AMA Arch Ophthalmol. 1959;61:88-92.
4. Okajima K, Yazaki M, Wada Y. Thymidine kinase activity in individuals with galactokinase deficiency. Am J Hum Genet. 1987;41:503-4.

1566. VON SALLMANN-PATON-WITKOP SYNDROME (HBID SYNDROME; HEREDITARY BENIGN INTRAEPITHELIAL DYSKERATOSIS; WITKOP-VON SALLMANN SYNDROME) CORNEAL VASCULARIZATION

General

Autosomal dominant; conjunctival and oral lesions; found in whites.

Ocular

Foamy gelatinous plaques located in a typical horseshoe fashion at 3 and 9 o'clock positions of the perilimbal area; superficial hyperemia of bulbar conjunctiva; corneal vascularization and consequent visual decrease.

Clinical

Thickening of oral mucosa with whitish plaques and folds of a spongy character (asymptomatic), with slow progression from birth into second decade of life.

Laboratory

Diagnosis is made by clinical findings.

Treatment

Dental evaluation and treatment.

Bibliography

1. McLean IW; Riddle PJ, Schruggs JH, et al. Hereditary benign intraepithelial dyskeratosis. A report of two cases from Texas. Ophthalmology. 1981;88:164-8.
2. Von Sallmann L, Paton D. Hereditary benign intraepithelial dyskeratosis. I. Ocular manifestations. Arch Ophthalmol. 1960;63:421-9.
3. Witkop CJ, Shankle CH, Graham JB, et al. Hereditary benign intraepithelial dyskeratosis. II. Oral manifestations and hereditary transmission. Arch Pathol. 1960;70:696-711.

1567. VON WILLEBRAND DISEASE

General

Autosomal inherited mucocutaneous bleeding disorder; caused by a deficiency of the protein termed von Willebrand factor (vWF).

Clinical

Easy bruising; prolonged bleeding after minor trauma to skin or mucous membrane; severe hemorrhage after major surgery; heavy bleeding after tooth extraction; menorrhagia.

Ocular

Ocular bleeding.

Laboratory

Prothrombin time; ristocetin cofactor activity; vWF antigen.

Treatment

DDAVP is the treatment of choice of most individuals; platelet transfusion is reserved for individuals with more severe cases of the disease.

Additional Resource

1. Pollak ES (2012). von Willebrand Disease. [online] Available from http://www.emedicine.medscape.com/article/206996-overview [Accessed April, 2012].

1568. WAARDENBURG SYNDROME (EMBRYONIC FIXATION SYNDROME; INTEROCULO-IRIDODERMATO-AUDITIVE DYSPLASIA; PIEBALDISM; VAN DER HOEVE-HALBERSTAM-WAARDENBURG SYNDROME; WAARDENBURG-KLEIN SYNDROME) HYPERTELORISM

General

Irregular dominant inheritance; developmental fault in neural crest with absence of the organ of Corti, aplasia of the spiral ganglion, and pigmentary changes; no sex preference; onset at birth.

Ocular

Hyperplasia of the medial portions of the eyebrows; hypertelorism; blepharophimosis; strabismus; heterochromia iridis; aniridia; microcornea; cornea plana; microphakia; abnormal fundus pigmentation; hypoplasia of optic nerve; synophrys; poliosis; hypopigmentation and hypoplasia of retina and choroid; epicanthus; lateral displacement of inferior puncta; lenticonus; underdevelopment of orbital bones; lateral displacement of inner canthi; hypopigmented iris.

Clinical

Congenital deafness; unilateral deafness or deaf-mutism; broad and high nasal root with absent nasofrontal angle; albinotic hair strain (unilateral); faint patches of skin pigmentation; pituitary tumor; nasal atresia; white forelock.

Laboratory

Molecular testing and audiology.

Treatment

Genetic counseling, audiology and otolaryngology management.

Additional Resource

1. Schwartz RA (2011). Genetics of Waardenburg Syndrome. [online] Available from http://www.emedicine.com/ped/TOPIC2422.HTM [Accessed April, 2012].

1569. WAGNER SYNDROME (CLEFTING SYNDROME; FAVRE HYALOIDEORETINAL DEGENERATION; GOLDMANN-FAVRE SYNDROME; HEREDITARY HYALOIDEORETINAL DEGENERATION AND PALATOSCHISIS; HYALOIDEORETINAL DEGENERATION; RETINOSCHISIS WITH EARLY HEMERALOPIA) NYSTAGMUS

General

Irregular dominant inheritance; both sexes affected.

Ocular

Epicanthus; nystagmus; myopia; iris atrophy; vitreous opacities with dense streaks and folds in posterior hyaloid membrane; corneal degeneration, including band-shaped keratopathy; cataracts; hyaloideoretinal degeneration (usually apparent after 15 years); narrowing of retinal vessels; pigmentary changes; type of retinal degeneration varies from case to case; retinal detachment and avascular preretinal membranes; marked choroidal sclerosis; pale optic disk; Bergmeister papilla.

Clinical

Palatoschisis; genua valga; facial anomalies; hypoplastic maxilla; saddle nose; hyperextensible fingers, elbows and knees; tapering fingers.

Laboratory

Diagnosis is made by clinical findings.

Treatment

Nystagmus: See-saw nystagmus—visual field to consider neoplastic or vascular etiologies. Upbeat nystagmus—may indicate multiple sclerosis, cerebellar degeneration, tumors or infarcts. Treatment is directed toward identification and resolution of underlying cause. Downbeat nystagmus—affects the cerebellum or craniocervical junction including Arnold-Chiari malformation, multiple sclerosis, trauma, tumor, infarction and many toxic metabolic entities. MRI may indicate a surgically correctable lesion. Periodic alternating nystagmus is continuous horizontal nystagmus from stroke, tumor, multiple sclerosis, trauma, infection and drug intoxication. Can occur from cataract, vitreous hemorrhage or optic atrophy.

Corneal opacity: Medical treatment includes the use of hyperosmotic drops, nonsteroidal and steroid eye drops. Corneal transplant may be necessary.

Cataract: Change in glasses can sometimes improve a patient's visual function temporarily; however, the most common treatment is cataract surgery.

Bibliography

1. Black GC, Perveen R, Wiszniewski W, et al. A novel hereditary developmental vitreoretinopathy with multiple ocular abnormalities localizing to a 5-cM region of chromosome 5q13-q14. Ophthalmology. 1999;106:2074-81.
2. Frandsen E. Hereditary hyaloideoretinal degeneration (Wagner) in a Danish family. Arch Ophthalmol. 1966;74:223-32.
3. Hirose T, Lee KY, Schepens CL. Wagner's hereditary vitreoretinal degeneration and retinal detachment. Arch Ophthalmol. 1973;89:176-85.
4. Kaiser-Kupfer M. Ectrodactyly, ectodermal dysplasia, and clefting syndrome. Am J Ophthalmol. 1973;76:992-8.
5. Wagner H. Ein Bisher Unbekanntes Erbleiden des Auges (Degeneratio Hyaloideo Hereditaria), Beobachtet im Kanton Zurich. Klin Monatsbl Augenheilkd. 1938;100:840-57.

1570. WALDENSTRÖM SYNDROME (MACROGLOBULINEMIA)

General

Occurs mainly in males over age 50 years; chromosomal abnormalities were reported, with most of the cells having 47 chromosomes.

Ocular

Sludging of conjunctival vessels; crystalline deposits in conjunctiva and cornea; keratoconjunctivitis sicca; retinal venous thrombosis; hemorrhagic glaucoma; papilledema; retinal microaneurysms; cotton-wool spots; dry eye.

Clinical

Adenopathy; hepatosplenomegaly; weakness; fatigue; pallor; dyspnea; weight loss; lymphoid orbital tumor.

Laboratory

Chromsomal evaluation.

Treatment

Consult hematologist.

Bibliography

1. Cordido M, Fernández-Lago C, Fernández-Vigo J, et al. Dry eye in Waldenstrom's macroglobulinemia. Improvement after systemic chemotherapy. Cornea. 1995;14:210-1.
2. Ettl AR, Birbamer GG, Philipp W. Orbital involvement in Waldenstrom's macroglobulinemia: ultrasound, computed tomography and magnetic resonance findings. Ophthalmologica. 1992;205:40-5.
3. Feman SS, Stein RS. Waldenstrom's macroglobulinemia, a hyperviscosity manifestation of venous

stasis retinopathy. Int Ophthalmol. 1981;4: 107-12.

4. Friedman AH, Marchevsky A, Odel JG, et al. Immunofluorescent studies of the eye in Waldenstrom's macroglobulinemia. Arch Ophthalmol. 1980;98:743-6.

5. Lu LW, Carbone AO, Katzman B. Sjögren's syndrome and benign hyperglobulinemic purpura of Waldenstrom. Ann Ophthalmol. 1981;13:1285-7.

6. Sen HN, Chan CC, Caruso RC, et al. Waldenstrom's macroglobulinemia-associated retinopathy. Ophthalmology. 2004;111:535-9.

1571. WALKER-CLODIUS SYNDROME (LOBSTER CLAW DEFORMITY WITH NASOLACRIMAL OBSTRUCTION; EEC; ECTRODACTYLY, ECTODERMAL DYSPLASIA, AND CLEFT LIP/PALATE)

General

Autosomal dominant; both sexes affected; onset from birth; association with chromosome 7 abnormalities.

Ocular

Hypertelorism; nasolacrimal obstruction with constant epiphora; mucopurulent conjunctival discharge; keratitis; nanocanalization of the lacrimal duct.

Clinical

Deformities of hands and feet ("lobster claw"); absence of both index and middle fingers and second metacarpals with rudimentary third metacarpals; syndactylism; cleft palate and lips; deafness; ear malformation; renal anomalies.

Laboratory

Chromosomal evaluation.

Treatment

Consult specialist for general body problems.

Bibliography

1. Fukushima Y, Ohashi H, Hasegawa T. The breakpoints of the EEC syndrome (ectrodactyly, ectodermal dysplasia, and cleft lip/palate) confirmed to 7q11.21 and 9p12 by fluorescence in situ hybridization. Clin Genet. 1993;44:50.

2. Walker JC, Clodius L. The syndromes of cleft lip, cleft palate and lobster-claw deformities of hands and feet. Plast Reconstr Surg. 1963;32:627-36.

3. Wiegmann OA, Walker FA. The syndrome of lobster claw deformity and nasolacrimal obstruction. J Pediatr Ophthalmol. 1970;7:79-85.

1572. WALKER-WARBURG SYNDROME (CEREBRO-OCULAR DYSPLASIA-MUSCULAR DYSTROPHY; COD-MD SYNDROME; FUKUYAMA CONGENITAL MUSCULAR DYSTROPHY; HARD + OR - E SYNDROME; WARBURG SYNDROME) CATARACT

General

Rare; encompassing a triad of brain, eye and muscle abnormalities; probably autosomal recessive.

Ocular

Microphthalmia; cataract; immature anterior chamber angle; retinal dysplasia; retinal detachment; persistent hyperplastic primary vitreous; optic nerve hypoplasia; iris coloboma; opaque cornea; myopia; orbicularis weakness; irregular gray subretinal mottling; optic atrophy.

Clinical

Cerebral and cerebellar agyria-micropolygyria; cortical disorganization; glialmesodermal proliferation; neuronal heterotopias; hypoplasia of nerve tracts; hydrocephalus; encephalocele; muscular dystrophy; seizures; mental retardation; hypotonia; abnormal facies.

Laboratory

Magnetic resonance imaging (MRI), creatine kinase levels, electromyography and nerve conduction study.

Treatment

No specific treatment is available.

Additional Resource

1. Lopate G (2011). Congenital Muscular Dystrophy. [online] Available from http://www.emedicine.com/neuro/TOPIC549.HTM [Accessed April, 2012].

1573. WALLENBERG SYNDROME (DORSOLATERAL MEDULLARY SYNDROME; LATERAL BULBAR SYNDROME) PTOSIS

General

Occlusion of the posterior inferior cerebellar artery; onset after age 40 years; similar to Babinski-Nageotte syndrome but crossed hemiparesis is absent; nystagmus is produced by involvement of the vestibular nuclei or posterior longitudinal bundle.

Ocular

Enophthalmos; ptosis; spontaneous homolateral or contralateral horizontal or torsional nystagmus; miosis; Horner syndrome; skew deviation; impaired contralateral pursuit; saccadic abnormalities; gaze-holding abnormalities.

Clinical

Nausea; vertigo; difficulty in swallowing and speaking; ipsilateral ataxia; muscular hypotonicity; ipsilateral loss of pain and temperature sense of the face; neurotrophic skin ulcers; contralateral hypalgesia; facial weakness.

Laboratory

Computed tomography (CT) scan.

Treatment

Seek neurological assistance. Ptosis evaluation.

Bibliography

1. Brazis PW. Ocular motor abnormalities in Wallenberg's lateral medullary syndrome. Mayo Clin Proc. 1992;67:365-8.
2. Hornsten G. Wallenberg's syndrome. I. General symptomatology, with special reference to visual disturbances and imbalance. Acta Neurol Scand. 1974;50:434-46.
3. Marcoux C, Malfait Y, Pirard C, et al. Neurotrophic ulcer following Wallenberg's syndrome. Dermatology. 1993;186:301-2.
4. Sacco RL, Freddo L, Bello JA, et al. Wallenberg's lateral medullary syndrome. Clinical-magnetic resonance imaging correlations. Arch Neurol. 1993;50:609-14.
5. Silfverskiold BP. Skew deviation in Wallenberg's syndrome. Acta Neurol Scand. 1966;41:381-6.
6. Wallenberg A. Anatomische Befunde in Einem als "Akute Bulbaraffektion (Embolie der Arteria Cerebellar. Post. Inf. Sinist.)" Beschriebenen Falle. Arch F Psychiatr. 1901;34.

1574. WARD SYNDROME (EPITHELIOMATOUS PHAKOMATOSIS; NEVUS-JAW CYST SYNDROME) HYPERTELORISM

General

Autosomal dominant.

Ocular

Hypertelorism; dystopia canthorum; nevi of eyelids; congenital cataracts; congenital corneal opacities; colobomata.

Clinical

Basal cell nevi with multiple basalomatous nodules on face, neck and trunk; epithelioma adenoides cysticum.

Laboratory

Diagnosis is made by clinical findings.

Treatment

Dermatologic evaluation.

Bibliography

1. Font RL, Ferry AP. The phakomatoses. Int Ophthalmol Clin. 1972;12:1-50.
2. Gorlin RJ, Goltz RW. Multiple nevoid basal-cell epithelioma, jaw cysts and bifid ribs. A syndrome. N Engl J Med. 1960;262:908-12.

1575. WATER INTOXICATION SYNDROME (OVERHYDRATION SYNDROME)

General

Administration of water in excess of kidney excretion capacity; psychogenic water drinker; may be chronic, with slow accumulation of water, or acute.

Ocular

Lacrimation

Clinical

Chronic symptoms include weakness, sleepiness, apathy, anorexia, nausea, vomiting, sialorrhea, diarrhea, perspiration, behavioral changes, seizures and coma, tendon hyporeflexia, pitting edema, hemiplegia, pulmonary edema and congestive heart failure; acute symptoms include tendon hyporeflexia, decreased attention, confusion, aphasia, muscle twitching, hemiplegia, incoordination, apathy, violent behavior and marked muscle weakness.

Laboratory

Diagnosis is made by clinical findings.

Treatment

General medical evaluation.

Bibliography

1. Magalini SI, Scrascia E. Dictionary of Medical Syndromes, 2nd edition. Philadelphia: JB Lippincott; 1981.

1576. WEBER-CHRISTIAN SYNDROME (PFEIFFER-WEBER-CHRISTIAN SYNDROME) UVEITIS

General

Etiology unknown; subcutaneous inflammatory lesions; occurs at any age; no gender dominance.

Ocular

Secondary glaucoma; anterior uveitis; acute exudative central choroiditis.

Clinical

Generalized distribution of subcutaneous nodular lesions that vary in size and are located predominantly on the trunk, arms and legs; recurrent attacks of fever; anorexia; hepatosplenomegaly; malaise; oropharyngeal infections; myocardosis; liver cirrhosis; retroperitoneal fibrosis; ulcerative colitis; myalgia; cardiac dilatation with congestive heart failure.

Laboratory

Liver function test, CBC, electrolyte levels and erythrocyte sedimentation rate. Chest radiograph to rule out autoimmune disease.

Treatment

No specific therapy for Weber-Christian syndrome exists.

Additional Resource

1. Giardino AP (2010). Weber-Christian Disease. [online] Available from http://www.emedicine.com/ped/TOPIC2429.HTM [Accessed April, 2012].

1577. WEBER SYNDROME (ALTERNATING OCULOMOTOR PARALYSIS; CEREBELLAR PEDUNCLE SYNDROME; VENTRAL MEDIAL MIDBRAIN SYNDROME; WEBER-DUBLER SYNDROME) PTOSIS

General

Lesion of the peduncle (crus), pons or medulla, which interrupts the third nerve before it emerges from the peduncle and interrupts fibers in the pyramidal tract above the level of the third nuclei; hemorrhage and thrombosis; tumor of the pituitary region, extending posteriorly; also may result secondary to cerebrovascular disease.

Ocular

Ptosis; homolateral III nerve palsy (usually complete); fixed, dilated pupil.

Clinical

Contralateral hemiplegia; contralateral paralysis of face and tongue (supranuclear type).

Laboratory

Diagnosis is made by clinical findings.

Treatment

Ptosis: If visual acuity is affected most cases require surgical correction, and there are several procedures that may be used including levator resection, repair or advancement and Fasanella-Servat.

Bibliography

1. Kistler JP, Ropper AH, Martin JB. Cerebrovascular diseases. In: Isselbacher KJ et al. (Eds). Harrison's Principles of Internal Medicine, 13th edition. New York: McGraw-Hill; 1994. p. 2242.
2. Newman NJ. Third, fourth and sixth-nerve lesions and the cavernous sinus. In: Albert DM, Jakobiec FA (Eds). Principles and Practice of Ophthalmology. Philadelphia: WB Saunders; 1994. p. 2451.
3. Miller NR (Ed). Walsh and Hoyt's Clinical Neuro-Ophthalmology, 6th edition. Baltimore: Williams & Wilkins; 2004. p. 2384.
4. Weber H. A contribution to the pathology of the crura cerebri. Med Chir Trans. 1863;46:121-140.1.
5. Wolf BS, Newman CM, Khilnani MT. The posterior inferior cerebellar artery on vertebral angiography. Am J Roentgenol Radium Ther Nucl Med. 1962;87:322-37.

1578. WEBINO SYNDROME (WALL-EYED BILATERAL INTERNUCLEAR OPHTHALMOPLEGIA)

General

Differential diagnosis includes demyelinating disease, arteriosclerotic cerebrovascular disease, trauma, Arnold-Chiari malformation, syphilis, periarteritis nodosa, glioma, cryptococcal meningitis, and premature infants; usually represents midline involvement of oculomotor nucleus.

Ocular

Wall-eyed internuclear ophthalmoplegia (bilateral internuclear ophthalmoplegia with exotropia).

Clinical

Depends on cause; association with multiple sclerosis in young patients.

Laboratory

Diagnosis is made by clinical findings.

Treatment

Evaluate internuclear ophthalmoplegia.

Bibliography

1. Daroff RE, Hoyt WE. Supranuclear disorders of ocular control systems in man. In: Bach-Y-Rita P, Collins CC (Eds). The control of eye movements. Orlando, FL: Academic Press; 1971. p. 223.
2. Lepore FE, Nissenblatt MJ. Bilateral internuclear ophthalmoplegia after intrathecal chemotherapy and cranial irradiation. Am J Ophthalmol. 1981;92:851-3.
3. Miller NR (Ed). Walsh and Hoyt's Clinical Neuro-Ophthalmology, 6th edition. Baltimore: Williams & Wilkins; 2004. p. 4323.

1579. WEGENER SYNDROME (WEGENER GRANULOMATOSIS)

General

Etiology unknown; occurs in the fourth and fifth decades of life; persistent rhinitis or sinusitis; three characteristic features are: (1) necrotizing granulomatous lesions in the respiratory tract, (2) generalized focal arthritis and (3) necrotizing thrombotic glomerulitis.

Ocular

Exophthalmos; lid and conjunctival chemosis; papillitis; conjunctivitis; corneal ulcer; corneal abscess; optic atrophy; optic neuritis; orbital cellulitis; episcleritis; sclerokeratitis; cataract; peripheral ring corneal ulcers; ptosis; dacryocystitis; retinal periphlebitis; cotton-wool spots; retinal and vitreous hemorrhages; rubeosis iridis; neovascular glaucoma.

Clinical

Severe sinusitis; pulmonary inflammation; arteritis; weakness; fever; weight loss; bony destruction; granulomatous vasculitis of the upper and lower respiratory tracts; glomerulonephritis; diffuse pulmonary infiltrates; lymphadenopathy; diffuse pulmonary hemorrhage; overlap with giant cell arteritis.

Laboratory

Histopathology—necrotizing, granulomatous vasculitis with infiltrating neutrophils, lymphocytes and giant cells; urine—proteinuria, hematuria and urinary casts.

Treatment

Topical eye lubricants, ophthalmic antibiotic solution or ointment and corticosteroid drops may prove to be beneficial. Orbital decompression needed when medical treatment is unresponsive to treat optic nerve compression.

Bibliography

1. Collins JF. Handbook of Clinical Ophthalmology. New York: Masson; 1982.
2. Flach AJ. Ocular manifestations of Wegener's granulomatosis. JAMA. 1995;274:1199-200.
3. Roy FH, Fraunfelder FW, Fraunfelder FT. Roy and Fraunfelder's Current Ocular Therapy, 6th edition. Philadelphia: WB Saunders; 2008.
4. Haynes BF, Fishman ML, Fauci AS, et al. The ocular manifestations of Wegener's granulomatosis. Fifteen years' experience and review of the literature. Am J Med. 1977;63:131-41.
5. Leavitt RY, Fauci AS. Less common manifestations and presentations of Wegener's granulomatosis. Curr Opin Rheumatol. 1992;4:16-22.
6. Robinson MR, Lee SS, Sneller MC, et al. Tarsal-conjunctival disease associated with Wegener's granulomatosis. Ophthalmology. 2003;110:1770-80.
7. Straatsma BR. Ocular manifestations of Wegener's granulomatosis. Am J Ophthalmol. 1957;44: 789-99.

1580. WEIL DISEASE (LEPTOSPIROSIS)

General

Acute severe infection caused by *Leptospira* transmitted by ingestion of food contaminated by the reservoir bacterium.

Ocular

Acute conjunctivitis; episcleritis; fibrinous iridocyclitis with vitreal haze; hypopyon; keratitis; pain on ocular movement; uveitis; optic neuritis; cataract; hemorrhagic retinitis; ptosis.

Clinical

Jaundice; fever; headaches; chills; vomiting; anemia; psychologic disturbances.

Laboratory

Complete blood count, urinalysis and isolation of organism in blood, urine or cerebrospinal fluid.

Treatment

Intravenous penicillin G for a week. Ceftriaxone can also be used.

Additional Resource

1. Hickey PW (2010). Pediatric Leptospirosis. [online] Available from http://www.emedicine.com/ped/TOPIC1298.HTM [Accessed April, 2012].

1581. WEISSENBACHER-ZWEYMULLER SYNDROME (MYOPIA)

General

Probably neonatal expression of Stickler syndrome; autosomal dominant.

Ocular

Myopia; congenital glaucoma; cloudy cornea; buphthalmos; Descemet's membrane tears; retinal detachment; cataracts.

Clinical

Flattened occiput; flat facies; low nasal bridge; anteverted nostrils; flat vascular nevus-covered glabellar area; small mouth with protruding tip of tongue; high-arched palate; short neck; limbs shorter proximally; dumbbell-shaped long bones; posterior defects in vertebral bodies thoracic region; platyspondylic evidence of coronal cleft lumbar area; deafness; small size at birth; mid face hypoplasia; parieto-occipital encephalocele; hearing loss; dwarfism.

Laboratory

Diagnosis is made by clinical findings.

Treatment

Glaucoma: Its medication should be the first plan of action. If medication is unsuccessful, a filtering surgical procedure with or without antimetabolites may be beneficial.

Cataract: Change in glasses can sometimes improve a patient's visual function temporarily; however, the most common treatment is cataract surgery.

Bibliography

1. Galil A, Carmi R, Goldstein E, et al. Weissenbacher-Zweymuller syndrome: long-term follow-up of growth and psychomotor development. Dev Med Child Neurol. 1991;33:1104-9.
2. Ramer JC, Eggli K, Rogan PK, et al. Identical twins with Weissenbacher-Zweymuller syndrome and neural tube defect. Am J Med Genet. 1993;45:614-8.
3. Scribanu N, O'Neill J, Rimoin D. The Weissenbacher-Zweymuller phenotype in the neonatal period as an expression in the continuum of manifestations of the hereditary arthro-ophthalmopathies. Ophthalmic Paediatr Genet. 1987;8:159-63.
4. Weissenbacher G, Zweymuller E. Gleichzeitiges Vorkommen Eines Syndroms von Pierro Robin und einer Fetalen Chondrodysplasie. Mschr Kinderheilkd. 1964;112:315-7.
5. Winter RM, Baraitser M, Laurence KM, et al. The Weissenbacher-Zweymuller, Stickler, and Marshall syndromes: further evidence for their identity. Am J Med Genet. 1983;16:189-99.

1582. WERLHOF DISEASE (HEMOPHILIA AND THROMBOCYTOPENIC PURPURA)

General

Hemorrhagic disease of unknown etiology.

Ocular

Retinal hemorrhages; degeneration or severe intraocular hemorrhages with resultant retinitis proliferans.

Clinical

Petechiae and ecchymoses of skin and mucous membranes; tendency to bruise; decreased level of circulating platelets with a normal clotting time.

Laboratory

Diagnosis is made by clinical findings.

Treatment

Consult hemotologist.

Bibliography

1. Kobayashi H, Honda Y. Intraocular hemorrhage in a patient with hemophilia. Metab Ophthalmol. 1985;8:27-30.
2. Pau H. Differential Diagnosis of Eye Diseases. New York: Thieme; 1987.
3. Werlhof PG. Disquisitio Medica et Philogica de Variolis et Anthracibus. Brunswick. 1735.

1583. WERMER SYNDROME (ENDOCRINE ADENOMA-PEPTIC ULCER COMPLEX; MULTIPLE ENDOCRINE NEOPLASIA 1; MEN1; MULTIPLE ENDOCRINE ADENOMATOSIS 1; MEA1; PLURIGLANDULAR ADENOMATOSIS N) VISUAL FIELD DEFECT

General

Autosomal dominant; high degree of penetrance; both sexes affected; onset after the first decade of life (Zollinger-Ellison Syndrome).

Ocular

Visual field defects secondary to pituitary adenoma.

Clinical

Parathyroid adenomas or hyperplasia; pancreatic adenomas; pituitary adenomas; thyroid adenomas; adrenocortical adenomas; subcutaneous lipomas; hypoglycemic crisis; headaches; amenorrhea; diarrhea; weight loss; acromegaly; Cushing syndrome; hyperthyroidism; ulcer; cerebral aneurysm.

Laboratory

pH probe to measure gastric acid, fasting hypoglycemia test, elevated serum glucagons levels, vasoactive intestinal polypeptide and serotonin. Assess growth hormone levels.

Treatment

Surgery is the treatment of choice.

Additional Resource

1. Lendel I (2010). Wermer Syndrome (MEN Type 1). [online] Available from http://www.emedicine. com/med/TOPIC2404.HTM [Accessed April, 2012].

1584. WERNER SYNDROME (PROGERIA OF ADULTS) BLUE SCLERA

General

Etiology unknown; recessive inheritance; consanguinity; occurs in the second and third decades of life; possible mechanisms have been proposed to explain mutation of a gene causing inhibition of DNA synthesis and early cellular senescence.

Ocular

Absence of eyelashes and scanty eyebrows; blue sclera; juvenile cataracts; bullous keratitis; trophic corneal defects; paramacular retinal degeneration; proptosis; telangiectasia of lid; astigmatism; nystagmus; presbyopia; uveitis.

Clinical

Leanness; short stature (160 cm maximum); thin limbs; short, deformed fingers; small mouth; early baldness; stretched, atrophic skin (scleropoikiloderma); telangiectasia and trophic indolent ulcers on toes, heels and ankles; arteriosclerosis with secondary heart failure.

Laboratory

Fasting blood glucose test, oral glucose tolerance test, triiodothyronine, levothyroxine and thyrotropin test.

Treatment

No specific treatment exist.

Additional Resource

1. Janniger CK (2012). Werner Syndrome. [online] Available from http://www.emedicine.com/derm/ TOPIC697.HTM [Accessed April, 2012].

1585. WERNICKE SYNDROME I (AVITAMINOSIS B; BERIBERI; ENCEPHALITIS HEMORRHAGICA SUPERIORIS; GAYET-WERNICKE SYNDROME; HEMORRHAGIC POLIOENCEPHALITIS SUPERIOR SYNDROME; SUPERIOR HEMORRHAGIC POLIOENCEPHALOPATHIC SYNDROME; THIAMINE DEFICIENCY; WERNICKE-KORSAKOFF SYNDROME) PTOSIS

General

Lack of vitamin B or thiamine; focal vascular lesions in the gray matter around third and fourth ventricles and sylvian aqueduct; alcoholics (adults); beriberi of all ages.

Ocular

Ptosis; acute bilateral nuclear ophthalmoplegia; complete ophthalmoplegia; retinal hemorrhages; optic atrophy; optic neuritis; conjunctivitis; blepharitis; nutritional amblyopia; central scotoma; papilledema; nystagmus; absolute pupillary paralysis or Argyll Robertson pupils; accommodative palsy.

Clinical

Early prostration; lethargy; irritability; stupor; delirium; mental disturbances to Korsakoff psychosis; ataxia; tremors; peripheral neuritis; anorexia; vomiting; insomnia; perspiration; tachycardia; hallucinations; retrograde amnesia; apathy; anxiety; fear; defective concentration; cardiomyopathy.

Laboratory

Electrolyte studies, serum thiamine levels, CBC. Evaluation of hypoxemia, hypercarbia, acidosis or alkalosis. Serum/urine toxin drug screen and liver enzymes.

Treatment

Parenteral thiamine is the treatment of choice.

Additional Resource

1. Xiong GL (2011). Wernicke-Korsakoff Syndrome. [online] Available from http://www.emedicine.com/med/TOPIC2405.HTM [Accessed April, 2012].

1586. WEST NILE VIRUS INFECTION (PHOTOPHOBIA)

General

Zoonotic disease transmitted by a mosquito vector with wild birds serving as its reservoir; seen worldwide but first seen in North America in 1999.

Ocular

Photophobia; chorioretinal lesions; mild vitreous inflammatory reaction; retinal hemorrhage; optic disk swelling.

Clinical

Muscle rigidity; meningeal inflammation; encephalitis; poliomyelitis; acute flaccid paralysis.

Laboratory

Complete blood count, CSF analysis and serologic testing.

Treatment

Treatments must be individualized because of the different degrees of infecton. Physical therapy, occupational therapy and speech therapy.

Additional Resource

1. Salinas JD (2012). West Nile Virus. [online] Available from http://www.emedicine.com/pmr/TOPIC236.HTM [Accessed April, 2012].

1587. WEST SYNDROME (MASSIVE MYOCLONIA; JACKKNIFE CONVULSION) NYSTAGMUS

General

Brain damage from trauma, anoxia, degenerative and metabolic factors and infective agents; onset in the first year of life.

Ocular

Nystagmus

Clinical

Convulsion; nodding of head; opisthotonos; mental retardation.

Laboratory

Complete blood count, metabolic workup, blood, urine and cerebrospinal fluid cultures if infecton is suspected. MRI, CT scan, electroencephalogram and lumbar puncture.

Treatment

Adrenocorticotropic hormone (ACTH) and conventional antiepileptic medications, cortico-steroids and hormonal agents.

Additional Resource

1. Glauser TA (2012). Infantile Spasm (West Syndrome). [online] Available from http://www.emedicine.com/neuro/TOPIC171.HTM [Accessed April, 2012].

1588. WESTPHAL-STRUMPELL DISEASE (PSEUDOSCLEROSIS OF BASAL GANGLION)

General

Part of Wilson disease; mostly in men; onset age is 11–25 years (Wilson Disease).

Ocular

Brown-yellow-green ring in Descemet's membrane, about 2 mm wide, which begins directly at the limbus and fades away toward the center; deposition of copper.

Clinical

Jaundice; difficulty in swallowing, speaking and mastication; extensive muscular rigidity; coarse tremors.

Laboratory

Copper studies.

Treatment

Consult specialist.

Bibliography

1. Roy FH, Fraunfelder FW, Fraunfelder FT. Roy and Fraunfelder's Current Ocular Therapy, 6th edition. Philadelphia: WB Saunders; 2008.

2. Pau H. Differential Diagnosis of Eye Diseases. New York: Thieme; 1987.

1589. WEYERS SYNDROME (2) (DENTOIRIDEAL DYSPLASIA; DYSGENESIS IRIDODENTALIS; DYSGENESIS MESODERMALIS CORNEAE ET IRIDES WITH DIGODONTIA; IRIDODENTAL DYSPLASIA; WEYERS IV SYNDROME) CORNEAL OPACITY

General

Present from birth; hereditary; etiology unknown.

Ocular

Dysplasia; small perforation of iris; pupillary synechiae; microphthalmia; corneal opacity.

Clinical

Dwarfism; myotonic dystrophy; microdontia; oligodontia; hypoplasia of dental enamel.

Laboratory

Diagnosis is made by clinical findings.

Treatment

None

Bibliography

1. Magalini SI, Scrascia E. Dictionary of Medical Syndromes, 2nd edition. Philadelphia: JB Lippincott; 1981. p. 864.

2. Weyers H. Dysgenesis Irido-dentalis. Ein Neues Syndrome mit obweichdendem Chromosomalen Geschlecht bei Weiblichen Merkmalträgern. Presented at the Meeting of Deutsche Gessellschaft fuer Kinderheilkunde, Kassel, Germany: 1960.

1590. WHIPPLE DISEASE (INTESTINAL LIPODYSTROPHY) PAPILLEDEMA

General

Multisystem disorder; prominent in males; onset between the fourth and seventh decades of life; etiology unknown.

Ocular

Ophthalmoplegia (vertical gaze involved more than horizontal gaze); papilledema; intraocular inflammation; vitreous opacities; bilateral pan-uveitis; small, round grayish retinal lesions; chemosis; supranuclear ophthalmoplegia; myoclonic ocular jerks; pendular nystagmus.

Clinicalm

Pneumonia; pleurisy; tonsillitis; sinusitis; cystitis; arthritis; fever; leukocytosis; diarrhea; malabsorption; death; dyspnea; weight loss; lymphadenopathy; polyserositis; gray pigmentation of skin; dementia; facial jerks; rhythmic movement of the mouth, jaw and extremities.

Laboratory

The following test may be useful to screen for the presence of malabsorption but they are not specific for the disease: Sudan stain of stool, serum carotene, serum albumin, prothrombin time, and CT scan may be helpful.

Treatment

Antibiotic therapy.

Additional Resource

1. Roberts IM (2011). Whipple Disease. [online] Available from http://www.emedicine.com/med/TOPIC2409.HTM [Accessed April, 2012].

1591. WHITE DOT SYNDROME

General

Acquired diseases that cause inflammation and multifocal lesion at the level of the outer retina, retinal pigment epithelium and inner choroid.

Clinical

None

Ocular

Unilateral mild decrease in vision, choroidal neovascular membrane, photopsia, scotomata.

Laboratory

Diagnosis is made by clinical findings.

Treatment

No treatment is required.

Additional Resource

1. Tewari A (2012). White Dot Syndromes. [online] Available from http://www.emedicine.com/oph/TOPIC749.HTM [Accessed April, 2012].

1592. WILDERVANCK SYNDROME (CERVICO-OCULO-ACOUSTICUS SYNDROME; CERVICO-OCULO-FACIAL DYSMORPHIA; CERVICOOCULOFACIAL SYNDROME; FRANCESCHETTI-KLEIN-WILDERVANCK SYNDROME; WILDERVANCK-WAARDENBURG SYNDROME) NYSTAGMUS

General

Etiology unknown; female preponderance; similarities to Klippel-Feil syndrome; onset at birth.

Ocular

Abducens paresis; nystagmus; heterochromia iridis.

Clinical

Deafness or deaf-mutism; torticollis with short, webbed neck; epilepsy; mental retardation; cleft palate; scoliosis; ventricular septal defect; ectopic kidney; hydrocephalus; hypoplastic thumb and growth retardation.

Laboratory

Diagnosis is made by clinical findings.

Treatment

Tape or base-out prism on one eyeglass may be useful, botulinum toxin type A into the antagonist medial rectus muscle, if no improvement after

6–12 months—recess/resect of medial and lateral rectus.

Bibliography

1. Geeraets WJ. Ocular Syndromes, 3rd edition. Philadelphia: Lea & Febiger; 1976.
2. Jensen J, Rovsing H. Dysplasia of the cochlea in a case of Wildervanck's syndrome. Adv Otorhinolaryngol. 1974;21:32-9.
3. Kose G, Ozkan H, Ozdamar F, et al. Cholelithiasis in cervico-oculo-acoustic (Wildervanck's) syndrome. Acta Paediatr. 1993;82:890-1.
4. Wildervanck LS. A cervico-oculo-acoustic nerve syndrome. Ned Tijdschr Geneeskd. 1960;104: 2600-5.

1593. WILLIAMS-BEUREN SYNDROME (BEUREN ELFIN FACE; HYPERCALCEMIA SUPRAVALVULAR AORTIC STENOSIS; HYPERCALCEMIC FACE; SUPRAVALVULAR AORTIC STENOSIS) HYPERTELORISM

General

Onset at birth or early infancy; occurs in both sexes; etiology unknown; possible abnormality of vitamin D metabolism.

Ocular

Bilateral corneal opacities; hypertelorism; prominent epicanthal folds; strabismus.

Clinical

Anorexia; slow weight gain; retarded physical and mental development; elfin face; absent aortic systolic click; harsh ejection systolic murmur; tooth enamel hypoplasia; malocclusion; cavities.

Laboratory

Fluorescent in situ hybridization (FISH) for the 7q11.23 elastin gene deletion, serum calcium, blood urea nitrogen and creatine levels. Thyroid-stimulating hormone levels, baseline echocardiogram and renal ultrasound.

Treatment

Treatment is done on a patient-to-patient basis with multiple health care professionals are involved.

Additional Resource

1. Khan A (2012). Williams Syndrome. [online] Available from http://www.emedicine.com/ped/TOPIC2439.HTM [Accessed April, 2012].

1594. WILSON DISEASE (HEPATOLENTICULAR DEGENERATION) NIGHT BLINDNESS

General

Lesion in the putamen and lenticular nucleus; familial; occurs in the first decade of life; reduced liver function; increase in copper content in tissue.

Ocular

Night blindness; golden, grayish-green or ruby-red peripheral posterior corneal stromal deposit (Kayser-Fleischer ring); sunflower cataract (same as with retention of copper foreign body); nystagmus; extraocular muscle palsies.

Clinical

Liver cirrhosis; jaundice (early); difficulties in speaking (early); difficulties in swallowing and mastication; extensive muscular rigidity; mouth usually open with salivation ("fixed grin"); coarse tremor.

Laboratory

Serum ceruloplasmin levels, total serum copper levels and increased urinary copper excretion. CT scan may be beneficial.

Treatment

Copper-chelating medications.

Additional Resource

1. Carter BA (2009). Genetics of Wilson Disease. [online] Available from http://www.emedicine.com/ped/TOPIC2441.HTM [Accessed April, 2012].

1595. WINDSHIELD WIPER SYNDROME

General

Following cataract extraction with a posterior chamber J-loop intraocular lens; intraocular lens too short and moves from side to side with the same motion as windshield wipers.

Ocular

Ruptured zonules; lateral intraocular lens tilt; lateral decentration of intraocular lens; decreased visual acuity; glare.

Clinical

None

Laboratory

Diagnosis is made by clinical findings.

Treatment

Change the intraocular lens to another intraocular lens.

Bibliography

1. Simcoe CW. Simcoe Posterior chamber lens: theory, techniques and results. J Am Intraocul Implant Soc. 1981;7:154-7.
2. Smith SG, Lindstrom RL. Malpositioned posterior chamber lenses: etiology, prevention, and management. J Am Intraocul Implant Soc. 1985; 11:584-91.

1596. WISKOTT-ALDRICH SYNDROME (CORNEAL ULCER)

General

Sex-linked recessive; early infancy with death in the first decade of life; abnormal immune responses; expression of CD43 is defective in this X chromosome-linked immunodeficiency disorder, suggesting that CD43 might have a role in T-cell activation.

Ocular

Periorbital hemorrhages; vesicular skin eruptions; blepharitis; lid nodules; episcleritis; scleral icterus; conjunctival hemorrhages and purulent discharge; corneal ulcers; retinal hemorrhages; papilledema; peripapillary hemorrhages.

Clinical

Eczema; epistaxis; purpura; hematemesis; bloody diarrhea; otitis media.

Laboratory

Complete blood count, delayed-type hypersensitivity (DTH) skin test and chest radiographs.

Treatment

Stem cell reconstitution is the main stream of therapy.

Additional Resource

1. Schwartz RA (2011). Pediatric Wiskott-Aldrich Syndrome. [online] Available from http://www.emedicine.com/ped/TOPIC2443.HTM [Accessed April, 2012].

1597. WOLF-HIRSCHHORN SYNDROME (NYSTAGMUS)

General

Partial deletion of the short arm of chromosome 4 (4p).

Ocular

Exodeviation; nasolacrimal obstruction; foveal hypoplasia; upperlid coloboma; optic disk anomalies; microcornea; hypertelorism; nystagmus; chorioretinal coloboma.

Clinical

Developmental delay; microcephaly; seizures; craniofacial anomalies; mental retardation; cardiac defects.

Laboratory

High-resolution cytogenetic studies, conventional cytogenetic, fluorescence in situ hybridization.

Treatment

No known treatment exists for the underlying disorder.

Additional Resource

1. Chen H (2011). Wolf-Hirschhorn Syndrome. [online] Available from http://www.emedicine.com/ped/TOPIC2446.HTM [Accessed April, 2012].

1598. WOLF SYNDROME (CHROMOSOME 4 PARTIAL DELETION SYNDROME; HIRSCHHORN-COOPER SYNDROME; MONOSOMY 4 PARTIAL SYNDROME) PTOSIS

General

Partial deletion of chromosome 4 of the B group; short life expectancy; present from birth (Cri-du-Chat Syndrome).

Ocular

Hypertelorism; antimongoloid slanting of palpebral fissures; ptosis; nystagmus; strabismus; iris coloboma; retinal coloboma.

Clinical

Microcephaly; mental retardation; seizures; ear malformations; hypospadias; beaked nose; broad nasal root; cleft lip and palate; hypotonia.

Laboratory

High-resolution cytogenetic studies, conventional cytogenetic, fluorescence in situ hybridization.

Treatment

No known treatment exists for the underlying disorder.

Additional Resource

1. Chen H (2011). Wolf-Hirschhorn Syndrome. [online] Available from http://www.emedicine. com/ped/TOPIC2446.HTM [Accessed April, 2012].

1599. WOODY-GHADIMI SYNDROME (GHADIMI-WOODY SYNDROME; HYPERLYSINEMIA, PERSISTENT) EXOTROPIA

General

Inherited probably autosomal dominant; affects both sexes; age of detection from infancy to early adulthood.

Ocular

Strabismus; ectopia lentis.

Clinical

Severe mental retardation; convulsions; laxity of joints; absence of secondary sex characteristics; hepatosplenomegaly; altered facial features.

Laboratory

Check for hyperlysinemia.

Treatment

Strabismus: Equalized vision with correct refractive error; surgery may be helpful in patient with diplopia.

Ectopia lentis: Repair of an impending dissecting aortic aneurysm, treatment of glaucoma, lensectomy.

Bibliography

1. Ghadimi H, Binnington VI, Pecora P. Hyperlysinemia associated with retardation. N Engl J Med. 1965;273:723-9.
2. Magalini SI, Scrascia E. Dictionary of Medical Syndromes, 2nd edition. Philadelphia: JB Lippincott; 1981.
3. McKusick VA. Mendelian Inheritance in Man: A Catalog of Human Genes and Genetic Disorders, 12th edition. Baltimore: The Johns Hopkins University Press; 1998.
4. McKusick-Nathans Institute for Genetic Medicine, Johns Hopkins University and National Center for Biotechnology Information, National Library of Medicine. (2007). Online Mendelian Inheritance in Man (OMIM). [online] Available from http://www. ncbi.nlm.nih.gov/omim [Accessed April, 2012].
5. Woody NC. Hyperlysinemia. Proceedings of the American Pediatric Society VII Annual Meeting, Seattle, Washington, 1964:33(abst).

1600. WRINKLY SKIN SYNDROME (OPTIC ATROPHY)

General

Autosomal recessive; consanguinity; similar to pseudoxanthoma elasticum and Ehlers-Danlos syndrome; onset from birth.

Ocular

Myopia; chorioretinitis; partial optic atrophy; microphthalmia; blepharophimosis; cataract.

Clinical

Dry skin with many wrinkles, including the dorsal surfaces of hands and feet; many creases of palms and soles; loss of skin elasticity; no abnormal wrinkles or creases about the face; prominent venous pattern over the chest wall; mental retardation; dwarfism; kyphosis; delayed growth; small size at birth; retarded growth and development; microcephaly; craniofacial dysmorphism; skeletal anomalies.

Laboratory

Skin biopsy.

Treatment

Consult dermatologist.

Bibliography

1. Gazit E, Goodman RM, Katznelson MB, et al. The wrinkly skin syndrome: a new heritable disorder of connective tissue. Clin Genet. 1973;4:186-92.
2. Geeraets WJ. Ocular Syndromes, 3rd edition. Philadelphia: Lea & Febiger; 1976.
3. Goodman RM, Katznelson MB, Frydman M. Evolution of palmar skin creases in the Ehlers-Danlos syndrome. Clin Genet. 1972;3:67-72.
4. Kreuz FR, Wittwer BH. Del(2q)—cause of the wrinkly skin syndrome? Clin Genet. 1993;43:132-8.

1601. X CHROMOSOMAL DELETION (OPTIC ATROPHY)

General

Deletion of proximal part of long arm of the X chromosome; deletion covers part of region Xq21.1–Xq21.31, the locus for choroideremia; congenital deafness; probable mental retardation.

Ocular

Choroideremia, translucent pigment epithelium; peripheral hyperpigmentation; diffuse choriocapillary layer and retinal pigment epithelium; decreased night vision; optic atrophy; excessive myopia; nystagmus.

Clinical

Congenital deafness; mental retardation; corpus callosum agenesia; cleft lip and palate; anhidrotic ectodermal dysplasia; agammaglobulinemia.

Laboratory

Chromosome studies.

Treatment

None

Bibliography

1. Bleeker-Wagemakers LM, Friedrich U, Gal A, et al. Close linkage between Norrie disease, a cloned DNA sequence from the proximal short arm, and the centromere of the X chromosome. Hum Genet. 1985;71:211-4.
2. Rosenberg T, Niebuhr E, Yang HM, et al. Choroideremia, congenital deafness and mental retardation in a family with an X chromosomal deletion. Ophthalmic Paediatr Genet. 1987;8:139-43.

1602. X-LINKED CONE DYSFUNCTION SYNDROME (MYOPIA)

General

X-linked pattern of inheritance; stationary cone dysfunction.

Ocular

Myopia; visual loss; color vision abnormality.

Laboratory

Diagnosis is made by clinical findings.

Treatment

None

Bibliography

1. Michaelides M, Johnson S, Bradshaw K, et al. X-linked cone dysfunction syndrome with myopia and protanopia. Ophthalmology. 2005;112:1448-54.

1603. X-LINKED MENTAL RETARDATION SYNDROME (XLMR) GLAUCOMA

General

X-linked mental retardation syndrome, of which many types may exist.

Ocular

Glaucoma may be found in some patients; optic atrophy has been noted.

Clinical

Short stature; small hands and feet; seizures; cleft palate; "coarse" facial appearance; brachydactyly.

Laboratory

Diagnosis is made by clinical findings.

Treatment

Glaucoma: Its medication should be the first plan of action. If medication is unsuccessful, a filtering surgical procedure with or without antimetabolites may be beneficial.

Bibliography

1. Armfield K, Nelson R, Lubs HA, et al. X-linked mental retardation syndrome with short stature, small hands and feet, seizures, cleft palate, and glaucoma is linked to Xq28. Am J Med Genet. 1999;85:236-42.
2. Carpenter NJ, Qu Y, Curtis M, et al. X-linked mental retardation syndrome with characteristic "coarse" facial appearance, brachydactyly, and short stature maps to proximal Xq. Am J Med Genet. 1999;85:230-5.

1604. XANTHELASMA (XANTHELASMA PALPEBRARUM)

General

Hereditary, isolated disorder associated with aging and hormonal changes. May occur as a result of hyperlipemia.

Clinical

Hyperlipemia, hypercholesterolemia, obesity, cardiovascular changes.

Ocular

Soft, yellow, plague-like, velvety lesion usually in the medial canthus area.

Laboratory

Lipid profile.

Treatment

Dietary restrictions for obesity and increased triglycerides, dermatologic—trichloroacetic acid, blepharoplasty incision and laser—CO_2 laser.

Bibliography

http://www.emedicine.medscape.com/article/1213423-overview

1605. XANTHISM (RUFOUS ALBINISM)

General

Autosomal recessive; occurs in Blacks.

Ocular

Lack of color in iris.

Clinical

Bright copper-red color of skin and hair.

Laboratory

Diagnosis is made by clinical findings.

Treatment

None

Bibliography

1. Barnicot NA. Human pigmentation. Man. 1957;57:114-20.
2. McKusick VA. Mendelian Inheritance in Man: A Catalog of Human Genes and Genetic Disorders, 12th edition. Baltimore: The Johns Hopkins University Press; 1998.
3. McKusick-Nathans Institute for Genetic Medicine, Johns Hopkins University and National Center for Biotechnology Information, National Library of Medicine. (2007). Online Mendelian Inheritance in Man (OMIM). [online] Available from http://www.ncbi.nlm.nih.gov/omim [Accessed April, 2012].

1606. XERODERMA PIGMENTOSUM (SYMBLEPHARON)

General

Rare, autosomal recessive disorder characterized by extreme cutaneous photosensitivity; both sexes affected; onset in infancy or early childhood.

Ocular

Conjunctivitis; symblepharon; keratitis; corneal ulcer; blepharitis; uveitis; malignancies of conjunctiva, cornea, eyelids and iris; ectropion; keratoconus; lid freckles; chronic conjunctival congestion; corneal opacification; bilateral pterygium; epibulbar and palpebral squamous cell corneal carcinoma.

Clinical

Neurologic abnormalities and cutaneous malignancies of ectodermal origin; speech disorders; spastic paralysis; convulsions; mental deficiency; gonadal hypoplasia; stunted growth; carcinoma of tongue.

Laboratory

No consistent laboratory studies.

Treatment

Sunlight protection, treatment of any malignancies, sunscreens, protective clothing, sunglasses and hats.

Additional Resource

1. Diwan AH (2011). Xeroderma Pigmentosum. [online] Available from http://www.emedicine.com/derm/TOPIC462.HTM [Accessed April, 2012].

1607. XXXXX SYNDROME (PENTA X SYNDROME, TETRA X SYNDROME) HYPERTELORISM

General

Congenital syndrome due to aneuploidy.

Ocular

Epicanthal folds; hypertelorism; antimongoloid (upward slant) of palpebral fissures.

Clinical

Growth retardation, bilateral.

Laboratory

Urine microscopic analysis, blood test for creatinine, urea and electrolytes, renal ultrasonography.

Treatment

No drug therapy is currently available for this condition.

Additional Resource

1. Swiatecka-Urban A (2011). Multicystic Renal Dysplasia. [online] Available from http://www.emedicine.com/ped/TOPIC1493.HTM [Accessed April, 2012].

1608. XXXXY SYNDROME (HYPERTELORISM)

General

49 chromosome anomaly; characterized by mental retardation; hypoplastic male genitalia; proximal radioulnar synostosis.

Ocular

Upward slanting of palpebral fissures; strabismus; hypertelorism.

Clinical

Microcephaly; mongoloid facies; high-arched palate; cubitus valgus; in-curving fifth fingers and toes; depressed nasal bridge; nasal speech; prominent lower lip; broad chin; round face configuration; small chest; depressed sternum; wide-spaced nipples; genu valgum; flat feet; no facial or pubic hair; small testes; poor scrotal development; girdle obesity; tremor; excessive dribbling; withdrawal; irritability; proximal radioulnar synostosis; vertebral anomalies; parkinsonism.

Laboratory

Chromosome studies.

Treatment

Strabismus: Equalized vision with correct refractive error; surgery may be helpful in patient with diplopia.

Bibliography

1. Hecht F. Observation on the natural history of 49,XXXXY individuals. Am J Med Genet. 1982;13:335-6.
2. Singh TH, Rajkowa S. 49,XXXXY chromosome anomaly: an unusual variant of Klinefelter's syndrome. Br J Psychiatry. 1986;148:209-10.

1609. XYY SYNDROME

General

Y chromosome polysomy syndrome.

Ocular

Colobomata

Clinical

Mild mental retardation; autism; impulsiveness; aggressive behavior; developmental motor and language delays; excessive height for age; frequent antisocial behavior.

Laboratory

Chromosome studies.

Treatment

None

Bibliography

1. Onwochei BC, Simon JW, Bateman JB, et al. Ocular colobomata. Surv Ophthalmol. 2000;45: 175-94.
2. von Gontard A, Hillig U. Ein Kind mit XYY-Syndrom im Erleben seiner Mutter. Ein Bericht nach Tagebuchaufzeichnungen (A child with XYY syndrome as experienced by his mother. A report of daily journal recordings). Z Kinder Jugendpsychiatr. 1992;20:46-53.

1610. Y SYNDROME (EXOTROPIA)

General

Etiology unknown.

Ocular

Partial V-pattern strabismus seen only in superior gaze; a partial A-syndrome with the deviation only occurring in down gaze can be considered an inverted Y-syndrome; occurs primarily with exodeviation.

Clinical

None

Laboratory

Diagnosis is made by clinical findings.

Treatment

Strabismus: Equalized vision with correct refractive error; surgery may be helpful in patient with diplopia.

Bibliography

1. Pau H. Differential Diagnosis of Eye Diseases. New York: Thieme; 1987.

1611. YAWS (FRAMBESIA) KERATITIS

General

Chronic infectious disease of childhood; causative agent is *Treponema pertenue*; incubation period 3–4 weeks; factors include poor hygiene, humidity and scanty clothing; infectious cutaneous relapses occur during the first 5 years of life.

Ocular

Conjunctivitis; lid granulomas; keratitis; iridocyclitis; lid ulceration; corneal leukomata; cicatricial ectropion.

Clinical

Skin lesion and relapsing secondary lesion of skin and bone; painful papules of soles of the feet; crablike gait; fever; lymphadenopathy; nocturnal bone pain; periostitis; gummas of skin and long bones; hyperkeratoses of soles and palms; osteitis; periosteitis; hydrarthrosis.

Laboratory

Diagnosis is made by clinical findings.

Treatment

Antibiotics

Additional Resource

1. Klein NC (2011). Yaws. [online] Available from http://www.emedicine.com/med/TOPIC2431. HTM [Accessed April, 2012].

1612. YELLOW FEVER

General

Acute infectious disease of short duration and extremely variable severity.

Ocular

Lid edema; orbital pain; subconjunctival, vitreal and anterior chamber hemorrhages; mydriasis; optic neuritis; partial optic atrophy.

Clinical

Fever; headache; nausea; epistaxis; relative bradycardia; albuminuria; convulsions; tongue shows red margins with white furred center; copious hemorrhages; anuria; delirium; slow pulse; jaundice; "black vomit"; hematemesis; coma; death.

Laboratory

Complete blood count, coagulation studies, urinalysis, chest X-ray, PCR assay, monoclonal enzyme immunoassay.

Treatment

No specific treatment is available.

Additional Resource

1. Busowski MT (2011). Yellow Fever. [online] Available from http://www.emedicine.com/med/TOPIC2432.HTM [Accessed April, 2012].

1613. YERSINIOSIS

General

Infection with one of the invasive rod-shaped Yersinia bacteria.

Clinical

Gastroenteritis; high fever; acute terminal ileitis.

Ocular

Corneal perforation, panophthalmitis, anterior uveitis, photophobia, lacrimation, pericorneal ciliary injection, aqueous flare and cell, keratic precipitates and macular edema.

Laboratory

Small, nonmotile, Gram-negative coccobacilli found in stool samples and conjunctiva.

Treatment

Tetracycline or Chloramphenicol is the drug of choice.

Bibliography

1. Roy FH, Fraunfelder FW, Fraunfelder FT. Roy and Fraunfelder's Current Ocular Therapy, 6th edition. Philadelphia: WB Saunders; 2008.

1614. YOUNG-SIMPSON SYNDROME (BLEPHAROPHIMOSIS)

General

Rare congenital syndrome.

Ocular

Blepharophimosis

Clinical

Congenital hypothyroidism; congenital heart defects; facial dysmorphism (microcephaly, bulbous nose, low-set ears, micrognathia); cryptorchidism in males; hypotonia; mental retardation; postnatal growth retardation.

Laboratory

Diagnosis is made by clinical findings.

Treatment

The ptosis is corrected by frontalis fixation at an early age. Canthoplasties may be performed to improve the blepharophimosis. The considerable epicanthus is usually best left until early adolescence, since the degree of this problem tends to diminish with time, and the skin becomes more easy to move.

Bibliography

1. Bonthron DT, Barlow KM, Burt AM, et al. Parental consanguinity in the blepharophimosis, heart defect, hypothyroidism, mental retardation syndrome (Young-Simpson syndrome). J Med Genet. 1993;30:255-6.
2. Nakamura T, Noma S. A Japanese boy with Young-Simpson syndrome. Acta Paediatr Jpn. 1997;39:472-4.
3. Masuno M, Imaizumi K, Okada T, et al. Young-Simpson syndrome: further delineation of a distinct syndrome with congenital hypothyroidism, congenital heart defects, facial dysmorphism, and mental retardation. Am J Med Genet. 1999;84: 8-11.

1615. Z SYNDROME

General

Occurs with hinged accommodating intraocular lens (IOL), such as the Crystalens, the capsule contracts and causes long-axis compression resulting in the asymmetric folding; Z syndrome— so named because the shape of the distorted IOL resembles a stretched-out "z".

Ocular

Increase myopia and astigmatism; coma aberration; tilting of the IOL optic; striae/fibrosis of posterior capsule.

Laboratory

Diagnosis is made by clinical observation.

Treatment

Yttrium-aluminum-garnet (YAG) capsulotomy is the treatment of choice and works well unless there is a gap between the posterior capsule and any part of the IOL. If there is a gap, a surgical procedure to reposition the IOL or in severe cases removal of the IOL may be necessary.

Bibliography

1. Yuen L, Trattler W, Boxer Wachler BS. Two cases of Z syndrome with the Crystalens after uneventful cataract surgery. J Cataract Refract Surg. 2008;34:1986-9.

1616. ZELLWEGER SYNDROME (CEREBROHEPATORENAL SYNDROME OF ZELLWEGER)

General

Rare; congenital; lethal disease; prevalent in females; demyelination of cerebral white matter, spinal cord and peripheral nerves; enzymatic defects cause myelin deficiency (Smith-Lemli-Opitz Syndrome); severe multisystem disorder resulting from defective biogenesis of the peroxisome causes death within the first year.

Ocular

Hypertelorism; microphthalmia; nystagmus; glaucoma; hemimydriasis; corneal opacities; cataract; narrowing of retinal vessels; pigment irregularities and areas of depigmentation; retinal holes without detachment; tapetoretinal degeneration; irregular border-lined optic disks; gray-colored disks; hypoplastic supraorbital ridges; optic atrophy.

Clinical

Hypotony; hepatomegaly; albuminuria; mental retardation; failure to thrive; vomiting; seizures; low birth weight; jaundice; short stature; broad nose; hypospadias; cryptorchidism; septal defect; craniofacial dysmorphic features; high forehead; renal cyst; psychomotor retardation; hepatosplenomegaly; severe hearing impairment.

Laboratory

Diagnosis is made by clinical findings.

Treatment

Multisystem disorder will involve separate specialities to treat the specific disorders.

Bibliography

1. Fenichel GM. Cerebrohepatorenal syndrome (Zellweger syndrone). In: Fenichel GM (Ed). Clinical Pediatric Neurology, 2nd edition. Philadelphia: WB Saunders; 1993. p. 151.
2. Bowen P, Lee CS, Zellweger H, et al. A familial syndrome of multiple congenital defects. Bull Johns Hopkins Hosp. 1964;114:402-14.

1617. ZIEVE SYNDROME (HYPERLIPEMIA-HEMOLYTIC ANEMIA-ICTERUS SYNDROME)

General

Unknown etiology; pancreatitis; prevalent in middle-aged males with history of recent alcohol intake; insidious onset.

Ocular

Moderate-to-marked icterus; cloudy cornea; corneal ulcers; retinal lipemia.

Clinical

Anorexia; nausea and vomiting; epigastric pain; diarrhea; weight loss; fatigue; weakness; jaundice; hepatomegaly.

Laboratory

Serum amylase and lipase; serum electrolytes; CBC; C-reactive protein.

Treatment

Stop alcohol intake; kidney dialysis may be necessary.

Additional Resource

1. de Alarcon PA (2011). Acanthocytosis. [online] Available from http://www.emedicine.com/ped/ TOPIC2.HTM [Accessed April, 2012].

1618. ZINSSER-ENGMAN-COLE SYNDROME (COLE-RAUSCHKOLB-TOOMEY SYNDROME; DYSKERATOSIS CONGENITA WITH PIGMENTATION) ECTROPION

General

Variant of Fanconi familial aplastic anemia; recessively inherited with male linkage; consanguinity; onset between the ages of 5 and 13 years.

Ocular

Ectropion; chronic blepharitis; obstruction of lacrimal puncta; conjunctival keratinization; bullous conjunctivitis; epiphora; nasolacrimal duct obstruction; loss of eyelashes; cataract; glaucoma; strabismus; abnormal fundi.

Clinical

Congenital dyskeratosis with pigmentation of "marble" configuration or "gun metal" appearance; atrophic areas and telangiectasis; dystrophy of nails; vesicular and bullous lesions of oral cavity followed by ulceration; mucosal atrophy; leukoplakia; aplastic anemia; defect of teeth; physical and mental development may be retarded; tufts of hairs on the limbs; keratinized basal cell; papillomas on the trunk.

Laboratory

Screen for bone marrow, neurologic, pulmonary and mucosal malignancies. CBC, chest radiography, pulmonary function test and stool test for occult blood. Mutation analysis test.

Treatment

Anabolic steroids for bone marrow failure. Stem cell transplantation is the long-term curative option.

Additional Resource

1. Robles DT (2011). Dyskeratosis Congenita. [online] Available from http://www.emedicine.com/derm/ TOPIC111.HTM [Accessed April, 2012].

1619. ZIPRKOWSKI SYNDROME

General

X-linked recessive albinism.

Ocular

Ocular albinism.

Clinical

Albinism generalized.

Laboratory

Test for hearing loss.

Treatment

Consult ENT specialist and dermatologist.

Bibliography

1. Francois J. Albinism. Ophthalmologica. 1979;178: 19-31.

1620. ZOLLINGER-ELLISON SYNDROME (MULTIPLE ENDOCRINE ADENOMATOSIS PARTIAL SYNDROME; POLYGLANDULAR ADENOMATOSIS SYNDROME) OPTIC ATROPHY

General

Autosomal dominant; more frequent in males (2:1); etiology is islet cell adenoma of pancreas secreting a gastrin-like material; onset in the third to fifth decade of life (Werner Syndrome).

Ocular

Scotomata according to size and position of pituitary tumors; optic nerve atrophy; papilledema; bilateral extraocular muscle metastases.

Clinical

Enteritis and/or peptic ulcers; malignant or benign tumor of islet cell of pancreas; hypersecretion; vomiting; diarrhea; polyglandular adenomatosis; endocrine involvement.

Laboratory

Fasting serum gastrin levels, secretin stimulation test, levels of basal acid output, endoscopic ultrasonography.

Treatment

Proton pump inhibitors (PPIs) are the first line of treatment for Zollinger-Ellison syndrome (ZES).

Additional Resource

1. Guandalini S (2011). Pediatric Zollinger-Ellison Syndrome. [online] Available from http://www. emedicine.com/ped/TOPIC2472.HTM [Accessed April, 2012].

Index